Gastrointestinal Eponymic Signs

Steven H. Yale • Halil Tekiner
Eileen S. Yale • Ryan C. Yale

Gastrointestinal Eponymic Signs

Bedside Approach to the Physical Examination

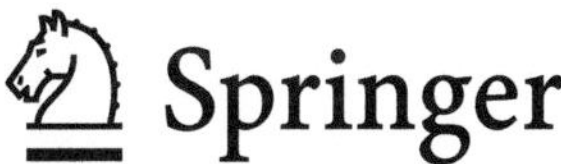

Springer

Steven H. Yale
College of Medicine
University of Central Florida
Orlando, FL, USA

Eileen S. Yale
College of Medicine
University of Florida
Gainesville, FL, USA

Halil Tekiner
School of Medicine
Erciyes University
Kayseri, Türkiye

Ryan C. Yale
The Home Mag
Ponte Vedra, FL, USA

ISBN 978-3-031-33675-1   ISBN 978-3-031-33673-7   (eBook)
https://doi.org/10.1007/978-3-031-33673-7

This Springer imprint is published by the registered company Springer Nature Switzerland AG
The registered company address is: Gewerbestrasse 11, 6330 Cham, Switzerland

Paper in this product is recyclable.

To Joseph J. Mazza, MD, MACP, former emeritus researcher at Marshfield Clinic Research Institute, Marshfield, Wisconsin. He is a true master clinician who passed on his unwavering enthusiasm and true joy in learning. He inspired me to listen and think critically while always keeping the patient's best interest in mind.

To John R. Schmeltzer, Ph.D., former Director and Health Economist-Health Services Research at the Marshfield Clinic Research Institute, Marshfield, Wisconsin, who passed on his unique gifts of passive listening, silent leadership skills, and providing clarity even to the most complex issues.
Steven H. Yale, MD

To the beautiful memory of my grandparents, Şengül and Halil Has, who reunited before this book was completed. They will forever continue inspiring my academic paths.
Halil Tekiner, PhD

To the memory of my parents, Thomas and Eileen Scott, for their unconditional and unwavering love and support they provided to my family and I throughout our lives.
Eileen S. Yale, MD

Foreword

We were initially unsure whether to include a foreword to accompany this book. We asked about its purpose, goal, and what we hope to gain. The message had to say something that would titillate or inspire the reader. Most importantly, who should write it? There are many inspiring, prominent medical historians in the field, but the bygones of those who left indelible marks on the physical examination have since passed. These include such persons as Elmer L. DeGowin, M.D. (1901–1980), and his son Richard L. DeGowin, M.D. (1934–2021), coauthoring *Bedside Diagnostic Examination* in 1969, as well as Barbara Bates, M.D. (1928–2002), authoring *A Guide to Physical Examination and History Taking* in 1974. Regarding physical signs, Hamilton Bailey, M.D. (1894–1961), authoring *Demonstrations of Physical Signs in Clinical Surgery* in 1942, remains the time-honored name of clinical examination and diagnosis benchmark.

Learning the physical examination is a rite of passage in medical school. The physical examination is taught as a series of steps by which students are expected to master their sense of observation, auscultation, palpation, and percussion and are assessed based on how well they apply and perfect these skills. Unfortunately, these skills are not surprisingly lost over time since they are neither routinely used nor reinforced. It is always perplexing to hear when the learner reports that the physical examination is normal in the presence of a mountain of pathological abnormalities.

The realization that signs of the physical examination can provide so much more information serving as an additional potential mechanism for diagnosing disease sparked our interest and passion for understanding them further. This "hands-on" approach through these signs now has meaning and significance and may tell you something about what is going on with the patient.

This book fills the gaps in the literature and misattribution about the correct use of these signs. We argue that they should only be dismissed from medical discourse once they have been appropriately vetted or studied. We recognize that the signs could only be studied in their correct form once a standard description was available as told in the authors' own words. For reasons that are not entirely clear, many of these signs deviate from the authors' initial descriptions, thus making any inference about their significance impossible.

The other challenge we faced was how to guide instructors to teach these signs and simultaneously stimulate the learner's interest. We recognize that one of the most enjoyable ways of learning is through storytelling. Morning report, an inquisitive exercise where cases are presented, is a time-honored traditional exercise of storytelling in medicine. The audience, generally consisting of medical students, residents, and faculty, applies the Socratic method to foster critical thinking skills. The stories we told in our books were about these physicians whose accomplishments, in many cases, left an indelible mark on the next generation of their students and humankind. As you read the stories, you realize that they are more than just their name on a sign ascribed to them postmortem. Many of these physicians were prominent leaders in their hospitals and societies and pioneers in medicine and surgery, designing tools and devising techniques to move the field further. Unfortunately, we learn that a few of these physicians committed atrocities against humanity. Furthermore, because of the war and antisemitism, some physicians were forced to leave their posts and flee to another country.

The antagonist will argue that the world has evolved, and this information is antiquated and no longer required in patient care. Patients are now frequently whisked away for laboratory and imaging tests before the physician has taken an appropriate history or placed their hands on the patient. Suppose no abnormality or an unexpected finding is found. In that case, the physician finds themselves having to start over again to identify what they missed—a costly error not only in terms of expense but inconvenience and delayed diagnosis for the patient. It would be difficult to argue that this is a cost-effective or appropriate evidence-based approach to patient care.

So why should a medical student, resident, or faculty read this book and our prior one, *Cardiovascular Eponymic Signs: Diagnostic Skills Applied During the Physical Examination?* We hope that these books become an essential addition to the libraries of the history of medicine and physical examination and that the information they contain be further studied so that we can learn about the significance of these signs. In the interim, we believe that the sign augments the physical examination and provides a more rational way of approaching testing and diagnosis.

Steven H. Yale, MD
College of Medicine
University of Central Florida
Orlando, FL, USA

Halil Tekiner, PhD
School of Medicine
Erciyes University
Kayseri, Türkiye

Eileen S. Yale, MD
College of Medicine
University of Florida
Gainesville, FL, USA

Preface

Over the past five years, the authors have written collaboratively on a variety of topics related to medical eponyms. We had just completed our first book titled *Cardiovascular Eponymic Signs: Diagnostic Skills Applied During the Physical Examination* and were now interested in telling the stories about those physicians who described signs involving diseases of the gastrointestinal tract. Our goal was to pass on this knowledge so that others could appreciate how their lives impacted medicine and how others benefited from their presence. Additionally, we sought to provide the learner with an appreciation for how these bedside physical examination techniques afford a richer perspective on the pathophysiology and diagnosis of disease.

Medicine continues to progress and will undoubtedly become even more technologically advanced in the future. However, despite these advancements, one aspect remains constant: the best physicians are still those who have skillfully perfected the *ars medicinae* which requires excellence in patient history and a physical examination as a prerequisite for sound clinical reasoning and diagnosis. Technological advancements have made medical care delivery more sophisticated and costly. Moreover, it seems it has also resulted in a less personalized doctor-patient relationship as technology substitutes for, rather than complements, doctor-patient interactions. Is it any wonder then that physical examination skills decline in disuse? Or that there appear to be adverse consequences caused by the incongruency between what should be done for patients and what is actually being done to them.

We recognize that many signs are not taught, given only cursory attention during medical education, and have not been well studied. Hence, their reliability, validity, and utility in diagnosis in many cases are limited or currently unknown. Furthermore, the description of how to perform the sign may depart from the way it was originally intended, further contributing to misattribution, misinformation, and misunderstanding. In this regard, medical eponyms are akin to folklore, where information is modified over time such that the meaning of the sign may now differ from its original text.

This book intends to clarify inconsistencies and imperfections within the medical literature and provide an accurate account of the description of the sign by quoting the original text. Thus, we wrote this book to demonstrate to students and physicians that the skills of observation, palpation, percussion, and auscultation applied at the bedside through the conduit of what is named "signs" is the method that makes inferences in diagnosis. Moreover, the sign as a critical aspect of the physical examination provides an additional benefit of connecting the patient with the physician, which is fundamental to the goal of patient-centeredness. We intend this book to fill some of those gaps and titillate discussion and interest in further studying these signs.

Orlando, FL, USA   Steven H. Yale
Kayseri, Türkiye   Halil Tekiner
Gainesville, FL, USA   Eileen S. Yale
Ponte Vedra, FL, USA   Ryan C. Yale

Acknowledgments

Writing a book is a tremendous undertaking for those so adventurous to assume such a task. We were inspired by our students and other learners who maintain a zest for acquiring new knowledge while understanding the relevance of the bedside physical examination to the art of medicine.

We thank the University of Central Florida librarian staff for obtaining the original manuscripts. Without their work, this book would never have been possible. We thank Ryan Yale BFA, graphic designer, for his clear and precise illustrations, which brought to life these bedside techniques. We acknowledge Allison Yale, who reviewed the manuscript and provided her grammatical expertise, and Rekhta Muthusamy, Project Coordinator at Springer Nature, who supported us throughout the publishing process.

Eileen & Steven Yale, MDs

This book could not have been possible without the assistance of many scholarly friends, colleagues, and staff of several libraries, scientific institutes, and national academies of medicine and surgery in more than a dozen countries. I would especially like to express my gratitude to Dr. Bruno Bonnemain, President of the French Society for the History of Pharmacy; Arne Pflüger, Deputy Head of Business Development Department at the Library of Marburg Philipps University in Germany; and Laura N. Braga, librarian at the National Library of Argentina, for their extraordinary cooperation and precious guidance in assembling some difficult-to-obtain sources in French, German, and Spanish.

I am grateful for the intellectually stimulating and collaborative working environment I have been afforded for the last 10 years at Erciyes University in Kayseri, Turkey. I thank the Rector, Prof. Dr. Fatih Altun, and my colleagues and friends at the Schools of Medicine and Pharmacy for their continuous encouragement and unwavering support. I feel deeply indebted to my dear family members—Emel, İrfan, Sibel, and Kasım—and my beautiful Three-B(ee) nieces—Beren, Beste, and Buse—for not only being helpful and patient but also indulgent for the limited time I was able to spend with them during the preparations of this book.

Halil Tekiner, PhD

The authors also wish to acknowledge the journal *Clinical Medicine & Research*, which published an earlier version of a portion of this work that now presents a novel approach in its current form.

- Rastogi V, Singh D, Tekiner H, Ye F, Kirchenko N, Mazza JJ, Yale SH. Abdominal physical signs and medical eponyms, part I: physical examination of palpation, 1876–1907. Clin Med Res. 2018;16(3–4):83–91. https://doi.org/10.3121/cmr.2018.1423.
- Rastogi V, Singh D, Tekiner H, Ye F, Mazza JJ, Yale SH. Abdominal physical signs and medical eponyms: movements and compression. Clin Med Res. 2018;16(3–4):76–82. https://doi.org/10.3121/cmr.2018.1422.
- Rastogi V, Singh D, Tekiner H, Ye F, Mazza JJ, Yale SH. Abdominal physical signs and medical eponyms, part II: physical examination of palpation, 1907–1926. Clin Med Res. 2019;17(1–2):47–54. https://doi.org/10.3121/cmr.2018.1426.
- Rastogi V, Singh D, Tekiner H, Ye F, Mazza JJ, Yale SH. Abdominal physical signs of inspection and medical eponyms. Clin Med Res. 2019;17(3–4):115–26. https://doi.org/10.3121/cmr.2019.1420.
- Rastogi V, Singh D, Tekiner H, Ye F, Mazza JJ, Yale SH. Abdominal physical signs and medical eponyms, part III: physical examination of palpation, 1926–1976. Clin Med Res. 2019;17(3–4):107–14. https://doi.org/10.3121/cmr.2018.1427.
- Rastogi V, Singh D, Tekiner H, Ye F, Mazza JJ, Yale SH. Abdominal physical signs and medical eponyms, part I: percussion, 1871–1900. Clin Med Res. 2020;18(1):42–7. https://doi.org/10.3121/cmr.2018.1428.
- Rastogi V, Singh D, Tekiner H, Ye F, Mazza JJ, Yale SH. Abdominal physical signs and medical eponyms, part II: percussion and auscultation, 1924–1980. Clin Med Res. 2020;18(2–3):102–8. https://doi.org/10.3121/cmr.2018.1429.

About This Book

The word eponym is derived from Greek origin, meaning "named after." It is traditionally bestowed posthumously to honor an individual(s) contribution to the art of medicine and humanity. Eponyms remain controversial and contentious, and there has been a move to replace them in lieu of more descriptive terms. We acknowledge the limitations of eponyms, including issues related to misattribution and misclassification. Interestingly, despite their long-standing presence in medicine and medical discourse, there has been limited interest and attempts to identify ways to teach and study them. Often lost is the failure to recognize that signs intended to provide a better means to identify ways to diagnose and understand disease at a time when physicians only had available at their disposal the powers of observation, palpation, percussion, and auscultation. Thus, signs provide the means to diagnose; they make an inference about a disease. By doing so, a sign, in some cases, also explains the pathophysiologic disease process. We believe this essential art must be preserved, learned, and studied further.

This book serves as the source text for learners, teachers, practicing physicians, and medical historians interested in learning physical examination signs of the gastrointestinal tract. The focus is on the historical aspect of the named signs and pathophysiologic mechanisms required to elicit a positive test. We propose that eponyms be taught so learners can better associate the name with the sign. The approach we outlined in this book involves providing historical information chronologically about that person(s)'s accomplishment and the sign in a manner that gives meaning and significance and thereby titillates a learner's interest for further study. Our goal is to guide the reader to appreciate how these bedside signs provide a more profound understanding of the mechanism of disease. They become more than simply rote memorization but a fundamental tool for applying a direct hands-on assessment that involves how observing, engaging, listening, and touching the patient aids in diagnosis. These techniques also provide the additional benefit of better connecting the practitioner to the patients and maintaining the art of medicine, which has unfortunately rapidly lost its foothold within the medical community. In summary, the book intends to pass on this knowledge to students and advanced learners in order for them to appreciate further the fundamental and time-honored aspects of the patient-physician interaction.

Signs are quoted as initially described and translated to English from the original references in French, German, Spanish, Polish, or Russian. Testimonies about the person's character who described the sign, if available, were intended to give the reader an appreciation and perspective for those authors' humanistic qualities that are of utmost relevance to the art of medicine. We included information about these physicians' other accomplishments, acknowledging that the sign represented a minor role in their overall contribution(s) to medicine and society at large. If available, the sign's sensitivity, specificity, and predictive value in clinical practice were included.

We envision a scenario whereby students are taught these signs and techniques as demonstrated by the teacher. The learner practices and demonstrates the method with feedback provided by the teacher. Students learn to perfect the technique through training and are later reassessed. The teacher also provides information regarding the pathophysiologic mechanism required for a positive test and an opportunity to assess their knowledge and understanding of the role of the sign in clinical practice. Illustrations within the text provide a visual representation of the correct location and demonstrate how to perform the sign. We believe that this method of teaching and learning is more meaningful to the student in that they will be able to associate the name with the person's historical features, the sign, and its pathophysiologic mechanism(s). This teaching method thus provides a more meaningful learning experience in an applied learning environment whereby the learner understands the application of the physical examination in diagnostic decision-making.

The book covers the entire alimentary canal and intra-abdominal organs. The signs are presented chronologically in each chapter based on the year of publication. A table at the end of each chapter includes the name, the date the sign was first presented or published, and a summary of how the learner should perform the signs as the method for diagnosing. We intended this structure to serve as a quick resource for clinicians and students, whereby the information is more accessible without having to read that section of the book. Eponymic signs are organized based on the organ the disease primarily affects. For example, the Kayser-Fleischer sign is an ocular finding seen in patients with Wilson disease—a condition that primarily affects the liver and other organ systems (e.g., red blood cells and kidneys). The eponym, in this case, is found within the chapter on liver disease. This book represents a compilation of eponymic signs on the components of the gastrointestinal tract arranged sequentially using an organ system approach. The oral cavity is the first chapter since it represents the entry to the gastrointestinal tract.

Signs are rarely pathognomonic and should be thought of as a tool to supplement and not supplant other more advanced imaging or laboratory tests. We recommend that these signs be studied pragmatically prior to expunging them from medical discourse. Once we better understand their validity and utility, further research can be conducted to identify the best teaching method for learners. Teachers and learners can use this book to guide students to advance their diagnostic skills. It is also a valuable guide for academic clinical researchers interested in advancing the science of medicine to study these signs further to fully understand their role in clinical practice.

Contents

List of Figures

List of Tables

Chapter 1
Oral Cavity Signs

1.1 Introduction

The noun "mouth" has its origins from the middle to modern English adjective *oralis*, while the term "cavity" comes from the Latin *cavitatem* or hollowness [1, 2]. Thus, the oral cavity refers to the open space within the mouth. It is the initial portion of the alimentary tract (digestive tube) or gastrointestinal tract. Various diseases are found within the oral cavity and involve the soft tissues of the mucosa; tonsillar, pharyngeal, glandular, and lymph tissues; and the firmer tissues of the teeth, tongue, and palate, which may interfere with chewing (mastication) and swallowing (deglutition).

The physical examination of the oral cavity requires the examiner to apply their sense of vision, hearing, and touch through palpation and percussion, a light source, and a wooden spatula. The oral cavity, like the skin, provides visual information about the systemic nature of internal disease. Unfortunately, it is often neglected and given only cursory attention during the physical examination. This may reflect that the oral examination is not thoroughly taught, studied, or emphasized during medical education. Physicians thereby lack appropriate education, and skills, regarding their ability to recognize abnormalities and knowledge that heavy metals toxicity (e.g., lead) or infections (e.g., syphilis) may also occur or have their origins within the mouth.

Since the early nineteenth century, various signs have been described in the oral cavity. This chapter is devoted to presenting those signs by describing the persons and signs as initially reported and their role in current clinical practice. If available, we include tributes regarding their character and the impact that their presence had on others' lives. Most remarkable is that some of the oral cavity eponymic signs include the names of Corrigan, Trélat, Mueller, Fournier, Escherich, Gorlin, and Marfan—these eponymic names that most physicians and historians are familiar with are not the ones attributed to the oral cavity. By learning these signs and

© The Author(s), under exclusive license to Springer Nature Switzerland AG 2023
S. H. Yale et al., *Gastrointestinal Eponymic Signs*,
https://doi.org/10.1007/978-3-031-33673-7_1

historical information about the eponym, students and physicians can begin to appreciate the critical role that the oral cavity plays in disease diagnosis.

1.2 Eponymously Named Signs of the Oral Cavity

1.2.1 Burton Sign

Henry Burton (1799–1849) received his Bachelor of Medicine degree in 1826, a medical degree from Gonville and Caius College, Cambridge, in 1831, and a fellowship from the Royal College of Physicians (FRCP) in 1832 [3]. He served within the Royal College of Physicians (RCP) as censor in 1838 and consiliarius in 1843 [3]. Burton practiced at St. Thomas's Hospital throughout his career, rising from the ranks of an assistant physician and lecturer on chemistry and materia medica to senior physician [3, 4].

Burton described a finding observed on the gingiva of persons who ingested lead:

> The edges of the gums attached to the neck of two or more teeth of either jaw, were distinctly bordered by a narrow leaden-blue line, about the one-twentieth part of an inch in width, whilst the substance of the gum apparently retained its ordinary colour and condition, so far as could be determined by comparing the gums of these patients with those of other patients of the same class in the hospital [5, p. 66]. (…) For the discolouration is very permanent; it has endured through months and until death, and having been once observed may be afterwards easily recognize [5, p. 68]. The time required to produce the blue line varies in general with the amount of the dose, but not always, and, *coeteris paribus*, large doses affect the gums sooner than small [5, p. 77–78].

Thus, Burton sign refers to a narrow blue line at the gingival margin involving two or more teeth in the maxilla or mandible caused by lead poisoning (Table 1.1).

1.2.2 Carabelli Sign

Georg Carabelli (György Karabéla) (1787–1842) was born in Pest (currently Budapest, Hungary) and received his doctorate at Josefsakad [6]. He practiced dentistry in Vienna from 1809 to 1813, where he also served as court dentist to Franz Joseph I (1830–1916), the Emperor of Austria [6, 7]. At the University of Vienna, he was a professor and cofounder of the stomatological clinic [7].

Carabelli described a supernumerary tubercule found on the lingual (median) side to the mesial wall of the maxillary molar tooth as reported in his book *Systematisches Handbuch der Zahnheilkunde* (Systematic Manual of Dentistry) published in 1844, two years posthumously:

> Sometimes on the inner wall of the molars, especially on the first, there is an enameled hump (tuberculus anomalous), the base of which arises from the neck of the tooth and the tip of which stands free in the great oral cavity, somewhat remote from the crown [8, p. 107].

This anomalous accessory cusp, often called Carabelli cusp or cusp of Carabelli, is typically found in the maxillary permanent first molar and may be identified on the maxillary primary second molar [9] (Table 1.1). Their main significance is that the groove in this tooth predisposes to caries and may present challenges when placing orthodontic bands [4]. A genetic etiology has been proposed involving the PAX9 and MSX1 genes [10].

1.2.3   Corrigan Sign

Sir Dominic John Corrigan (1802–1880) was born in Dublin, Ireland, and received his medical degree from the University of Edinburgh, Scotland, in 1825 [11–15]. He was a physician at the Meath-Street Dispensary, Cork-Street Fever Hospital, and later Jervis-Street Hospital in 1831, and to the House of Industry Hospitals (Whitworth Medical, Hardwicke Fever, and Richmond Hospital—later renamed Carmichael Hospital) in 1840 [11, 12, 15–18]. Corrigan served as a professor of medicine at the Digges-Street School, Peter-Street School, and Richmond Hospital College of Medicine [11]. He was a member of the Royal College of Surgeons, England, in 1843 and received his honorary medical degree from the University of Dublin in 1849 [11, 14]. He was appointed physician to the College of Maynooth, an honorary physician in ordinary to Queen Victoria of Ireland in 1879, and com-missioners of National Education in Ireland [11]. He was anointed Baronet of Cappagh and Inniscorrig, Dublin, in 1866 [11, 12, 15, 19, 20].

Among his other appointments and accomplishments, he was the founder of the Dublin Pathological Society in 1838, later serving as president; a member of the Senate of the Queen's University in Ireland in 1841; fellow of the Royal College of Physicians, Ireland, in 1856; and representative on the Medical Council in 1859. Notably, he was elected president of the Royal College of Physicians, Ireland, in 1859; president of the Royal Zoological Society; and president of the Pharmaceutical Society of Ireland [13]. He served as vice-chancellor of the Queen's University, Ireland, in 1871 and president of the King and Queen's College of Physicians [11, 20]. He held a seat as a member of the House of Parliament at Westminster for the city of Dublin from 1870 to 1874 [11, 12, 21, 22].

As to his character:

> As a practitioner, he exhibited in a striking manner the distinguishing traits of his character, decision and boldness; tempered, however, with kindness and tenderness towards the sick, and guided by the most scrupulous honour in his professional relationship. (…) In debate he was at his best. Always fluent and impressive, and capable of marshalling his facts with a skill possessed by few public men, he was occasionally eloquent. To these qualities, enhanced in no small degree by his easy and dignified action, his fine erect figure and intel-lectual countenance, which, when he rose to the full height of the occasion, glowed with enthusiasm and conscious power, lent considerable force [11, p. 227].

These represent a glimpse of the plethora of his honorary achievements. Despite his enduring accomplishments, his name is undoubtedly best recognized and entrenched in the medical literature in the association of the sign related to aortic insufficiency, eponymously named the "Corrigan pulse" or "Corrigan sign." He published this finding in 1832 in the *Edinburgh Medical and Surgical Journal* and was titled "On permanent patency of the mouth of the aorta, or inadequacy of the aortic valves," where he stated:

> Visible pulsation of the arteries of the head and superior extremities: (…) When a patient affected by the disease is stripped, the arterial trunks of the head, neck, and superior extremities immediately catch the eye of their singular pulsation. At each diastole the subclavian, carotid, temporal, brachial, and in some cases even the palmar arteries, are suddenly thrown from their bed, bounding up under the skin. The pulsations of these arteries may be observed in a healthy person through a considerable portion of their tract, and become still more marked after exercise or exertion but in the disease now under consideration, the degree to which the vessels are thrown out is excessive. Though a moment before unmarked, they are at each pulsation thrown out on the surface in the strongest relief. From its singular and striking appearance, the name of *visible pulsation* is given to the beating of the arteries [23, p. 227].

Thus, one eponymous sign ascribed to Corrigan refers to the visible pulsation observed in the head, neck, and upper extremities. Corrigan also described a finding found in patients with chronic exposure to copper:

> In all cases of copper-poisoning which have come under my notice there was exhibited a very peculiar feature, which does not appear to have been previously noticed, viz., an edging of rich purple on the margin of the gums of the incisor, canine, and bicuspid teeth of both jaws. (…) In many of the cases of copper-poisoning, the effects have been produced by handling old or dirty copper, on which the carbonate has accidentally formed [24, p. 229].

Thus, Corrigan sign also refers to the purple-colored line occurring at the junction or margins between the teeth (incisor, canine, and bicuspid) and gingiva (Table 1.1).

1.2.4   Trélat Sign

Ulysse Trélat (1828–1890) was born in Paris, France, served as a hospital intern in Paris in 1849, and received his medical degree based on the thesis titled *Des fractures de l'extrémité inférieure du fémur* (Fractures of the distal femur) in 1854 [25]. He was an associate of anatomy at the École Pratique from 1853 to 1857, agrégé of the Faculty of Medicine in Paris, based on the thesis titled *De la nécrose causée par le phosphore* (Necrosis caused by phosphorous) in 1857, and lectured on congenital surgical diseases and surgery from 1859 to 1861 [25–27]. He was appointed surgeon at the Central Bureau in 1860, rose to the rank of chief of Maternité surgeon in 1864, followed by appointments at Saint-Antoine Hospital in 1867, Saint-Louis Hospital in 1868, Pitié Hospital in 1869, and Charité Hospital in 1872; the later as professor of external surgical pathology [25, 27].

During the Franco-Prussian War of 1870, he was chief surgeon of the fifth ambulance of the Society for the Relief of the Military Wounded [25, 28]. After the war, he was appointed surgeon and professor of pathology at Charité in Paris, followed by professor and chair of the surgical clinics at Hôpital Necker in 1880, and subsequently professor of clinical surgery at Charité in 1884. Trélat was passionately involved in issues involving public and occupational health and assistance [25, 27].

He was a member of the Society of Surgery in 1864 (president in 1872), the Academy of Medicine in 1874 (president in 1886), the Society of Public Medicine (chairman in 1885), the Superior Council of Public Assistance, the Council for Hygiene and Sanitation of Seine in 1874, and decorated as Commander of the Legion of Honor in 1889 [25]. His lectures were posthumously published by his former student Pierre Delbet (1861–1957) in 1891 in the two-volume book titled *Clinique Chirurgicale* (Surgical Clinic) [28, 29].

In the words of Professor Tarnier as to a description of his character:

> Throughout his life, he hated banality, loving only beauty and authenticity. His efforts were directed toward specific goals and relentlessly advanced toward achieving those goals. His intelligence was so keen and his power of assimilation so great that his knowledge seemed vast. We often admired the insight and marvelous intuition with which he approached the most difficult problems of surgery, hygiene, and administration [25, p. 14].

One of his former students, Dr. Paul Segond, described Trélat as:

> Incomparable teacher, marvelous worker, and clinician who was as judicious as wise. He possessed all of the great qualities of common sense, righteousness, and balance that have made French surgery famous. In short, you were the master for us, the one we listen to, admired, respected and loved—But that's not all. Those who would only remember your operative dexterity, your penetrating eloquence, your profound knowledge, the wary care you always took to pursue progress as the truth, your marvelous abilities to synthesize, clarify or summarize the most obscure scientific questions would still know you imperfectly. They would be unaware that you were not only a great surgeon and that you possessed within you many other qualities of the heart and mind [25, p. 23–24].

Trélat presented at the French Academy on 27 November 1869 an observed finding in the oral cavity in patients with tuberculosis (Table 1.1):

> It now remains for me to reveal a finding that I regard as pathognomonic. It occurs early, but as these ulcers progress, they are almost always persistent findings that enable us to recognize them since they are invasive. Tuberculosis ulcers of the mouth develop in the following way: one finds on the mucous membrane a spot, a barely protruding plate, round, 1 to 3 or 4 millimeters in width, with its surface covered with epithelium, and one or more follicular orifices. This spot is light yellow, similar to that of phlegmonous pus. After a few days, the epithelium is destroyed and soon leaves behind an ulcerated surface. Instead of one spot, we observe several of them at different stages of evolution. The patient whose history I have related had, the first time I saw him, new ulceration for a long time until towards the end of his life, the whole tongue was ulcerated [30, p. 44–45].

Thus, Trélat sign refers to tiny superficial light-yellow spots (abscesses) on the surface of a tuberculous lesion in the mouth progressing to form a large tuberculous ulcer (Table 1.1).

His name is undoubtedly best recognized in regard to the sign he described in 1883 and independently by Edmund Lesser (1852–1918) in 1901 (Lesser-Trélat sign). Lesser's description and reporting of cherry angiomas associated with various internal malignancies were similar to the findings discussed in Trélat lectures as early as 1883 [31, 32]. However, it was Hollander in 1900 who described the seborrhea keratosis associated with internal malignancy:

> The second form of the observed skin abnormality, which itself, as is known, tends to malignant degeneration, is formed by seborrheic warts, like those similar here as well verrucae seniles. Especially in young cancer patients, I have observed that the abdomen and breast are covered by these seborrheic, flat, shiny, sometimes somewhat pigmented lesions [33, p. 485].

Thus, Hollander described the findings of seborrheic keratosis occurring with internal malignancy (most commonly gastrointestinal malignancies). What Lesser-Trélat described were cherry angiomas (Table 1.1).

1.2.5   Clarke Sign

William Fairlie Clarke (1833–1884) was born in Calcutta, West Bengal, India, and received his Master of Arts (M.A.) and Medical Baccalaureate (M.B.) degree from Oxford in 1862 [34–38]. He was a house surgeon and assistant demonstrator in anatomy at King's College Hospital, earning a fellowship to the College of Surgeons in 1863 [34, 35, 38].

He served as clinical assistant to Sir William Bowman (1816–1892) in Moorfields, London, for 3 years, followed by sequential appointments as surgeon to the St. George and St. James Dispensaries, assistant surgeon to the West London Hospital, and assistant surgeon at Charing Cross Hospital from 1871 to 1877 [34, 38]. He received his medical degree from Oxford in 1876 in worked as a general practitioner in Southborough, near Tunbridge Wells in Kent 1877 [36–38].

Clarke was elected fellow of the Medico-Chirurgical Society in 1866 [34, 38]. He authored the *Manual of the Practice of Surgery* in 1865 and the monograph *Diseases of the Tongue* in 1873 [34, 36–38]. He was a cofounder of the London Medical Missionary Society [35].

As to his character:

> He thought much and wrote well on hospital out-patient reform, on the provident dispensary system, on Poor-law relief, on the improvement of the dwellings of the poor (long before its importance was so fully recognized as it is now), on medical missions, and on temperance. (…) Dr. Clarke was a man of amiable and refined nature whose high culture and endowments lent an additional grace to a character firmly based upon deep religious conviction [39, p. 919].

Clarke described the fissuring of the tongue in cases of syphilis (Table 1.1):

> It may be asked, are we to regard all cases of fissured tongues as of syphilitic origin? Before I answer this question let me point out the distinction between a fissured and a wrinkled tongue, for to the superficial observer their appearances are sometimes very similar. A fissure goes deeply into the substance of the organ, but rugae are confined to the mucosa. This may be demonstrated at once by taking the tongue between the fingers, and gently stretching it. The rugae can be obliterated with the greatest case, while no impression is produced on the fissures. Their sides may be separated, but they cannot be obliterated. Almost every tongue presents some wrinkles and folds in its mucous membrane. These may be very

marked, if the patient's health has been such as to produce a temporary enlargement with a subsequent diminution, in the size of the organ. Thus, a period of indigestion or debility may give rise to a pale and swollen tongue—a tongue which readily takes the impression of the teeth. But when a better state of the general health is brought about, when the muscular fibres recover their tone, the stretched mucous membrane falls into folds, and it is of some time before this condition passes away, and the organ resumes its natural firmness. A rugous tongue is, therefore, a very simple affair, and may be the results of nothing more than a little dyspepsia. But, as far as my experience goes, the vast majority of fissured tongues are due to syphilis, and are characteristic of the later stages of that disease [40, p. 150–151].

Thus, Clarke sign refers to the presence of a fissured tongue in cases of syphilis (Table 1.1).

1.2.6 Drummond Sign

Sir David Drummond (1852–1932) was born in Dublin, Ireland, and received his M.B. and M.Ch. degrees from Trinity College, Dublin, in 1874 and a medical degree in 1876 after completing his studies in Prague, Vienna, and Strasbourg [41]. He served as an assistant physician at the Children's Hospital in Newcastle, England, and as an honorary staff pathologist and assistant physician at the Royal Victoria Infirmary from 1878 to 1912, followed by consulting physician in 1912 [41]. From 1911 to 1924, he was a professor of the Principles and Practice of Medicine at the University of Durham College of Medicine, Newcastle-on-Tyne, England [41].

Among his numerous accolades, he received the Knight Commander of the Order of the British Empire (C.B.E.), disambiguation in 1920, and was knighted in 1923 [41, 42]. He received the honorary degree D.C.L. from the University of Newcastle and was elected honorary fellow from the Royal Academy of Medicine, Ireland. He was nominated president of the North of England Branch of the British Medical Association and Northumberland and Durham Medical Society from 1921 to 1922. He later served as president of the Association of Physicians of Great Britain and Ireland [42].

As to his character as described by a colleague:

No appreciation of "Physician Drummond" as he was known throughout the North, would be adequate without a reference to his invariable and unstudied courtesy, his consideration for others, his genuine sympathy, and generous help to all in need of it. Apart from the justified confidence in his professional attainments, these qualities won for him the respect and love of many friends. No man consistently held to higher ideals of the duty of a consulting physician in relation to medical ethics none had greater pride in his profession. His skill and intuition in diagnosis remain a traditional memory among students of the Newcastle school, based as they were on accurate observation and treasured experience. He was at his best with the senior student and young graduate, for it was not always that the junior could follow the rapid steps which led to final diagnosis and prognosis [41, p. 865].

In the words of Professor George Grey Turner (1877–1951):

Sir David Drummond will always be gratefully remembered by a numerous succession of men, now scattered all over the world, who came under his influence either as students or house-physicians or young practitioners, and each will remember him for his sound teaching, genial personality, and kindly influence and timely help rendered in one way or another. Drummond was a great clinician and clinical teacher, who constantly taught and urged the importance of actual contact with patients [41, p. 866].

The marginal artery of Drummond or arteria marginalis coli is frequently misattributed to David Drummond. In fact, his son, Hamilton Drummond, first reported the significance of this arteria in 1913.

> In order to prove the value of this so-called marginal artery, which runs along the mesenteric edge of the large intestine, I carried out a series of post-mortem investigations with ligatures applied on the main trunk of the large intestine vessels in the course of this anastomosis. I found by injecting the ileocolic artery at its origin from the superior mesenteric vessel, and with ligatures placed on the right middle and left colic, and the sigmoid branches at points near their origin, that the vessels forming the marginal artery from the caecum to the middle of the pelvic colon were well filled. An additional ligature was applied to the branch of the superior mesenteric which supplies the lower end of ileum in order to prevent the injection reaching the aorta by way of the superior mesenteric artery. Again, with the main trunks ligatured as before, and an additional ligature applied to the line of the marginal artery, where the junction of the middle and left colic arteries meet in the region of the splenic flexure, the injection travelled no farther than the descending colon, the vessels of the iliac and pelvic colons not being injected. As a rule, before the injection carried farther than the point ligatured on the marginal artery the vessels burst as the result of injecting at too high a pressure [43, p. 188].

Thus, the marginal artery represents a common anastomotic site or collateral artery between the right and middle colic arteries and the left colic and sigmoid arteries running along the mesenteric border of the colon [43, 44].

David Drummond described an auscultatory finding in patients with thoracic aortic aneurysms (Table 1.1):

> Briefly, the oral whiff, which I may call the sign I am now referring to, can be detected in the following manner in cases of aortic aneurysm. The patient is directed, whilst lying on his back, to breathe as quietly as possible through the widely open mouth; the oval piece of the binaural stethoscope is then introduced into the mouth to receive the expired air. Should, then, the sign be present, the expiration will appear to be interrupted at each beat of the heart by a whiff, which, in some cases, is very loud, whilst, in others, it is only detected at the end of expiration, an indication that it is but feebly marked. In certain cases, especially if the aneurysm be large, a diastolic whiff can be heard as well as a systolic. In cases in which the sign is well marked, it can be plainly heard in the trachea during quiet expirations, or when the patient is holding his breath, with the mouth open and the tongue depressed, so as to allow the gaping glottis to communicate freely with the buccal cavity. In very well marked cases, the whiff is audible in the trachea with the mouth closed, but it at once disappears when the nostrils are compressed by the fingers. In seeking for the sign, it is most important to avoid cardiac excitement; hence it should only be sought for after the patient has lain in the recumbent position for a short while, and after the reasons for inserting such a formidable looking instrument as the binaural stethoscope into the mouth have been fully explained. It is well, indeed, to school the patient accurately before commencing the examination, for nervous, interrupted respiration on the one hand, and forcible or nasal breathing on the other, will defeat the object of the examination [45, p. 773].

Drummond reported that in 22 patients with thoracic aneurysm, the whiff sign was loud in 17 and soft in 3 [45]. Thus, Drummond sign refers to the presence of a whiff or "puff" auscultated at the opening of the mouth during expiration in patients with an aortic aneurysm.

1.2.7 Mueller (Müller) Sign

Friedrich von Mueller (Müller) (1858–1941) was born in Augsburg, Germany, received his medical training in Augsburg, Munich, Tübingen, and Würzburg, and completed his medical state examination in Munich in 1881 [46, 47]. He was an assistant at Carl Adolph Christian Jacob (Karl Adolf Christian Jakob) Gerhardt (1833–1902) Clinic at the University of Würzburg in 1882 and accompanied him to Charité Clinic at the Friedrich-Wilhelms University, Berlin, in 1885, habilitating in 1887 [46–48]. During this time, he published with Heinrich Wilhelm Otto Seifert (1853–1933) *Taschenbuch der medizinisch-klinischen Diagnostik* (Pocket Book of Medical-Clinical Diagnostics) with the first edition appearing in 1886 [46].

He was appointed professor at the University of Bonn in 1889, where he taught laryngology for 1 year, after which he accepted a position as professor of laryngology in Breslau, Germany [46]. He moved to Marburg, Germany, where he served the polyclinic and rose to dean of the faculty from 1892 to 1899 [46, 47]. He accepted a position in the Department of Internal Medicine in Basel, Switzerland, in 1899, was appointed chair of the Second Medical Clinic in 1902, and rector in 1914 until his retirement at the University of Munich in 1937 [46]. He was elected president of the Congress of Internal Medicine in 1908, the International Medical Congress in 1913, and the German Academy in 1927 [47, 49].

As to his character:

> He remained throughout passionately devoted to Germany and to its mode of life, but it was a devotion we can all admire, without any trace of self-interest, full of appreciation of the achievements of others and deeply valuing their friendship. There have been few greater ambassadors for medicine and for its highest ideals. For all those who are interested in the teaching of medicine his life deserves careful study, for they will find in him the rare combination of a great clinical teacher and a great clinician. If they can convey to their students something of the spirit which inspired Friedrich Müller they will not have taught in vain [46, p. 342].

Although his name is perhaps best recognized in association with his description of the physical finding of uvula pulsation in patients with aortic insufficiency, it is important to recognize that his interests and contribution were vast, including the study of the intermediate products of metabolism and coining the term "nephrosis" at the Meran, Germany, meeting of the German Pathological Society in 1905 [50, 51].

Mueller reported the oral finding first observed in a 22-year-old female with pulmonary and aortic insufficiency (Table 1.1):

> The inflamed, reddened tonsils and the anterior and posterior palatine arches moved somewhat medially synchronously with each carotid pulse; pulsation was also noted on the soft palate, the free edge being moved downwards with the uvula. In this way, the palatine arches and tonsils' contraction and the deepening of the soft palate and uvula with each pulse resulted in narrowing of the palate. Observed is a rhythmic intensification and reddening of the palate. As the discomfort resolved, the strength of the palatal pulsation became slightly diminished but did not entirely disappear, persisting as long as the patient was hospitalized [52, p. 251].

The discovery was made in three of six patients with aortic insufficiency at the Second Medical Clinic. Two patients had aortic insufficiency, while the third had mitral and aortic insufficiency. Thus, Mueller sign refers to the presence of rhythmic pulsation of the soft palate and uvula and erythema of the soft palate synchronous with the cardiac cycle.

1.2.8 Shelly Sign

Charles Edward Shelly (1854–1935) was born in Nuneaton, England, received his medical training at St. Bartholomew Hospital, qualifying as a member of the Royal College of Surgeons (M.R.C.S.), and received the Medical Baccalaureate (M.B.) degree from Cambridge in 1879 [53]. Shelly was appointed medical officer at Haileybury College in 1880 and Hertford County Hospital in 1884 [53]. He received his medical degree in 1890 and was appointed a member of the Royal College of Physicians (M.R.C.P) in 1894 [53]. Shelly was a consulting physician at Hertford County Hospital in 1917 and was appointed as consulting physician to Hertford and Ware Joint Isolation Hospital and Haileybury College [53].

Shelly served as president of the Association of School Medical Officers, a member of the British Medical Association, and vice-president of the Metropolitan Counties Branch in 1920 [53]. He was editor of the *Transaction of the Seventh International Congress of Hygiene and Demography* in 1891 [54].

Shelly observed on the soft palate of patients with influenza that it was (Table 1.1):

> [c]ompletely studded with minute translucent lenticular elevations, somewhat resembling tiny well-boiled grains of sago. They varied in size, being in most cases about 0.5 mm, and hardly ever exceeding 1 mm in diameter. They gave the idea of small localized distensions of a thin layer of transparent epithelium, and their lens-like appearance was increased by the fact that occasionally a minute blood vessels lying beneath one of them became magnified to quite considerable proportions, although it might be impossible to observe any other part of its course as it entered or left the vesicle on either side. These vesicles were most abundant about the soft palpate above the root of the uvula; but in some cases-and these were generally of the more sever type-they occupied a much larger areas being visible over the greater part of the roof of the mouth; but being always most marked and most abundant in the situation first mentioned [55, p. 791].

Although Shelly identified these findings in patients with influenza, he recognized that they were not pathognomonic for this disease.

1.2.9 Fournier Sign

Jean Alfred Fournier (1832–1914) was born in Paris, France, and received his medical degree from the University of Paris Medical School in 1860 [56, 57]. He was appointed professor agrégé in the Faculty of Medicine of Paris in 1863; and chief of service to Lourcine Hospital in 1868 and St. Louis Hospital in 1876 [56]. He was elected to the Academy of Medicine in 1879 and was chair of Syphilology and Cutaneous Diseases at the University of Paris in 1880 [56–58].

Fournier's primary area of research interest and expertise was the study of syphilis. His pursuit of the field of venereology was sparked during his internship with Philippe Ricord (1800–1889) at the Hôpital du Mid, Paris, in 1855 [57]. His name and eponym are best recognized for his description of rapidly spreading fulminant gangrene involving the perineum and scrotum with widespread purpuric cutaneous findings in a young man with diabetes (Fournier gangrene or necrotizing fasciitis of the perineum) [56].

Among his other accomplishments and contributions was that he served as president and founder of the French Society of Dermatology and Syphilography (currently French Society of Dermatology and Sexually Transmitted Diseases) in 1889, president and founder of the French Society of Sanitary and Moral Prophylaxis in 1901, and recipient of the Commander of the Legion of Honor and Order of Leopold of Belgium [56–59].

As to his character:

> Few men have had the style and talent for teaching to the same degree like the master of Lourcine and Saint-Louis Hospital. Inculcating in his students the truths to which his experience had led him was not enough for him; he constantly strove to deduce from it the necessary consequences and rules of practical conduct. He, therefore, sought not merely to instruct but to persuade. It has been said that most of his lectures and almost all of his academic speeches are genuine pleas. His facility of speech, correctness, and elegance of his style was quite remarkable. To be confident of rendering his thought with all its nuances and better penetrating his listeners' minds, he liked to use synonyms, gradation, and superposition of analogous terms. The disposition of his speeches, their architecture if one can say so, did not seem to him unworthy of his care. He had a gift of visual memory and mental representation such that he could recite the text of his lessons, glancing at it infrequently, almost taking on the tone of improvisation as he leafed through it in front of him [57, p. 527].

Fournier described in 1894 findings in the oral mucosa that provide clues as to the presence of hereditary syphilis:

> It is very common for hereditary syphilis to cause disease involving the skin and mucous membrane during infancy. If the forms of the disease are superficial, they leave no trace after healing; but if they are deep or ulcerative, they must, of course, be followed by a visible scar, leaving an indestructible mark [60, p. 36]. Now, what are the scars that make their location suspicious? We will get to know four of these types: 1. Scars on the lip commissures (one could also say scars on the corners of the mouth because they occupy the angle formed by the lip commissure). In newborn or hereditary syphilitic children, syphilide on the lip commissures is one of the most common manifestations. There are actually few syphilitic children who are not affected by this disease. The syphilides which reside in this place are erosions, decomposed papules, or ulcers. They occupy only the commissure and encroach somewhat, on rare occasions, on the surrounding skin. In and of themselves, they are not deep. However, tears almost always appear at the corners of the mouth. They form rhagades, ulcerous streaks, which tear repeatedly, hollow out more and more, become deeper, heal only slowly and with difficulty and consequently leave behind persistent, always visible scars. In this way, even after many years, one finds, like a posthumous witness, a pronounced scar occupying the lip commissure and adjacent skin. This scar usually takes the form of a small whitish line that is elongated, running transversely or slightly obliquely from top to bottom. They may be barely visible on the mucosa (it is known that diseases of the mucous membrane heal less conspicuously than those of the skin), but a distinct and noticeable skin scar always remains. Rarely are scars of this type found around

the lips [60, p. 38–39]. (…) 2. Scars of the nose. (…) 3. Scars in the lumbar-buttocks region and posterior thigh. 4. Scars on the soft palpate and pharynx. The palate and pharynx, like the nose, are especially prone to produce gummata. It is almost superfluous to add that these gummata, which, moreover, are often misunderstood as to their nature. In a large number of cases they partially or completely attack, mutilate, and sometime destroy the soft palate, the palatine arches, and the pharynx [60, p. 39].

Thus, Fournier sign refers to the presence of scars located at the corner of the mouth in congenital syphilis (Table 1.1).

1.2.10 Krisowski (Krisovki) Sign

There is limited information on Max Krisowski (Krisovki) (1895–?). He was born in the district of Görlitz, Silesia, Prussia. Krisowski worked at the dermatologic clinic of Max Joseph (1860–1933), Berlin, in the 1890s and practiced medicine at Schwerin from 1895 to 1897, returning to practice there in 1900 [61]. His scientific work was primarily devoted to children's diseases and hygiene. He published the book *Unsere Schätze, unsere Kinder: für Ärzte, Lehrer und Eltern* (Our Treasures, Our Children: For Doctors, Teachers, and Parents) in 1899 [62].

In his paper published in 1895, Krisowski reported from Dr. Max Joseph's Dermatologic Clinic in Berlin a physical finding around the mouth in patients with hereditary syphilis:

> These scars are not commonly found succinctly and extensively throughout the mouth as in the present case. However, in two other previously published cases, namely, the ones mentioned above by von Robinson and Parrot, their extent and numbers are irrelevant since they did not emphasize their diagnostic significance. The characteristic finding is based on this feature, accounting for the severity and extent of the processes involved. Their linear shape, radial position, localization around the mouth, and separation from one another by normal skin characterize these scars. In hereditary syphilis, this finding occurs at the corner of the mouth [63, p. 896].

Thus, Krisowski sign refers to linear radial cicatricial lines located around the mouth in congenital syphilis (Table 1.1).

1.2.11 Koplik (Spot) Sign

Henry Koplik (1858–1927) was born in New York, USA, and received his medical degree from the College of Physicians and Surgeons of Columbia University (currently Columbia University Vagelos College of Physicians and Surgeons) in 1881 [64, 65]. He completed an internship at Bellevue Hospital in New York, and what was traditional at that time furthered his studies in Berlin, Vienna, and Prague [64, 66]. He was appointed attending physician of the Good Samaritan Dispensary Clinic in 1887. He established the first pasteurized milk depot in the United States and a baby health station providing formula, infant, and pediatric clinical services for the indigent [64–68].

He served as an adjunct visiting physician to the Children's Ward, eventually culminating in an appointment as an attending physician of pediatrics followed by consulting physician at Mt. Sinai Hospital, New York [64, 65]. His other appointments included attending physician to St. John's Guild, Hebrew Orphan Asylum, Hospital for Deformities, and the Jewish Maternity Hospital. He published his book titled *The Diseases of Infancy and Childhood: Designed for Students and Practitioners of Medicine* in 1902 [65, 68, 69].

Although his name is most widely recognized in association with the early oral mucosal sign in patients with measles, he is also credited for identifying, growing on media enriched with human blood, the etiologic bacteria responsible for whooping cough previously described by Bordet and Gengou [67, 68].

Koplik was a founder and served as president of the American Pediatric Society. He was a member of the Association of American Physicians, the New York Academy of Medicine, an honorary member of the Vienna and Budapest Medical Societies, and the Permanent Commission of the International Association of Child Welfare [65, 67–69].

As to his character:

> Personally Dr. Koplik was a man of distinguished appearance and dignified bearing. Whenever he discussed a presentation at a meeting, all eyes were at once turned to him, and all realized that they would hear a carefully-worded and authoritatively expressed statement based upon his own experience and his own views. In more intimate contacts one was impressed and attracted by his sparkling mind, his great knowledge and his goodly store of anecdotes and humorous stories. He was himself the kind of man concerning whom numerous anecdotes spring up. Some of these will no doubt be preserved [65, p. 670].

Koplik described a finding discovered at the Good Samaritan Dispensary involving the buccal mucosa in early measles (Table 1.1):

> On the buccal mucous membrane and the inside of the lips, we invariably see a distinct eruption. It consists of small, irregular spots, of a bright red color. In the centre of each spot, there is noted, in strong daylight, a minute bluish white speck. These red spots, with accompanying specks of a bluish white color, are absolutely pathognomonic of beginning measles, and when seen can be relied upon as the forerunner of the skin eruption [70, p. 919–920]. No one, however, has to my knowledge called attention to the pathognomonic nature of these small bluish white specks, and their background of red irregular shaped spots. (…) That being the case it will be seen that the buccal eruption is of greatest diagnostic value at the outset of the disease *before* the appearance of the skin eruption and at the outset and height of the skin eruption [70, p. 920].

The pathognomonic nature of this finding has been questioned as it has been found in cases of Echovirus 9 (ECHO-9), parvovirus B19 (PV-B19), and Coxsackievirus A16 (CV-A16) infections [71–73].

It is of interest that Richard Hazeltine reported in 1804 about a measles outbreak occurring in Berwick, Maine:

> I notice no phenomenon which I could call a precursor of the disease, except the early
> appearance of the eruption in the internal fauces might be called one. In almost every
> instance where the commencement of the disease came in my knowledge, this appearance
> was to be observed at least 36, and in some cases 48 hours before the eruption appeared
> externally. (…) I was informed by some persons, that they had pretty constantly observed a
> pale military eruption on the gums two or three days previous to the cuticular eruption; and
> I think I saw a case or two of this kind myself [74, p. 349].

Furthermore, Belsky reported a similar phenomenon involving the buccal mucosa in
1890 and Filatov in 1895 (see Filatov sign). Thus, Koplik sign refers to the presence
of small red spots containing in its center a minute blue-white speck in patients with
early measles.

1.2.12 Silex Sign

Paul Silex (1858–1929) was born in Gorgast, Küstriner Vorland, Germany, studied
medicine in Halle, Berlin, and Breslau (Wroclaw), receiving his doctorate from the
latter in 1883 [75–78]. He was appointed assistant to the Ludwig Laquer (1839–1909)
Ophthalmology Clinic in Strasbourg, followed by additional training under Karl
Ernst Theodor Schweigger (1830–1905) in 1890 in Berlin [77, 78].

He was a Privatdozent in 1890, an extraordinary professor of ophthalmology in
1897 at the Friedrich-Wilhelm University, Berlin, and member of the Secret Medical
Council in 1914 [76–79]. He published the book *Ueber Chorea adulforum und
Tremor* (About Chorea Adulforum and Tremor) in 1883 and *Compendium der
Augenheilkunde* (Compendium of Ophthalmology) in 1891 [76, 77].

Silex, in his discussion on the characteristic signs found in congenital syphilis,
spoke of a cutaneous finding on the face:

> Single scars on the corners of the mouth and on the lips are very suspicious and multiple
> pseudoscars occurring on the lips is nearly diagnostic of syphilis (I have observed excep-
> tions). However, scars and furrows on the face, radiating to the chin are a pathognomonic
> symptom of congenital syphilis [80, p. 165].

As to the pathogenesis of these findings:

> It is probable that we are dealing with a retraction of the skin caused by the pulling of the
> muscles. The concept of retraction is suggestive to us because we have a trouble finding the
> furrows on the specimen that are easy seen macroscopically. But this much is evident from
> the examination, and I stress this, that the majority of these lines that anyone calls scars are
> not scars in the anatomical sense. I therefore refer to them as pseudoscars in literature [80,
> p. 165].

Thus, Silex sign refers to the presence of multiple scars (pseudoscars) and furrows
radiating from the corner to the mouth to the chin in patients with congenital syphilis (Table 1.1). The same finding was observed and reported by Krisowski in 1895
(see Krisowski sign).

1.2.13 Forchheimer Sign

Frederick Forchheimer (1853–1913) was born in Cincinnati, Ohio, and received his medical degree from the College of Physicians and Surgeons (currently Columbia University Vagelos College of Physicians and Surgeons), New York, in 1873 [81–83]. After graduation, he studied abroad at the Universities of Vienna, Würzburg, and Strasburg [82]. He returned to Cincinnati as a private practitioner, followed by appointments at the Ohio Medical College as a lecturer on pathological anatomy from 1876 to 1877, chair of Medical Chemistry from 1877 to 1879, and professor of Physiology and Clinical Diseases of Children beginning in 1881 [81, 82].

Forchheimer was appointed professor of diseases of children from 1894 to 1897, chair of the practice of medicine and diseases of children from 1897 to 1901, professor of theory and practice of medicine from 1901 to 1909, and professor of internal medicine beginning in 1909 [82]. He served as dean at the Ohio Medical College in 1905. He retained this position after the merger of Ohio Medical College and Miami Medical College (currently named Ohio-Miami Medical College of the University of Cincinnati) in 1909 [82]. Forchheimer's other appointments, included being a staff physician at the Good Samaritan City Hospital (1887–1897 and 1908–1913), a physician in chief at the Home for Sick Children, and consulting physician at the Jewish Hospital from 1887 to 1913 [82].

He served as president of the American Pediatric Society in 1895 and the Association of American Physicians [81, 82]. He authored *Diseases of the Mouth in Children* in 1892 and *The Prophylaxis and Treatment of Internal Diseases* in 1906 and served as editor of the *Therapeutics of Internal Diseases* in 1913 [81, 82]. He was the recipient of the honorary degree of Doctor of Science from Harvard University [81, 82].

As to his character:

> Frederick Forchheimer was a devoted, friend, a great leader, a profound scholar, and a wise teacher, but above all these he was a physician, or, as he loved to say, a "practitioner" of medicine. With that big heart of his, he took a deep, personal interest in every patient, regarding him not merely as an object of scientific study, but as a human being with the power of thinking, feeling, and acting. For the troubles and trial of each one he had sympathy and advice; for he labored not only to comfort, to cure, and to strengthen, but also to help each man to live his life and to do his work in the world [84, p. 7].

Forchheimer described at the American Pediatric Society Tenth Annual Meeting in Cincinnati, Ohio, a characteristic exanthem occurring in German measles, which:

> [c]onsists of a macular, distinctly rose-red eruption upon the velum of the palate and the uvula, extending to, but not upon the hard palate. The spots are arranged irregularly, not crescentically, are about the size of a large pinhead and raised slightly elevated above the level of the mucous membrane. They do not induce any reaction [85, p. 16].

The enanthem and exanthem occur concurrently, fading within 24 h. Thus, Forchheimer sign refers to the small, irregularly arranged erythematous maculopapular lesions located on the velum of the palate and uvula.

1.2.14   Comby Sign

Jules Comby (1853–1947) was born in Pompadour, Corrèz, France, and received his doctorate from the University of Paris in 1881. He was a physician at the Trousseau Hospital in 1894 and director of the Hospital for Sick Children, Paris, from 1894 to 1919 [86–88].

His life work involved the care and study of childhood diseases. He was editor-in-chief of *La Médecine Infantile* (Children's Medicine) in 1894 and co-editor of *Archives de Médecine des Enfants* (Archives of Children's Medicine) from 1898 to 1922. He authored several books, including *Traité des Maladies de l'Enfance* (Treatise of the Diseases of Childhood) in 1892, and *Les Médicaments chez les Enfants* (Medications for Children) and *Formulaire Thérapeutique et Prophylaxie des Maladies des Enfants* (Therapeutic Formulary and Prophylaxis of Children's Diseases) in 1900 [89–92].

He described a family of four children who developed a measles rash (Table 1.1):

> All four had an oral enanthem early in the disease course, which I emphasized a few years ago with erythema and swelling of the gums and a pultaceous (exudative) coating of the mucous membrane [93, p. 421].

The measles rash was preceded by erythematous tonsillar enlargement, white spots (exudative pharyngitis), and cervical lymphadenopathy in two of the four children. Thus, Comby sign refers to an exudate swelling of the gingival and buccal mucosal and white spots on the tonsils in early measles.

1.2.15   Tresilian Sign

Frederick James Tresilian (1862–1926) was born in London, UK, and received his medical degree from Queen's College, Cork, with first-class honors in 1885, membership of the Royal College of Physicians (M.R.C.P.) in 1887, a fellowship of the Medical Society of London in 1897, and fellowship of the Royal College of Physicians (F.R.C.P.) in 1902 [94–96]. He practiced medicine in Enfield, London, throughout his career. Initially, he served as a clinical assistant to the ear-nose-throat, and eye departments at the Prince of Wales's General Hospital, Tottenham, and Central London Throat, Nose, and Ear Hospital [94]. At the Enfield War Hospital, he was appointed Honorary Medical Officer. He also served as president of the North-East Clinical Society and Prudential Assurance Company [94].

Tresilian described an oral finding in children with mumps:

> The point I wish to put is, that generally the opening of Stensen duct on the inner surface of the cheek outside the second upper molar is hard to discover in children; in most of these cases of mumps it was a bright red papilla, and lasted as such for a week or more. Salivation likewise occurred in many cases. I could not discover any similar papillary enlargement of Wharton's duct, the common opening of the submaxillary and sublingual glands [97, p. 889].

Thus, Tresilian sign refers to erythema and edema involving the papilla of Stensen duct (Table 1.1).

1.2.16 Castellani-Low Sign

Aldo Luigi Mario Castellani (1874–1971) was born in Florence, Italy, and received his medical degree magna cum laude from the University of Florence in 1899 [98–101]. He studied under Walter Kruse (1864–1943), most recognized for his work on *Shigella dysenteriae* at the Hygiene Institute at the University of Bonn, Germany, where he discovered in 1902 an agglutination (absorption) reaction that assisted in differentiating and diagnosing these bacteria [99, 101–104].

Castellani served under the aegis of Sir Patrick Manson (1844–1922) within the Foreign Office at the School of Tropical Medicine, London, beginning in 1901 and was recommended by Manson to study sleeping sickness epidemic in equatorial Africa, a commission established by the Royal Society of Physicians [99, 104]. George Michael Low and C. Christie accompanied Castellani during the expedition. While stationed at Entebbe, Uganda, in 1902, he is believed to be the first to identify the parasite trypanosome in the cerebrospinal fluid and determine the causal association between this organism and the disease sleeping sickness. This accreditation was contemptuous because of uncertainty whether he had accomplished this solely or in consultation and collaboration with Lieutenant-Colonel Sir David Bruce (1855–1931) [98, 99, 105].

He subsequently served as director of the Bacteriological Institute, professor of tropical medicine, and lecturer on dermatology, at the Medical College of Colombo, Ceylon, Sri Lanka, from 1903 to 1915 [98, 101]. His other appointments during that time included the director of the Colombo Clinic for Tropical Diseases and physician to the seamen's ward at the Colombo General Hospital [98]. During his tenure at the institute, he identified the causative agent of Framboesia or yaws (*Treponema pallidum subsp. pertenue*) and its treatment with salvarsan; and the species *Bacillus ceylonensis,* later named *Shigella sonnei,* an organism responsible for the disease bacillary dysentery [99, 104, 106]. In collaboration with Albert J. Chalmers, he and Castellani published the *Manual of Tropical Medicine* with the first edition in print in 1910 [101, 107]. Additionally, he discovered many dermatophyte (e.g., *Trichophyton rubrum)* and yeast (*Torulopsis estoeilensis*) species [108]. He was instrumental in developing the polyvalent typhoid-paratyphoid vaccine (TAB) and typhoid-paratyphoid cholera vaccine (TABC), and a solution (carbol fuschin) used in the treatment of mycotic infections (Castellani paint) [106]. Overall, the depth of his expertise was broad, spanning the fields of bacteriology, mycology, and parasitology [109].

He served during and after World War I as an Italian medical officer in the Balkans. Castellani was appointed junior Italian representative at the International Office of Public Hygiene in London and Paris and interallied Sanitary Commission in Poland after the war [99, 104]. He established with Sir William Simpson

(1855–1931) the Ross Institute of Tropical Medicine in London, named in honor of Sir Ronald Ross (1857–1932), Noble Prize laureate for his discovery of malaria transmission, in 1923. He was appointed Director of Tropical Medicine and Dermatology and later Director of Mycology and Mycotic Disease when the Ross Institute became part of the London School of Hygiene and Tropical Medicine in 1934 [98, 99, 101, 104, 110]. He was the editor of the *Journal of Tropical Medicine and Hygiene* [99, 100]. Castellani described and named the benign cutaneous condition dermatosis papulosa nigra while in Jamaica and Central America in 1925. He served as chair and was responsible for developing the School of Tropical Medicine at Tulane University in New Orleans, Louisiana, in 1926, later resigning from this position and was appointed Professor at Louisiana State University [98, 101]. He also served as chair of the Institute of Tropical Medicine at the University of Rome, Italy, in 1930 [98, 101, 104, 111].

He served as surgeon general to the Italian army during the Ethiopian War from 1935 to 1936 and as a professor at the Tropical Disease Institute, Lisbon, Portugal, in 1947 [101, 104]. He cofounded, along with Frederick Reiss, the International Society of Tropical Dermatology in 1959 (currently the International Society of Dermatology since 1999) and served as its first president from 1960 to 1964 [101, 112]. Professor Kasuke Ito established the Castellani-Riess Medal and Award in their honor, which is:

> [t]he highest honor given by the Society in memory of its founders, Aldo Castellani and Frederick Reiss. It is awarded every five years at the time of the International Congresses to that individual who has demonstrated exceptional services to the advancement of the study of international dermatology and services to humanity as envisioned by our founders [112, p. 23].

He was also the recipient of the Serbian White Eagle, Legion of Honor from France, Ordronzenia Order by Poland, Italian Military Cross, Knight Order of St. Michael and St. George (KCMG) by King George V by the British in 1927, and Italian Count of Kisimaio by King Vittorio Emanuele III in 1935 [98–101, 104].

As a description of his character by Kaue Ito, emeritus professor at Gifu University School of Medicine in Gifu City, Japan:

> His "investigating mania," as he called it, had led him to explore the then unknown world of bacteria and pathogenic fungi in the tropics. It was still with him a few months before he died. However, he was not isolated or imprisoned in a laboratory of academic thought, he loved the company of human beings. He could "mix with kings without losing the common touch." We find him mixing easily with royalty, but at the same time mourning the death of his former illiterate servant in Africa, and enjoying his encounters with his patients in remote parts of Ceylon [104, p. 1026].

George Carmichael Low (1872–1952) was born in Monifieth, Forfarshire, Scotland. He received his medical degree with first-class honors from Edinburgh University in 1897 and a medical degree with a gold medal in 1910 [113–116]. He worked with Patrick Manson, head of the London School of Tropical Medicine housed within the Royal Albert Dock (Seamen's) Hospital, Greenwich, which led to the discovery that larval *Filaria bancrofti* is transmitted through the proboscis of *Culex fatigans* (*Culex quinquefasciatus*) mosquito, later confirming it to be the etiology of lymphatic filariasis [113, 117]. He was instrumental in establishing the relationship between *Filaria bancrofti* to the disease elephantiasis (lymphatic filariasis) and *Plasmodium vivax*-infected mosquitoes to human malaria [113, 114]. He accompanied Aldo Castellani and Cuthbert Christy (1863–1932) in 1902 during an expedition to Entebbe, Uganda, which led to the discovery of the cause of sleeping sickness [116].

He was appointed superintendent at the London School of Tropical Medicine from 1903 to 1905, an assistant physician at the Albert Dock Seaman Hospital in 1912, a pathologist at the West London Hospital from 1906 to 1909, consulting pathologist and lecturer at the London School of Tropical Medicine from 1910 to 1912, and assistant director of Tropical Diseases Bureau in 1912 [113–116, 118]. During World War I, he was a major in the India Medical Services (I.M.S.) at the Albert Dock Hospital. After the war, he was a full physician in 1918 and a senior physician in 1919 at the Hospital for Tropical Diseases and Seamen's Hospital [114, 116, 118, 119].

The London School of Tropical Medicine relocated to Endsleigh Gardens, Bloomsbury district of central London, in 1920 to become the Hospital for Tropical Disease, where Low was appointed senior physician until 1937 [114, 115, 118]. The London School of Tropical Medicine merged with the London School of Hygiene and renamed the London School of Hygiene and Tropical Medicine, where Low served as Director of the Division of Clinical Tropical Medicine from 1929 to 1937 [113, 114, 118].

Along with Sir James Cantlie (1851–1926), he was a cofounder of the Society of Tropical Medicine and Hygiene, established in 1907, later renamed with the suffix the Royal Society of Tropical Medicine and Hygiene [113, 116]. He also served for two terms, beginning as the 12th President of the Royal Society of Tropical Medicine and Hygiene from 1929 to 1933 [114, 118]. He is the recipient of numerous awards, including the Edinburgh University Straits Settlements Gold Medal in Tropical Medicine in 1912 and the Mary Kingsley Medal from the Liverpool School of Tropical Medicine in 1929 [114, 116]. He was appointed an honorary member of the French Society of Tropical Medicine and a corresponding member of the Society of Exotic Pathology, Paris [113].

As a description of his character by Sir Neil Fairley:

> He was a man of great intellectual honesty, said what he thought and adopted a justifiably critical and somewhat conservative attitude to things medical which were "not proven." He was a strict disciplinarian with patients and post-graduate students alike, sound in judgment, and full of that most valuable asset—common sense. Socially, he was a charming and delightful colleague, and those of us who were privileged to enjoy his friendship know what kindness, dry humour and sterling lay behind the rugged exterior he sometime presented [114, p. 573].

Castellani and Low divided sleeping sickness into three clinical stages. During the second stage:

> Abnormal muscular movements are perhaps the most striking features of the disease; fine tremor in the tongue is very constant, and a somewhat coarser tremor is also usual in the

hands and arms, any purposeful movements, as lifting a cup to the lips, often increasing it [120, p. 29].

Thus, Castellani-Low sign refers to the fine tremor of the tongue occurring in patients during the second stage of sleeping sickness (Table 1.1).

1.2.17 Schultze Sign

Friedrich Schultze (1848–1934) was born in Ranthenow, Brandenburg, Germany, completed his medical studies in Berlin and Bonn, and received his medical degree from the University of Heidelberg in 1871 [121]. That same year, he was appointed assistant to Nikolaus Friedreich (1825–1882) at the Heidelberg Internal Medicine Clinic [122]. Schultze habilitated in internal medicine in Heidelberg in 1876, was appointed associate professor in 1880, and was a professor and director of the medical clinics at Dorpat University in 1887 and the University of Bonn in 1888 [122]. He cofounded the journal *Deutsche Zeitschrift für Nervenheilkunde* (German Journal of Neurology) and along with Hermann Oppenheim (1858–1919), Wilhelm Heinrich Erb (1840–1921), and Adolph Strümpell (1853–1925) the Society of German Neurologists [122].

Schultze developed expertise in pediatric neurology, promoting the correlation of the clinical, anatomical, physiologic, and pathological aspects of neurologic disorders [121, 122]. He described a finding occurring in patients with tetany:

> The mechanical excitability of the muscles shows the typical changes precisely, especially when tapping the muscles of the thenar, gastrocnemius, deltoid, and extensor of the forearms. The muscle contraction was prolonged, with or without concavity formations. The most exquisite indentation occurred when tapping the half-protruding tongue, with the musculature taking an unusual form [123, p. 4].

Thus, Schultze sign refers to the presence of a concave depression formed by tapping on the tongue in patients with latent tetany (Table 1.1).

1.2.18 Miécamp (Mirchamp) Sign

We could only identify limited historical information on Etienne-Louis Miécamp (Mirchamp). He received his medical degree at the University of Montpellier, France. He published his book *Pathogénie de l'Oedème Aigu du Poumon* (Pathogenesis of Acute Pulmonary Edema) in 1900 and *Un signe de Diagnostic Précoce des Oreillons* (An early diagnostic sign of mumps) in *Le Caducée*, a French journal of military surgery and medicine in 1903 [124, 125]. He was an aide-major physician of the first class in 1906, an aide-major physician of the second class in June 1911, and a recipient of a military prize during his service in North Africa [126]. Miécamp described a finding found in patients with early mumps parotitis:

> Now, the outcomes from his research show that in the early phase of mumps parotitis, as soon as the swelling occurs, contact on the tongue with a sapid substance causes painful secretory reflex salivation. This painful reflex secretion is always more commonly found on the more swollen side. (…) To obtain this secretion, dilute acetic acid or vinegar is used. In any case, the patient must be advised to make an effort to swallow, for it is only at that moment that the painful secretory reflex is more commonly produced. Mr. Miécamp thinks this sign could nearly always detect mumps or confirm the diagnosis in uncertain cases. Moreover, suppose its finding does not lead to the diagnosis. In that case, we can always observe the patient with and without this sign and determine which one develops or does not develop mumps parotitis. There is no doubt that further studies will confirm the clinical importance of this finding [127, p. 313–314].

His name is frequently misspelled as Mirchamp in the English literature. Thus, Miécamp sign, as an early sign of mumps, refers to the presence of a painful salivary reflex after a sapid substance (dilute acetic acid or vinegar) is placed on the tongue (Table 1.1).

1.2.19   Filatov (Filatoff) Sign

Nil Fedorovich Filatov (Filatoff) (1847–1902) was born in Penza region, Saransk district of village Mikhailovka, Russia, and received his medical degree from Moscow State University Faculty of Medicine in 1869. He practiced in the Saransk district, Prague, Vienna, and Heidelberg [128]. Filatov served as an Associate Professor at Moscow Sofia Children's Hospital in the Department of Children's and Women's Disease and Obstetrics in 1875, rising to the rank of Professor and Director of the Department of Children's Disease at Children's Hospital at Moscow University in 1891 [128]. He was chair of the Society of Pediatrics of Moscow in 1892 [128, 129].

Filatov is considered the founder of pediatrics in Russia and made significant contributions to this specialty [128]. Filatov-Dukes disease, later described by Clement Dukes (1845–1925) in 1900, was originally called scarlet rubella by Filatov. He also described idiopathic inflammation of the cervical lymph nodes or Filatov disease, now recognized as infectious mononucleosis. Filatov described in 1895 the dotted grayish-white rash involving the buccal mucosa occurring one day prior to the measles rash, the same finding reported by Koplick in 1896 [128].

Filatov reported in 1904 the cutaneous findings in children with scarlet fever:

> Some authors erroneously hold that the scarlatinal rash spares the face. In most cases, the skin of the face is changed peculiarly in scarlet fever so that this disease is promptly recognized directly from the patient's face, without even undressing him or taking the history. The peculiarity consists in the pronounced paleness of the lips and of the surrounding skin in contrast with the bright redness of the cheeks [130, p. 646].

Thus, Filatov sign refers to a circumoral pallor of the lips in scarlet fever (Table 1.1). The paper by Filatov titled "Letsii ob Ostrich Infektsionnikh Boliez64nyakh u Dietei" (Lectures of acute infectious diseases in children), published in 1887, has been cited as containing the first description of the sign. We were unable to access this publication.

1.2.20   Marfan Sign

Antoine Bernard-Jean Marfan (1858–1942) was born in Castelnaudary, Languedoc-Roussillon, France, and initially received his medical training at the Faculty of Medicine in Toulouse, and subsequently in Paris, qualifying in 1887. He was chief of the clinic at Necker Hospital from 1889 to 1891 [131]. He served as agrégé at the Sick Children's Clinic in 1892 and directed the diphtheria ward at the Sick Children's Hospital in the Rue de Sèvres in 1901 [132, 133]. Marfan was appointed physician of the Hospitals of Paris in 1902, professor of therapeutics at the Faculty of Medicine, Paris, in 1908, chair of infantile hygiene at the Clinic of Early Childhood Diseases, Paris, in 1914, and chair at the Hospice for Sick-Assisted Children in 1920. There he also established the Institute of Childcare [132, 133].

Marfan is considered the founder of pediatric education in France and undoubtedly best recognized for the syndrome which he described in 1896 in his paper titled, "Un cas de déformation congénitale des quatre membres, plus prononcée aux extrémités, caractérisée par l'allongement des os avec un certain degré d'amincissement" (A case of congenital deformity of the four limbs, more pronounced at the extremities, characterized by elongation of the bones with some degree of thinning) [134]. His other areas of interest and publication involved infant feeding and nutrition, diphtheria, typhoid fever, and disease of infants. He co-edited with Jules Comby (1853–1947) and Jacques-Joseph Grancher (1843–1907) *Traité des Maladies de l'Enfance* (Treatise on Children's Diseases) in 1897 and with Jean Martin Charcot (1825–1893), Charles Jacques Bouchard (1837–1915), and Edouard Brissaud (1852–1909) *Traité de Médecine* (Treatise on Medicine) second edition in 1901 [135].

Among his other services and accomplishments, he founded the journal *Le Nourrisson* (The Infant) in 1913 and served as president of the National Committee for Childhood [132]. He was selected as a member of the French Academy of Medicine, section of medical pathology, in 1914, decorated with the Legion of Honor in 1922, and honorary fellow of the Royal Society of Medicine in 1934 [133]. As a description of his character:

> Marfan particularly admired the virtues which were his own: the austerity of private life, the uprightness of character, the firmness of convictions, the contempt of intrigues, the disdain of compromises, leading him in all circumstances and whatever may happen to conform his acts to his mature opinion [132, p. 270].

Grancher writes in the second edition of their book *Traité des Maladies de l'Enfance* published in 1907:

> Before going any further, I would like to express to Mr. Marfan, whose authority in the matter of pediatrics is so well known and so esteemed, all the regret that his retirement inspires in us. For entirely personal reasons, Mr. Marfan did not believe he could continue his collaboration with us. It is, therefore, under my name and that of M. Comby alone that this edition will appear [136, p. i-ii].

As described by Mery in the second edition of *Traité des Maladies de l'Enfance* in their discussion on typhoid fever:

> Mr. Marfan reported a triangle-shaped peeling tongue extending from tip to base. The
> tongue has the characteristic red and thin appearance at the edges and at the tip, covered in
> the middle with a more or less thick saburral coating. In severe forms, the tongue dries and
> covers itself, as well as the lips, with fuliginous [136, p. 492].

Thus, Marfan sign is found in patients with typhoid fever. It refers to the red and thin
appearance of the tongue at the tip and edges, along with a yellowish-white plaque
with slightly elongated filiform papilla (saburral coating) in the middle—the triangular-shaped denuded region extends from the tip to the base of the tongue
(Table 1.1).

1.2.21   Escherich Sign

Theodor Escherich (1857–1911) was born in Ansbach, Bavaria, Germany, studied
medicine at Strasbourg, Würzburg, Kiel, and Berlin, and received his medical
degree in Munich in 1881 [137–140]. He practiced at the medical clinic in Würzburg
as an assistant under the auspices of Carl Adolph Christian Jacob (Karl Adolf
Christian Jakob) Gerhardt (1833–1902) in Juliusspital (Julius Hospital) in the
Department of Internal Medicine from 1882 to 1884, rising to the rank of first assistant [138–140]. He sought further training in pediatrics in Paris and Vienna at St.
Anna Children's Hospital in 1884, the latter to which he returned more than a
decade later [138, 141]. At the Vienna Pathological Institute, he conducted bacteriological studies on breast milk [142].

Escherich conducted further bacteriologic studies in Munich beginning in 1884.
He was a clinical assistant in the Children's Polyclinic of the Reisingerianum and
Hauner Children's Hospital in Munich under Heinrich von Ranke (1830–1909) in
1885 and Associate Professor in pediatrics at the Ludwig-Maximillian University,
Munich, in 1887 [137, 139, 141, 143]. At the University of Graz, Austria, he was
appointed extraordinary professor and chair of pediatrics of the K.K. Children's
Clinic in 1890 and ordinary professor in 1894, followed by a professorship of pedi-
atrics and chair at the University of Vienna and St. Anna's Children's Hospital,
Vienna, Austria in 1902 [137–141, 144].

He made substantial contributions to infectious diseases in children, including
diphtheria, croup, tetany, and tuberculosis [144]. His name is best recognized in
conjunction with the colonic bacteria *Bacterium coli commune*, now named
Escherichia coli, first discovered in 1885 and published in 1886 in the text *Die
Darmbakterien des Säuglings und ihre Beziehungen zur Physiologie der Verdauung*
(The Intestinal Bacteria of the Infant and their Relations to the Physiology of
Digestion) [144, 145]. He served as president of the Austrian Society for Children's
Research in 1908 and was instrumental in constructing the Imperial Institute of
Maternal and Child Care [142].

As a description of his character:

> His energy for work was tremendous, and his disposition strenuous and masterful. He is
> described as impulsive, uncommonly strict, strong-willed, faithful, severe with himself but

kindly towards others. That the children, his patients, loved him, is evidence that he loved them and therefore, had a good heart [138, p. 474].

He described a finding in patients with tetany termed idiopathic tetany in childhood, attributed to rickets and hypoparathyroidism:

> On the other hand, I am inclined to regard what I have described as mouth phenomena similar to the true facial reflex. It is most easily recognized in healthy, well-developed children almost regularly during the first two months of life, especially those who are breastfed. In some cases, it occurs longer if the mouth or an adjacent area is percussed with a finger or a hammer during deep sleep. A sharpening and protrusion of the lips occur as if grasping the nipples, which disappears quickly, sometimes followed by sucking movements. The fact that the amplitude of the muscle contractions is more clearly perceptible on the non-percussed side is based on the obvious mechanical conditions. The phenomenon cannot be triggered in the waking state. In agreement with Thomsen, I consider it probable that this is a process related to the sucking reflex, and conclude from this fact that it is only present in very young and sleeping children, and in later age only in pathological cases, and that the same is often successfully triggered only after prolonged regularity percussion attempts. Hence, this phenomenon is not found exclusively in tetany [146, p. 57].

Thus, Escherich sign refers to the protrusion of the lips when tapping the mouth or adjacent areas (lips or tongue) in patients with tetany or latent tetany secondary to hypoparathyroidism (Table 1.1).

1.2.22 *Gaucher Sign*

Charles Phillipe Ernest Gaucher (1854–1918) was born in Champlemy, Nièvre, France, studied medicine at the Faculty of Medicine, Paris, and served as an intern of the Paris Hospitals in 1877 and histology technician in 1880 [147–149]. He received his medical degree at the Faculty of Medicine, Paris, in 1882 based on his thesis *De l'épithélioma primitif de la rate* (On Primary Epithelioma of the Spleen) later eponymously recognized as Gaucher disease [147, 149–151], and chief of the medical clinic at Charité Hospital from 1882 to 1884 [150]. He was appointed physician to the Paris Hospitals in 1886, physician of the Hospital Saint-Antoine, and professor agrégé of the Faculty of Medicine in 1892 [148, 150]. He served as clinical professor and chair of Cutaneous and Syphilitic Disease at the Saint-Louis Hospital in 1902 [147–151]. During World War I, he was appointed chief physician of the Military Hospital, Villemin [147, 148, 150, 151].

Gaucher founded the journal *Annales des Maladies Vénériennes* (Annals of Venereal Diseases) in 1906. He was elected member of the Paris Academy of Medicine in 1910 and president of the General Association of Doctors of France and the Medical Society of the Hospitals of Paris [147, 148, 150]. He was anointed Officer of the Legion of Honor in 1917 in recognition of his contributions at the Villemin Hospital during World War I [150, 151].

According to Georges Baudouin:

> Under a somewhat rough exterior, which made those who knew him but slightly judge him unjustly, there were hidden an excellent heart, an upright character, and absolute professional rectitude. Especially kind and considerate to the unfortunate, he unstintingly gave his charitable soul and zealously devoted himself to the organization and development of the Medical War Fund (Caisse Médicale de Guerre) which was established for the assistance of the unfortunate confrères and of the widows and children of physician who had been cruelly stricken by the war [148, p. 573].

Gaucher reported in a series of 16 patients an unusual partition of the incisors in patients with congenital syphilis:

> To draw from the previous presentation the lesson it contains, I would like you to remember that in addition to the numerous stigmata of hereditary-syphilis today well known and, particularly in addition to the classic dental dystrophies, so well described by Hutchinson, by Fournier and by Parrot, there is one whose special value is not known, the importance of which I have just demonstrated to you and to which I call the attention of physicians, namely the separation of the upper middle incisors [152, p. 823].

Gaucher noted that the separation of the upper middle incisors might occur as an isolated finding or along with other stigmata of congenital syphilis.

1.2.23   *Hathcock Sign (Hathchock Sign)*

Thomas Alexander Hathcock Jr. (1865–1943) was born in Albemarie, North Carolina, USA, and received his medical education at the Baltimore Medical College, University of Maryland, Baltimore, graduating in 1894 [153]. He practiced in Norwood, North Carolina, and served in public office as county commissioner, mayor, school committee, and board of commissioners [154]. During World War I, he served as First Lieutenant at Medical Officers Training Camps in Greenleaf, Chickamauga Park (Fort Oglethorpe), Georgia, later transferring to the Base Hospital at Camp Wheeler Macon, Georgia [153, 154].

He described his eponymously named sign at Camp Wheeler during a Mumps epidemic. He was promoted to captain in 1918 and discharged as major that same year [153]. After the war, he returned and served as superintendent at Norwood Methodist Church and president of Stanley Oil, Riverview Milling, Norwood Electric and Water, Norwood Development, Bank of Norwood, and surgeon to Southern Norfolk-Southern railroads [153]. As reported by Lieutenant M.J. Radin in 1918 (Fig. 1.1):

> The most diagnostic prodromal sign, pathognomonic, in fact, was first noted by Lieutenant Hathcock, who has personally observed and treated over 2000 cases, and who is, from the standpoint of knowledge gained by close clinical observation of the disease, probably the best authority on mumps in the United States. The sign is tenderness just beyond the angle of the jaw on running the finger toward the angle, under the mandible. If the parotid gland is at all involved, the patient winces with pain. This occurs before any swelling can be made out. It is proper and fitting—much as eponyms are held by some to be improper—that this sign go down in the literature as Hathcock's sign. It is almost constant, it is early, it is definite and it is exclusive; therefore, it is diagnostic, like Koplik's spots in measles [155, p. 360].

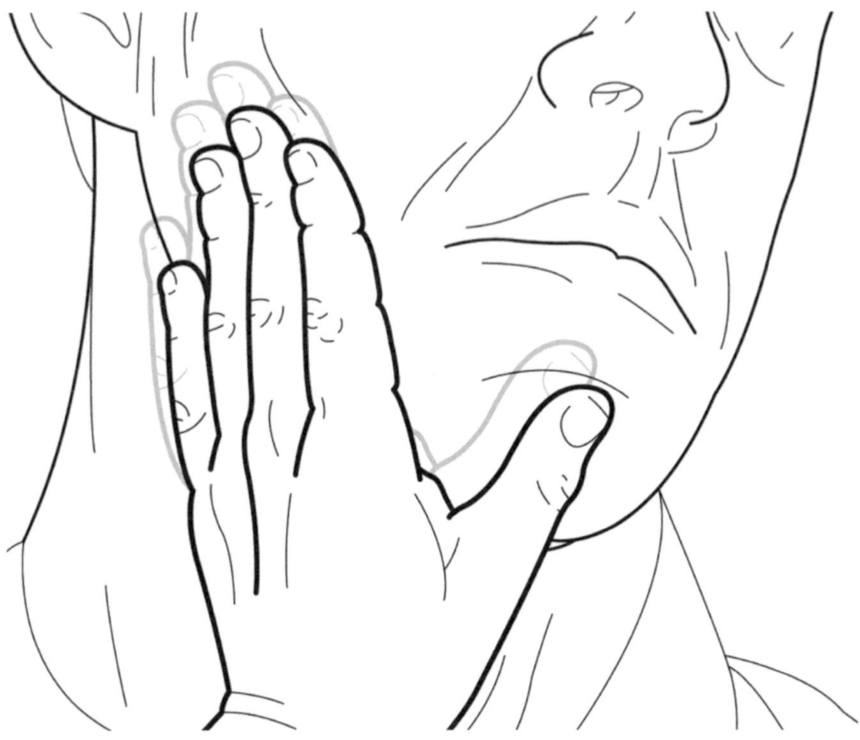

Fig. 1.1 Hathcock sign (by Ryan Yale)

Thus, Hathcock sign refers to palpatory tenderness beyond the mandibular angle found on running the finger along the mandible toward its angle (Table 1.1).

1.2.24   Sterling-Okuniewski Sign

Stefan Adam Sterling-Okuniewski (1884–1934) was born in Warsaw, Poland, and received his medical degree and Doctor of Philosophy degree from the University of Zurich, Switzerland, and medical degree from the Faculty of Medicine, Wroclaw; Breslau, Germany (currently Poland) in 1910 [156]. He served as a senior assistant at the Serological and Bacteriological Institute at Warsaw Scientific Society, followed by the chief of the Municipal Bacteriological Library. He founded the first cancer clinic in *Łódź*, Poland, in 1918 and served as senior clerk of the Ministry of Public Health, Warsaw [156]. During the Polish-Bolshevik War, he conducted research on typhus and was commander of the Czerniakowski Hospital of Infectious Disease and Military Hospital no. V in Warsaw, and a Hygiene Officer at D.O.K.I. in 1921 [156]. Sterling-Okuniewski obtained his habilitation in pathology and internal medicine, lecturing on infectious diseases in 1924 [156]. He was appointed physician for terminally ill cancer patients at St. Lazarus Hospital in Warsaw in 1927 and associate professor and head of the Ujazdowski Hospital, Warsaw, in 1928 [156]. He cofounded the Polish Anti-Cancer Committee in 1921 and was editor of the *Biuletyn Polskiego Komitetu do Zwalczania Raka* (Bulletin of the Polish Anti-Cancer Committee), renamed the *Nowotwory Journal* in 1923 [156, 157].

Sterling-Okuniewski described a finding in patients with typhus:

> Sometimes the patient cannot protrude the tongue when requested by the physician. (…) Various authors have long noticed this symptom. Nevertheless, Malcz writes: "On the second day, the layers of the throat and tongue swell, and yet, the patient is still able to speak. On day three, the speech was impeded, and the tongue was slowly being pulled back when talking" [158, p. 225]. In fact, there are cases where the patient cannot stick out the tongue. If this is present, it can be a serious symptom in the diagnosis of typhus. However, there is no way of accepting Renilinger's view that this symptom always occurs (within three years, "we do not remember […] ever seeing the sign of the faulty tongue"). After reading the article by the French author, I checked his observations on a hundred or more cases in different periods of the disease, and only in a few cases was it difficult for the patient to protrude the tongue. Once a sick person, at my request, was unable to protrude his tongue but was able, with a few fingers of his right hand, to pull it out with some effort [158, p. 226].

Thus, Sterling-Okuniewski sign refers to the inability of a patient to protrude his tongue on command (Table 1.1). The pathogenesis is postulated to be caused by perivascular infiltration involving the hypoglossal nucleus and nerve. This sign was believed to be beneficial as a clinical test to differentiate epidemic louse-borne typhus fever from enteric fever [159].

1.2.25   Jackson Sign

Chevalier Quixote Jackson (1865–1958) was born in Pittsburg, Pennsylvania, and received his medical degree from Jefferson Medical College, Philadelphia, in 1886 [160–162]. He received further training in laryngology under the auspices of Morell Mackenzie (1837–1892) in England, returning to Pittsburg in 1887 to practice this specialty [160, 163]. He designed an esophagoscope prior to 1890 and subsequently worked on a bronchoscope whose purpose was foreign body extraction [160]. His later work demonstrated the safety and usefulness of these instruments in diagnosing and treating diseases in infants and adults, including esophageal stricture [160, 164]. He was appointed professor of laryngology at the University of Pittsburgh Medical School and director of the bronchoscopic clinic at Pittsburgh Children's Hospital beginning in 1912 [160, 161, 163]. Jackson published his first text titled *Tracheo-Bronchoscopy, Esophagoscopy, and Gastroscopy* in 1907 and *Peroral Endoscopy and Laryngeal Surgery* in 1914 [160, 162, 164].

He accepted an appointment as a professor of laryngology at Jefferson Medical College, Philadelphia, Pennsylvania, in 1916 [162, 164]. He served as chair of Bronchoscopy and Esophagoscopy at the University of Pennsylvania, Graduate School of Medicine, in 1919. He held a similar position at Jefferson Medical College, Temple University, where he developed the Chevalier Jackson

Bronchoscopy Clinic of Temple University and Medical School and at Woman's Medical College of Pennsylvania [160, 163, 164]. He was appointed president of the latter institution from 1935 until 1941 [160]. Another significant and perhaps less well-recognized achievement was that he was instrumental in promoting the passage of the Federal Caustic Act in Congress, signed by President Coolidge in 1927, requiring all manufactures to label and print the antidote for poisonous caustic or corrosive substances [160, 162, 164].

He served as president of the American Laryngological, Rhinological, and Otological Society in 1911, founding member of the American College of Surgeons in 1913, and as president of the American Laryngological Society in 1926. He received the chevalier rank of the Legion of Honor from France and the chevalier rank of the Order of Leopold from Belgium in 1927 [160]. He received many other awards and accolades throughout his career, including the Distinguished Service Medal of the American Medical Association and meritorious services from the American College of Chest Physicians in 1952 [160, 161].

As to his character as described by Holinger:

> The great modesty, sincerity and singleness of purpose of this man who lived through almost a century of medicine can hardly be realized. He developed a specialty through keen observation, consummate skill and great perseverance. (…) His kindness, gentleness, and courtesy pervaded all his actions and these basic attitudes commanded the greatest respect from his patients and the colleagues who worked with him. (…) Those few who had the privilege of a visit to "The Mill" where he lived in the beautiful countryside outside of Philadelphia saw a man keenly interested in nature and humble in his appreciation of the beauty of his surroundings. (…) Chevalier Jackson's influence in medicine will continue to be felt far beyond the borders of his country and the span of his life. Modern medicine as well as his individual patients pay great homage to this man who did so much more than his part "as his turn came round" [160, p. 569].

In the words of Maxwell Ellis:

> There could have been no more single-minded man in the history of medicine. He sighted his goal early in life; he moved towards it unerringly and steadily for over half a century; and in the end he saw his work become an integral part of the practice of medicine [161, p. 568].

Jackson described the following findings found in patients with a foreign body:

> Tracheal Foreign Body. (1) "Audible slap", (2) "palpatory thud", (3) "asthmatoid wheeze" are pathognomonic. The "tracheal flutter" has been observed by McCrae. Cough, hoarseness, dyspnea and cyanosis are often present. Diagnosis is established by roentgen ray, auscultation, palpation, bronchoscopy. Listen long for "audible slap," best heard at open mouth during cough. The "asthmatoid wheeze" is heard with the ear or stethoscope bell (McCrae) at the patient's open mouth. History of initial chocking, gagging, and wheezing is important if elicited by is valueless negatively [165, p. 316].

Thus, (Chevalier) Jackson sign refers to the ability to hear a wheezing sound over the open mouth in a patient with a foreign body within the trachea or bronchus (Table 1.1).

1.2.26 Biederman Sign

Joseph B. Biederman (1907–1984) was born in Mazowieckie, Poland, and received his medical degree from the University of Cincinnati College of Medicine in 1932 [166, 167]. He practiced medicine at the Cincinnati General Hospital Allergy Clinic at the University of Cincinnati Medical College. He patented several products, including a mask to prevent and relieve respiratory allergy symptoms and a respiratory filtering device [168].

He was a recipient in 1983 of the American College of Allergy, Asthma, and Immunology Award of Merit, which stated:

> To qualify for the award, candidates must have demonstrated outstanding performance in the field of clinical allergy and immunology, be Fellows of recognized national organizations of allergy and immunology, reached the age of 70 and have practiced in the field for at least 25 years [169, p. 3].

Biederman described in patients with latent syphilis that:

> The anterior tonsillar pillars frequently present a dark dusky red color in a well-defined congested area. This area begins at the base of the pillars and extends upward ½ to 2½ cm and is approximately 6 to 10 mm in breadth. The appearance is that of a definite vascular congestion. In the examination of 469 syphilitic patients this sign was present in 324 or 69.1 per cent. Not every case of syphilis presented this sign, nor could every patient having this sign be proved to have syphilis [170, p. 305].

Thus, Biederman sign refers to the dark red color involving the anterior tonsillar pillars of the tonsillar fauces in late syphilis (Table 1.1).

1.2.27 Gorlin Sign

Robert James Gorlin (1923–2006) was born in Hudson, New York, and received his Doctor of Dental Surgeons (DDS) degree from the Washington University School of Dentistry, St. Louis, in 1947, followed by a medical and surgical pathology fellowship at the National Institute of Health and Columbia Presbyterian Medical Center from 1947 to 1951 [171–175]. During this time, he also had appointments as an instructor in medical pathology at Columbia Presbyterian Hospital and oral pathology at Bronx Veterans Administration Hospital [175]. At the State University of Iowa (currently the University of Iowa), he taught a medical pathology course to dental students while advancing his education, receiving a master's degree in chemistry in 1956 [175]. He was appointed associate professor and chairman of the Division of Oral Pathology and held faculty appointments in the departments of pediatrics, laboratory medicine and pathology, and dermatology in 1971; and in the departments of obstetrics and gynecology and otolaryngology at the University of Minnesota in 1973 [173, 175, 176]. From the University of Minnesota, he was appointed Regents Professor of Oral Pathology and Genetics in 1978, professor emeritus in 1993, Reagent Professor Emeritus in 2000, and Honorary Doctor of Science in 2002 [171, 173, 177, 178].

His career and research interests spanned the fields of dentistry, oral and maxillofacial pathology, otolaryngology, obstetrics, craniofacial and orofacial genetic malformations, hereditary hearing loss, pediatrics, and dermatology [171, 172, 177]. His primary area of interest was in delineating the cause of congenital malformation affecting the head and neck, culminating in the description of more than 100 syndromes, 11 eponymously named craniofacial syndromes (Gorlin syndrome or basal cell nevus syndrome), one sign (Gorlin sign), and benign odontogenic cysts (Gorlin cyst) ascribed to honor and acknowledge his keen insights and observations. As further testimony to his accomplishments, he was instrumental in identifying the gene responsible for some of these syndromes and diseases [171].

Robert James Gorlin and Jens Jørgen Pindborg (1921–1995) published their highly acclaimed medical reference book *Syndromes of the Head and Neck* in 1964; the second edition published in 1976 included Michael M. Cohen, Jr. (1937–2008) as co-editor. The third edition, published in 1990, was authored by Gorlin, Michael M. Cohen (1937–2018), and L. Stefan Levin, and the fourth by Gorlin, Cohen, and Raoul C.M. Hennekam, published in 2002 [179].

Gorlin had an impressive list of honors and accomplishments. He cofounded and was elected diplomate of the American Board of Medical Genetics, president of the International Association for Dental Research and American Academy of Oral Pathology, and was a senior fellow of the Institute of Medicine of the National Academy of Science, Premio Phoenix Anni Verdi Award from the Italian Genetics Society to name a few [171, 175]. He also received an Honorary Doctorate in Science from the Universities of Athens and Thessalonica, Greece [180]. He was the editor of oral pathology in the *Journal of Oral Surgery, Oral Medicine and Oral Pathology* [180].

As to his character, he was described as:

> A larger-than-life presence in oral pathology for over 50 years, he was a man of enormous intellect and curiosity, thoughtful deliberation, and infinite compassion and kindness [176].

Gorlin made the following statement regarding his perception about eponyms assigned to the syndromes and diseases which bear his name:

> I am personally opposed to eponyms since they say nothing about the disorder, frequently give rise to argument regarding priority of discovery, and may be chauvinistic and unfair to those whose contributions to knowledge of the syndrome far exceed those of the individual for whom the disorder is named. Perhaps, at some distant time a nifty system for an International Nomenclature of Syndromes will be devised and universally accepted, but I doubt it [175, p. 323].

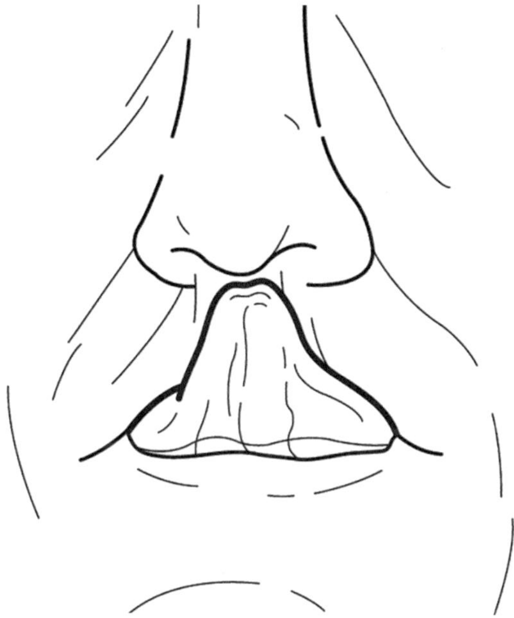

Fig. 1.2 Gorlin sign (by Ryan Yale)

As described by Michael M. Cohen:

> He was a very warm human being who had an engaging way with everyone. He loved people from all walks of life and had a wide array of friends. He was a loving husband, a wonderful father, a consummate and caring clinician, and an astounding humorist. (…) With patients, Bob was an empathetic listener. The more troubled a patient was, the more sensitive and caring he became and the more time he would spend. He had a warm way of making a patient feel less isolated and better about himself or herself. He often hugged men, women, and children. He had a special way of communicating with the distraught parents of an affected child [181].

Gorlin and Pindborg described a finding in patients with Ehlers-Danlos syndrome; 50% of persons with Ehlers-Danlos syndrome "have the ability to touch the nose with the tongue, an ability manifested by about 8–10 per cent of ostensibly normal person" [182, p. 197]. Thus, Gorlin sign refers to the ability to touch the tip of the nose by the protruded tongue in patients with Ehlers-Danlos syndrome (Table 1.1 and Fig. 1.2).

Table 1.1 Oral cavity signs

Name	Year	Description of sign	Method	Etiology
Burton [5]	1840	The margins of the gums at the neck of two or more teeth in the maxilla or mandible are distinctly bordered by a narrow lead-blue line	Inspection	Lead
Carabelli [8]	1844	On the first median wall of the molars, there is an enameled hump (tuberculus anomalous), the base of which arises from the neck of the tooth, and the tip stands free in the oral cavity, somewhat remote from the crown	Inspection	Hereditary
Corrigan [24]	1854	There is a purple color on the margin of the gums, incisor, canine, and bicuspid teeth of the maxilla and mandible	Inspection	Copper
Trélat [30]	1870	Tuberculosis ulcers of the mouth develop in the following way: one finds on the mucous membrane a spot, a barely protruding plate, which is round and wide from 1 to 3 or 4 mm and revealing on its surface still covered with epithelium, one or more several follicular orifices. This spot is light yellow, similar to that of phlegmonous pus. The epithelium is destroyed after a few days leaving an ulcerated surface. Instead of one spot, several are observed at different stages of development	Inspection	Tuberculosis
Clarke [40]	1873	A fissure transverses deeply into the tongue, while rugae are confined to the mucosa. This fissure is best demonstrated by taking the tongue between the fingers and gently stretching it. The rugae can be obliterated in these cases, while no change occurs on the fissures—their sides may be separated, but they cannot be obliterated	Inspection	Syphilis
Drummond [45]	1882	While in the supine position, the patient is told to breathe as quietly as possible through the wide open mouth. The oval piece of the binaural stethoscope is introduced into the mouth. If the sign is present, expiration will appear interrupted at each beat of the heart by a "whiff," which, in some cases, is very loud, while, in others, it is detected only at the end of expiration. In some instances, especially if the aneurysm is large, a diastolic whiff can be heard as well as a systolic. In cases where the sign is well marked, it is heard in the trachea during quiet expirations or when the patient is holding his breath with the mouth open and the tongue depressed to allow the gaping glottis to communicate freely with the buccal cavity. In very well-marked cases, the whiff is audible in the trachea with the mouth closed and disappears when the fingers compress the nostrils. It is crucial to avoid cardiac excitement; hence it should only be sought after the patient has lain in the recumbent position for a short while and after the reasons for inserting the binaural stethoscope into the mouth have been fully explained. Indeed, it is well to explain to the patient accurately before commencing the examination, for nervous, interrupted respiration, and forcible or nasal breathing defeat the reason for the examination	Auscultatory	Thoracic aneurysm

Mueller [52]	1889	The inflamed, reddened tonsils and the anterior and posterior palatine arches moved somewhat medially synchronously with each carotid pulse; pulsation was also noted on the soft palate, and the free edge moved downwards with the uvula. In this way, the palatine arches and tonsils' contraction and the soft palate and uvula deepen with each pulse resulting in a narrowing of the palate. A rhythmic intensification of the reddening of the palate is also observed	Inspection	Thoracic aneurysm
Shelly [55]	1893	The soft palate is completely studded with minute translucent lenticular elevations varying in size, in most cases about 0.5 mm, and hardly ever exceeding 1 mm in diameter. They gave the impression of small localized distensions of a thin layer of transparent epithelium. Their lens-like appearance is increased so that a minute blood vessel lying beneath one of them occasionally becomes magnified. However, it might be impossible to observe any other part of its course as it entered or left the vesicle on either side. These vesicles were most abundant about the soft palpate above the root of the uvula. However, in some cases—and, these were generally of the more severe type—they occupied a much larger area being visible over the greater part of the roof of the mouth, but being always most marked and most abundant at the soft palate	Inspection	Influenza
Fournier [60]	1894	One of the most common manifestations of newborn or congenital syphilis occurs on the lip commissures (one could also say scars on the corners of the mouth because they occupy the angle formed by the lip commissure). The diseases in this place are erosions, decomposed papules, or ulcers. They only occur at the commissure, encroaching on the surrounding skin on rare occasions. In and of themselves, they remain superficial, with tears almost always appearing at the level of the corners of the mouth. Here they form rhagades, ulcerous streaks that repeatedly tear one after the other, hollow out more and more, become deeper, heal slowly and with difficulty, and leave behind persistent, always visible scars. This scar usually forms a small whitish line drawn out, elongated, and running transversely or slightly obliquely from top to bottom. It may be that they are barely visible on the mucosa. (It is known that diseases of the mucous membrane heal less conspicuously than those of the skin.) However, there always remains a distinct and noticeable skin scar. Rarely are scars of this type found around the lips	Inspection	Congenital syphilis

(continued)

Table 1.1 (continued)

Name	Year	Description of sign	Method	Etiology
Krisowski [63]	1895	Linear-shaped and radial-positioned scars occur at the corner of the mouth, separated by normal-appearing skin	Inspection	Congenital syphilis
Koplik [70]	1896	There is invariably a distinct eruption on the buccal mucous membrane and the inside of the lips. It consists of small, irregular spots of bright red color. In the center of each spot, there is a minute bluish-white speck. These red spots, with accompanying specks of a bluish-white color, are pathognomonic of early measles and, when seen, can be relied upon as the forerunner of the skin eruption. The buccal eruption is of greatest diagnostic value at the outset of the disease *before* the appearance of the skin eruption and at the outset and height of the skin eruption	Inspection	Measles
Silex [80]	1896	Multiple scars (pseudoscars) and furrows located on the corners of the mouth and radiating to the chin	Inspection	Congenital Syphilis
Forchheimer [85]	1898	Erythematous maculopapular lesion located on the velum of the palate and the uvula, extending to, but not upon, the hard palate. The spots are arranged irregularly and are the size of large pinheads	Inspection	German measles (Rubella)
Comby [93]	1900	Oral enanthema and erythema with swelling of the gums and an exudative coating involve the mucous membrane	Inspection	Measles
Tresilian [97]	1901	A bright red papilla is observed at the opening of Stensen duct (buccal mucosa at the second upper molar), along with excess salivation	Inspection	Mumps
Castellani-Low [120]	1903	Persistent fine and coarse tremors in the tongue	Inspection	Sleeping sickness
Schultze [123]	1903	Indentation occurs on the tongue when percussing one-half of a protruded tongue	Percussion	Tetany
Miécamp [127]	1903	In early mumps parotitis, a sapid substance (dilute acetic acid or vinegar) is placed on the tongue, and the patient is told to swallow. Painful salivation more commonly occurs on the side of parotid swelling	Inspection	Mumps
Filatov [130]	1904	Circumoral pallor	Inspection	Scarlet fever
Marfan [136]	1907	A triangle-shaped peeling tongue extends from tip to base. The tongue has a characteristic red and thin appearance at the edges and tip, covered in the middle with a more or less thick saburral coating. In severe forms, the tongue dries and covers itself and the lips with fuliginosity	Inspection	Typhoid

Eponym	Year	Description	Method	Disease
Escherich [146]	1909	A sharpening and protrusion of the mouth occur as if grasping the nipples, which disappears quickly, sometimes followed by sucking movements. The fact that the amplitude of the muscle contractions is more clearly perceptible on the non-percussed side is based on the obvious mechanical conditions. The phenomenon cannot be triggered in the waking state	Inspection	Tetany
Gaucher [152]	1913	Separation of the upper middle incisors	Inspection	Congenital syphilis
Hathcock [155]	1918	Palpatory tenderness is located near the angle of the mandible	Palpation	Mumps
Sterling-Okuniewski [158]	1922	Inability to voluntarily protrude the tongue	Inspection	Typhus
Jackson [165]	1923	An audible slap, palpatory thud, and asthmatoid wheeze are pathognomonic of a tracheal foreign body. Cough, hoarseness, dyspnea, and cyanosis are often present. The audible slap is best heard by asking the patient to keep the mouth open during cough. The "asthmatoid wheeze" is heard with the ear or stethoscope bell at the patient's open mouth	Auscultatory	Foreign body
Biederman [170]	1934	Anterior tonsillar pillars are dark dusky red in a well-defined area that begins at the pillars' base, extends ½–2½ cm upward, and is approximately 6–10 mm in width	Inspection	Syphilis
Gorlin [182]	1964	Touch the nose with the tongue	Inspection	Ehlers-Danlos syndrome

1.3 Conclusion

Signs of the oral cavity were discovered and named eponymously for dentists (e.g., Carabelli, Gorlin) and physicians, with the majority caused by infectious diseases. Although we intended for the historical background of these persons to be brief, it was undoubtedly difficult in many cases, given the depth and breadth of their overall accomplishments extending far beyond their named signs. Some of these signs illustrate the limitations of eponyms; the names may be attributed to more than one sign (e.g., Corrigan), or the same name may refer to different authors (e.g., Jackson). These signs were primarily identified through observation, emphasizing the importance of inspection, the first step of the physical examination, when evaluating an organ or structure. They provide additional supporting evidence for a systemic disease process and reinforce to clinicians how a meticulously performed beside physical examination aids in diagnosis. They are often found early in the disease process and are easily overlooked, particularly if the oral examination is given only brief attention.

References

1. Skinner HA. The origin of medical terms. Baltimore: The Williams & Wilkins Company; 1949.
2. Cavity. Online etymology dictionary. https://www.etymonline.com/word/cavity. Accessed 3 Jan 2022.
3. Burton H. Royal College of Physicians. RCP Museum. 2019. https://history.rcplondon.ac.uk/inspiring-physicians/henry-burton. Accessed 3 Jan 2022.
4. [No author]. Obituary. Med News. 1849;20:149.
5. Burton H. A remarkable effect upon the human gums produced by the absorption of lead. Med Chir Trans. 1840;23:63–79.
6. Carabelli-Lunkaszprie. Österreichisches Biographisches Lexikon. https://www.biographien.ac.at/oebl/oebl_C/Carabelli-Lunkaszprie_Georg_1787_1842.xml?frames=yes. Accessed 3 Jan 2022.
7. Carabelli von Lunkaszprie, Georg. Deutsche Nationalbibliothek. https://d-nb.info/gnd/11029775X. Accessed 4 Jan 2022.
8. Carabelli G. Specielle Beschreibung der anomalen Zähne des Oberkiefera. In: Systematisches Handbuch der Zahnheilkunde, Bd. 1. Wien: Braumüller und Seidel; 1844. p. 97–109.
9. Sarpangala M, Devasya A. Occurrence of cusp of Carabelli in primary second molar series of three cases. J Clin Diagn Res. 2017;11:ZR01–2.
10. Sedano HO, Ocampo-Acosta F, Naranjo-Corona RI, Torres-Arellano ME. Multiple dens invaginatus, mulberry molar and conical teeth: case report and genetic considerations. Med Oral Patol Oral Cir Bucal. 2009;14:E69–72.
11. [No author]. Obituary: Sir Dominic John Corrigan, Bart MD. Br Med J. 1880;1:227–8.
12. [No author]. Obituary: Sir Dominic J. Corrigan, Bart MD Edin. Lancet. 1880;118:268–9.
13. [No author]. Sir Dominic John Corrigan. JAMA. 1962;180:406–7.
14. Agnew RAL. The achievement of Dominic John Corrigan. Med Hist. 1965;9:230–40.
15. Willius FA, Keys TE. Sir Dominic John Corrigan (1802–1880). In: Classics of cardiology, vol. 2. New York: Dover Publications; 1941. p. 419–22.
16. Major RH. Dominic John Corrigan (1802–1880). In: Classic descriptions of disease with biographical sketches of the authors. 3rd ed. Springfield: Charles C. Thomas; 1932. p. 352–6.
17. Mapother ED. Sir Dominic Corrigan. Irish Monthly. 1889;3:160–71.

18. Stone J. Sir Dominic John Corrigan. In: Hurst JW, Conti CR, Fye WB, editors. Profiles in cardiology. New Jersey: Foundations for Advances in Medicine and Science; 2003. p. 64–7.
19. Mair RH. Debrett's Illustrated Baronetage and Knightage (and Companionage) of the United Kingdom of Great Britain and Ireland. London: Dean & Son Publishers; 1880.
20. Williamson RT. Sir Dominic Corrigan. Ann Med Hist. 1925;7:354–61.
21. O'Brien ET. The man behind the eponym: Sir Dominic John Corrigan (1802–1880). NEJM. 1981;304:365–6.
22. [No author]. In memoriam: Sir Dominic John Corrigan. Dublin J M Sc. 1880;69:268–72.
23. Corrigan DJ. On permanent patency of the mouth of the aorta, or inadequacy of the aortic valves. Edinb Med Surg J. 1832;37:224–45.
24. Corrigan DJ. Cases of slow copper-poisoning, with observations. Dublin Hosp Gaz. 1854;1:229–32.
25. [No author]. Obsèques du Professeur Ulysse Trélat, 31 mars 1890. Paris: Bureaux du Progrès Médical; 1890.
26. [No author]. Death of Trélat. Med Rec. 1890;37:455.
27. Pagel J. Biographisches Lexikon hervorragender Ärzte des neunzehnten Jahrhunderts. Berlin: Urban & Schwarzenberg; 1901.
28. Péan J, Guérin A, Floderer A, Wauthier A, Delmas B. Trélat Ulysses. Comité des travaux historiques et scientifiques. https://cths.fr/an/savant.php?id=106002#. Accessed 15 Jan 2022.
29. Trélat U. Clinique Chirurgicale. Paris: Libraire J.B. Baillière et Fils; 1891.
30. Trélat U. Note sur l'ulcère tuberculeux de la bouche et en particulier de la langue. Arch Gén de Méd. 1870;15:35–47.
31. Leser E. Über ein die Krebskrankheit beim Menschen häufig begleitendes, noch wenig gekanntes Syndrom. München med Wochenschr. 1901;51:2035–6.
32. Denucé M. Un symptôme de malignité (signe des naevi de Trélat) applicable aux tumeurs profondes de l'abdomen et du basin. Rev Mal Cancér. 1899;4–6:146–56.
33. Hollander EV. Beitrage zur Frühdiagnose des Darmcarcinomas (Hereditatsverhaltnisse und Hautveranderungen). Dtsche med Wochenschr. 1900;26:483–5.
34. [No author]. Obituary: Dr. William Fairlie Clarke. Med Chir Tr. 1885;68:14–6.
35. [No author]. Obituary: W. Fairlie Clarke. Br Med J. 1884;1:975–6.
36. Clarke, William Fairlie (1833–1884). Royal College of Surgeons of England. Plarr's Lives of the Fellows. https://livesonline.rcseng.ac.uk/client/en_GB/lives/search/detailnonmodal/ent:$002f$002fSD_ASSET$002f0$002fSD_ASSET:373372/one?qu=%22rcs%3A+E001189%22&rt=false%7C%7C%7CIDENTIFIER%7C%7C%7CResource+Identifier. Accessed 21 Aug 2022.
37. Greenhill WA. Clarke, William Fairlie. Dictionary of National Biography. https://en.wikisource.org/wiki/Dictionary_of_National_Biography,_1885-1900/Clarke,_William_Fairlie. Accessed 11 Sept 2022.
38. Johnson G. Dr. William Fairlie Clarke. Med Chir Tr. 1885;68:14–5.
39. [No author]. W. Fairlie Clarke, MD, FRCS. Lancet. 1884;1:918–9.
40. Clarke WF. Syphilis as it affects the tongue. In: A treatise on the diseases of the tongue. London: Henry Renshaw; 1873. p. 141–70.
41. [No author]. Obituary: Sir David Drummond MD, DCL. Br Med J. 1932;1:865–6.
42. [No author]. Central Chancery of the Order of Knighthood. Lond Gaz. 1920:1237.
43. Drummond H. Some points relating to the surgical anatomy of the arterial supply of the large intestine. Proc R Soc Med Proctol. 1913;7:185–93.
44. Drummond H. The arterial supply of the rectum and pelvic colon. Br J Surg. 1913;1:677–85.
45. Drummond D. On auscultation of the trachea and mouth in thoracic disease. Br Med J. 1882;2:773–4.
46. Souttar H. Friedrich von Müller. Br Med J. 1951;2:340–2.
47. Wormer EJ. Müller, Friedrich von. In: Neue Deutsche Biographie, Bd. 18. München: Bayerische Akademie der Wissenschaften; 1997. p. 379–81.
48. Biografie, Friedrich von Muller. Wissenschaftliche Sammlungen. Teil-Katalog der wissenschaftlichen Sammlungen. Humboldt-Universität zu Berlin. https://www.sammlungen.hu-berlin.de/objekte/-/17224/. Accessed 21 Jan 2022.

49. [No author]. Friedrich von Muller and William Osler. NEJM. 1955;252:76–7.
50. Müller F. Morbus Brightii. Verh Deutsch Path Ges. 1905;9:64–9.
51. Castiglioni A. A history of medicine (trans: E.B. Krumbhaar). New York: Alfred A. Knopf; 1941.
52. Müller F. Pulsation des Gaumens bei Aorteninsuffizienz. In: Charité-Annalen, Bd. 14. Berlin: Verlag von August Hirschwald; 1889. p. 251–2.
53. [No author]. Dr. Charles Edward Shelly. Br Med J. 1935;2:708–9.
54. Shelly CE. Transactions of the seventh international congress of hygiene and demography, London, August 10-17th, 1891. London: Eyre & Spottiswoode; 1892.
55. Shelly CE. Vesicular eruption in the palate a sign of influenza. Br Med J. 1893;1:791–2.
56. Coleman ML, Fournier JA. Gangrène foudroyante de la verge. Semaine Méd. 1883;3:345.
57. Darier J. Alfred Fournier (1832–1914). Paris: Imprimerie Durand; 1915.
58. Waugh MA. Alfred Fournier, 1832–1914: his influence on venerology. Br J Vener Dis. 1974;50:232.
59. Toodayan N. Jean Alfred Fournier (1832–1914): his contributions to dermatology. Our Dermatol Online. 2015;6:486–91.
60. Fournier A. Vorlesungen über Syphilis hereditaria tarda. Leipzig: Franz Deuticke; 1894.
61. Blanck GFA, Wilhelmi AST. Die mecklenburgischen Ärzte von den ältesten Zeiten bis zur Gegenwart. Schwerin I.M. Eduard Herberg's Hofbuchdruckerei und Verlagshandlung; 1901. p. 246.
62. Krisowski M. Unsere Schätze, unsere Kinder: für Ärzte, Lehrer und Eltern. Berlin: Verlag von Streisand; 1899.
63. Krisowski M. Über ein bisher wenig beachtetes: Symptom der hereditären Lues. Berl klin Wochenschr. 1895;32:893–6.
64. Bass MH. Henry Koplik, 1858–1927. J Pediatr. 1955;46:119–25.
65. Libman E. Obituary: Dr. Henry Koplik. Bull N Y Acad Med. 1927;3:667–71.
66. Good Samaritan Dispensary. New York Times. 22 June 1897. http://tenement-museum.blogspot.com/2010/02/modified-milk-and-lower-east-side.html. Accessed 11 Feb 2022.
67. Dr. Henry Koplik, scientist, dies. The Sentinel. 13 May 1927. https://www.nli.org.il/en/newspapers/cgs/1927/05/13/01/?&. Accessed 11 Feb 2022.
68. Koplik H. Archives & special collections. Catalogue of the Alumni, Officers and Fellows, 1807–1891. https://www.library-archives.cumc.columbia.edu/obit/henry-koplik. Accessed 14 Feb 2022.
69. [No author]. Dr. Henry Koplick, noted physician, dies at age of 69. Jewish Daily Bulletin; 3 May 1927, p. 4.
70. Koplik H. The diagnosis of the invasion of measles from a study of the exanthema as it appears on the buccal mucous membrane. Arch Pediatr. 1896;13:918–22.
71. Artesnstein MS, Demis DJ. Recent advances in the diagnosis and treatment of viral diseases of the skin. NEJM. 1964;270:1101–11.
72. Hoeprich PD. Infectious diseases: a modern treatise of infectious processes. New York: Harper & Row; 1972.
73. Evans LM, Grossman ME, Gregory N. Koplik spots and a purpuric eruption associated with parvovirus B19 infection. J Am Acad Dermatol. 1992;27:466–7.
74. Hazeltine R. An account of the measles, as it appeared in Berwick, County of York, District of Maine, during a part of the years 1802 and 1803. M Reposit. 1804;1:348–57.
75. Silex P. Deutsche Digitale Bibliothek. https://www.deutsche-digitale-bibliothek.de/person/gnd/117629758. Accessed 12 Aug 2022.
76. Biografied, Paul Silex. Wissenschaftliche Sammlungen. https://www.lautarchiv.hu-berlin.de/objekte/-/18731/. Accessed 2 Sep 2022.
77. Ausgabe V. Silex, Paul. In: Who's who in Germany – Wer ist's?, Bd. 5. Leipzig: Verlag von H.A. Ludwig Degener; 1911. p. 1371–2.
78. Silex P. Handbuch der Gesamten Augenheilkunde, Bd. 15. Berlin: Verlag von J. Springer; 1918, p. 185.

79. [No author]. Dr. Paul Silex. Br Med J. 1929;1:377.
80. Silex P. Pathognomonische Kennzeichen der congenitalen Lues. Berl klin Wochenschr. 1896;33:162–5.
81. [No author]. Frederick Forchheimer, 1853–1913. Boston Med Sci J. 1913;169:71–2.
82. Collective. Forchheimer, Frederick. In: The National Cyclopedia of American Biography, vol. 16. New York: J.T. White; 1918. p. 388.
83. Otto J. In memoriam Frederick Forchheimer. Cincinnati: Cincinnati & Hamilton County Public Library; 1914.
84. [No author]. Address by President Charles William Dabney. In: Inauguration of the Frederick Forchheimer Chair of Medicine. Cincinnati: University of Cincinnati; 1916. p. 5–11.
85. [No author]. The enanthem of German measles. Phila Med J. 1898;2:15–6.
86. Comby J. Reial Acadèmia de Medicina de Catalunya. http://ramc.cat/biblioteca/medicina-doccitania/biografies-mediques/jules-comby/. Accessed 15 Feb 2021.
87. Garrison FH. History of pediatrics. Philadelphia: W.B. Saunders; 1923.
88. Corbella J. Comby, Jules. In: Metges i Medicina d'Occitània. Barcelona: Institut d'Estudis Catalans; 2012. p. 285.
89. [No author]. News of the week: Dr. Jules Comby. Med Rec. 1894;46:141.
90. Comby J. Traité des Maladies de l'Enfance. Paris: J. Rueff; 1892.
91. Comby J. Les Médicaments chez les Enfants. Paris: J. Rueff; 1900.
92. Comby J. Formulaire Thérapeutique et Prophylaxie des Maladies des Enfants. Paris: J. Rueff; 1900.
93. Comby J. Quatre cas de rougeole dans la même famille particularités cliniques. Arch méd enf. 1900;3:421–4.
94. [No author]. Dr. F.J. Tresilian. Br Med J. 1926;1:459.
95. [No author]. Editorial and personal. Student's J & Hosp Gaz. 1885;13:180.
96. [No author]. Tresilian, Frederick James. Trans Med Soc Lond. 1901;24:41.
97. Tresilian F. A sign of mumps. Br Med J. 1901;1:889.
98. Dr. Aldo Castellani, a specialist on sleeping sickness, is dead. New York Times. 5 Oct 1971. https://www.nytimes.com/1971/10/05/archives/l-dr-a-ldo-castellani-a-specialist-on-sleeping-sickness-is-dead.html. Accessed 11 Feb 2022.
99. [No author]. Aldo Castellani MD, FRCP, FACP. Br Med J. 1971;4:175.
100. Parish LC. Reflections on Aldo Castellani and tropical dermatology. Trans R Soc Trop Med Hyg. 2018;112:155–7.
101. Ito K. A synopsis of the life of Aldo Castellani. Int J Dermatol. 1972;11:192–6.
102. Firkin BG, Whitworth JA. Dictionary of medical eponyms. New York: The Parthenon Publishing Group; 1987.
103. Castiglioni A. Clinical medicine. In: A history of medicine (trans: EB Krumbharr). New York: Alfred A. Knopf; 1941. p. 818–35.
104. Ito K. Aldo Castellani, 1874–1971. Bull NY Acad Med. 1984;60:1011–29.
105. Boyd J. Sleeping sickness: the Castellani-Bruce controversy. Notes Rec R Soc Lond. 1973;28:93–110.
106. Cipollaro VA. Euphoria et cacophoria-anecdotes, reminiscences and controversies of Aldo Castellani; and "who let Castellani go"? Int J Dermatol. 2007;46:439–42.
107. Castellani A, Chalmers AJ. Manual of tropical medicine. London: Baillière, Tindall and Cox; 1910.
108. Castellani A. A short preliminary note on a probably new Torulopsis found in two cases of chronic purulent-ulcerative affection of the fingers. Mykosen. 1969;12:507–8.
109. [No author]. Obituaries: Aldo Castellani, MD, FRCP; FACP. Med Mycol. 1972;10:103.
110. Papers of Castellani, Sir Aldo (1877–1971). London School of Hygiene and Tropical Medicine Archives. GB 809 CASTELLANI' on the Archives Hub. https://archiveshub.jisc.ac.uk/data/gb809-castellani. Accessed 1 Feb 2022.
111. Sebastiani A, Serarcangeli C. Aldo Castellani (1874–1971): un viaggio scientifico lungo un secolo. Medicina nei Secoli Arte e Scienza. 2003;15:469–500.

112. Cipollaro VA. The history of the International Society of Dermatology. 2018. https://www.intsocderm.org/files/ISD%20Golden%20Jubilee_WEB.pdf. Accessed 30 Jan 2022.
113. Cook GC. George Carmichael Low, FRCP: an underrated figure in British tropical medicine. J R Coll Physicians Lond. 1993;27:81–2.
114. Fairely NH. Obituary: George Carmichael Low, MA, MD, CM, FRCP. Trans R Soc Trop Med Hyg. 1952;46:571–3.
115. [No author]. Obituary: George Carmichael Low, MA, MD, CM, FRCP. Br Med J. 1952;2:341–4.
116. Brown GH. George Carmichael low. Royal College of Physicians. https://history.rcplondon.ac.uk/inspiring-physicians/george-carmichael-low. Accessed 2 Feb 2022.
117. Low GC. A recent observation on Filaria nocturna in Culex: probable mode of infection of man. Br Med J. 1900;1:1456–7.
118. Cook GC. Royal Society of Tropical Medicine and Hygiene Meeting at Manson House, London, 10 December 1992. George Carmichael Low FRCP: twelfth President of the Society and underrated pioneer of tropical medicine. Trans R Soc Trop Med Hyg. 1993;87:355–60.
119. Parliamentary Papers. Great Britain, Parliament, House of Commons. 1904. https://www.google.com/books/edition/Parliamentary_Papers/4pIOAQAAIAAJ?hl=en&gbpv=0. Accessed 11 Feb 2022.
120. Low GC, Castellani A. Report on sleeping sickness from its clinical aspects. In: Reports of the Sleeping Sickness Commission. London: Harrison and Sons; 1903. p. 14–63.
121. Ashwal S, Schultze F. Child neurology: its origin, founders, growth and evolution. 2nd ed. London: Elsevier Science; 2021. p. 281–3.
122. Kreuter A. Deutschsprachige Neurologen und Psychiater: ein biographisch-bibliographisches Lexikon von den Vorläufern bis zur Mitte des 20. Jahrhunderts. München: K.G. Saur; 1996.
123. Schiefferdecker P, Schultze F. Beiträge zur Kenntnis der Myotonia Congenita, der Tetanie mit myotonischen Symptomen, der Paralysis agitans und einiger anderer Muskelkrankheiten, zur Kenntnis der Aktivitäts-Hypertrophie und des Normalen Muskelbaues. Dtsche Ztschr Nervenh. 1903;25:1–9.
124. Miécamp L. Pathogénie de l'Oedéme Aigu du Poumon. Lyon: Imprimerie Perrellon; 1900.
125. Miécamp L. Un signe de diagnostic précoce des oreillons. Le Caducée. 1903;3:77.
126. Miécamp EL. Annuaire Official de l'Armée Française. Paris: Berger-Levrault et Cie; 1906.
127. Miécamp L. Signe diagnostic précoce des oreillons. J Méd Chir Prat. 1903;74:313–4.
128. Morgoshiia TS. [Professor Nil Fedorovich Filatov (1847–1902): innovative pediatrician, clinician and teacher (on the occasion of his 170th birthday)]. Epidemiologija i Infekcionnye Bolezni. 2018;23:260–3.
129. Filatov N. Praebook. https://prabook.com/web/nil.filatov/2105256. Accessed 12 Feb 2022.
130. Filatov NF. Febrile disease. In: Semeiology and diagnosis of diseases of children, vol. 2. Cleveland: Cleveland Press; 1904. p. 644–70.
131. [No author]. Bernard Jean Antonin Marfan, MD, 1858–1942. Am J Dis Child. 1942;6:354–5.
132. Renault J. Notice nécrologique sur M. Marfan. Bull Acad Nat Med. 1942;126:267–70.
133. [No author]. Professor Marfan. Br Med J. 1942;2:175.
134. Marfan AB. Un cas de déformation congénitale des quatre membres, plus prononcée aux extrémités, caractérisée par l'allongement des os avec un certain degré d'amincissement. Bull Mém Soc Méd Hôp Paris. 1896;13:220–6.
135. Bouchard C, Brissaud E, Charcot JM. Traité de Médecine: Maladies Chroniques du Poumon, tome 7. Paris: Masson et Cie; 1901.
136. Grancher J, Comby J. Traité des maladies de l'enfance, tome 1. 2e éd. Paris: Masson et Cie; 1907.
137. [No author]. Obituary: Professor Theodor Escherich. Br Med J. 1911;1:472.
138. [No author]. Obituary: Theodor Escherich, MD. Boston Med Sci J. 1911;164:474–5.
139. Pfaundler M. Theodor Escherich. München med Wochenschr. 1911;58:521–3.
140. Katner W. Escherich, Theodor. In: Neue Deutsche Biographie, Bd. 4. Berlin: Duncker & Humblot; 1959. p. 649–50.

141. Schulman ST, Friedmann HC, Sims RH. Theodor Escherich: the first pediatric infectious diseases physician? Clin Infect Dis. 2007;45:1025–9.
142. Friedmann HC. Escherich and Escherichia. American Society for Microbiology. 2014. https://journals.asm.org/doi/epub/10.1128/ecosalplus.ESP-0025-2013. Accessed 30 Jan 2022.
143. [No author]. Death of Professor Escherich. Lancet. 1911;1:626.
144. Hamburger F. Theodor Escherich. Wien klin Wochenschr. 1911;24:263–6.
145. Escherich T. Die Darmbakterien des Säuglings und ihre Beziehungen zur Physiologie der Verdauung. Stuttgart: Verlag von Ferdinand Enke; 1886.
146. Eschreich T. Die Tetanie der Kinder. Wien: Holder; 1909.
147. [No author]. Medical news: death of Gaucher. JAMA. 1918;70:639.
148. Baudouin G. Professor Charles Philippe Ernest Gaucher (trans: John E. Lane). Am J Syphilis. 1918;2:571–3.
149. [No author]. Nécrologie: le professeur Ernest Gaucher. Paris Méd. 1918;28:95.
150. [No author]. Le professeur Ernest Gaucher. Paris Méd. 1918;28:60.
151. [No author]. Ernest Gaucher, 1854–1918. J Cutan Dis Syph. 1918;36:493–4.
152. Gaucher E. L'Écartement des incisives médians supérieures dystrophie hérédo-syphilitique: sa valeur comme stigmate d'hérédité syphilitique. Ann Mal Vén. 1913;1:801–23.
153. Gwen's Genealogy Village. 29 July 2016. http://gwensgenealogyvillage.blogspot.com/2016/07/big-daddy-hathcock-thomas-alexander.html. Accessed 15 Jan 2022.
154. Efird OO. The history and genealogy of the Efird Family. Madison: The University of Wisconsin; 1964.
155. Radin MJ. The epidemic of mumps at Camp Wheeler, October 1917 – March 1918. Arch Intern Med. 1918;22:354–69.
156. [No author]. Ś.p. Docent Dr. Stefan Sterling-Okuniewski. Lekarz Polski. 1934;10:121.
157. Towpik E, Wysocki WM. The Nowotowry Journal over the last 95 years (1923–2018). Nowotory J Oncol. 2017;67:321–35.
158. Sterling-Okuniewski S. Dur Wysypkowy (Tyfus plamisty) (typhys exanthematicus, febris petechialis). Lwów-Warszama: Ksiaznica Polska Towarżystwa-Nauczycieli Szól Wyższych; 1922.
159. Kryszek H, Cracow MD. Tongue sign in louse-borne typhus fever. Br Med J. 1942;1:2469.
160. Holinger PH. Chevalier Jackson, MD, ScD; LLD; LHD; FACS, 1865–1958. Chest. 1959;36:567–9.
161. [No author]. Obituary: Chevalier Jackson, MD, FACS. Br Med J. 1958;2:568–9.
162. Chevalier Jackson (1865–1958). JMC Class of 1886. Notable Jefferson Alumni of the Past. Thomas Jefferson University. https://library.jefferson.edu/archives/exhibits/notable_alumni/chevalier_jackson.cfm. Accessed 4 July 2022.
163. Boyd AD. Chevalier Jackson: the father of American bronchoesophagoscopy. Ann Thorac Surg. 1994;57:502–5.
164. Nguyen PD, Cowan SW, Yeo CJ, Evans N. Chevalier Jackson, MD (1865–1958): il ne se repose jamais. Am Surg. 2013;79:454–6.
165. Jackson C. The mechanism of physical signs with especial reference of foreign bodies in the bronchi. Am J Med Sci. 1923;165:313–20.
166. Joseph B. Biederman. Ancestry. https://www.ancestry.com/search/categories/42/?name=Joseph+_Pitrman&death=_OH. Accessed 10 Feb 2022.
167. [No author]. Obituary: Biederman, Joseph B. JAMA. 1984;25:1199–201.
168. Patent Office. Inventor: Joseph B. Biederman. https://patents.google.com/?inventor=Joseph+B+Biederman. Accessed 10 Feb 2022.
169. ACA President's Newsletter. Award of merit presented to 29 ACA members. March 1983. https://college.acaai.org/sites/default/files/Advantage/HistoricalNewsletters/aca_news_1983.pdf. Accessed 10 Feb 2022.
170. Biederman JB. Diagnostic sign: a preliminary report of another. Am J Syph Neurol. 1934;18:305.

171. Hoyle J. Dr. Robert J Gorlin, world-renowned oral pathologist, dies at 83. JADA. 2006;137:1371–2.
172. Oransky I. Robert Gorlin. Lancet. 2006;368:1414.
173. Cohen MM, Robert J. Gorlin, 1923–2006: evolution of his phenotype. Am J Hum Genet. 2007;80:585–7.
174. Eng C, Robert J, Gorlin DDS. MS (1923–2006): a geneticist for all seasons. J Med Genet. 2007;44:478–9.
175. Gorlin RJ. Living history-biography: from oral pathology to craniofacial genetics. Am J Med Genet. 1993;46:317–34.
176. Rohrer M. Robert J. Gorlin, 1923–2006. American Academy of Oral and Maxillofacial Pathology. https://www.aaomp.org/wp-content/uploads/2016/12/AAOMP_Fall_2006_Newsletter.pdf. Accessed 12 Jan 2022.
177. Jeremy Pearce: Robert Gorlin, 83, pathologist and expert on facial malformations, is dead. The New York Times. 14 Sept 2006. https://www.nytimes.com/2006/09/14/obituaries/14gorlin.html. Accessed 12 Jan 2022.
178. Gorlin RJ. Star Tribune. 30 Aug 2006. https://www.startribune.com/obituaries/detail/8499324/. Accessed 12 Jan 2022.
179. Balci S. To the memory of Robert J. Gorlin. Genet Med. 2007;9:195.
180. Robert J. Gorlin - 1997 distinguished Alumnus. Alumni Newsletter School of Dental Medicine. Winter, 1997–1998, vol. 30, no. 1. St. Louis: Washington University. https://static1.squarespace.com/static/5c59e470e6666952cedc924e/t/5c5bc6064785d3fecc1be8ab/1549518350225/WudaaAlumniNewletter_Winter1997-98.pdf. Accessed 12 Jan 2022.
181. Cohen MM. Robert J. Gorlin, 1923–2006: a remembrance. Am J Med Genet. 2006;140:2516–20.
182. Gorlin RJ, Pindborg JJ. Syndromes of the head and neck. New York: McGraw-Hill; 1964.

Chapter 2
Oropharynx and Esophagus Signs

2.1 Introduction

The British English "oesophagus" or American English "esophagus" terms originated from the ancient Greek word οἰσοφάγος (oisophagos), meaning gullet, which bears or carries food to swallow [1]. The gullet refers to the tube that transports food from the pharynx to the stomach [1]. Early eponymic signs reported in the late nineteen century described delayed auscultatory sounds to distinguish obstructive disorders of the esophagus. With the advent of oral barium contrast, it is now possible to visualize the esophagus and, by its appearance, the means to distinguish esophageal stricture from esophageal carcinoma. Other findings in the early twentieth century involved using a palpatory technique to diagnose pharyngeal diverticulum or Zenker diverticulum, named for Friedrich Albert von Zenker (1825–1898), who first described this pathological entity in 1867 [2]. The most significant advancement in the study of the esophagus came about with the development of the endoscope and illumination devices which now allowed direct visualization of this organ and the flexible fiberoptic endoscopy by Basil Hirschowitz (1925–2013) and his student Larry Curtiss in 1958 [3].

2.2 Eponymic Signs

2.2.1 Meltzer Sign

Samuel James Meltzer (1851–1920) was born in Ponevyeh, Curland, Russia, and received his medical degree from the University of Berlin in 1882 [4, 5]. He emigrated to the United States in 1883, worked as a private practitioner, and conducted research at the Welch Laboratory at Bellevue and Curtis Laboratory at Columbia

S. H. Yale et al., *Gastrointestinal Eponymic Signs*,
https://doi.org/10.1007/978-3-031-33673-7_2

University College of Physicians and Surgeons (currently Columbia University Vagelos College of Physicians and Surgeons) [5]. He was appointed director of the Department of Physiology and Pharmacology at the Rockefeller Institute for Medical Research in 1906 [4, 6]. During World War I, he was a major in the Army Medical Reserve Corps of the United States. His research focus involved the science of physiology and the practical application of clinical medicine [4, 6].

He was a cofounder and served as the first president of the American Association for Thoracic Surgery in 1918; president of numerous societies and organizations, including, among others, the American Physiological Society in 1888, the Association for the Advancement of Clinical Research in 1909, the American Society for Clinical Investigation in 1912, the Society for Experimental Biology and Medicine, the American Gastro-Enterological Society, the Harvey Society, Association of American Physicians, the Society for Experimental Pathology, the American Philosophical Society, the National Academy of Sciences, and the American Association of Pathology and Bacteriology [4–8].

As a tribute to his character by the staff of the Rockefeller Institute for Medical Research:

> His leadership and his contributions are second to the contributions of no other man in their significance for this generation of medical men. Dr. Meltzer's interest in humanity transcended the field of his medical activities. In the spirit of human cooperation, he desired to include all men, so that there might glow, across the boundaries of nations, a desire for progress in the direction of universal ideals. These great interests were recognized, not only in this country, but in Europe as well, and gave Dr. Meltzer a unique position as a lover of his kind [8, p. 88].

Meltzer describes the movement of food into the esophagus during the act of swallowing (Table 2.1):

> When auscultating at the epigastrium or near the xiphoid process, a sound is heard in almost all cases during swallowing, indicating that the swallowed mass (preferably liquid) has entered the stomach. A study of more than 100 persons on this subject produced the following results: In most cases examined, a long noise was heard 6–7 seconds after swallowing began, as if air or liquid was being pushed through a previously closed sphincter. I call this sound a Durchpreßgeräusch [pressing noise]. In a minority of cases, a distinct hissing sound is heard immediately after the first moment of swallowing, often as if the swallowed liquid was running into the stethoscope. One has the impression that the swallowed liquid is immediately squirted into the stomach without hindrance. Where this noise was present, there was no pressing sound. In some cases, the former was present only more or less suggestively, and afterward, the latter was heard but weak; only in a few cases was the sound absent [9, p. 2]. (…) In most cases, one hears in the epigastrium a constant pressing noise occurring 6–7 seconds after the start of swallowing. From this, we conclude that the cardia is normally closed and that the mass for the individual swallowing arrives 6–7 seconds above the cardia. A distinct squeezing sound is heard immediately after swallowing when the cardia is quiet. I bear no hesitation in pointing out that the distinct presence of the sound is a sure symptom of esophageal insufficiency [9, p. 4].

Thus, Meltzer found that the second sound is either delayed or absent in cases of esophageal obstruction.

2.2.2 *Roger Sign*

Georges Eugène Henri Roger (1860–1946) was born in Paris, France, and served as an extern in 1881 and intern at the Hospitals of Paris in 1883 [10, 11]. He was a physician at Concours du Bureau Central Hospital and earned his agrégé in 1892 [12]. He was appointed physician to the Contagious Hospital at Porte d'Aubervilliers and head of the laboratory from 1895 to 1903 and the Charité Hospital in 1903, followed by the Hôtel-Dieu Hospital [10–12]. He was appointed professor of the Department of Experimental and Comparative Pathology of the Faculty of Medicine, the University of Paris in 1904, professor at the Institute of Colonial Medicine in 1905, and dean of the Faculty of Medicine from 1917 to 1930 [10–12].

Roger co-founded the journal *La Presse Médicale* and received honorary doctorates from Edinburgh, England; Cluj, Romania; and Vilnius, Lithuania [11]. He was president of the Association of General Medicine in 1890 and the National Academy of Medicine in 1910 [11, 12]. He was knighted in 1908 and elected member of the Academy of Medicine of Paris for the section of pathological anatomy in 1910, as well as the Academies of Milan, Warsaw, Turin, Madrid, and Buenos Aires [10–12]. He was Commander of the Legion of Honor in 1923 and was crowned from Italy, Romania, and Poland. He was appointed a foreign correspondence in 1924 and Foreign Honorary Member in 1926 [10].

As to a description of his character by Bénard:

> He was one of the greatest intellects of his time, with a mind open to all knowledge. A man of science and a fine scholar in love with art, history, and philosophy—in a word, with the most varied culture. Such is the memory left behind by the distinguished personality of Henri Roger [13, p. 651].

Roger was the first to describe the esophago-salivary reflex (Table 2.1):

> The significance of the esophago-salivary reflex is obvious. When a large food bolus stops within the esophagus, the flow of saliva facilitates its progression. M. Carnot has observed that in humans, catheterization of the esophagus causes a flow of saliva, sometimes so abundant that the liquid flows freely out of the mouth. It is important, says this author quite rightly, when carrying out this gastric chemistry test, tilts the subject's head forward to avoid swallowing saliva and diluting the gastric juice [14, p. 150–151]. (…) In summary, the excitations of the esophagus depends on the function of the salivary and glands within the mouth. They provoke an abundant secretion, and the liquid produced by them stimulates the pharynx and, consequently, promotes esophageal contractions. It is by a circuitous mechanism that the esophagus responds to excitations. Incapable of contracting effectively, the esophagus facilitates the pharynx's excitability by stimulating the buccal secretions. This set of reflexes stimulates esophageal movement resetting the reflex to its starting point [14, p. 156].

Roger also recognized the presence of a gastro-salivary reflex caused by increased acid within the stomach due to hyperacidity:

> The meaning of this flow of saliva seems obvious to me. Saliva is an alkaline liquid. In cases of gastric hyperacidity, it neutralizes the contents of the stomach and prevents both the action of fermentation acids and the action of hydrochloric acid. All physicians who have observed hyperchlorhydrics know how frequently sialorrhea occurs in these patients. As

M. Linossier points out, in three cases, sometimes the saliva produced in excess is swallowed and neutralizes the gastric contents. At other times it flows outside the mouth or, as a consequence of a spasm of the cardia, accumulates in the lower part of the esophagus to be rejected later in the form of aqueous pseudo-vomiting. Thus, the neutral or alkaline vomiting of hyperchlorhydrics is explained [14, p. 161–162].

Thus, Roger sign refers to the esophago-salivary and gastro-salivary reflexes.

2.2.3 *Frimaudeau Sign*

There is limited historical information on Achille-Henri-Louis Anastase Frimaudeau (1886–?). He served as a provisional intern of the Hospitals of Bordeaux and Medical Electricity Service and was a laureate of the hospital [15, 16]. He received his medical degree based on the thesis titled "Diagnostic et étude des rétrécissements de l'œsophage par la radioscopie" (Diagnosis and study of esophageal strictures by radioscopy) in 1911 [15]. He was an officer in the Military Health Services in 1911 [16].

Frimaudeau described the appearance of the esophagus in patients with esophageal stricture and cancer (Table 2.1):

The various stenoses are preceded by dilatations of different shapes, which aid in the underlying diagnosis. Thus, cancerous strictures assume a cup shape dilation of the esophagus, which contains a regular and round bottom. Cicatricial stenoses, on the contrary, are complicated by conical dilation. We explain the fact in this way: most cancerous stenoses are due to the increase in the volume of neoplasm starting from one esophageal wall and growing towards the esophageal lumen. Neoplastic infiltration never extends far upstream from the stenosis. Above the neoplasm, the esophageal walls are flexible, easily dilated, and round in shape under the pressure of the bismuth liquid. On the contrary, cicatricial stenoses lie between the completely sclerotic zone and normal walls and an intermediate zone of semi-sclerosis whose dilatability decreases from top to bottom, causing this to dilate in a funnel shape [17, p. 542–543].

Thus, Frimaudeau sign refers to the "cup-shape" esophagus in patients with a stricture secondary to esophageal carcinoma and "funnel-shape" in cases of esophageal stricture caused by fibrosis.

2.2.4 *Boyce Sign*

John Welch Boyce (1871–1930) was born in Sligo, Pennsylvania, USA, and served on the staff of West Penn and South Side Hospitals [18]. He was a consulting physician for the Eye and Ear Hospital and visiting physician for the Mayview City Hospital, Pennsylvania. Boyce was a major in the Medical Reserve Corps at Camp Jackson's medical department [18, 19]. He served as president of the Allegheny County Medical Society. He also studied law and was admitted to the Allegheny County Bar [18].

Chevalier Jackson (1865–1958) attributed Boyce sign to Dr. John W. Boyce, a consultant, and colleague of Jackson. In Jackson's book *Peroral Endoscopy and Laryngeal Surgery*, published in 1915, he reported a finding described by Boyce in patients with a pharyngeal diverticulum (Table 2.1):

> The chief symptoms are cough, regurgitation of food, gurgling sound and subjective sensation on swallowing, a peculiar sour odor to the breath, and difficulty of swallowing. Boyce's sign can usually be elicited immediately after swallowing. It consists in a gurgling sound produced by pressure of the hand on the side of the neck. A fresh swallowing movement without food or water is needed for each test. The sound is probably made by forcing out of air and bubbles of secretion from the sac. All symptoms are valueless diagnostically, but they are urgent indications for esophagoscopy [20, p. 544–545].

Interestingly, Albert Boyce Barrow and Joseph Cunning described the case in 1905 of a 55-year-old woman who:

> During the previous six months there was a marked increase in the difficulty of swallowing solid food. She volunteered the information that she had regurgitated, not vomited food quite unchanged as long as three days after taking it. As instances, she gave a pickled onion and portions of rabbit. She also complained that stooping caused regurgitation and that she made a curious noise on swallowing. The patient looked so thin and half-starved that several surgeons who saw her were tempted to say, "Oh! She looks as if she had a malignant disease." On examination of the neck no swelling or enlargement of the glands could be detected, but on bilateral pressure over the oesophagus just below the level of the cricoid cartilage, a certain amount of gas could be squeezed up into the mouth. On swallowing two- or three-times gas could again be squeezed up. A medium sized bougie stopped eight inches from the teeth and could be felt to the left of the trachea. A small bougie could be passed into the stomach. As an oesophageal pouch was now suspected from the history of regurgitation of unchanged food and from being able to squeeze up gas on pressure at the base of the neck two bougies were passed together. The first went into the pouch, the second into the stomach [21, p. 928–929].

Thus, Boyce sign refers to a gurgling sound auscultated on the side of the neck when pressure is applied in cases of an esophageal diverticulum.

2.2.5 *Clerf Sign*

There is limited historical information on Louis H. Clerf. He was a fellow of the College of Physicians of Philadelphia, USA, in December 1931 [22]. At that time, he was an instructor in bronchoscopy and esophagoscopy and a demonstrator of laryngology at Jefferson Medical College in Philadelphia, Pennsylvania. His other appointments included being an assistant professor in the Department of Bronchoscopy and Esophagoscopy at the Graduate School of Medicine at the University of Pennsylvania. He was also a chief clinical assistant in the Department of Bronchoscopy and Esophagoscopy at Jefferson Hospital and an assistant in Bronchoscopy and Esophagoscopy at the University Hospital Philadelphia, Pennsylvania [22].

He and Chevalier Jackson described the method of diagnosing an esophageal diverticulum (Table 2.1):

> A tentative diagnosis of diverticulum can be made from the symptoms and the Boyce and Clerf signs. The patient is asked to swallow, which puts air in the diverticulum. Pressure with the fingers low on the neck will force out the air and cause a gurgling sound heard at the patient's open mouth (Boyce sign). If, by indirect mirror laryngoscopy, the laryngeal mirror be watched, bubbles will be seen to emerge from one or other pyriform sinus [23, p. 295–296].

Thus, Clerf sign refers to the presence of air bubbles seen on indirect laryngoscopy in patients with pharyngeal diverticulum.

2.2.6 Heimlich Sign

Henry Judath Heimlich (1920–2016) was born in Wilmington, Delaware, USA, and received his medical degree from Cornell Medical College, New York City, in 1943 [24, 25]. He served in the Navy during World War II and, upon his return, was a thoracic surgical resident in New York City, including the Veterans Administration Hospital from 1946 to 1947, Mount Sinai Hospital from 1947 to 1948, Bellevue Hospital from 1948 to 1949, and Triboro Hospital from 1949 to 1950 [26]. He was an attending surgeon and director at Montefiore Hospital, Bronx, from 1950 to 1968 [24, 26]. Heimlich was appointed director of surgery at the Jewish Hospital, Cincinnati, Ohio, until 1977 and professor of Advanced Clinical Sciences at Xavier University in 1977 [24].

He received the Lasker Award in 1984 and an honorary Doctor of Science degree from Wilmington College in Delaware in 1981; the Adelphi University, New York, in 1982; the Rider College, New Jersey, in 1983; and the Alfred University, New York, in 1993 [26]. Heimlich founded and served as president of the Heimlich Institute in Cincinnati, Ohio (located at the Deaconess Hospital), from 1977 to 1989 [26]. He was the inventor of a valve named the Heimlich chest drain valve used to remove pleural fluid [24, 25]. His maneuver and other aspects of his professional career remain controversial and contentious.

Heimlich described a sign and maneuver to recognize and prevent choking on food. Heimlich proposed that the chocking victim use this sign as a way to notify others that he/she is chocking (Table 2.1):

> It is necessary, therefore, to introduce a universal signal that the victim can use and that a rescuer can recognize to indicate that this accident has occurred. I recommend that the victim grasp his neck between the thumb and index finger of one hand to signal he is choking on food [27, p. 398].

The abdominal infradiaphragmatic pressure maneuver was first published in June 1974 in *Emergency Medicine* in a paper titled "Pop goes the café coronary" as a method for dislodging food occluding the oropharynx or trachea [28]. The maneuver, named in honor of Heimlich, who was the first to describe the technique, is performed with the victim standing or sitting or if in a supine position [29]. In the standing or sitting position:

> Standing behind the victim, the rescuer puts both arms around him just above the belt line, allowing head, arms, and upper torso to hang forward. Then, grasping his own right wrist with his left hand, the rescuer rapidly and strongly presses into the victim's abdomen, forcing the diaphragm upward, compressing the lungs, and expelling the obstructing bolus. The same effect can be observed with the victim lying face down on the floor, the rescuer silting astride (the victim's lower torso or buttocks). If, however, the victim is already lying on his back, he needn't be moved. The rescuer merely sits astride him and suddenly presses both hands—one on top of the other—forcefully into the upper subdiaphragmatic abdominal region [28, p. 154].

The 2020 guidelines for managing a foreign body obstructing the airway recommend that in children and adults, back slaps be used when the victim has an ineffective cough. When back slaps are ineffective than in adults and children (>1 year), an abdominal thrust is applied [30].

Table 2.1 Oropharynx and esophagus signs

Name	Year	Description of sign	Significance
Meltzer [9]	1883	When auscultating at the epigastrium or near the xiphoid process, the first sound (pressing sound) is heard 6–7 s after swallowing, indicating that the swallowed mass (preferably liquid) has entered the stomach. Sometimes, a distinct second hissing sound is heard immediately after the first swallowing sound. The second sound is weak and may be absent in esophageal insufficiency	Esophageal dysmotility
Roger [14]	1907	When a large food bolus stops within the esophagus, a flow of saliva occurs, facilitating its progression	Esophago-salivary reflex
Frimaudeau [17]	1911	Cancerous strictures are preceded by cup shape dilation of the esophagus—a dilation with a very regular and round bottom. Cicatricial stenoses assume a conical dilation	Shape of esophagus on barium esophagram
Boyce [20]	1915	A gurgling sound occurs while pressing on the side of the neck after swallowing	Pharyngeal diverticulum
Clerf [23]	1926	The patient is asked to swallow. Pressing low on the neck force air out, causing a gurgling sound at the patient's open mouth (Boyce sign). By indirect mirror laryngoscopy, bubbles emerge from one or other pyriform sinus	Pharyngeal diverticulum
Heimlich [28]	1974	The victim grasps his neck between the thumb and index finger of one hand	Chocking

2.3 Conclusion

There are a few signs referable to the esophagus. Interestingly, Albert Boyce Barrow and John Welch Boyce described a gurgling sound occurring after pressing on the side of the neck. Included is the Heimlich sign, which, in 1975, received widespread notoriety for the universal description of choking, which involved the victim to grasp his neck between the thumb and index finger of one hand as a method of informing others that he/she is choking. As widely recognized, he described the maneuver for aiding choking victims, which has since been replaced by an alternative method.

References

1. Skinner HA. The origin of medical terms. Baltimore: Williams & Wilkins; 1949. p. 1110.
2. Zenker FA, von Ziemssen HW. Krankheiten des Oesophagus. Leipzig: F.C. Vogel; 1867.
3. Hirschowitz BI, Curtiss LE, Peters CW, Pollard HM. Demonstration of a new gastroscope, the fiberscope. Gastroenterology. 1958;35:50–3.
4. [No author]. Obituary: Samuel J. Meltzer, MD. Med Rec. 1920;98:824.
5. Howell WH. Biographical memoir: Samuel James Meltzer, 1851–1920. Mem Nat Acad Sci. 1926;21:1–20.
6. Meltzer SJ. The Rockefeller University. Digital Commons. https://digitalcommons.rockefeller.edu/faculty-members/49/. Accessed 3 Nov 2022.
7. Brainard ER. History of the American Society for Clinical Investigation, 1909–1959. J Clin Invest. 1959;38:1784–837.
8. [No author]. Samuel J. Meltzer. Science. 1921;53:88.
9. Meltzer SJ. Schluckgeräusche im Scrobiculus cordis und ihre physiologische Bedeutung. Centralbl med Wissensch. 1883;21:1–4.
10. Roger H. Académie royale de Médecine de Belgique. Fédération Wallonie-Bruxelles. http://old.armb.be/index.php?id=4500. Accessed 10 Nov 2022.
11. Rouvillois H, Trémolières F, Hennet S, Wauthier A. Roger GEH. Comité des travaux historiques et scientifiques; 15 Dec 2020. https://cths.fr/an/savant.php?id=4637. Accessed 10 Nov 2022.
12. [No author]. Élections: Henri Roger. Bull Acad Méd. 1861–1862;27:684.
13. Bénard H. Éloge de Henri Roger (1860–1946). Bull Acad Méd. 1966;150:651–6.
14. Roger GH. Alimentation et digestion. Paris: Masson Cie; 1907.
15. [No author]. Frimaudeau AHLA. In: Bibliographie de la France. Paris: Cercle de la Librairie; 1911. p. 318.
16. [No author]. Annuaire Officiel de l'Armée Française, Troupes Métropolitaines et Troupes Coloniales pour 1913. Paris: Berger-Levrault; 1912.
17. Frimaudeau A. Étude et diagnostic des sténoses de l'œsophage par la radioscopie. Arch électr méd. 1911;19:542–52.
18. [No author]. Dr. John W. Boyce dies in hospital. The Pittsburgh Press; 24 Nov 1930. p. 8.
19. [No author]. Medical Officers Reserve Corps Majors: John W. Boyce. Mil Surg. 1917;41:548.
20. Jackson C. Peroral endoscopy and laryngeal surgery. Saint Louis: Laryngoscope Co.; 1915.
21. Barrow AB, Cunning J. A case of oesophageal pouch successfully treated by excision. Lancet. 1905;1:928–9.
22. [No author]. Fellows of the College of the Physicians of Philadelphia. Tr Coll Phys Phila. 1931;53:xviii.

23. Jackson C, Clerf LH. Diseases of the oesophagus. In: Osler W. Modern medicine, its theory and practice, vol. 3: Diseases of metabolism, diseases of the digestive system. Philadelphia: Lea & Febiger; 1926. p. 283–302.
24. McFadden RD. Dr. Henry J. Heimlich, famous for antichocking techniques, dies at 96. New York Times; 17 Dec 2016. https://www.nytimes.com/2016/12/17/us/dr-henry-j-heimlich-famous-for-antichoking-technique-dies-at-96.html. Accessed 6 Nov 2022.
25. Roehr B. Henry Heimlich. Br Med J. 2017;356:j118.
26. Shampo MA, Kyle RA. Henry Heimlich: Heimlich maneuver. Mayo Clin Proc. 2000;75:474.
27. Heimlich HJ. A life-saving maneuver to prevent food-chocking. JAMA. 1975;234:398–401.
28. Heimlich HJ. Pop goes the café coronary. Emerg Med. 1974;6:154–5.
29. [No author]. Simple method relieves café coronary. JAMA. 1974;229:746–7.
30. Olasveengen TM, Mancini ME, Perkins GD, et al. Adult basic life support: international consensus on cardiopulmonary resuscitation and emergency cardiovascular care science with treatment recommendations. Resuscitation. 2020;156:A35–79.

Chapter 3
Stomach Signs

3.1 Introduction

Ibn Sina (Avicenna) (980–1037), a Persian philosopher and physician, is credited for being the first to describe symptoms of gastric ulcers. Regarding tenderness of the pylorus, he makes the following statement in his famous medical encyclopedia titled *al-Qanun fi al-Tibb* (*The Canon of Medicine*): "One knows that this tenderness is present because pain is felt during the passage of acrid substances through it" [1, p. 502]. Giovanni Battista Morgagni (1682–1771), in 1737, was the first to record the pathological findings of stomach and duodenum ulcers in a 50-year-old female:

> Its mucous coat was ulcerated in several places, and the ulcers appeared recent, and exhibited a gangrenous blackness. Near the pylorus they were minute and crowed, and in the fundus of the stomach they were larger and more dispersed; but at that part where the stomach begins to expand itself from the termination of the oseophagus, they were of a greater extent than at any other part [2, p. 34].

Jean Cruveilhier (1791–1874) first described and illustrated the clinical symptoms and macroscopic pathological appearance of gastric ulcers in his two-volume atlas *Anatomie Pathologique du Corps Humain* (Pathological Anatomy of the Human Body), published from 1829 to 1842 [3]. Georges Maurice Debove (1845–1920), in 1866, presumably the first eponymous sign ascribed to the stomach, assessed for the presence of hydrochloric acid in the stomach as a method for differentiating gastric ulcer from gastric carcinoma. With the advent of radiographic technique and contrast, the shift in better understanding peptic ulcers occurred in the first quarter of the twentieth century: Lewis G. Cole (1874–1954) in 1908, Martin Haudek (1880–1931) in 1910, and Russell D. Carman (1875–1926) in 1921 identified specific pathologic features or signs to differentiate benign from gastric ulcers. Gastroscopy allowed Norbert K. Henning (1896–1985) to directly visualize the stomach to assist in the diagnosis of benign gastric ulcer. Other signs were attributed

S. H. Yale et al., *Gastrointestinal Eponymic Signs*, https://doi.org/10.1007/978-3-031-33673-7_3

to conditions that directly or indirectly involved the stomach. Described are the eponymously named signs of the stomach as initially reported, listed chronically starting from the earliest report.

3.2   Eponymous Signs

3.2.1   Chaussier Sign

François Chaussier (1746–1828) was born in Dijon, France, and served as prosector under the aegis of Raphaël Bienvenu Sabatier (1732–1811) in Paris [4]. He was a surgeon in the hospital and prison and a forensic scientist for the courts of Dijon [5, 6]. He lectured on anatomy and comparative anatomy beginning in 1769. The chair of professor of anatomy was endowed in his honor by the citizens of the State of Burgundy in 1780 [5, 6].

Chaussier was requested by the government to assist in the organization of medical education for Paris in 1874 [4, 5]. He returned to Paris and was appointed professor of anatomy and later physician to the École Polytechnique and chief obstetrician to the Hospices de la Maternité (Maternity Hospices) in 1804 [4, 5]. He was professor of physiology, anatomy, and medical jurisprudence for the district at the Faculty of Paris until 1822. He was also elected member of the National Academy of Sciences and the Academy of Medicine [4, 6].

As to a description of his character by a colleague:

> Chaussier's reputation was immense and rightly meritorious. He touched almost all points of science; anatomic, medicine, surgery; legal medicine, and accouchements proving that he was a truly superior man in all areas. (…) His work in forensic medicine is stamped with the corner of great science, great insight, and profound and sagacious attention, and bears in many places the imprint of a great heart and a truly good man [6, p. 574].

Chaussier described an early finding found in women with puerperal convulsion (eclampsia) (Table 3.1):

> Considering the seizure and the subsequent development of these symptoms, it is evident that all characterize nervous irritation and congestion of the blood in the brain. What must be noted is that these severe cerebral symptoms, the results of a general disorder of the circulation, are the secondary or sympathetic effect of an irritation which arises in the abdominal viscera. Nearly almost before the seizure, the patient experience epigastric pain followed by a heaviness in the stomach and derangements in the digestive functions, which propagate to the uterus and extend to the brain. Sometimes we have seen women who, during a seizure, automatically place their hands on the epigastrium, strike this region hard, and try to tear it with their nails. However, at other times the irritation seems to begin in the uterus and thence spread to the stomach and to the nervous system, resulting from the intimate and reciprocal connection between all the parts of the body. Whatever the organ is the primary seat of the irritation, the uterus is always in a particular state which ought to fix all the attention. If we place the hand on the abdomen and keep it there for some time, we feel through its walls that the uterus experiences a tonic, permanent contraction, which, however, increases on the return of the convulsive attacks [7, p. 344–345].

Thus, Chaussier described the clinical symptoms of the disease, later named eclampsia.

3.2.2 *Fenwick Sign*

Samuel Fenwick (1821–1902) was born in Earlsdon House, Northumberland, near Newcastle-on-Tyne, England, in 1821 and received his medical degree from St. Andrews University, Scotland, in 1846 [8–12]. He was a general practitioner at North Shields, followed by appointments as lecturer on pathological anatomy and later examiner in medicine at Newcastle-on-Tyne, the University of Durham Medical School in 1861 [13]. He received an honorary doctorate from Durham University, England, in 1859 [11].

Fenwick served as a consulting physician at Harley Street, London, in 1862 [9–11, 14]. He was appointed lecturer of medicine at the London Hospital Medical College and assistant physician to the City of London (Victoria Park) Hospital for the Diseases of the Chest and later the same staff appointment at the London Hospital [10]. He was appointed full physician at the London Hospital in 1879 [14].

He was elected fellow of the Royal Medical and Chirurgical Society of London in 1863; a fellow of the Royal College of Physicians, London, in 1870; and a member of the Pathological Society [9]. His two books, *The Student's Guide to Medical Diagnosis*, first published in 1869, and *Outlines of Medical Treatment*, published in 1879, have endured multiple editions [9, 10].

As to his character:

> If I were asked to name the feeling with which he inspired us, I should say it was reverence. He was our revered teacher, for these reasons: his great clinical wisdom and his unique power of imparting his knowledge to the least of us evoked our admiration; while his courteous, kindly manner to his patients and ourselves won our affection [10, p. 673].

Fenwick first reported and described the case in a 45-year-old male whom he diagnosed with atrophy of the stomach (Table 3.1). He wrote:

> I am, however, not aware that any cases have been published in which the whole of the secreting structures of the stomach was found after death to be in a state of atrophy, and in which the symptoms were sufficiently well marked to admit of an accurate diagnosis being made during the life of the patient [15, p. 78].

Histological examination found:

> The whole of the glandular structure of the organ was in a state of atrophy; in no part could I succeed in procuring a section of normal tissue. In the pyloric and middle regions the secreting tubes seemed to be converted into a mass of connective tissue, (…) and it was only near the cardiac end that a trace of gland structure could be observed [15, p. 79].

It is now well-recognized that chronic atrophic gastritis is associated with vitamin B12 and iron deficiency anemia. Interestingly, Fenwick noted the resemblance of symptoms found in his patients to idiopathic anemia described by Dr. Thomas Addison (1793–1860). Based on these findings, he recommended histologic examination of the stomach and intestines in patients with Addison disease [15, p. 80].

3.2.3 *Trousseau Sign*

Armand Trousseau (1801–1867) was born in Tours, France, and received his medical degree from School of Medicine in Paris in 1825. He was appointed physician to the Bureau Central in 1831, was an assistant at Récamier Clinic, Hôtel-Dieu, and physician to Saint-Antoine Hospital, Sainte-Marguerite Hospital, and eventually Necker Hospital [16]. He was appointed chair of therapeutics and materia medica of the Paris Faculty of Medicine in 1839 and professor and chair of clinical medicine at Hôtel-Dieu in 1852 [17–19].

Trousseau published his three-volume books, *Traité de Thérapeutique et de Matière Médicale* (Treatise on Therapeutics and Materia Medica) from 1836 to 1839. He was recognized by the French Academy of Medicine in 1837, being the recipient of the grand prize for his work titled "Traité pratique de la phthisic laryngée, de la laryngite chronique et des maladies de la voix" (Practical treatise on laryngeal phthisis, chronic laryngitis and diseases of the voice) and elected member of the National Academy of Medicine in 1856. His other significant accomplishments include tracheotomy in croup and thoracentesis in pleural effusions [17, 19].

It should be noted that Armand Trousseau (1856–1919), chief of the clinic of Hôpital des Quinze-Vingts (Hospital of the Three Hundred [Beds]) and the Rothschild Eye Institute, was the grandson of Armand Trousseau (1801–1867) [20].

As to a description of his character:

> Mr. Trousseau remains as one of the grand medical figures of our time. If he had not genius to discover, he had it to apply. The fortunate chances of his medical education were happily joined to his natural disposition. A rare quickness of impression, a greater delicacy of perception, perfected by study, the gift of seeing everything and foreseeing everything, rendered him quick to seize and to fix that which was difficult of attainment, and even more quick to deduce therefrom practical percepts. He lived penetrated with this thought, that in an epoch of transition such as ours, the physician has nothing better to do than to take refuge, as well as possible, in the unfinished edifice of medicine. Full off work of the day, men like Mr. Trousseau are in their lives more useful perhaps than others, but in their death we have a double loss [21, p. 552].

Trousseau sign is one of the few "signs" for which it is appropriate to use the possessive form (Trousseau's) since he described the physical finding or disease which he had acquired in association with a gastric tumor: "[i]t is all up with me, the appearance of a patch of phlebitis last night leaves no loophole for doubt as to the nature of my illness" [22, p. 836]. In patients with thrombosis and advanced tuberculosis, uterine and visceral cancer, Trousseau described the occurrence of spontaneous coagulation and phlegmasia alba dolens or painful white inflammation (Table 3.1):

> I have long been struck with the frequency with which cancerous patients are affected with painful edema in the superior or inferior extremities, *whether one or other was the seat of cancer*. This frequent concurrence of phlegmasia alba dolens with an appreciable cancerous tumor, led me to the inquiry whether a relationship of cause and effect did not exist between the two, and whether the phlegmasia was not the consequence of the cancerous cachexia. (…) I have thus been led to the conclusion, that when there is a cachectic state not attributable to the tuberculous diathesis nor to the puerperal state, there is most probably a cancerous tumor in some organ [23, p. 287].

The occurrence of spontaneous, migratory, painful thrombosis involving the superficial and deep vein occurring in patients with cancer defines this sign. Trousseau described his symptoms in association with gastric cancer.

3.2.4 Lucas Sign

Richard Clement Lucas (1846–1915) was born in Oaklands, Sussex, England, and received his medical training at Guy Hospital and the University of London [24–26]. He was a member of the Royal College of Surgeons England, licentiate of the Royal College of Physicians in 1868, and received his Bachelor of Medicine degree, gold medal, and fellowship to the Royal College of Surgeons in 1871 [24, 26, 27].

He spent his entire medical career at Guy Hospital. His first appointment was assistant demonstrator of anatomy in 1872, followed by senior demonstrator in 1874, assistant surgeon in 1875, demonstrator or practical surgery in 1877 [24–27], full surgeon and lecturer in anatomy from 1888 to 1900, lecturer in surgery from 1900 to 1914, and consulting surgeon upon his retirement in 1906 [26–28].

He was elected president of the Hunterian Society from 1888 to 1890; examiner in anatomy for the Conjoint Board in 1892 (including the University of London); member of Council of the Royal College of Surgeons from 1901 to 1914, and vice-president of the College from 1909 to 1911; and delivered the Bradshaw lecture in 1911 [24, 25, 27].

His character was described as:

> Hearty—almost bluff—in expression, he was the staunchest and firmest friend one could have; and where the occasion happened that he could show practical interest in a friend's welfare, he would so in a way that was as sincere as it was delicately undertaken. He never knowingly hurt anyone's feelings, and was straightforward in word and deed [29, p. 97].

Lucas, in a discussion about the pathology of rickets, described a symptom he believed was commonly found in this disease (Table 3.1):

> I refer to the distended abdomen; and I would ask the gentlemen present whether they have ever seen rickets without a distended abdomen; for in my experience it is a constant, and an indication of the bad digestion and mal-assimilation in which the disease takes origin. I think, perhaps, too much stress has been laid on the enlargement of the solids organs a cause of this distention. (…) By far the chief cause, however, of the enlarged abdomen is the distention of the stomach and intestine with flatus, consequent upon injudicious feeding [30, p. 356].

Thus, Lucas sign refers to abdominal distension occurring during the early stages of rickets.

3.2.5 Reichmann Sign

Mikołaj Reichmann (Reichman or Rejchman) (1851–1918) was born in Warsaw, Poland, and received his medical degree from Warsaw University in 1873 [31–33].

He was appointed as a hospital and later prison physician in Irkutsk, Russia, and volunteered to provide medical care for Poles exiled to Russia. He received specialized training in gastroenterology in Paris in 1879 and was a private practitioner in Warsaw in 1880 [32, 33].

Reichmann developed a solubility test of gastric secretions in 1881 and a quantitative method for identifying peptone by colorimetry [31]. He established and served as president of the Polish Committee for the Study and Control of Cancer at the Warsaw Hygiene Society in 1906. He founded and served as the first president of the Polish Society of Gastroenterology from 1909 to 1918. He was an honorary member of the Warsaw Medical Society in 1913 [32, 33].

In his description of a 27-year-old male with probable gastric outlet obstruction, he postulated that "Considering everything said so far, we must conclude that the root cause of all these disorders is a pathologically increased section of gastric fluid" (Table 3.1) [34, p. 608]. As reported by Einhorn in 1896, 5 of 6 cases of stomach dilation reported by Reichmann were presumably caused by pyloric stenosis [35]. It is possible that one of Reichmann's cases of gastric hypersecretion was caused by a gastrinoma, a condition recognized by Zollinger and Ellison in 1955 that would later become known as Zollinger-Ellison syndrome. The term gastrosuccorrhoea continua chronica was coined to define the condition described by Reichmann, involving a continuous flow of gastric secretions occurring even in an empty stomach in the absence of external stimuli [35].

3.2.6 Debove Sign

Georges Maurice Debove (1845–1920) was born in Clignancourt, Paris, France. He was a hospital intern in 1869 and received his medical degree from the Faculty of Medicine, Paris, in 1873 [36]. He was appointed head of the Germain Sée Clinic, followed by appointment as a hospital physician in 1877, agrégé in 1878, and professor in 1890. At the Faculty of Medicine, he was a professor of pathology from 1890 to 1900 and became dean in 1906 [36]. He held appointments as a physician at Bicêtre Hospital and Tournelles Hospital (later renamed Andral Hospital), and became chair of pathology at the Charité Hospital in 1901. For the remainder of his career, he was a physician at medical clinic at Beaujon Hospital [36].

Debove was a member of the French Academy of Medicine in 1893 and was elected as perpetual secretary in 1913. He was honorary president of the Superior Council of Hygiene, president of the Anti-alcohol League and the League for the Rescue of Childhood, and president of the Medical Society of Hospitals in 1897 [36].

His interests as an internist and pathologist extended to diverse subject matters and therapeutic areas. He was best recognized for his work on splenomegaly (Debove disease), and histologically described the thin layer between the epithelium and tunic propria of the trachea, bronchi, and intestinal mucous membrane (Debove membrane). He developed a tube for gastric lavage, which assisted in diagnosing gastric cancer [37].

Debove also described a method for diagnosing gastric carcinoma (Table 3.1):

> I have examined many stomach diseases, including gastritis, ulcers, dyspepsia, dilatations, cancers, etc. Whenever this examination was performed during the digestive period, I found hydrochloric acid and lactic acid or hydrochloric acid alone in non-cancerous diseases. Hydrochloric acid was never present in any cases of cancer [38, p. 510]. (…) This observation seemed worthy of presentation because it clearly shows the importance of obtaining stomach acid. I hope that in a short time, the experience of our colleagues will confirm the value of this diagnostic sign [38, p. 511].

Thus, Debove sign refers to the absence of gastric hydrochloric or lactic acid in gastric carcinoma.

3.2.7 Troisier Sign

Charles Émile Troisier (1844–1919) was born in Sévigny-Waleppe, Ardennes, France, and received his doctorate in medicine in 1874 from the Paris Medical School for his work titled "Recherches sur lymphangites pulmonaires" (Research on pulmonary lymphangitis), currently referred to as pulmonary lymphangitic carcinomatosis [39, 40]. He was appointed hospital doctor in 1874 and professor of the chair of pathology and therapeutics in 1880 [39]. He was a physician at Tenon, La Pitié, Lariboisière, and Beaujon Hospitals [39].

Troisier was anointed knight of the Legion of Honor in 1890 and elected to the French Academy of Medicine, section of medical pathology in 1901, and a member of the Anatomical Society and vice-president of the Society of Biology. His other accomplishments included his description of phlegmasia alba dolens and bronzed diabetes or hemochromatosis, eponymically referred to as Troisier-Hanot-Chauffard syndrome [39, 40].

Troisier described three cases in 1886 of supraclavicular lymph node enlargement in patients with carcinoma of the stomach (Table 3.1):

> The facts I have just communicated to you seem to show that stomach cancer spreads to the supraclavicular fossa's ganglia. It results from three observations and the two facts reported with some details, one by Henoch, the other by Friedreich, that this secondary alteration of the ganglions affects especially the left side of the neck. It is proof of the spread of cancer, but with an important point. What surprises me is not the distance separating the ganglia from the initially injured organ nor the absence of alteration of the ganglia or intermediate organs. However, it is this precise localization in the supra-clavicular node. In conclusion, the diagnosis must rest on this anatomical fact [41, p. 398].

Troisier acknowledged in his paper this finding by Henoch:

> When M. Charcot was president of the Anatomical Society, I had often heard him say that Henoch, in his *Clinique des maladies du bas-center*, had pointed out the spread of cancer of the stomach to the nodes of the supraclavicular fossa (in particular, *The Bulletins of the Year 1876*, p. 460). This is how my attention was drawn to this point, and since that time, I have never neglected to seek this propagation [41, p. 395].

It is of historical interest that Virchow, in his publication "Zur Diagnose der Krebse im Unterleibe" (On the diagnosis of cancer of the abdomen) in 1848, described:

> We have repeatedly shown that cancer in the abdominal organs spreads and can be found on examination in the jugular nodes. A recent case again confirmed this sign: the relationship between the abdominal organs and lymph nodes. (…) [o]ne sees, especially in cancers of the stomach, pancreas, ovaries, etc., that as the disease progresses, it spreads from the lymph glands of the abdomen to the posterior mediastinum adjacent to the thoracic duct and finally around the jugular glands around the junction of the thoracic duct (left supraclavicular fossa). (…) It must be taken into account that the disease does not spread to the jugular lymph nodes in every case where an abdominal organ contains cancer. The absence of a supraclavicular lymph node enlargement proves nothing against the presence of a carcinomatous process in the abdomen [42, p. 248].

Troisier acknowledges a previous description in a treatise by Leube, published in *Die Krankheiten des Magens und Darmes* (The Diseases of the Stomach and Intestines) in 1876:

> An already more certain index of the existence of stomach cancer is cachexia and swelling of the peripheral lymph nodes, particularly those in the supraclavicular region (Virchow). However, it is often missing and can naturally be due to other causes. As we see, Leube attributes to Virchow, and not to Henoch, the merit of mentioning this alteration of the cervical ganglia in stomach cancer. I need to find out what is grounded in this assertion. I have searched for this mention in the *Treatise on Tumors*. For us, this propagation is neither reported in the classic books of internal pathology nor in monographs [41, p. 396–397].

In a tribute to Troisier, Maurice Letulle wrote:

> The left supraclavicular neoplastic lymphadenopathy has even passed into the common domain, under the term of "ganglion of Troisier"; supreme glory and just consecration of a life of work, which assures our friend regretted the durability of his name [43, p. 35].

Thus, Troisier sign refers to the presence of a left supraclavicular lymphadenopathy in patients with gastric cancer.

3.2.8 *Rosenheim Sign*

Theodor Rosenheim (1868–1939) was born in Bromberg (Bydgoszcz), Poland, and received his medical degree from the University of Berlin in 1884 [44–46]. He was appointed assistant to Paul Walther Fürbringer (1849–1930) in the Department of Internal Medicine at Friedrichshain Municipal Hospital, Berlin, from 1885 to 1888 and from 1888 to 1896, was a junior physician under the tutelage of Hermann Senator (1834–1911) at the III. Medical University Polyclinic in Charité, Berlin [44–46]. He habilitated in internal medicine at the Friedrich-Wilhelms University of Berlin in 1889 and was a titular professor in 1897 at the University of Berlin [44–46].

Rosenheim founded a polyclinic and private hospital for gastrointestinal disease in Berlin in 1896. He was named associate professor of medicine at Friedrich-Wilhelms University in 1921. His teaching license was revoked during national socialism because of his Jewish heritage [44, 45].

Rosenheim described a method for diagnosing perigastritis (Table 3.1):

> The objective proof of perigastritis is usually very difficult or impossible. Extensive extreme tenderness in the epigastrium, primarily when it extends to the right beyond the stomach borders, indicates a serosa affection on the anterior gastric wall, even if there is no dullness. A large, irregularly shaped dull zone in the region of the spleen is found, where exudate has formed on the left side. Simple adhesions are found here by the severe pain caused when the lower left side is pressed laterally, and the edge of the thorax is pulled upward somewhat abruptly. Finally, postperigastritis manifests as sensitivity to the left of the first and second lumbar vertebrae on percussion and palpation. Sometimes localized pain in an unusual place provides a clue [47, p. 48].

Thus, Rosenheim sign refers to the clinical features of perigastritis, including pain on the left side due to adhesion elicited when pressure is exerted laterally at the splenic region and the thorax is pulled abruptly superiorly.

3.2.9 Mendel Sign

Felix Frederick Mendel (1862–1925) was born in Essen, North Rhine-Westphalia, Germany, and received his medical degree at Leipzig University in 1884. He was a general practitioner and medical officer in Essen, Germany [48].

Mendel was instrumental in introducing several alternative drug delivery methods, including prelingual and intravenous injections. He recognized the therapeutic value of a low-salt diet [49]. He was also the first to study the diagnostic value and application of the tuberculin skin test in diagnosing tuberculosis. He clarified in his 1921 paper entitled "Die Intrakutanreaktion" (The intracutaneous reaction) the appropriate attribution to his work as being the first to discover the tuberculin reaction:

> As early as 1909, in Brauer's contribution to the clinical diagnosis of tuberculosis, I provided detailed proof published in the *Med Klin* 1908, no. 12, of the application and diagnostic value of tuberculin in the diagnosis of tuberculosis which was given the name "intracutaneous reaction" which remains generally accepted today. Moussu and Mantoux only announced the same reaction on August 10, 1908, i.e., more than a half year later, in the Academy of Sciences in Paris and coined the linguistically impossible name of the "intradermoreaction". (…) If the author's name refers to the intracutaneous reaction, historical justice demands that it be called Mendelian rather than Mantoux's intracutaneous reaction [50, p. 852].

Hence, Mendel reported the intracutaneous reaction to tuberculin in 1908, while Moussu and Mantoux reported their intradermal reaction later that year [50]. Since the intradermal or subcutaneous application provided more consistent and reproducible results when read at 48 to 72 hours, it became the standard for determining persons exposed to tuberculosis.

Mendel described a percussion method for detecting the presence of a gastric ulcer (Table 3.1, Fig. 3.1):

It must therefore be our endeavor to find an examination method that not only secures the diagnosis of gastric ulcer in doubtful cases but also enables us to monitor the success of our treatment at any time. Suppose the percussion hammer lightly hits the epigastrium while the abdomen is as relaxed as possible. In that case, even the most sensitive patient will not feel any pain as long as the stomach or its neighborhood is healthy. However, if the patient suffers from gastric ulcer, the percussion performed in this way will soon reach a point where even the slightest blow is felt as intense pain, followed by a more or less persistent pain. Suppose we percuss the epigastrium, proceeding radially from all directions to the designated pain point first found to be sensitive to pain. In that case, we will then connect all these points; in most cases, there is a circular area. Within this sharply defined zone, even the slightest percussion is painful, while outside its boundary line, even heavier blows cause no pain. Of course, this zone of pain does not have to correspond in position and size to the existing ulcer. However, in those cases where all other examination methods fail, it still proves that disease processes start somewhere in the stomach, from which the percussion emits a pain-producing stimulus. An ulcer located on the anterior stomach wall is relatively rare. In that case, the vibration of the abdominal wall, produced by percussion is transmitted directly to the anterior stomach wall, thereby exerting a mechanical stimulus on the ulcer surface. If the ulcer is at the pylorus, one of the predilection sites for ulcers covered by the left lobe of the liver, percussion of the abdominal wall will propagate to the firm liver tissue and, from there to the stomach. If the ulcer is in the posterior gastric wall the wave motion caused by percussion is transmitted from the anterior stomach wall through the stomach contents to the posterior wall causing a painful stimulus wherever it encounters an inflammatory processes. (…) Very often, however, the ulcer cannot be reached by palpation due to its anatomical location. Consequently, the symptom of pressure pain, which is important for the diagnosis, cannot be detected using the examination methods. The shock, however, produced by the direct percussion of the epigastrium, propagates in waves in all directions, and reaches the gastric ulcer, wherever it may be producing pain. Let us now mark the border of that area from which we can exert a painful stimulus on an existing ulcer by direct percussion of the epigastrium. In this way, we project the image of the gastric ulcer onto the abdominal wall [51, p. 554–555].

In his discussion on duodenal ulcers:

An equally valuable tool is direct percussion of the epigastrium for diagnosing duodenal ulcer, a condition much more common than is commonly thought but also more often overlooked for various reasons than gastric ulcer. (…) By direct percussion of the epigastrium, we will be able to confirm the diagnosis even if palpation does not reveal a pressure-sensitive area corresponding to the duodenum's anatomical position. Directly to the right of the linea alba, slightly below the midpoint between the costal arch and umbilicus, is a sharply defined area of pain, usually the size of a two-marrow piece. This examination method is used in all cases of duodenal ulcers, similarly to that used in the evaluation of gastric ulcers [51, p. 555].

Thus, Mendel sign refers to epigastric abdominal wall tenderness in gastric ulcers and an area to the right of the linea alba between the costal arch and umbilicus in duodenal ulcers.

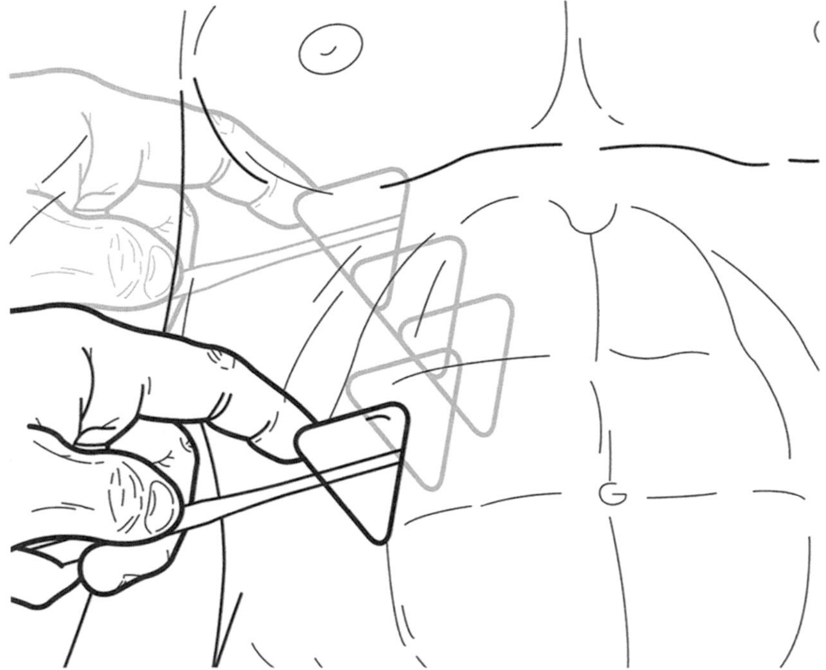

Fig. 3.1 Mendel sign (by Ryan Yale)

3.2.10 Bouchard Sign

Charles Jacques (Joseph) Bouchard (1837–1915) was born in Montier-en-Der, Haute-Marne, France, and received his medical training in Lyon, where he served as an intern in 1857 and extern in Paris in 1861 and intern from 1862 to 1865, receiving his medical degree in 1866 [52]. He was a house physician with Jean-Martin Charcot (1825–1893) at the Salpêtrière Hospital whose affiliation led to the doctoral thesis titled "Études sur quelques points de la pathogénie des hémorragies cérébrales" (Studies on some points of the pathogenesis of cerebral hemorrhages) which demonstrated that inflammation of the blood vessels preceded the development of cerebral aneurysm—later eponymously named Charcot-Bouchard aneurysms [53, 54].

Bouchard was chief of the clinic in 1868 and became agrégé in 1868 [52]. He was appointed chair of general pathology and therapeutics at the Faculty of Medicine in Paris in 1879 [53]. He cofounded the journals *Revue de la Tuberculose* in 1887 and *Journal de Physiologie et de Pathologie Générale* in 1899. He was appointed honorary doctor of the hospital in 1902 [53].

Bouchard was elected member of the French Academy of Medicine in 1886 and Academy of Sciences in 1887 [52]. He was president of the Second French Congress of Medicine in 1895, Society of Biology in 1896, and French Academy of Sciences in 1910. He was the recipient of the Grand Cross of the Legion of Honor in 1914 [52, 53].

Bouchard described the physical finding of a splashing sound found in a patient with gastric dilation (Table 3.1):

> In order to elicit the sound, the patient must be fasting and consume one-third of a glass of water. If you do not hear it at first, you should not assume that the stomach is not dilated as it may be flattened and fall flabbily behind the abdominal wall, like an apron. If you introduce one-third of a glass of water into a dilated stomach, you will immediately hear splashing over a region larger in extent than expected. This phenomenon is not present in the healthy man 15 h after a meal. I still believe it is necessary to hear the splashing sound at a point of a line drawn from the umbilicus to the border of the left costal arch. However, in reality, this line is of little importance. Every stomach not retracted when it is empty is a dilated stomach. Dilatation is not distension. A dilated stomach is a stretched stomach, the cavity of which is apparent only when it is empty because even though its walls touch each other, it is no longer capable of reducing its size by retraction. It is insufficient only to know that the stomach is dilated. It is essential to know precisely the dimensions of this dilated stomach, its extreme limit below and to the right of the median line, to listen for splashing until it disappears from above downward and from left to right, and to establish its limits by two lines, traced upon the limits of the zone where we observe splashing-one of these lines is horizontal, the other vertical and parallel and to the right of the median line [55, p. 165].

Thus, Bouchard sign refers to the presence of a "splashing sound" in patients with gastric dilation.

3.2.11 Tansini Sign

Iginio Tansini (1855–1943) was born in Milan, Italy, and received his medical degree from the University of Pavia in 1878. He served as the first assistant of the surgical clinic of Pavia, followed by director and chief surgeon at the Maggiore Hospital in Lodi from 1882 to 1888, and then professor of surgery at the University of Modena from 1888 until 1892. He served as director of the surgical clinic at the University of Palermo from 1898 to 1903 and Pavia from 1903 to 1931 [56]. During the First World War, he served as president of the regional health committee and surgeon consultant of the Milan corps [57]. He developed new surgical techniques and novel therapeutic concepts in the fields of abdominal, urologic, and plastic surgery. In Italy, he was the first surgeon in 1887 to successfully perform a pylorogastric resection with a partial hepatic resection for gastric cancer [58]. He recommended cauterization of nerve stumps in peripheral neurectomies, a compound musculocutaneous scapular flap for breast reconstruction in cases of radical mastectomy for breast cancer in 1896, and anastomosis of the portal vein into the vena cava in cases of portal vein obstruction in 1902 [56, 59, 60].

Nino Della Mano, in his 1924 paper entitled "Il valore del 'Segno di Tansini' per la diagnosi di metastasi intestinale nel cancro del piloro" *(The value of 'Tansini sign' for the diagnosis of intestinal metastasis in pyloric cancer),* wrote about Tansini's sign (Table 3.1):

> It was in 1906 that, for the first time, Professor Tansini spoke about it at a conference of the Milan Health Association, on the theme *stomach cancer in surgery.* On that occasion, Professor Tansini illustrated some phenomena which can contraindicate even a simple exploratory laparotomy [61, p. 66–67]. (…) Another fact which I have not seen mentioned in the treatises and which I observed twice is a certain swelling of the abdomen; because it must be assumed that, in this case, there are metastases in the lower intestine from the stomach of those with stomach cancer with pyloric stenosis. The two times I observed the protruded abdomen, this fact persuaded me to abstain from any intervention. I found at autopsy cancer in the splenic fissure in one case, in the ascending colon in the other [61, p. 67].

He also noted that if cancer is localized to the pylorus without metastases, the abdomen is flat, without ascites [58].

Tansini believed that if the sign when confirmed would add a new criterion for the operative indications and prognosis of gastric cancer. Della Mano postulated that:

> Professor Tansini, bringing this finding to the physicians' attention, believed that the protruded abdomen in patients with gastric cancer indicates the extensive metastatic spread of the neoplasm in the abdominal without specifying the precise location of the metastases. This is the only helpful conclusion I bring to my observation of the value of the Sign of Tansini. (…) I believe that this "sign" can be advantageous to the clinician, as it allows him to formulate a prognosis in all its gravity and evaluate whether or not to subject the patient to surgery. Before deciding whether to operate on the patient, it is crucial to know whether the neoplasm is widely diffuse and the operating difficulties that it will have to overcome— sometimes, to not allow any radical palliative intervention [61, p. 81–82].

Thus, Tansini recognized that the abdomen is protuberant in cases of metastatic gastric carcinoma while it is scaphoid in carcinoma confined to the pylorus.

3.2.12 Jonas Sign

There is limited historical information on Siegfried Jonas (1874–1926). At the time of the publication of his sign in 1906, Jonas worked in the laboratory of radiology and diagnostics at the Vienna General Hospital under the aegis of associate professor Guido Holzknecht (1872–1931) [62]. Holzknecht was the first to diagnose stomach cancer radiographically and, with Jonas, published their work on diagnosing gastric and extragastric tumors in 1908 [63]. Jonas was also associate professor at the University of Vienna Medical School in 1912 [64].

Jonas described and reported on the findings in six cases of reverse peristalsis or antiperistalsis, usually following normal direct peristalsis of the stomach, five of which were diagnosed with pyloric stenosis (Table 3.1):

> [a]s shown in cases 1 and 2 by stiffening and fasting residue, in cases 2 and 4 during operation, in cases 3, 4, and 5 by palpation and fluoroscopy, and in cases 5 during an autopsy, which indicated pyloric obstruction. In case 6, fluoroscopy revealed several findings which did not correspond to the behavior of a normal pars pylorica. So in this situation, if antiperistalsis due to torsion of the stomach caused by meteorism of the intestines is ruled out, the pars pylorica is presumably responsible for the antiperistalsis. Thus, a causal connection between pyloric stenosis and antiperistalsis may well be assumed. However, because there are numerous causes of stenosis without antiperistalsis, another phenomenon and unknown

factor are involved in triggering antiperistalsis. In conclusion, it should be pointed out that the phenomenon of antiperistalsis of the stomach has been observed clinically, first in a lecture by Dr. Wechsberg in case 2. It will undoubtedly be found more frequently if one pays attention to it. Particularly notable are those cases of pyloric stenosis in which, in addition to peristaltic waves coming from the left costal arch, we also see bulges that arise in the pars pylorica and seem to stop there [62, p. 919].

Thus, Jonas recognized the presence of reverse peristalsis of the stomach in patients with pyloric stenosis.

3.2.13 Dubard Sign

There is limited historical information on Pierre-Marie-Maurice Dubard (1862–1941). He was born in Côte-D'Or, Bourgogne, France, and served as professor at the school of medicine in Dijon and was appointed chair of pathology and medicine clinics at the Dijon School of Medicine [65, 66]. He was appointed as a physician to the National Association against Tuberculosis and was instrumental in developing a center for treating and educating patients with tuberculosis [67].

Huchon, in a thesis conducted at Lyon, proposed a pathogenesis for a gastric ulcer that assists in the diagnosis and prognosis. Dubard recognized the relationship between pulmonary tuberculosis and gastric ulcer and proposed that a "[c]hronic lesion of the lung irritates the pneumogastric nerves' pulmonary terminals, resulting in neuritis or neuralgia of this nerve. The neuritis, in turn, leads to a trophic disturbance on the side of the stomach and, consequently, a gastric ulcer" (Table 3.1) [68, p. 903].

Huchon called this association between pneumogastric neuritis and simple gastric ulcer "Dubard sign." Huchon believed that in addition to tuberculosis, other conditions can cause a similar phenomenon, including an aneurysm and cancer of the lung if the pneumogastric nerve is involved. Furthermore, Huchon found that in patients with a confirmed benign ulcer, pressure exerted at the neck always shows either one or both nerves sensitive, which was absent in those with gastric cancer.

3.2.14 Cole Sign

Lewis Gregory Cole (1874–1954) was born in Mahopac, New York, USA, and received his medical degree from the College of Physicians and Surgeons (currently Columbia University Vagelos College of Physicians and Surgeons) in 1898 [69, 70]. He was an intern at Roosevelt Hospital in New York, followed by general clinical practice at Roosevelt Hospital [69]. He was major and chairman of the Committee of Roentgenology of the Medical Advisory Board of the National Council of Defense [71]. He served on staff at the French and Memorial Hospitals in New York and St. Mary's Hospital in Orange, New Jersey. He was professor of roentgenology at Cornell University Medical College from 1913 to 1921 [70].

Cole pioneered techniques in studying gastrointestinal diseases and was a staunch advocate for the use of lung radiography to diagnose tuberculosis. He designed a unique table for the direct roentgenographic evaluation of duodenal ulcers [72]. His work on the pathophysiologic correlates of gastric ulcer and gastric cancer led to an enhanced understanding of the natural history, the cause, mechanisms, and surgical treatment of disease. He served as director of silicosis research. His work with his son William Gregory Cole and other pathologists and radiologists led to the publication of the book titled *Pneumoconiosis (Silicosis): The Story of Dusty Lungs—A Preliminary Report* in 1940 [73]. He also studied the effects of irradiation on tissues from atomic bomb casualties [69].

Among his numerous accolades, he is the recipient of the James Ewing Award, the fifth Julius Friendenwald Medal of the American Gastroenterological Association, and the first Gold Medal of the Radiological Society of North America in 1922 for his studies on X-ray diagnosis of the stomach and duodenum [69, 74].

As to his character as described by Orndoff:

> [a] lifetime characterized by sustained interest, enthusiasm, and a truly scientific mind that swayed, revamped, and broadened the thinking of so great a number of medical teachers and radiological students. Know-how, coupled with confidence and tenacity, enabled Dr. Cole to meet difficult problems and assignments. Lewis Gregory Cole forged his way through many and adverse situations to win the acclaim of American medicine as a pioneer, an independent thinker, and a great radiologist [75, p. 599].

Cole described the roentgenographic method for detecting small round ulcers and mucosal and submucosal gastric ulcers (Table 3.1):

> The small, round ulcers and the mucosal or submucosal ulcers may be shown in the prone posture and not in the erect or oblique films, or vice versa. They may be shown in the films made immediately after the ingestion of the barium meals, or not until the two hour period, or vice versa. In 1915, I demonstrated this type of ulcer, and I note that in Carman and Miller's latest book they show this type of ulcer. In these cases the stomach is singularly free from the gross deformities referred to in the previous type of ulcers; there is no deep sulcus on the greater curvature opposite the ulcer; the stomach is freely movable and not adhered to the under surface of the liver; in many cases the deformity is so slight that it can be differentiated from a double peristaltic sulcus only the by the use of serial roentgenography and matching each film of the series over the other. (…) These ulcer occur most frequently on the lesser curative above the sulcus of the angle, or about half way between the pylorus and the esophagus [76, p. 266].

Thus, Cole sign refers to the presence of gastric ulcers detected radiographically by deformity of the contour of the stomach, located above the sulcus of the angle on the lesser curvature of the stomach.

3.2.15 *Haudek Sign*

Martin Haudek (1880–1931) was born in Vienna, Austria, and received his medical training at Hermann Nothnagel (1841–1905) Clinic at the I. Medical Clinic of University and Anton Weichselbaum (1845–1920) at the Pathological-Anatomical

Institute, Vienna, in 1905 [77, 78]. He served as acting director of the Frisch Department of Internal Medicine at the Vienna General Hospital in 1907 and at the Guido Holzknecht Institute in 1908 [77, 79]. He headed the radiologic institute and several large hospitals during World War I and served as associate professor of medical radiology in 1915 [80]. Haudek was chair at the Roentgen Institute at the Wilhelminen Hospital, Vienna, in 1920 and titular associate professor in 1928 [77, 78].

Haudek was president of the Austrian General Associate for Physical Sport-Austrian National Olympic Committee and a member of the International Olympic Committee from 1924 to 1928. He promoted the institution of sports in the school curriculum [80, 81]. He served in the German Radiology Congress, as chairman of the German Radiology Society in 1926, and member of the Working Committee of the International Radiological Council at the Second International Radiological Congress, Stockholm [82].

Haudek, in his 1910 paper titled "Zur röntgenologischen Diagnose der Ulzerationen in der Pars media des Magens" (On the radiological diagnosis of ulcerations in the pars media des stomach) describes the niche as a radiologic feature of a gastric ulcer with the following caveats (Table 3.1):

> Abnormal circumscribed shadows on a radiograph of the stomach arise only from the deposition of bismuth in pathological niches of the stomach. (…) The assumption that a bismuth coating forms on a flat ulcer gives a shadow on radiographic images is incorrect. (…) A unique form of these niches is the penetrating gastric ulcer, seen on radiographs as a diverticulum-like bulge of the bismuth shadow with a gas bubble at the summit [83, p. 1589].

Thus, Haudek sign refers to the radiographic characteristic niche in benign gastric ulcers.

3.2.16   Günzburg Sign

Alfred Otto Günzburg (1861–1945) was born at Offenbach am Main, Germany, studied medicine in Heidelberg, Marburg, and Leipzig, and received his medical degree from the University of Leipzig in 1885 [84–86]. He served as a physician at the Jewish Community Hospital in Frankfurt am Main [84].

He founded the Gumpertz's Infirmary, a Jewish nursing home for the terminally ill, in Frankfurt in 1888 [85]. He was a chief physician in the Department of Internal Medicine at Königswart Hospital from 1909 to 1914 and then at the New Hospital at Frankfurt-am-Main from 1914 to 1935 [85, 87]. He cofounded the Jewish Nurses Association in Frankfurt in 1893, promoting nursing education [85–87]. He was expelled from Germany during national socialism and immigrated to Jerusalem in 1935 [85].

Günzburg developed a method for detecting hydrochloric acid in gastric fluid, eponymously named the "Günzburg test" as well as the "Günzburg sign" in duodenal ulcers [88]. Günzburg described a palpatory method for diagnosing a duodenal ulcer (Table 3.1):

I want to discuss another sign I observed in the literature which I have not mentioned—the tympanitic zone described above in the area of the quadratus lobe of the liver. When this "percussion phenomenon" struck me, I did not attach any importance to it. However, since I have often found the sign again, I think I should speak of it so that others can confirm this finding. According to the anatomical manuals, the upper horizontal duodenal crura runs behind the quadrate lobe of the liver, forming an impression. I had the opportunity to thoroughly examine the duodenum in a case where the percussion became quite tympanic after opening the abdominal cavity. Significant distention and gas tension within the duodenum was found. A short time after creating an anastomosis between the stomach and the lower duodenum, the percussion conditions remained as found before the operation. However, a few weeks later, when the patient had fully recovered, and blood was no longer detectable in the stool, the percussion phenomenon could no longer be detected. The conclusion is that the upper duodenal crus dilation has been eliminated by the chyme making its way through the anastomosis. I surmise, then, that the tympanitic tone mentioned is found in chronic duodenal ulcers with moderate stenosis, just as the prepyloric portion is found enlarged in narrowing of the pylorus. (…) It hardly needs to be mentioned that the percussion tone described is found in only some cases. It can only be detected when the liver is in a normal position and, secondly, when the left lobe of the liver is detected by percussion, the dull sound of which one learns to distinguish with careful attention from cardiac dullness. However, when the liver is canted, the tympanitic tone of the enlarged duodenum cannot be distinguished from that of the adjacent bowel loops; nor does one obtain the characteristic finding when the duodenum develops enteroptosis. Percussion to the right of the lobe quadrat is the colic impression. If the colon is distended, the bowel must be emptied thoroughly before the percussion phenomenon discussed can be ascertained with certainty [89, p. 1319].

Thus, Günzburg sign refers to a tympanitic zone located in an area of the liver's quadrant lobe in patients with duodenal ulcers.

3.2.17 *Pottenger Sign*

Francis Marion Pottenger Sr. (1869–1961) was born in Sater, Ohio, USA, received his medical training at Medical College of Ohio from 1892 to 1893 and Cincinnati College of Medicine and Surgery from 1893 to 1894, and medical degree, with first gold medal honor, in 1894. His son, Francis Marion Pottenger Jr. (1901–1967), also received his medical degree from the University of Cincinnati College of Medicine [90–92].

After graduation, he studied abroad in Vienna, Berlin, Munich, and London and returned to Ohio, later earning an appointment as assistant to the chair of surgery at the Cincinnati College of Medicine and Surgery in 1895 [90, 91].

He practiced in Monrovia, California, from 1895 to 1896 and after returning in 1898 after a brief return to Germantown, Ohio, moved back to Monrovia as a private practitioner, where the scope of his practice was devoted to treating tuberculosis [90, 91]. He was faculty at the University of Southern California in 1903, a lecturer on tuberculosis and climatology from 1904 to 1905, and professor of clinical medicine in the medical department of the University of Southern California [92].

He founded the Pottenger Sanatorium for Diseases of the Lungs and Throat in Monrovia, California, in 1903. He received his AM degree in 1907 and honorary

LLD degree from Otterbein University Westerville, Ohio [90–92]. He served as president of the Los Angeles County Medical Association, American Therapeutic Society, and the Southern California Anti-Tuberculosis League in 1902 and chairman of the Tuberculosis Committee of the California State Medical Society, among others [90, 91].

Pottenger described a new physical sign using light palpation as a method for delineating organs especially within the chest (heart, mediastinal tumors, infiltrations of the lung—tuberculosis, pneumonia, actinomycosis, syphilis, or cancer, and pleural effusion) and abdomen (liver, stomach within 2–3 h after eating and fasting, tumors, and peritoneal effusion) (Table 3.1):

> The fact that by a touch so light that it scarcely indents the skin, one can outline organs whose borders are at a distance from the surface of the body, is of great import in further developing physical diagnosis [93, p. 87]. (…) We have been in the habit of looking upon light palpation as a method suited to examining the surface only and have thought of it as depending entirely on the sense of touch; but we are now convinced that even a very light touch sets up vibrations in the tissues which not only penetrate deeply, but which are able to penetrate several different tissues of different density [93, p. 88].

He described the method for light palpation:

> In employing light touch palpation considerable care is necessary at first, until the examiner is fully aware of what he is attempting to feel. He should remember that he is attempting to recognize slight differences. In outlining organs of differences in density of tissues, I have found it better to examine the part which is presumably of lesser density first, and pass from it to the organ or part of greater density [93, p. 89]. (1) Always palpate wholly, either in the intercostal spaces or over the ribs. This can be applied to the liver and spleen, as well as the heart, because of the oblique direction of the ribs. (2) Begin palpating beyond the border of the organ and approach it slowly. When the border is reached an increased resistance is at once noted, the degree varying in different chests. (3) The palpating finger must not be moved too rapidly, or confusion will result. Sufficient time must be allowed to concentrate the mind on the sensation produced at each touch [93, p. 91].

Thus Pottenger sign refers to the light touch palpatory method for determining the dimension of an organ.

3.2.18 Zugsmith Sign

Edwin Zugsmith (1875–1939) was born in Allegheny, Pennsylvania, USA, and received his medical degree from the University of Pennsylvania in 1896 [94, 95]. He received several awards at his medical school commencement, including the alumni medal (highest general average in examination), Thoma-Zeis blood corpuscle counting apparatus and Fleischl Hämometer (best clinical reports), and Treve's *Operative Surgery* book for outstanding performance in one of the four surgical ward class sections [94–96]. ·

Zugsmith was a staff physician at the Pittsburgh Tuberculosis Hospital and general practitioner in Allegheny and Pittsburgh, Pennsylvania, a delegate to the state society of the Allegheny County Pennsylvania Medical Society in 1913, and a fellow to the American Academy of Medicine in 1915 [95, 97, 98].

Zugsmith presented a sign found in patients with benign and malignant gastric ulcers at the general meeting at the Medical Society of the State of Pennsylvania, Harrisburg Session on September 23, 1911 (Table 3.1):

> The sign of which I speak is an abnormal dullness to percussion in the second interspace extending for a variable distance on both sides of the sternum. In observations extending over a period of a year, I have noted the presence of this sign in cases of gastric ulcer and much more positively in cases of gastric cancer. It is present in the absence of all heart, vessel and mediastinal disease, as it must be to be of value in abdominal diagnosis. On account of the normal relationship of the heart to the surface of the chest, the dullness found on the right is perhaps of more value. Normally the one half inch adjacent to the sternum is rather dull to percussion; the dullness to which I am referring is continuous with this and extends toward the axilla for one, two or more inches [99, p. 436].

Zugsmith emphasized that light percussion be applied when performing this maneuver. He postulated that dullness is caused by lymphatic enlargement along the sternum, specifically at the second intercostal space above the area of cardiac dullness and outside the region of the large vessels.

3.2.19 Brenner Sign

Alexander Brenner (1859–1936) was born in Vienna, Austria, and studied medicine at the University of Vienna; served as a student demonstrator in anatomy to the chair, Karl Langer, Ritter von Edenberg (1819–1887), and received his medical degree in 1882 [100]. From 1884 to 1886, he obtained his surgical training under Theodor Billroth (1829–1894) and later served as an assistant to Leopold Ritter von Dittel (1815–1898), considered the founder of urology [100]. Here Brenner was the first resident physician in the surgical department. He was one of the first to catheterize the female ureter and added a single urethral catheter channel to the Nitze-Leiter direct-view cystoscope to irrigate the bladder [101]. He was chair of the Department of Surgery in Lanz and appointed head of the surgical department of the General Hospital in Lanz in 1888, a position which he retained throughout the remainder of his career [100, 102]. He served as the medical administrative chair to the hospital from 1904 to 1914 and consultant surgeon in Lanz and Upper Austria from 1914 to 1918 during World War I [100].

Among his other accolades, he was a member of the upper Austrian State Medical Council beginning in 1909, president of the Upper Austrian Medical Association, a position which he served from 1893 to 1899, and corresponding member of the Society of Physicians, Vienna [100]. He was an honorary member of the Society for Urology, the Viennese Urological Society, and the Upper Austrian Medical Association. He founded the academic gymnastic club in Vienna and was appointed deputy chairman in 1889, an honorary member in 1912, and chairman from 1914 to 1927 [100].

Regarding his character:

> He would often turn up at the bedside in the middle of the night, his hand on his pulse like a faithful watchman. It is, therefore, a natural expression of gratitude if today the federal government and the city, all his students, and the crowd of his patients work together in the

endeavor to tell this man in cedar in every imaginable form how valuable his work was as a doctor and human being for so many individuals and the general public [100].

Brenner described at a meeting of the German Natural Scientists and Physicians in Vienna in 1913 an early finding in five of six patients with gastric perforation (Table 3.1):

> It is a metallic-sounding rubbing sound below the diaphragmatic border, caused by the rubbing of gastric fluid mixed with air between the diaphragm and the balloon-like swollen stomach [103, p. 1973]. Only the rubbing that is noticeable in the first few hours after the perforation can be interpreted as a symptom of escaping gastric fluid, while later, the fibrinous-purulent coating of the inflamed peritoneum of the organs below the diaphragm can also cause this rubbing [103, p. 1974].

Brenner believed that perforation of the anterior wall of the stomach or duodenum causes fluid to move cephalad toward the diaphragm when the patient assumes a supine position resulting from severe pain.

3.2.20   Prével Sign

We were unable to identify any historical information on Prével. He observed that the pulse increases when moving from the supine to the upright position: He postulated that this phenomenon of orthostatic cardiac acceleration or the abdominal-cardiac reflex was a pathological condition caused by the movement of the intestines, in particular the stomach (Table 3.1):

> The inverted position causes some subjects to have a slower pulse. The pulse beats slower than in the supine position (In the inverted position, the fall of the abdominal mass towards the pelvis is corrected as much as possible). In the sitting position, where the stomach and the intestinal mass are only partially removed from the action of gravity, an intermediate number of pulsations are obtained between those obtained in the supine position (the slowest) and in the standing position (the fastest). Without modifying the upright position or applying a tight belt to the hypogastric region to raise the abdominal mass towards the diaphragm, the acceleration due to standing diminishes or disappears [104, p. 138].

He concluded, based on his case analyses, the stomach was the primary cause of this condition and proposed the following three reasons to account for this explanation based on his case studies:

> (1) The stomach, as a result of its conformation and its role as an intermittent reservoir of the alimentary mass, is that of the abdominal organs, which most easily obeys the stresses of gravity. (2) Orthostatic acceleration is much clearer after a meal and tends to diminish towards the time of complete emptying of the stomach; it disappears during fasting in certain subjects; (3) Acceleration decreases when dyspeptic phenomena improve [104, p. 139].

As to the pathophysiology of the abdominal-cardiac reflex, he concluded:

> Orthostatic cardiac acceleration or the abdominal, cardiac reflex should be considered a pathological phenomenon related to the movement of the abdominal organ, particularly the stomach. This imbalance most often depends on two main factors, reacting alternately with each other. The overwork of the stomach causes this by an excessively large food mass and

the muscular insufficiency of the abdominal wall. In this connection, it is curious to see the obvious relationship between the drooping of the abdomen with sub-umbilical protrusion and the extent of the abdominal-cardiac reflex [104, p. 140–141]. (…) As a consequence of this notion that the abdominal-cardiac reflex depends on an abnormal state, our concept of the physiological pulse, at least regarding its many causes, must be slightly modified [104, p. 142].

Thus, Prével sign refers to the abdominal-cardiac reflex whereby the pulse change based on the patients position and whether the stomach is empty or full after a meal.

3.2.21 Carman Sign

Russell Daniel Carman (1875–1926) was born in Iroquois, Ontario, Canada, received his medical training at the University of Minnesota and Marion Sims College of Medicine, St. Louis, Missouri (currently St. Louis University), and medical degree in 1901 [105, 106]. He pursued graduate studies at Johns Hopkins Medical School, Baltimore, Maryland, from 1901 to 1902 and Harvard Medical College in orthopedics in 1903, then returned to St. Louis as a general practitioner, developing expertise in gas X-ray tubes used for imaging [105, 107, 108].

Carman was appointed assistant in surgery from 1902 to 1907, assistant of roentgenology at Marion Sims-Beaumont Medical College from 1907 to 1909, and an assistant professor of roentgenology from 1909 to 1910 [107]. He was a special lecturer in roentgenology at Washington University School of Medicine from 1910 to 1913, later served as chief of the section of roentgenology and professor of roentgenology at the Mayo Clinic, Rochester, Minnesota, beginning in 1913 [105, 107, 109–111]. Here he was appointed professor of roentgenology at the Mayo Foundation Graduate School at the University of Minnesota. His primary area of interest was the imaging of the gastrointestinal tract [108].

Among his many memberships and associations, he served as president of the Radiological Society of North America in 1923 and the American Roentgen Ray Society in 1925 [105]. The Greater St. Louis Society of Radiologists established a memorial in Carman honor for excellence by establishing the Annual Carman Lecture [112].

As a description of his character:

> More important were his solid, constant attributes: extraordinary keenness of observation; abundant common sense; conservative, trustworthy, professional judgment; unflagging industry coupled with a marvelous capacity for work an eager wish for the truth, the whole truth and nothing but the truth in his chosen field. These were the characteristics of Carman the man, the roentgenologist, which earned him leadership. Outstanding, too, was his warm goodwill toward men, his hearty friendliness [106, p. 54].

Carman described what he identified as a pathognomonic finding on fluoroscopic examination of large malignant gastric ulcer which ranged in size from 3 to 8 cm or more with deep crater, elevated or overhanging margins and whose appearance depends on the site of the abnormality (Table 3.1):

When the ulcer is on the vertical portion of the lesser curvature or on the posterior wall near the lesser curvature, approximation of the walls of the stomach by palpation causes a dark, slightly crescentic shadow of the barium-filled crater to appear on the screen. In these situations the convexity of the crescent is toward the gastric wall and the concavity toward the gastric lumen. The resemblance to a meniscus is so obvious that the word aptly applies to the sign. If the ulcer saddles the lesser curvature distal to the incisura angularis of a fishhook stomach a meniscus is similarly revealed by palpation, but in this instance the base of the ulcer follows the bending line of the curvature and the concavity of the meniscus is toward the gastric wall. When the ulcer is on the posterior wall, well away from the curvature, thinning the barium by stroking pressure with the hand reveals the crater as a somewhat circular, dark shadow surrounded by a lighter zone. No meniscus is apparent because in this situation the examiner does not view the cavity of the ulcer in profile. Whether the lesion is situated on the lesser curvature or on the posterior wall, if it is large, a mass may be felt by careful, deep palpation. If the ulcer is high in the stomach, palpation is less effective in eliciting all the signs described, although the shadow of the crater may be seen. If the ulcer is on the posterior wall and its crater can be demonstrated in the anteroposterior view, but no niche can be seen in the oblique view, we believe that we are dealing with this particular type of malignant ulcer [113, p. 991–992].

Carman further recognized that in malignant ulcer barium is not easily emptied from the crater by palpation due to the presence of overhanging margins.

In summary, large malignant ulcers located on vertical portion of the lesser curvature or posterior wall of the curvature of the stomach resemble a meniscus (convexity toward the gastric wall and concavity position toward the lumen) fluoroscopically when the stomach walls are manually appositioned through palpation. A malignant ulcer saddles the lesser curative with the concavity positioned outward toward the gastric wall. Thus, Carman sign or the "meniscus sign" is a radiographic finding to assist in the diagnosis of ulcerating gastric carcinoma.

3.2.22   *Henning Sign*

Norbert Knudsen Henning (1896–1985) was born in Hundeshagen, Germany, and received medical training at the Universities of Leipzig, Göttingen, and Freiburg, beginning in 1918, and his medical degree in 1922 [114–116].

He was appointed medical doctor at the University of Freiburg in 1923 and associate professor habilitating in internal medicine at the University of Leipzig in 1929 [114, 115]. He was an extraordinary professor of internal medicine at the University of Leipzig from 1935 to 1949 and director of the medical clinics in Fürth, Bavaria, Germany [116]. Henning was an associate professor of internal medicine at the University of Würzberg from 1949 to 1953 and a full professor of internal medicine at the University of Erlangen from 1953 to 1966. He published *Lehrbuch der Gastroskopie* (Textbook of Gastroscopy) in 1935, and *Lehrbuch der Verdauungskrankheiten* (Textbook of Digestive Disease) in 1949 and with Siegfried Witte *Atlas der gastroenterologischen Zytodiagnostik* (Atlas of Gastroenterological Cytodiagnostics) in 1968 [114, 115].

Henning was a member of the German Academy of Natural Scientists, Leopoldina, and chairman of the Society for Digestive and Metabolic Diseases from

1953 to 1955. He is credited for modifying and improving the performance of the gastroscope by increasing the viewing angle, reducing the outer diameter, adding soft rubber balls to the tip to reduce the risk of perforation, and adding a biopsy port and method for photographic imaging and documentation of the stomach [117, 118]. He founded the German Society for Gastroenterological Endoscopy, served as editor of *Gastroenterologia,* and founded *Zeitschrift für Gastroenterologie* (Journal of Gastroenterology). He was president and chair of the World Congress for Gastroenterology in 1962 [116].

He was a member of the Nationalsozialistische Deutsche Arbeiterpartei (NSDAP, National Socialist German Worker's Party) and Sturmbannarzt (Chief Medical Officer of a Sturmbann unit) of the Sturmabteilung (SA, the paramilitary unit of the NSDAP) beginning in 1933. His affiliation with NSDAP, if so confirmed, would exclude him from receiving any eponymously named term or other awards in his namesake as eponyms are terms used to honor one's accomplishments [115].

Henning described a finding to assist in the diagnosis of a benign gastric ulcer (Table 3.1):

> An important indirect sign of an ulcer, which I have described, is deformity of the angulus. Instead of being the usual rounded arch it is pointed. This sign is always seen when the ulcer lies close to the angulus, and is produced by the folds converging toward the ulcer [119, p. 77]. (…) If the ulcer is located immediately above or below the angulus, the parabolic curve of the angulus may be distorted in a characteristic way. It loses its roundness and acquires the form of a Gothic arch [119, p. 238].

Authors have coined the term "Gothic arch" in reference to the shape of the angulus (parabolic curve) of the stomach caused by ulcers located above or below the angulus [120].

3.2.23 Raw Sign

Stanley Collingwood Raw (1910–1994) was born in Spratton, Northamptonshire, England, and received his Medical Baccalaureate from Durham University in 1934. He continued his postgraduate training as a house physician, house surgeon, and resident surgical officer at the Royal Victoria Infirmary, Newcastle-upon-Tyne [121, 122]. He was a member of the Royal Army Medical Corps (RAMC) in 1942 and subsequently a lieutenant colonel in 1945. After World War II, he was appointed consultant at Farnham and Frimley Park Hospitals in 1948 [121, 122].

Raw described a way to differentiate pleuritis of thoracic origin from diaphragmatic pleuritis caused by perforated peptic ulcer disease (Table 3.1):

> In perforation the onset is nearly always dramatic, with little vomiting or change in pulse and temperature. The pain does not vary and the patient usually lies still. Breathing is short and thoracic in type. In pleurisy, rigidity may sometime be overcome by holding the breath; in colic, it is commonly removed by breathing; but in peroration it never disappears completely [123, p. 12].

Thus, Raw sign refers to persistent rigidity of the abdominal wall in cases of a perforated peptic ulcer.

Table 3.1 Stomach signs

Name	Year	Description of sign	Significance
Chaussier [7]	1823	Before the seizure, the patient experiences epigastric abdominal pain followed by a heaviness in the stomach and altered digestive functions that propagate to the uterus and extend to the brain. Sometimes during a seizure, the patient automatically places their hands on the epigastrium, strikes this region hard, and tries to tear it with their nails. However, at other times the irritation seems to begin in the uterus and thence spread to the stomach and the nervous system, resulting from the intimate and reciprocal connection between all the parts of the body. Place and maintain the hand on the abdomen over the uterus. A tonic, permanent contraction, is palpated and increases during the seizure	Eclampsia
Fenwick [15]	1870	Atrophy of stomach	Atrophic gastritis
Trousseau [23]	1873	Phlegmasia alba dolens occur in the upper and lower extremities in patients with cancer	Carcinoma and thrombosis involving the upper and lower extremities
Lucas [30]	1881	Abdominal distension	Rickets
Reichmann [34]	1882	Increased gastric secretion in patients with pyloric stenosis	Pyloric stenosis
Debove [38]	1886	Hydrochloric acid and lactic acid are present in the stomach during digestion in patients with benign gastric ulcers and absent in gastric cancer	Gastric carcinoma
Troisier [41]	1886	Supraclavicular lymphadenopathy	Metastatic gastric carcinoma
Rosenheim [47]	1895	A large, irregularly shaped dull zone is found in the region of the spleen. Exudate and simple adhesions are found here. Severe pain is caused when the lower left side is pressed laterally, and the edge of the thorax is pulled upward somewhat abruptly	Perforated gastric ulcer

(continued)

Mendel [51]	1903	*Gastric Ulcer* While the abdomen is relaxed, lightly percuss the epigastrium using a percussion hammer. Healthy persons do not experience pain. In patients with a gastric ulcer, percussion identifies a point on the abdomen where the slightest blow is felt as intense pain, followed by persistent pain. Percuss the epigastrium, proceeding radially from all directions to the designated pain point first found to be sensitive to pain. After connecting these points, a circular area, in most cases, will be defined. Within this sharply defined zone, even the slightest perfusion is painful, while outside its boundaries, even heavier blows cause no pain *Duodenal ulcers* Direct percussion of the abdomen in the epigastrium to confirm the diagnosis of a duodenal ulcer. Directly to the right of the linea alba and slightly below the middle between the costal arch and the navel, a sharply defined area of pain, usually, the size of two coins, is found in all cases of duodenal ulcers	Gastric and duodenal ulcers
Bouchard [55]	1906	A splashing sound is heard in persons with gastric dilation. To elicit the sound, the patient must be fasting and consume one-third of a glass of water. The stomach could be dilated even if the splashing sound is initially absent. In that case, the stomach may be flattened and fall flabbily like an apron behind the abdominal wall. Ask the patient to drink one-third of a glass of water. A splashing sound is heard over a larger region than expected in a dilated stomach. This phenomenon is never perceptible in a healthy person fifteen hours after a meal. The splashing sound is heard below the middle of a line drawn from the umbilicus to the point nearest to the border of the left coastal arch	Gastric dilation
Tansini [59]	1906	Protrusion of the lower abdomen caused by metastases in the lower section of the intestine from the stomach in patients with gastric carcinoma and pyloric stenosis. Cancer localized to the pylorus without metastases causes the abdomen to be scaphoid without ascites	Gastric carcinoma
Jonas [62]	1906	Reverse antiperistalsis of the stomach in pyloric stenosis	Gastric carcinoma
Dubard [68]	1907	Chronic lung lesion in patients with pulmonary tuberculosis irritates the pneumogastric nerves' pulmonary terminals, resulting in neuritis or neuralgia of this nerve, a trophic disturbance on the side of the stomach, resulting in a gastric ulcer	Gastric ulcer

(continued)

Table 3.1 (continued)

Name	Year	Description of sign	Significance
Cole [72]	1908	In the prone posture small round mucosal or submucosal ulcers are seen on oblique radiographs. This finding occurs either immediately after the ingestion of the barium meals or two hours later. In these cases, the stomach has no gross deformities or deep sulcus on the greater curvature opposite the ulcer. The stomach is freely movable and not adhered to the undersurface of the liver. These ulcers occur most frequently on the lesser curvature above the sulcus of the angle or about halfway between the pylorus and the esophagus	Gastric ulcer
Haudek [83]	1910	Abnormal circumscribed shadows on a radiograph of the stomach arise only from the deposition of bismuth in pathological niches of the stomach. A unique form of these niches is the penetrating gastric ulcer, seen on radiographs as a diverticulum-like bulge of the bismuth shadow with a gas bubble at the summit	Gastric ulcer
Günzburg [89]	1910	The tympanic percussion zone is found in an area at the quadratus lobe of the liver. This tone can only be detected when the liver is in a normal position and the left lobe is percussed	Duodenal ulcer
Pottenger [93]	1912	Light touch palpation to delineate the borders of an organ	Visceral organs
Zugsmith [99]	1912	Dullness to percussion is located at the second interspace extending for a variable distance on both sides of the sternum in gastric ulcers, especially gastric cancer. Usually, an area of one-half inch adjacent to the sternum is dull to percussion. However, the dullness in gastric cancer extends toward the axilla for one, two, or more inches	Gastric ulcer
Brenner [103]	1913	A metallic rubbing sound is heard behind and below the diaphragmatic border. It is caused by rubbing gastric fluid mixed with air between the diaphragm and the dilated, bloated stomach. The rubbing noticeable in the first few hours after the perforation is a symptom of escaping gastric fluid. Later the fibrinous-purulent coating of the inflamed peritoneum of the organs below the diaphragm can also cause this rubbing	Gastric perforation

Prével [104]	1917	In the sitting position, where the stomach and the intestinal mass are only partially removed from the action of gravity, an intermediate pulse is obtained. In contrast, the lowest pulses occur in the supine position, while the highest occur during standing. Without modifying the upright position and applying a tight belt to the hypogastric region to raise the stomach toward the diaphragm, the acceleration occurring during standing diminishes or disappears. Passive raising of the upper and lower body caused several subjects to slow their pulse (slower than in the supine position)	Orthostatic hypotension
Carman [113]	1921	When the ulcer is on the vertical portion of the lesser curvature or the posterior wall near the lesser curvature, approximation of the stomach walls by palpation causes a dark, slightly crescentic shadow of the barium-filled crater to appear on the screen. The convexity of the crescent is toward the gastric wall, and the concavity is toward the gastric lumen. The resemblance to a meniscus is so apparent that the word aptly applies to the sign. Suppose the ulcer saddles the lesser curvature distal to the incisura angularis of a fishhook stomach. In that case, the meniscus is found by palpation. However, in this instance, the base of the ulcer follows the bending line of the curvature and the concavity of the meniscus is toward the gastric wall	Gastric ulcer
Henning[a] [119]	1937	An indirect sign of an ulcer is a deformity of the angulus. This sign occurs when the ulcer lies close to the angulus and is produced by the folds converging toward the ulcer. Suppose the ulcer is located immediately above or below the angulus. Instead of being the usually rounded arch, it is pointed. In that case, the parabolic curve of the angulus is distorted by losing its roundness and acquires the form of a Gothic arch	Gastric ulcer
Raw [123]	1944	In perforation, the onset is nearly always dramatic, with little vomiting or change in pulse and temperature. The pain does not vary; the patient usually lies still, breathing is short and thoracic in type, and rigidity persists	Gastric and duodenal ulcer

[a] Denotes an individual who supported anti-Semitism, racial acts, or committed crimes against humanity

3.3 Conclusion

The majority of the signs of the stomach were designed to detect peptic ulcer disease and other benign conditions and, in some cases, to differentiate them from gastric carcinoma. Pottenger size is the palpatory method for outlining the borders of an organ and is not specific to the stomach. Prével believed that the position of the stomach was involved in a reflex accounting for changes in the pulse occurring with changes in position. Trousseau sign, another nonspecific sign of underlying malignancy, is included in this section as this was the disease that Trousseau had when he recognized phlegmasia alba dolens occurring within himself. The utility of these signs used during the physical examination is not well known since they have yet to be studied. Radiological techniques and endoscopy revolutionized the detection of peptic ulcers and carcinoma. With it came a novel set of signs that defined the characteristic and differentiating features of benign from malignant disease.

References

1. Avicenna. A treatise on the canon of medicine of Avicenna. New York: AMS Press Inc.; 1973.
2. Morgagni JB. The seats and causes of diseases, investigated by anatomy, vol. 2. Boston: Wells & Lilly; 1824.
3. Cruveilhier J. Anatomie pathologique du corps humain. Paris: J.-B. Baillière; 1842.
4. Pariset E. Éloge de Chaussier. In: Mémoires de l'Académie Royale de Médecine, tome 5. Paris: J.-B. Baillière; 1836. p. 5–40.
5. Peisse JL. M. Chaussier. In: Les médecins français contemporains. Paris: Gabon; 1827. p. 113–9.
6. Dechambre A. Chaussier. In: Dictionnaire encyclopédique des sciences médicales, tome 15. Paris: G. Masson, P. Asselin; 1874. p. 573–5.
7. Chaussier F. Considérations sur les convulsions qui attaquent les femmes enceintes. J Univ Sci Méd. 1823;32:340–52.
8. Gibbs DD. Samuel Fenwick, MD, FRCP (1821–1902): physician and gastroenterologist. Br Med J. 1970;3:339–42.
9. Willett A. Address of Alfred Willett, President, at the annual meeting, March 2nd 1903: Dr. Samuel Fenwick. Med Chir Trans. 1903;86:101.
10. [No author]. Obituary: Samuel Fenwick MD, FRCP. Med Press Circ. 1902;125:673.
11. Brown GH. Samuel Fenwick MD St Andrews and Durham FRCP. Br Med J. 1902;2:1973–4.
12. Brown GH. Samuel Fenwick, MD St And & Durh, FRCP Lond. Lancet. 1902;2:1729–30.
13. [No author]. Medical news. Med Times Gaz. 1861;2:420.
14. Samuel Fenwick. Royal College of Physicians. https://history.rcplondon.ac.uk/inspiring-physicians/samuel-fenwick. Accessed 24 Oct 2022.
15. Fenwick S. On atrophy of the stomach. Lancet. 1870;96:78–80.
16. [No author]. The doctor's page: Armand Trousseau, 1801–1867. J Organ Des. 1926;10:208–9.
17. Buck AH. A reference handbook of the medical sciences: embracing the entire range of scientific and practical medicine and allied science, vol. 8. New York: William Wood & Co.; 1889.
18. Garrison FH. Armand Trousseau: a master clinician. Philadelphia: J.B. Lippincott; 1916.
19. [No author]. Armand Trousseau. Lancet. 1919;104:610.
20. [No author]. Medical news: death of Armand Trousseau. JAMA. 1919;21:1822.

21. Béclard J, Éloge de M. Trousseau: prononcé dans la séance publique annuelle de l'Académie de Médecine du 11 Janvier 1870. Paris: J.-B. Baillière et fils; 1870.

22. Rolleston H. Diseases described by medical men who suffered from them. Lancet. 1921;197:836–8.

23. Trousseau A. Phlegmasia alba dolens. In: Lecture on clinical medicine: delivered at the Hôtel-Dieu, Paris, vol. 5. Philadelphia: Lindsay & Blakiston; 1873. p. 281–332.

24. [No author]. Richard Clement Lucas, MB, BS Lond. Br Med J. 1915;2:77–8.

25. [No author]. Obituary: Richard Clement Lucas MB, MS (Lond), FRCS (Eng). Boston Med Surg J. 1915;173:182–3.

26. [No author]. Richard Clement Lucas MB, BS Lond; FRCS. Guys Hosp Gaz. 1915;29:299.

27. Lucas, Richard Clement (1846–1915). Plarr's Lives of the Fellows. Royal College of Surgeons of England. https://livesonline.rcseng.ac.uk/client/en_GB/lives/search/detailnonmodal/ent:$002f$002fSD_ASSET$002f0$002fSD_ASSET:376533/one. Accessed 3 Oct 2022.

28. Lucas, Richard Clement (1846–1915). King's College London Archives: Catalogue (Summary). https://kingscollections.org/_assets/components/archiospdfbuilder/?docid=2115. Accessed 3 Apr 2022.

29. [No author]. Richard Clement Lucas MB, BS Lond; FRCS Eng. Lancet. 1915;3:96–8.

30. Lucas RC. Discussion on the pathology of Rickets on November 16th, December 7th and 16th, 1880. Tr Path Soc Lond. 1881;32:313–68.

31. Wulman L, Tenenbaum J. The Martyrdom of Jewish Physicians in Poland. New York: Medical Alliance-Association of Jewish Physicians from Poland; 1964.

32. Hanecki M. Mikołaj Rejchman, MD. Pol Med Sci Hist Bull. 1970;13:50–1.

33. Hanecki M. Mikołaj Rejchman (W 50 rocznice śmierci). Wiad Lek. 1969;22:959–62.

34. Reichmann M. Ein Fall von krankhaft gesteigerter Absonderung des Magensaftes. Berl klin Wochenschr. 1882;19:606–8.

35. Einhorn M. Diseases of the stomach. In: Stedman TL, editor. Twentieth century practice: an international encyclopedia of modern medical science, vol. 3. New York: William Wood & Co.; 1896. p. 276–82.

36. Achard C. Notice nécrologique: décès de M. Debove, secrétaire perpétuel. Bull Acad Méd Paris. 1920;84:238–42.

37. Debove V-RJ, Georges M. Enciclopedia Salvat de Ciencias Médicas. Barcelona: Salvat Editores; 1959. p. 245.

38. Debove GM. Diagnostic du cancer de l'estomac par l'examen chimique des sécrétions de cet organe. Bull Mém Soc Méd Hôp Paris. 1886;3:510–1.

39. Gilbert M. À propos du décès de M. Troisier. Bull Mém Soc Méd Hôp Paris. 1919;43:1089.

40. Troisier, Charles Emile. Comité des travaux historiques et scientifiques. http://cths.fr/an/savant.php?id=106003. Accessed 12 Apr 2022.

41. Troisier E. Les ganglions sus-claviculaires dans le cancer de l'estomac. Bull Mém Soc Méd Hôp Paris. 1886;3:394–8.

42. Virchow R. Zur Diagnose der Krebse im Unterleibe. Med Reform. 1848;10:248.

43. Letulle ME. Troisier (1844–1919). Presse Méd. 1920;28:33–5.

44. Killy W, Vierhaus R, Rosenheim T. Deutsche Biographische Enzyklopädie, Bd. 8. München: K.G. Saur; 2011. p. 425.

45. In Erinnerung an Prof. Dr. med. Theodor Rosenheim, 1860–1939. Deutsche Gesellschaft für Gastroenterologie, Verdauungs- und Stoffwechselkrankheiten. https://www.dgvs-gegen-das-vergessen.de/en/biografie/theodor-rosenheim/. Accessed 9 Nov 2022.

46. Rosenheim T. Biographisches Lexikon hervorragender Ärzte. http://www.zeno.org/Pagel-1901/A/Rosenheim,+Theodor. Accessed 9 Nov 2022.

47. Rosenheim T. Ueber die chirurgische Behandlung der Magenkrankheiten. Dtsch med Wochenschr. 1895;21:47–9.

48. Dr. med. Felix Frederick Mendel. Geni. 2020. https://www.geni.com/people/Dr-med-Felix-Mendel/6000000046229891107. Accessed 25 July 2022.

49. Feldberg WS. Mendel, 1897 to 1959. Biogr Mem Fellows R Soc. 1960;6:191–9.

50. Mendel F. Die Intrakutanreaktion. Münch med Wochenschr. 1921;22:852.

51. Mendel F. Die direkte Perkussion des Epigastrium, ein diagnostisches Hilfsmittel bei Ulcus ventriculi. Münch med Wochenschr. 1903;50:554–5.

52. Havelange I, Huguet F, Lebedeff B, Caplat G. Dictionnaire biographique, 1802–1914. Paris: Institut National de Recherche Pédagogique; 1986. p. 181–2.

53. [No author]. Charles Bouchard (1837–1915). Nature. 1937;140:457.

54. Bouchard CJ. Études sur quelques points de la pathogénie des hémorragies cérébrales. Thèse de doctorat. Paris: [n.a.]; 1867.

55. Bouchard C. Chronic gastro-intestinal auto-intoxication-dilation of the stomach. In: Oliver T, editor. Lectures on auto-intoxication in disease or self-poisoning of the individual. 2nd ed. Philadelphia: F.A. Davis; 1906. p. 162–84.

56. Ribuffo D, Cigna E, Gerald GL, et al. Iginio Tansini revisited. Eur Rev Med Pharmacol Sci. 2015;19:2477–81.

57. Collective. Enciclopedia Italiana di Scienze, Lettere ed Arti, vol. 33. Rome: Istituto Giovanni Treccani; 1937.

58. De Vecchi P. Modern Italian surgery and old universities of Italy. In: The University of Pavia. New York: Paul B. Hoever; 1921. p. 144–53.

59. Tansini I. Sopra il mio nuovo processo di amputazione della mammella. Gazz Med Ital. 1906;57:141–2.

60. Tansini I. Nuovo processo per l'amputazione della mammaella perla cancre. Riforma Med. 1896;12:3.

61. Della-Mano N. Il valore del 'Segno di Tansini' per la diagnosi di metastasi intestinale nel cancro del piloro. Il Policlinico. 1924;31:65–82.

62. Jonas S. Ueber Antiperistaltik des Magens. Dtsch med Wochenschr. 1906;32:916–9.

63. Holznecht G, Jonas S. Die radiologische Diagnostik der intra- und extra ventrikulären Tumoren und ihre spezielle Verwertung zur Frühdiagnose des Magenkarzinoms. Wien: Moritz Perles; 1908.

64. [No author]. Dr. Siegfried Jonas. Mitt Grenzgeb med Chir. 1912;15:641.

65. [No author]. Dubard, Pierre-Marie-Maurice, docteur en médecine. J Répub Fr. 1921;31:2466.

66. [No author]. Université de Lyon. In: Bulletin administratif du ministère de l'Instruction publique, tome 40. Paris: Impr. Nationale; 1896. p. 338.

67. [No author]. La lutte contre la tuberculose à Dijon. In: Pannwitz G, editor. Neunte Internationale Tuberkulose-Konferen Bericht: Brüssel, 6–8 Oktober 1910. Berlin-Charlottenburg: Internationale Vereinigung gegen die Tuberkulose; 1911. p. 406–8.

68. Huchon F. L'ulcère de l'estomac et la névrite du pneumogastrique. J Méd Chir Pract. 1907;78:903.

69. Andresen AF. Lewis Gregory Cole, 1874–1954. Gastroenterology. 1955;28:867–71.

70. Walsh JJ. Lewis Gregory Cole. In: History of medicine in New York: three centuries in medical progress, vol. 5. New York: National Americana Society Inc.; 1919. p. 357.

71. Brown L. Value of the Roentgen ray in diagnosis of pulmonary tuberculosis in war time. JAMA. 1918;70:516–9.

72. Cole LG. A new radiographic table. Trans Am Roent Ray Soc. 1908;9:274–6.

73. Cole LG, Cole WG. Pneumoconiosis (silicosis): the story of dusty lungs – a preliminary report. New York: John B. Pierce Foundation; 1940.

74. [No author]. Gold medal awards. Radiology. 1922;3:58.

75. Orndoff BH. Lewis Gregory Cole, MD, 1874–1954. Radiology. 1955;64:597–9.

76. Cole LG. Gastric ulcers. JAMA. 1923;81:261–9.

77. Collective. Haudek, Martin (1880–1931), Röntgenologe. In: Österreichisches Biographisches Lexikon (1815–1950), Bd. 2. Wien: Verlag der Österreichischen Akademie der Wissenschaften; 1958. s. 210.

78. Killy W, Vierhaus R, Haudek M. Deutsche Biographische Enzyklopädie. München: K.G. Saur Verlag; 1999. p. 437.

79. Schwarz G, Presser H. Vienna Roentgenologic Society. Radiology. 1932;18:1033–8.

80. Dr. Martin Haudek. Olympic museum. Members of the International Olympic Committee 1923-1932. https://olympic-museum.de/iocmembers/iocmembers1923.html. Accessed 30 Oct 2022.

81. Martin Haudek: biographical information. Olympedia. https://www.olympedia.org/athletes/899164. Accessed 21 Oct 2022.

82. [No author]. Martin Haudek. Acta Radiol. 1931;12:200.

83. Haudek M. Zur röntgenologischen Diagnose der Ulzerationen in der Pars media des Magens. Münch med Wochenschr. 1910;57:1587–91.

84. Koren N. Jewish physicians: a biographical index. Jerusalem: Israel Universities Press; 1973. p. 186.

85. Gumpertz' infirmary: biographical directory. Jüdische Pflege-geschichte. https://www.juedische-pflegegeschichte.de/gumpertz-infirmary-biographical-directory/. Accessed 10 Oct 2022.

86. Alfred Otto Günzburg. Deutsche Gesellschaft für Innere Medizin. https://www.dgim-history.de/en/biography/G%C3%BCnzburg;Alfred%20Otto;1552. Accessed 12 Oct 2022.

87. Sanitätsrat Dr. med. Alfred Otto Günzburg. Jüdische Pflege-geschichte. https://www.juedische-pflegegeschichte.de/recherche/?dataId=67345922910481&id=131724555879435&l=en&sid=1ce91ed16e34d921e697e0ac0c8b88d0. Accessed 12 Oct 2022.

88. Thomson WH. Diseases of the mouth, stomach, pancreas and liver. In: Sajous CE, editor. Annual of the universal medical sciences and analytical index: a yearly report of the progress of the general sanitary sciences throughout the world, vol. 1. Philadelphia: F.A. Davis; 1888. p. 290–342.

89. Günzburg A. Zur Diagnose der Duodenalgeschwüre. Dtsch med Wochenschr. 1910;28:1318–20.

90. Pottenger FM. Collective. In: The National Cyclopedia of American Biography, vol. 13. New York: James T. White Co.; 1906. p. 392.

91. Guinn JM. Dr. Francis Marion Pottenger. In: A history of California and an extended history of Los Angeles and Environs: also containing biographies of well-known citizens of the past and present, vol. 3. Los Angeles: Historic Record Company; 1915. p. 559–60.

92. Pottenger FM. Collective. In: Who's who in the Pacific Southwest: a compilation of authentic biographic sketches of citizens of Southern California and Arizona. Los Angeles: Times-Mirror; 1913. p. 299–300.

93. Pottenger FM. Light touch palpation. In: Muscle spasm and degeneration in intrathoracic inflammations and light touch palpation. St Louis: C.V. Mosby; 1912. p. 86–97.

94. [No author]. Catalogue of the University of Pennsylvania, 1896–1897. Philadelphia: University of Pennsylvania; 1896.

95. Maxwell WJ, Zugsmith E. General alumni catalogue of the University of Pennsylvania. Philadelphia: University of Pennsylvania General Alumni Society; 1917. p. 787.

96. [No author]. Alumni notes. Univ Pa Med Bull. 1911;23:805.

97. [No author]. Edwin Zugsmith. Bull Am Acad Med. 1915;16:31.

98. [No author]. News notes. Lancet. 1913;109:91.

99. Zugsmith E. A new sign in the diagnosis and treatment of ulcer and carcinoma of the stomach. Pa Med J. 1912;41:436–7.

100. Guggenberger E. Regierungsrat Doktor Alexander Brenner: 40 Jahre Primarius. Linz: NA; 1928.

101. Moran ME, Moll FH. History of cystoscopy. In: Patel SR, Moran ME, Nakada SY, editors. The history of technologic advancements in urology. Cham: Springer; 2018. p. 3–20.

102. Lesky E. The Vienna Medical School of the 19th century. Baltimore: Johns Hopkins University Press; 1976.

103. Brenner A. Das Zwerchfell reißen: ein Frühsymptom der Magenperforation. Wien klin Wochenschr. 1913;26:1973–4.

104. Prével M. Le réflexe abdomino-cardiaque: essai sur l'un des facteurs de l'accélération cardiaque orthostatique. Paris Méd. 1917;23:138–43.
105. Brown LR. A tribute to Russell Daniel Carman. Mayo Clin Proc. 1995;70:1215–7.
106. Miller A, Russell D. Carman, 1875–1926. Am J Roentgenol. 1926;16:53–5.
107. [No author]. Deaths: Russell Daniel Carman. JAMA. 1926;86:1991.
108. [No author]. Russell D. Carman. Radiology. 1926;7:170.
109. Russell D, Carman MD. Lecture Series sponsored by the Missouri Radiological Society. 10 Apr 2021. http://morads.org/wp-content/uploads/page/8/carman-2021-pdf.pdf. Accessed 5 Nov 2022.
110. Moore S. Obituary: Russell Daniel Carman. Br J Radiol. 2014;31:321–8.
111. [No author]. Russell Daniel Carman. Wash Univ Rec. 1911;7:5.
112. Carman Lecture: Russell Daniel Carman, MD. Missouri Radiological Society. https://morads.org/carman-lecture/. Accessed 22 Oct 2022.
113. Carman RD. A new roentgen-ray sign of ulcerating gastric cancer. JAMA. 1921;77:990–2.
114. Weber MF. Sven Effert (1922–2000): Leben und Werk. Kassel: Kassel University Press; 2018.
115. Prof. Dr. med. Norbert Henning. Professorenkatalog der Universität Leipzig/Catalogus Professorum Lipsiensium. Universität Leipzig. https://research.uni-leipzig.de/catalogus-professorum-lipsiensium/leipzig/Henning_471/. Accessed 3 Nov 2022.
116. Norbert Henning, 1896–1985. 100 Jahre DGVS. Deutsche Gesellschaft für Gastroenterologie, Verdauungs- und Stoffwechselkrankheiten. https://www.dgvs.de/epaper/100-jahre-dgvs/files/assets/basic-html/page71.html. Accessed 3 Nov 2022.
117. Sybodo Museum. Medical instruments and devices for nursing. https://www.kugener.com/de/humanmedizin/innere-medizin/55-artikel/3461-gastroskop.html. Accessed 2 Nov 2022.
118. Henning N, Keilhack H. Die gezielte Farbenphotographie in der Magenhöhle. Dtsch med Wochenschr. 1938;64:1392–3.
119. Rodgers HW. Henning's textbook of gastroscopy. London: Oxford University Press; 1937.
120. Sandweiss DJ. Peptic ulcer: clinical aspects, diagnosis, management. Philadelphia: W.B. Saunders; 1951.
121. Raw, Stanley Collingwood (1910–1994). Plarr's lives of the fellows. Royal College of Surgeons of England. 30 Sep 2015. https://www.google.com/books/edition/Lives_of_the_Fellows_of_the_Royal_Colleg/vw8gAQAAMAAJ?hl=en&gbpv=0. Accessed 20 Nov 2022.
122. Raw AJ. Stanley Collingwood Raw, MS, FRCS. Br Med J. 1994;38:1565.
123. Raw SC. Perforation of gastric and duodenal ulcers: a series of 312 cases. Lancet. 1944;243:12–4.

Chapter 4
Small and Large Bowel Signs

4.1 Introduction

The small intestines consist of three parts: duodenum, jejunum, and ileum. The first part, the *duodenum*, is the Latin word for twelve. It was named by Herophilus of Chalcedon (c. 335 BC–c. 280 BC) in reference to its length of twelve fingerbreadth [1]. The *jejunum*, the second part of the small intestines, was described by Aristotle (384 BC–322 BC) and named by Galen of Pergamon (129 AD–c. 216 AD). Galen referred to this section of the bowel as "fasting," translated into Latin as "jejunum," because of the absence of food in this portion of the intestines after death [1]. The final portion, the *ileum*, is the Greek term "twisted or to twist," also believed to be named by Galen [1]. Aulus Cornelius Celsus (c. 25 BC–c. 50 AD) was believed to use these terms in his work *De Medicina* (On Medicine), in the first century:

> The junction between the stomach and duodenum, the Greeks call pylorus, because it discharges the office of a door keeper to the lower intestines, by permitting the scape of such things, which were about to excrete. After the duodenum, begins the jejunum, not so much convoluted; which, as the name imports, never retains what it receives; but immediately transmits it into the inferior parts. Thence begins the smaller intestine, or ileum, highly convoluted; each of whose convulsions being held down by small connecting membranes; which being turned towards the right hypogastric region terminates in the great intestine, yet occupy more the superior parts [2, p. 242].

The origin of the term *colon* is unclear. The *caecum* is the Latin term for blind in reference to it being the blind gut or end of the large intestine. Celsus spoke about the large intestines:

> Afterwards, this intestine is joined by a thicker transverse one, which commences on the right side, is pervious and extends towards the left, forming an arch, which is not so towards the right, and for this reason is named the cæcum. But that portion which is open, being of large capacity and sinuous, less tendinous than the upper intestines, and arranged in various convolutions on each side, yet occupying the left and lower parts most, touches the liver and the stomach: then it is connected with some small membranes coming from the left kidney;

S. H. Yale et al., *Gastrointestinal Eponymic Signs*, https://doi.org/10.1007/978-3-031-33673-7_4

and taking a curve to the right forms the descending portion, where it excretes the faces, and on that account is there termed the straight gut or rectum [2, p. 243].

Signs of the small and large bowel describe those primarily caused by obstruction, volvulus, or intussusception. The development of fluoroscopy and barium contrast allowed visualization of the bowel and identification and delineation of the underlying process.

4.2 Eponymous Signs

4.2.1 Dance Sign

Jean-Baptiste Hippolyte Dance (1797–1832) was born at Saint-Pal-de-Chalencon, Haute-Loire, France, and was an extern in 1820 and intern in 1822 in medicine [3–6]. He received his medical degree from the University of Paris in 1826 and was an agrégé at the Faculty of Medicine, Paris, in 1826 [3–5]. Dance was a deputy physician to Leroux; chair of internal medicine at Cochin Hospital; the Charité Hospital in 1830; and appointed to the clinic at the Hôtel-Dieu in 1832, a position which he held for only a short time prior to his premature death from cholera [3–5]. He was a titular member of the Anatomical Society of Paris in 1827 [6].

Dance formulated a list of six rules of militant Cartesianism for students:

> (1) You must not accept as true what I tell you about the symptoms experienced by such a patient, only insofar as you have ascertained it for yourselves; (2) you will only have complete confidence about the symptom if you checked it several times yourself; (3) you will still be afraid of having made a mistake, even when the verification appears to be complete; (4) such a frame of mind will cause you to reconsider these things until you are entirely sure; (5) it will make you reject everything that does not carry with it the stamp of authenticity; (6) it will warn you against incomplete scientific observations. Has anyone ever said it better? [4, p. 19].

As to a description of his character by Dechambre:

> Dance was one of the most distinguished pathologists of our time. He was gifted with the most remarkable talent of observation, extreme sagacity, perseverance, and unfailing patience, supported by a sober and lucid judgment, a spirit of induction which, within the limited extent of experimental science, was without prejudice for or against the reigning doctrines. He possessed a rare independent and honest scientific faith without which the truth escapes the best intentions. Dance was easily recognized at a time when principles and opinions were often placed before facts [5, p. 385].

Dance described in three infants the following finding (Table 4.1):

> The cecum and the colon are displaced and reside in the sigmoid flexure. In these three cases, the shape of the abdomen is unusual. The absence of the ascending colon and cecum on the right side of the abdomen causes a depression. In contrast, intussusception produces a longitudinal enlarged voluminous mass on the left side [7, p. 211].

Thus, Dance sign refers to depression on the right side and protrusion on the left side of the abdomen caused by intussusception.

4.2.2 *Cruveilhier Sign*

Jean Cruveilhier (1791–1874) was born in Saint Martial, Limoges, France, and was an intern at Hôtel-Dieu under the tutelage of Guillaume Dupuytren (1777–1835) in 1811 [8]. Cruveilhier received his medical degree from the University of Paris in 1816 and became agrégé at the Faculty of Paris in 1823. He was appointed chair of operative medicine in Montpellier in 1824 [8, 9]. He returned to Paris to fill the position of professor of anatomy at the University of Paris School of Medicine in 1825, was deputy physician at the Maison Royale de Santé (also known as La Rochefoucauld Hospital) in 1828, and head physician of Maternity in 1830 [8–10]. Cruveilhier was chair of anatomy and subsequently chair of pathological anatomy in Paris from 1835 to 1865, head of the surgical department of Charité in 1847, and Salpêtrière in 1849 and an honorary doctor of the hospital in 1856 [11].

He was president of the Anatomical Society in 1826, elected to the Academy of Medicine in 1836 and served as its president in 1839, a member of the Advisory Committee on Hygiene at the Ministry of Agriculture and Commerce in 1848, president of the Imperial Academy of Medicine in 1859, and commander of the Legion of Honor in 1863 [11].

His character, as described by Després, was "modest, benevolent, and charitable" [9, p. 908]. Cruveilhier discussed the clinical characteristic of intussusception and stated that (Table 4.1):

> Intussusception is revealed by the symptoms of strangulation, identical to internal hernial strangulation caused by an organic constriction of the intestine, and generally causes severe pain. There are two characteristic signs of strangulation by intussusception: (1) the presence of considerable swelling formed by the invaginated portion of the intestine, a circumstance on which Dance rightly insisted, and; (2) expulsion through the anus of a large quantity of bloody mucus. This last sign is never lacking, and I consider it pathognomonic. In many cases, there is dysenteric tenesmus, so much so that one would be tempted to believe in the existence of dysentery if the symptoms of internal strangulation did not reveal the true character of the disease [12, p. 529].

Thus, Cruveilhier sign, as related to the intestines, refers to the bloody mucus in the stool in the case of intussusception. The Cruveilhier-Baumgarten sign consists of multiple dilated umbilical and paraumbilical veins on the abdominal wall (caput medusae) in patients with portal hypertension (see Chap. 11).

4.2.3 *Blatin Sign*

We believe that the sign is attributed to Juan-Bautista Blatin (1771–1835), born in Clermont-Ferrand. He was a surgeon major during the war of Savoy and Rhine [13]. Blatin published a treatise on uterine bleeding in 1802. He was a physician at Hôtel-Dieu and professor of materia medica at the Clermont-Ferrand School [13]. Blatin was a member of the Academy of Sciences; the Royal Academy of Medicine, Paris; and the Society of Clinical Medicine [13]. He was described as one who "has left among his compatriots the memory of beneficence and selflessness, very rare in the century in which we live" [13, p. 7].

Blatin described in a 28-year-old woman who was later diagnosed with hydatid cysts (Table 4.1):

> The abdomen was the volume of a 7 months pregnancy. It was without fluctuation. Percussion caused her abdomen to move with and tremble, similar to a gelatinous mass. The touch neither indicated either pregnancy nor an increase in uterine size. (…) Following an enema, she evacuated about seventeen pounds of hydatid cysts mixed with a large quantity of blood and stool within an hour and a half. The largest was the size of a small hazelnut, and the smallest was the size of a pea adhering to each other through filamentous tissue [14, p. 524–525].

According to Rolleston, the sign referred to as a "hydatid thrill" involves the perception of vibration on the left middle finger when percussed with the right hand over a hydatid cyst [15].

4.2.4 Cherchevsky Sign

We could only identify limited historical information on Mikhail Cherchevsky (Cherchevski). At the time of his publication of one of his signs in "Contributions à la pathologie des névroses intestinales" (Contributions to the pathology of intestinal neuroses) in 1883, he was a physician in Saint-Petersburg, Russia [16]. He also published a sign to determine the presence of atherosclerosis of the aortic arch titled "Sur un nouveau signe de sclérose de la crosse de l'aorte" (On a new sign of sclerosis of the arch of the aorta), when he was a medical consultant at Nicolas Hospital in Saint-Petersburg [17].

Cherchevsky reported exquisitely detailed symptoms and physical findings in six patients with a chronic history of an undefined recurrent intestinal neurosis characterized by diarrhea alternating with constipation, abdominal bloating and tenesmus, and various constitutional symptoms, including multiple tender points, dizziness, lower extremity weakness, insomnia, irritable bladder, and migraines (Table 4.1). As described in his first patient:

> The onset of the crisis, although always occurring unexpectedly when attentively observed, was far from spontaneous. In the shapes of the excrement, we found a very valuable clue that always enabled us to accurately predict the approaching onset of the spell. Almost from the onset of the disease, the volume or the stool's diameter had become noticeably smaller. This detail always astonished the patient, who remembers that the stool never returned to its former normal size and only underwent a slight increase in volume as during the state of perfect health. Before the attack, usually four or five days earlier, the evacuations became more frequent: instead of just one a day, there were two and even three bowel movements; usually molded into the shape of a sausage, the feces thinned out even more, and eventually broke off into distinct, rounded pieces from the size of a walnut to that of a hazelnut. This then degenerated into the form of ribbons somewhat thicker towards the middle and flattened towards the edges. Later the evacuations were only the thickness of a pencil, after which they became quite liquid and were expelled in the form of a very thin jet. Simultaneously with this final form, there usually appeared the painful sensation under the costal margins, as well as the pains described above, which indicated the beginning of the attack for the patient. These gradual changes in the form and consistency of the stools pre-

ceded the severe crises. They always presented exactly in this chronological order which we have just pointed out. Simultaneously with the onset of pain under the false ribs, the patient's face becomes pale and slightly cyanotic, breathing accelerated 26–28; the transverse diameter of the heart slightly exceeds the left parasternal line; the heart beats becomes rarer, the pulse drops from 70 to 60. The upper part of the abdomen is distended; the percussion makes a sonorous and tympanic noise heard with a metallic undertone. At the onset of the attack, the bloating, in most cases, is circumscribed, sometimes occupying the pit of the stomach, sometimes the right or left colonic flexures [16, p. 881–882].

Thus, Cherchevsky described the symptoms of the disease currently known as irritable bowel syndrome.

4.2.5   Wahl Sign

Eduard Georg von Wahl (1833–1890) was born in Vana-Pärnu (Pernau), Livonia (Estonia), and received his medical degree from the University of Dorpat in 1859 [18–20]. He continued his studies in Berlin and Paris and was a general practitioner in St. Petersburg, Russia, in 1860 [18–20]. He was an ordinate professor at Peter-Pauls Hospital from 1860 to 1862; Marien-Magdalenen Hospital from 1862 to 1865; senior physician at the Izmaylovsky Life Guards Regiment from 1865 to 1868; chief surgeon at the Prinz Peter von Oldenburg Children's Hospital; and consultant at the Maximillian Sanatorium, St. Petersburg, from 1869 to 1876 [18–22].

Wahl was appointed chair of state medicine at the University of Dorpat in 1876 and senior physician of the Evangelical Hospital in Sitowa, Bulgaria, in 1877 [18–21]. He was a professor of surgery at the University of Dorpat in 1878 and appointed *rector magnificus* at the University of Dorpat from 1881 to 1885 [18, 20].

Wahl described the appearance of the bowel in cases of strangulating bowel obstruction (Table 4.1):

> If the location of the obstruction has been approximately determined before the operation, which I consider a *sine qua non*, then there can be no question of aimless searching in the abdominal cavity. The darker color, increased gas, dilation, and congestion of the portion of the intestine above the obstruction lead in all circumstances to the constriction point. Once this part of the intestine is present in view after an abdominal incision, the nature of the obstruction is, in most cases, easily recognizable [23, p. 184].

Thus, Wahl sign refers to the appearance of the proximal distended portion of the bowel in strangulated intestinal obstruction.

4.2.6   Hirschsprung Sign

Harald Hirschsprung (1830–1916) was born in Copenhagen, Denmark. He worked as a student doctor during the cholera epidemic in 1853, qualified in medicine at the University of Copenhagen in 1855, and completed an internship at the Frederick Hospital and Fødselsstifftelsen (Royal Maternity Hospital) from 1857 to 1860 [24, 25]. He received a Master's degree in 1859 and completed his doctorate "Om mefødt

Tillunkning af Spiserør og Tyndtarm" (On Congenital Closure of the Esophagus and Small Intestines) in 1861 [24–26]. He was a reserve physician from 1862 to 1864 and visiting physician from 1864 to 1870 at Frederick Hospital, followed by an appointment at Bönehospitalet (Children's Hospital) in Rigensgades from 1870 to 1879 [24–26]. Hirschsprung was appointed professor at the University of Copenhagen in 1877 [24]. He was the founder and served as a chief medical officer at Queen Louise's Children's Hospital from 1879 to 1904 [24, 26]. He also was an associate professor in pediatrics at the University of Copenhagen, Denmark, in 1901 [24–26]. Hirschsprung served as an examiner for the medical office at the University of Copenhagen from 1866 to 1874. He was an honorary member of the Danish Pediatric Society in 1908 and the German Society of Pediatrics in 1912 [24, 26].

His character as described by Niels Thorkild Rovsing:

> As a person, Hirschsprung was brash and unassuming in appearance, humane and refined in thought, warm-hearted and open in his demeanor, and all in all, an uncommonly sympathetic personality that will be remembered with veneration and gratitude by all who knew him [24, p. 392].

There are several signs ascribed to Hirschsprung. In regard to intussusception:

> I had endeavored to show what was most characteristic of its clinical appearance, just as I had attempted in the accompanying plates, to provide information regarding the location of the mass, its size, mobility, or stability, as an aid in the differential diagnosis and for the determining the appropriate treatment. (…) [t]here is a fact here that deserves our full attention. The habitual sluggish opening in small children must certainly not be neglected. I cannot confidently say where the disease is most frequent [27, p. 564].

Thus, Hirschsprung was referring to the atony of the anal sphincter in cases of ileo-cecal invagination.

Hirschsprung presented another finding at the Society of Pediatrics in Berlin in 1886. He described two cases in infants where there was marked dilation and hypertrophy of the colon (Table 4.1):

> I present to this knowledgeable assembly two unique brief case histories and pathological specimens in the hope that this may lead to further reports of similar cases or pertinent remarks from the many colleagues present. I will present the first specimen to you immediately. It is a large intestine, as you can see, but of such dimensions it will surely surprise you to learn that it is from a child who was only 11 months old at death. It represents the intestinal loops of the sigmoid colon and the more dilated transverse colon. The other parts of the large intestine also appeared somewhat dilated; only the rectum was neither dilated nor narrowed. The parts of the intestine are not only distended, but the wall is also considerably thickened through all its layers, particularly the muscularis. In addition, the mucosa in the dilated parts has considerable erosions and ulcerations, which vary greatly in size and depth [28, p. 1]. (…) The fact that a finger could be inserted into the rectum with ease and that the rectum was very often full of feces on exploration, which, never emerged spontaneously, speaks against a narrowing lying deeper as well as higher in the intestinal tract. This finding seemed rather in favor of an atonic condition of the lower part of the intestinal canal [28, p. 3]. (…) [c]onsidering that the difficulties of defecation began early in life provides indisputable evidence that the underlying malady, brought from the womb, is imputable due to either a developmental anomaly or a morbid fetal process [28, p. 7].

Thus, this sign refers to congenital hypertrophic dilation of the colon.

4.2.7 *Gangolphe Sign*

Michel Gangolphe (1858–1919) was born in Lyon, France, and studied medicine at the Faculty of Medicine, Lyon, later serving as a hospital extern in 1876, anatomy assistant in 1877, hospital intern at Croix-Rousse Hospital in the surgical department in 1878, and preceptor at the Hôtel-Dieu [29, 30]. He served as head of Louis-Lépold Ollier (1830–1900) Clinic, was appointed chief surgeon at the Hôtel-Dieu from 1877 to 1908, agrégé in 1886, and professor agrégé in the Faculty of Pharmacy, Lyon, from 1889 to 1898 [29, 31].

Gangolphe was president of the Society of Medical Sciences of Lyon in 1896, a member of the Lyon Academy of Sciences, and a corresponding member of other Parisian societies [29, 32]. His areas of expertise were related to bone surgery and bone infection [32].

As a description of his character as told by Nové-Josserand:

> Gangolphe was my first master in surgery, and I was his first intern when he took up his post at the Croix-Rousse Hospital. He made me understand and love surgery, and I have remained deeply grateful to him. He was a valuable guide for young surgeons because he brought together the two qualities that make the nobility of our art: love of the patient and love of science. He taught daily by example that the end of surgery is not to perform brilliant operations but to cure the patient. The operative act was, therefore, for him, only the logical culmination of a meticulous clinical examination and a close discussion of its indications. In his mind, post-operative care was as critical as the intervention itself. However, these humanitarian considerations did not prevent him from being a man of science in the complete sense of the term. A prudent surgeon, he knew how to be bold and enterprising when necessary, as shown in particular by his conservative interventions in malignant tumors of the limbs. He also liked to research new facts, analyze and criticize them, and further classify them in order to promote their advancement [33, p. 613].

Gangolphe reported an observation as a way to distinguish a strangulated hernia from other causes of intestinal obstruction (Table 4.1):

> [I] thought that this sero-bloody fluid was characteristic of strangulation and made it possible to distinguish occlusions due to strangulation from occlusions due to any other cause. Experiments on dogs confirmed my view by showing that the constriction of an intestinal loop by a rubber ring results in causing this same sero-bloody liquid in the peritoneal cavity and intestines. The quantity of fluid was proportional to the extent of the trapped intestinal loop and the intensity of the constriction. This fact has some practical value. Unlike other forms of obstruction, intestinal obstruction due to strangulation is not amenable to medical treatment. The finding of dullness due to ascites requires the surgeon to intervene immediately and not to close the abdomen until the strangulation has been released. This sign is particularly valuable in females since the presence of ascites, even a small amount, is easy to identify by vaginal examination [34, p. 403–404].

Thus, Gangolphe sign refers to the presence of a serosanguinous ascitic fluid in cases of intestinal strangulation.

4.2.8   Schlange Sign

Hans Schlange (1856–1922) was born in Rittergut Schwaneberg, Uckermark, Germany, studied medicine at Georg-August University of Göttingen and Christian-Albrechts University in Kiel and received his medical degree in 1889 [35, 36]. He was an assistant to Friedrich Esmarch (1823–1908) at the University of Kiel from 1881 to 1885 and first assistant to Ernst von Bergmann (1836–1907) at the surgical clinic of the Charité University Hospital, Berlin, from 1866 to 1894, where he also habilitated [35, 36]. Schlange was a physician at Paul Gerhardt Stift Hospital, Berlin, from 1889 to 1894 and a senior physician and professor in the Department of Surgery at the Municipal Hospital in Hanover in 1894. He was appointed professor at the University of Berlin in 1895 [35, 36].

As to a description of his character as written by a former student:

> When I came to Bergmann's clinic in 1892, I was assigned to him. What I learned from him, who was already an excellent technician and diagnostician, significantly influenced my entire development. I will never forget him. (…) Above all, he was an encouraging, inspiring teacher at the time, whom numerous pupils almost enthusiastically adored, as did the entire staff of the clinic. He knew only one consideration in operations and medical operations: the patient's well-being [36, p. 49].

Schlange described a finding observed in patients with intestinal obstruction (Table 4.1):

> When the intestine is obstructed, the efferent portion of the intestine is always empty and collapses, while the afferent portion is filled. As long as there is no peritonitis, peristaltic movements of various intensities occur in the bloated intestine. The movements are strongest where constipation had slowly developed, i.e., with a gradually growing mass, with strictures, because here the muscularis of the proximal intestine has been trophically increased [37, p. 69–70]. (…) The sign for immediate surgery is now given with proof that a part of the intestine is bloated; the intestinal loop above the constriction also shows slight peristaltic movements. In this way, the intestinal distension in the assumed symptom complex acquires an enormously important diagnostic meaning. It is the first finding that falls into the mysterious concerns of the abdominal cavity and reveals its dangers to us; let us be careful not to unnecessarily cloud this purest source of knowledge or steer it in the wrong direction [37, p. 78].

Thus, Schlange sign refers to intestinal dilation and diminished peristaltic movements occurring above and collapsed intestine found below an area of obstruction in advanced stage of the disease.

4.2.9   Mya Sign

Giuseppe Mya (1857–1911) was born in Torino, Italy, and received his medical degree from the University of Turin in 1881 [38]. His first position after military service was as an assistant in the Turin Medical Clinic under the aegis of Camillo Bozzolo (1845–1920), Chair of the Medical Clinic [39, 40]. He was an extraordinary professor of the preparatory clinic at the University of Pisa in 1886 and lecturer in the propaedeutic clinic and special medical pathology at the University of Torino in 1887 [38, 39]. Mya was appointed head physician at the Hospital San Giovanni, Torino, in 1889 and an extraordinary professor of clinical medicine and special medical pathology at the University of Siena from 1890 to 1891 [38, 39, 41]. He accepted a special demonstrative pathologist position and was head of the pediatric clinic at the Higher Institute of Florence in 1891. Mya was a physician in this city throughout the remainder of his career, despite being offered more prestigious medical appointments because of his interest in childhood disease [38–40]. He was an ordinary professor of clinical pediatrics in 1899 and director of the new institute of children's disease at the Anna Mayer Hospital in Florence in 1901 [39, 40].

He cofounded with Luigi Concetti (1854–1920) the journal *Rivista di Clinica Pediatrica* (Journal of Pediatric Clinic) in 1903 and was co-editor of *Clinica Medica Italiana* (Italian Medical Clinic) and *Monatsschrift für Kinderheilkunde* (Pediatrics Monthly) [40, 42]. He was a founding member and vice-president of the Italian Society of Pediatrics in 1898 and later president in 1905 [40, 43].

As to his character as described by Picchi:

> I cannot close this brief mention of the scientific activity of Mya without reminding you how in all his works, he has shown a vast and solid culture, a common modernity of views, and a genius of conceptions, which, combined with a plain and easy exposition, but always scientific rigor, is the constant characteristic of his works. Mya did not write to give an uninspiring contribution or approval of others' ideas. However, he always tried to discover and develop novel methods in his works. Even when he dealt with topics from other treatises, he made personal contributions by breaking down concepts and theories he believed to be incorrect in order to fill the gaps. His scientific value was based not only on the versatility of his profound ingenuity and high intelligence but also on knowing how to discipline and perfect these natural gifts through indefatigable study and boundless enthusiasm, not only for pathology and the medical clinic but also for related sciences. His innate modesty made him shy away from seeking honors and popularity. However, his very high merits, nevertheless, largely conquered the souls of all those who love true knowledge with rectitude and goodness of the heart. (…) He was an excellent pathologist and clinician who wanted to devote himself to pediatrics and became such a teacher that his fame soon went beyond the borders of our homeland [40, p. 95].

Mya acknowledged the prior description of colonic dilation by Hirschsprung and articulated the purpose of his paper:

> Up to now, as far as I know, in Italy, there is no description of any case of this nature apart from that already mentioned by Faralli. Therefore, I thought it appropriate to enrich the history of this disease with two new observations, one of which is accompanied by the appropriate histological research, which I performed on anatomical pieces [43, p. 217].

He described two cases, and in one, he identified the morbid stage of the disease (Table 4.1):

> The lens under the microscope contains triple phosphate crystals, needle-like crystals of fat, and amorphous masses. (…) Among the phenomena experienced in this terminal period, we must first point out a rapid reduction of the abdomen, as had not been previously noticed. It was thus possible to ascertain through inspection 2 furrows directed from top to bottom and

from right to left. One is located 1 cm below the umbilical scar in the midline, the other at 6 cm above. These two sulci circumscribe an enormous intestinal loop. Above the superior sulcus, there is a 2nd tubular protrusion directed transversally. There is no indication of peritonitis. The median loop measured between the two grooves is 11 cm. The upper loop measures 6 cm. Another phenomenon is the previously absent febrile movement. (…) The terminal phase was interpreted as a severe form of acute enterocolitis involving the mucosa of the intestinal tract [43, p. 220].

Thus, Mya further described the clinical features of colonic dilation as initially reported by Hirschsprung.

4.2.10 Gersuny Sign

Robert Gersuny (1844–1924) was born in Teplitz-Schönau (Bohemia, Czech Republic) and received his medical degree from Charles-Ferdinand University, Prague, in 1866 [44–46]. He was appointed secondary assistant at the A. Jaksche Clinic at the Prague General Hospital and received his surgical training at the II. Surgical University Clinic under the auspices of Theodor Billroth (1829–1894) in Vienna in 1869 [44–46]. He served as a private assistant to Billroth in 1872, chief at Rudolfinerhaus Hospital, Döbling, in 1882, and chief surgeon to the Karolinen-Kinderspital (Children's Hospital) from 1880 to 1893 [44]. He succeeded Billroth as department chairman at the Rudolfinerhaus Hospital in Vienna in 1894 [44, 45].

Gersuny described a palpable abdominal finding in three patients with a fecal tumor (impacted fecal mass) (Table 4.1):

> The symptom is based on the fact that with intensive finger pressure, the intestinal mucosa sticks to the viscous mass of feces, forming a tumor, and detaches itself when the pressure is released. The preconditions for the development of the symptom, which for brevity I will call "sticking symptom," are a certain degree of dryness of the intestinal mucosa and indentation of the surface of the fecal tumor. If the fecal tumor is too hard, the sticky symptom only comes about when the tumor has softened somewhat on the surface (due to an oil chiasma). Finally, and this also seems to me to be the most important thing for the meaning of the "sticky symptom" — these include the intestinal gases, which are pushed away when pressure is applied to the fecal tumor, but when the pressure is relieved they inflate the intestine again at the pressed point and thus its wall detach from the surface of the tumor. The presence of the "sticky symptom" generally means that a solid, somewhat malleable mass, together with gas, is enclosed in a smooth-walled sack. Such conditions will not easily come about in the human body other than through a fecal tumor [47, p. 890].

He found in these cases that the disease began in early childhood with bowel irregularity and constipation relieved with purgatives and irrigation. Eventually, because of fecal impaction, chronic intestinal obstruction developed, and the large intestine became longer, wider, and contained a thickened wall resulting from hypertrophy. Thus, Gersuny sign refers to the presence of a palpable mass (impacted feces) found on abdominal palpation, which becomes detached when the finger is released. Gersuny was presumably unaware that Hirschsprung and Mya previously described this disease.

4.2.11 Bayer Sign

Carl Bayer (1854–1930) was born in Polná, Czech Republic, and received his medical degree from the University of Prague in 1879 [48]. He remained in Prague and was first appointed demonstrator at the Pathological-Anatomical Institute under Edwin Klebs (1834–1913), followed by an assistant at the surgical clinic under Carl Gussenbauer (1842–1903) from 1879 to 1887 [48, 49]. He habilitated at the University of Prague in 1886 and became a full professor of surgery in 1892 [48, 49]. Bayer served as head of the surgical department of the German Children's Hospital, Prague, from 1887 to 1918 and chief physician at the surgical department of the Barmherzige Brüder (Brothers of Charity) Hospital, Prague, from 1892 to 1929 [48, 49]. Bayer cofounded the Red Cross sanatorium in Korngasse from 1906 to 1929 [48, 49]. He was a corresponding member of the French Society of Surgery in Paris. Bayer was a writer of poems and short plays [48].

Bayer described the case of a 50-year-old man with a history of recurrent intestinal obstruction who presented with 5 days of severe pain, progressive abdominal distention, and an S-shaped bulge on the abdominal wall (Table 4.1). On physical examination:

> The patient's abdomen seemed to shift to the left in its upper half and to the right in its lower half. The overall impression was that of an S-shaped bead. The only unclear thing was that the oblique bulge ran diagonally from the top left to the bottom right, bending to the left again in the right hypogastrium and extending to the bottom right in the cecal region. It was stretched to the point of bursting and hemispherically round as to being felt like a bent knee. The saddle-shaped indentation on the left, at the border between the epigastrium and hypogastrium, is where the largest protrusion usually occurs with pronounced colon meteorism, conforming to the same protrusion of the opposite abdominal region. So the asymmetry and the overall oblique form of meteorism deviated from the usual type [50, p. 238–239]. (…) I interpreted this finding to mean that the lower part of the descending colon with the initial part of the sigmoid colon, or this latter alone, as a result of the complete obstruction and the maximum intestinal distension, would have protruded from the retro-abdominal space and folded over to the right on the small intestine. After opening the abdomen, which was performed immediately, I saw that the internal findings could have been read from the outer contours of the meteorism much more precisely than I thought possible. Looking side by side at the sketch of the meteorism and the picture of the inner finding, one must say that the latter resembles the former. In the event of a recurrence of this distinctive form of meteorism—assuming a similar state of the abdominal wall and intestinal tension—the precise diagnosis: of "sigmoid volvulus" would be possible. In our case, the S-sling was turned twice to the left (wrong clockwise); after removing the upper pole under the left costal arch, it spontaneously turned once to the right; a second right turn completed the detorsion [50, p. 240–241].

Thus, Bayer sign refers to the unique characteristic appearance of the abdominal wall caused by a sigmoid volvulus.

4.2.12 Bouveret Sign

Léon Bouveret (1850–1929) was born in Châtillon-sur-Chalaronne, Ain, France, studied medicine in Lyon and Paris, and was appointed intern of the Hospitals of Paris in 1873. He completed his medical degree in Paris in 1878 based on the thesis "Sur une tumeur osseuse généralisée à laquelle conviendrait le nom de tumeur à ostéoblasts" (On a generalized bone tumor to which the name osteoblast tumor would suit) [51, 52]. He returned to Lyon to serve as director of the clinic of the Faculty of Medicine, Lyon, under Raphaël Lépine (1840–1919) [53, 54]. In 1879 he was appointed doctor of the Hospital of Lyon and associate professor based on the thesis titled "Des sueurs morbides" (Morbid sweats) at the Hospitals of Lyon in 1880 [51, 53]. In 1885 he served patients during the cholera epidemic in the commune of Saint-Remèze [51, 52]. Bouveret was a member of the Lyon Academy of Sciences, Literature and Arts; the National Academy of Medicine, France; Society of Medical Sciences; and the Medical Society of Lyon [53].

In addition to the sign for his namesake, he is also credited for naming and describing a disease and syndrome. Bouveret disease is also known as tachycardie essentielle paroxystique (essential paroxysmal tachycardia), currently known as paroxysmal supraventricular tachycardia published in *Revue de Médecine* in 1889; and Bouveret syndrome, the obstruction of the stomach and duodenum caused by impaction of a gallstone that migrated through a biliogastric or bilioduodenal fistula in 1896 [54].

As a description of his character as articulated by Français:

> An observer and clinician of the first order, his hospital department had been a veritable school compelling both students and doctors. Everyone could appreciate his vast erudition, the clarity of his teaching, and his marvelous talent for diagnosis, which often astonished his listeners. They will piously preserve the memory of this excellent doctor, who was also a good man, endowed with the finest qualities of intelligence and heart [52, p. 313].

Bouveret described bowel obstruction involving the transverse colon, "the position of the intestine which the retraction of the gastrocolic omentum adheres to and fixes to the stomach. This kind of occlusion is not very rare; perhaps it is as common as occlusion by a neoplasm of the colon" [55, p. 326–327] (Table 4.1). In regard to the diagnosis, Bouveret wrote:

> Physical signs are much more important for the diagnosis. They must be carefully researched and are based on repeated frequent observation. Behind the obstacle of the transverse colon, the cecum and the ascending colon dilate and contract. In contrast, the descending colon and sigmoid retract and remain more or less immobile. This contrast between the two parts of the large intestine is the key to diagnosing transverse colon occlusion. Careful and repeated examination of the abdomen, by inspection and palpation, allows us to recognize this dilation and exaggeration peristalsis of the cecum and ascending colon. In previous work, I have already explained this diagnosis. Watch the patient's belly as he complains of colic, a strong, globular swelling lifts the abdominal wall in the right iliac fossa and hypochondrium and extends more or less to the epigastrium and the umbilicus, while the hypochondrium and the left iliac fossa remain soft, depressible, and maintain their normal configuration. In one patient at the time of a painful crisis, an oblique line extending from the middle of the right femoral arch to the left costal margin divided the abdomen into two parts: the right, which was often agitated by strong peristaltic contractions, and the left,

which did not participate in this agitation of the large intestine. For quite a long time, this exaggerated peristalsis remains limited to the colon; later, if the obstruction is complete, it can also involve the small intestine. At this moment, the sign no longer has the same value. However, generalized abdominal peristalsis starts and sometimes remains localized on the right side [55, p. 329]. (…) I have often found that the exaggerated peristalsis of the colon is more painful than that of the stomach. Also, patients with transverse colon stenosis following perigastritis ordinarily locate the maximum of their pain in the right iliac fossa [55, p. 331].

Thus Bouveret sign of the colon refers to observed and palpable globular swelling on the right iliac fossa and hypochondrium of the abdomen and soft, depressible hypochondrium and left iliac fossa on the left side of the abdomen in patients with obstruction involving the transverse colon.

4.2.13 Anschütz Sign

Alfred Wilhelm (Willy) Anschütz (1870–1954) was born in Halle (Saale), Germany, studied medicine in Halle, Marburg, and Tübingen, and received his medical degree from the latter in 1896 [56]. He was first appointed assistant in medicine in Halle from 1896 to 1897 and assistant to Johann von Mikulicz (1850–1905) and later senior physician in surgery at the Friedrich-Wilhelms University in Breslau (Wroclaw, Poland) from 1897 to 1902 [57, 58]. He was an associate professor in surgery in 1902 and at Friedrich-Wilhelms University in Breslau in 1906 [56–58]. Anschütz was appointed associate professor at the Philipps University in Marburg in 1906, followed by professor and deputy director of the surgery clinic at the Christian-Albrechts University of Kiel in Marburg the following year [56–58]. He was dean of medicine at the Christian-Albrechts University from 1919 to 1920 and director of the surgical clinic from 1945 to 1946 [57].

Anschütz was a member of the German Academy of Natural Scientists Leopoldina in Halle and president of the German Society of Surgery in 1930 [56, 57, 59]. He was co-editor of *Zentralblatt für Chirurgie* (Central Journal of Surgery) and *Deutsche Zeitschrift für Chirurgie* (German Journal of Surgery) [54]. Anschütz was also appointed Geheimer Medizinalrat (Privy Medical Counselor).

He was a member of the National Socialist German Workers' Party from 1933 to 1945 [57]. Eponymic names are honorific terms that highlight one's contribution to science and medicine. As such, they should not be used for individuals who support anti-Semitism, racial, or other crimes against humanity.

Anschütz described findings in patients with colon cancer causing intestinal obstruction and cecal dilation in the presence of a competent ileocecal valve (Table 4.1):

(1) There is a local meteorism due to overdistension observed at the cecum in low-lying colon obstruction. (2) The cause of this local flatulence and overstretching is the increased internal pressure in the closed colon tube with a resistant ileocecal valve. (3) The main cause of the local flatulence is found not only in differences in the resistance on the part of the intestinal wall but especially in the different widths of the large intestine sections. Tension at the cecum indicates the need for an operation [60, p. 220].

Thus, Anschütz sign refers to a closed-loop obstruction in patients with colon cancer in the presence of a competent ileocecal valve.

4.2.14 Nothnagel Sign

Carl Wilhelm Hermann Nothnagel (1841–1905) was born in Alt-Lietzegöricke, Brandenburg, Germany, and received his medical degree from Friedrich-Kaiser-Wilhelm Institute in 1863 [61–63]. He served as first assistant under Ernst Viktor von Leyden (1832–1910) at Königsberg from 1865 to 1868 and was an associate professor in internal medicine in 1867 [61, 63, 64]. He lectured in medicine at the University of Berlin from 1868 to 1870 and at the University of Breslau from 1870 to 1872 [61, 64]. Nothnagel was a professor of medicine and pharmacology in Freiburg in 1872, chair of special pathology and therapeutics in Jena in 1874, and professor of medicine at the University of Vienna in 1882. In Vienna, he completed *Die Specielle Pathologie und Therapie* (The Special Pathology and Therapy), a 20-volume collaborative work [61, 62, 64].

Nothnagel was a member of the German Academy of Natural Scientists, Leopoldina, in 1879; founded and served as the first president of the Vienna Society of Internal Medicine; appointed by the Emperor Member of the Austrian House of Lords in 1902; a member of the Academy of Sciences; and first chairman of the Society of Internal Medicine, Vienna. He cofounded with Leyden the journal *Zeitschrift für klinische Medizin* (Journal of Clinical Medicine) in 1880 [62].

As a description of his character and approach to disease:

> The brilliant diagnostician's goal was to train capable and conscientious physicians. He wanted to teach observation and examination of the patient and repeatedly reminded learners never to be blinded by symptoms, always examine the patient from head to toe, make observations without bias, avoid neglecting even the most minor details based on careful analysis, and derive relevant conclusions. He forgave ignorance but was intolerant of untruthfulness, recklessness, and lack of sense of duty in patient care and swiftly intervened with fire and sword when he identified the offender [65, p. 507].

Several signs of obstruction of the small and large bowel are attributed to Nothnagel. The first one is the ileal succession splash:

> In the case of stenosis of the bowel there is frequently a feeling of fluctuation on palpation, and occasionally distinct succussion-sounds can be produced, particularly above the stenosis. The presence of these two signs is natural, for fluctuation and succussion-sounds can always be produced in a dilated loop of intestine filled with a mixture of gas and liquid [66, p. 372].

Early in distal colon obstruction only the large intestine is distended with dilation occurring at the flanks:

> In stenosis of the sigmoid flexure complicated by meteorism from stasis, the upper and lateral aspects of the abdomen are usually distended. The distension of the lateral aspect of the abdomen is generally called flank meteorism. When the distension of the bowel is lim-

ited to certain sections of the colon, flank meteorism may be unilateral. This may occur even when stenosis is in the sigmoid flexure, for only a small segment of the bowel above the stricture may be distended [66, p. 605].

Percussion sound occurring at the same site as intestinal stenosis:

> In cases of stenosis of the bowel no definite and reliable information can be gained by percussion. (…) It is impossible, therefore, to formulate any definite rules with regard to the percutory phenomena observed in stenosis of the bowel. The information that can be obtained with regard to the clinical conditions existing is too general to be of value. Only one point is of diagnostic importance: it is that when local meteorism, strictly circumscribed to some one area of the bowel, can be discovered by percussion, we are justified in assuming that the stenosis is in this region; whenever this condition is found, all our efforts should be directed toward discovering other signs of constriction of the bowel in this particular area. Localized meteorism is of value only in the diagnosis of narrowing of the bowel per se when combined with other symptoms that point in the same direction [66, p. 372].

Thus, Nothnagel sign refers to (1) Palpatory fluctuation and auscultatory "succession splash" sound occur in the dilated bowel loop, (2) Colon dilation (meteorism) occurs at the flanks in stenosis of the sigmoid flexure, (3) Localized percussion sound identifies the areas of a stenotic bowel (Table 4.1).

4.2.15 Lane Sign

Sir William Arbuthnot Lane (1856–1943) was born at Fort George, Inverness, Scotland, and studied medicine at Guy Hospital, qualifying as a member of the Royal College of Surgeons in 1877 [67–69]. He received a Bachelor of Medicine and a Bachelor of Science with gold medals in anatomy and medicine in 1881 from the University of London. Lane accepted his first appointment as a house surgeon at the Victoria Hospital for Children, Chelsea. He returned to Guy Hospital as a demonstrator in anatomy in 1882 and was elected fellow in the Royal College of Surgeons, England, that same year. He received his Master of Surgery degree in 1883 [67–69].

Lane was appointed assistant surgeon, rising to the rank of consulting surgeon at Great Ormond Street Hospital for Sick Children from 1883 to 1888 [67–69]. He returned to Guy Hospital, where he was initially an assistant surgeon in 1888, a surgeon in 1903, and consulting surgeon in 1920 [67, 68]. He served on the Royal Army Medical Corps (RAMC) and, during World War I, was a consulting surgeon to Aldershot Command and organized the Queen Mary's Hospital, Sidcup, to treat facial injuries [67, 70]. In the Royal College of Surgeons, he was an examiner in elementary anatomy for the conjoint board (1887 to 1890) and served on the council (1908 to 1916) [67, 68].

He cofounded the Fellowship of Medicine in 1918 (the following year combined with the Post-Graduate Medical Association), serving as its president in 1923 [71]. He resigned his membership from the British Medical Association in 1925. That same year he founded the New Health Society and *New Health* journal the following year, whose purpose was to address issues of social medicine [67, 68, 72]. He was named first baronet of Cavendish Square in 1913, The Most Honorable Order of the Bath, Companion in 1917, and Chevalier of the Legion of Honor [67–69].

Lane's name is eponymously recognized in association with the technique for applying internal splints to fracture (Lane splints, screw, or plates); the disease (Lane disease or intestinal stasis); sign (Lane sign) found in intestinal stasis (also recognized as Lane bands, kinks, membrane) and its operative treatment (Lane operation or total or partial colectomy based on his theory of intestinal stasis and autointoxication); and surgical instruments and devices (holding clamp, holding forceps, catheter, dissector, elevator, mouth gag, needle, plates, rongeur, screwdriver, Murphy-Lane bone skid) [69, 71].

A description of his character:

> He holds a unique position among British surgeons and indeed among the surgeons of the world, in that he is an original thinker and has carried his views into practice in the face of opposition and prejudice. (…) Lane, however, possessed, as all men of his type possess, the courage of his convictions, and proceeded to demonstrate the wisdom and practicality of his opinions, without much regard to the opinions of his confreres [73, p. 654].

Lane described the etiology of chronic intestinal stasis of the ileum (Table 4.1):

> There develops on the under surface of the mesentery of the last few inches of the small intestines a new band, which at first forms part of the under surface of the mesentery. Later it forms a ligament distinct from the mesentery. The ligament contracts and deforms the ileum, producing a kink or obstruction of this portion of the trunk, especially in the erect posture of the trunk. In consequence of this kink the small intestines become very much dilated and this dilation may extend up as far as the pylorus. The symptoms produced by this obstruction are superficially very much like those of appendicitis [74, p. 496].

Thus, Lane sign refers to obstruction and dilation of the ileum by a ligament particularly when standing.

4.2.16   *Stierlin Sign*

Eduard Stierlin (1878–1919) was born in Zurich, Switzerland, studied medicine in Zurich, Bern, Berlin, Hamburg, and Tübingen, and completed his medical degree at the University of Zurich, passing his state examinations in 1903 [75]. He worked at the Women's Clinic at St. Gallen, Eppendorf, and Zurich Medical Clinic and subsequently was an assistant to Max Wilms (1867–1918) at the Surgical Clinic of Basel University in 1908 [75, 76]. He was a surgeon from 1912 to 1913 during the Balkan War (1912–1913). He was appointed first assistant in the Ferdinand Sauerbruch (1875–1951) Clinic in Zurich, where he habilitated in surgery, rising to the rank of a senior physician. He followed Sauerbruch to the Surgical Clinic of the University in Munich, where he continued his service as a senior physician at the surgical university clinic [75, 76].

Stierlin reported on eight patients with radiographic and pathological correlates of tuberculosis (four cases), cecal carcinoma (one patient), small intestinal stricture (two cases), and ulcerative colitis (one patient) of the large intestines (Table 4.1):

> Surgeons and internists may welcome a new diagnostic tool found radiographically for detecting earlier stages of ileocecal tuberculosis. In several clinically unclear cases, we have recently been able to use this method to determine strictures in the lower ileum and indurating and ulcerative processes in the wall of the cecum and ascending colon, thus pointing the way to the correct diagnosis [77, p. 1231].

He reported a method to diagnose tuberculous of the colon radiographically:

> Infiltrating, indurating, and ulcerative processes of the cecum and ascending colon are regularly identified radiographically by the absence of the physiological shadow in this colon section after 5–6 h in both the initial and advanced stages of the disease. Cecal tuberculosis is, therefore, the absence of the cecum—ascending colon—shadow between the lower ileum and transverse colon. With the help of radiography, the diagnosis is made in cases where it cannot be determined clinically. Ulcerative and infiltrates are seen in the rest of the colon in the skiagram by a gap corresponding to the diseased section [77, p. 1235].

Thus, Stierlin sign refers to the absence of a shadow in the cecum and ascending colon detected radiographically in infiltrating, indurating, and ulcerative bowel segments.

4.2.17 Cole Sign

Lewis Gregory Cole (1874–1954) was born in Lake Mahopac, New York, USA, and received his medical degree from the College of Physicians and Surgeons in 1898 [78–80]. He completed a year-long internship at Roosevelt Hospital, followed by general medical and surgical practice and clinical work at Roosevelt Hospital in 1899 [78–80]. He served as a professor of roentgenology at Cornell University Medical College from 1913 to 1921 [78, 80]. He advocated for the use of X-ray in the diagnosis of pulmonary tuberculosis, the differential diagnosis of gastric ulcers and gastric cancer, and the effects of radiation on tissue in atomic bomb casualties [78]. He also served as director of silicotic research within the John B. Pierce Foundation, which studied the effects of dust inhalation on the lung [78, 79].

He was a diplomate of the American Board of Radiology, a fellow of the American College of Radiology, and president of the American Roentgen Ray Society in 1917 [80]. Cole received numerous awards, including the James Ewing Award, the first Gold Medal of the Radiological Society of North America, and the Julius Friedenwald Medal from the American Gastroenterological Association [78–81].

As to a description of his character:

> Dr. Cole's brilliant, inquiring mind was devoted throughout his career to ferreting out the facts concerning controversial subjects which might be solved by radiological means. In the course of his studies he felt compelled to become expert in the fields of physiology, pathology and gastroenterology. He always entered into a discussion in a fighting mood, knowing

that he was going to be opposed and criticized, but in the end, he lived to see his work acclaimed [78, p. 870].

Cole applied the technique of serial radiography and roentgen-cinematography (upper gastrointestinal series) as the method for diagnosing pre-pyloric (duodenal) ulcers and found a (Table 4.1):

> [c]onstant deformity of the cap or sphincter, caused by the induration of cicatricial contraction surround the crater of an ulcer, or resulting therefrom. These findings are of extraordinary value if the radiographs of a large series are studied individually and collectively, and matched over each other or reproduced kinematographically. (…) The induration of an ulcer projects into the lumen of the cap, causing a displacement of bismuth as constant as one's finger-prints in a ball of putty. It may be so small as to present only a constant dent on side of the cap, or it may be so extensive as to distort the lumen of the cap beyond recognition. The process may involve one-half of the cap without distorting the other half [82, p. 1242].

Thus, Cole sign refers to a deformity of the duodenal cap or sphincter identified in an upper gastrointestinal series in patients with a duodenal ulcer.

4.2.18 Mathieu Sign

Albert Mathieu (1855–1917) was born in Thin-le-Moutier, Ardennes, France, and studied medicine in Paris at Midi, Hôtel-Dieu, Lariboisière, and St. Louis Hospital in 1882. He was an intern at the Pitié Salpêtrière Hospital under Ernest-Charles Lasègue (1816–1883) in 1878 and received his medical degree with the thesis "Sur les purpuras hémorragiques" (On hemorrhagic purpuras) in 1883 [83–85]. He worked at St. Louis Hospital under Charles-Philippe Lailler (1822–1893) in 1882 [84, 85]. He was head of the clinic of Professor Germain Sée (1818–1896) at the Hôtel-Dieu, Doctor of the Hospitals of Paris in 1891, head of the department of the Tenon Hospital in 1894, a physician at St. Andral Hospital in 1897, and later head of St. Antoine Hospital in 1907 [84, 85]. He cofounded with P. Le Gendre the French League of the School of Hygiene in 1902 and founded the *Archives des Maladies de l'Appareil digestif* (Archives of Diseases of Digestive System) in 1907 and appointed to the rank of Knight of the Legion of Honor in 1911 [85].

In a paper presented at the French Academy of Medicine on April 23, 1914, Mathieu described the finding of clapotage, or the splashing sound heard on succussion (false ascites), as a method of diagnosing intestinal stenosis (Table 4.1):

> Is it surprising that the findings of intestinal fluid and stasis accumulated upstream of the stenosis can be demonstrated by the external examination. It reveals itself by extensive clapotage and sloping dullness. It is surprising that the false ascites and abdominal clapotage occurring during the intestinal occlusion are often passed unnoticed [86, p. 303–304]. (…) M. Ricard made a communication on this subject to the Society of Surgery in June 1907, and the following year. I published in the *Archives des maladies de l'appareil digestif* a short study on the semiological value of clapotage and sloping dullness in incomplete occlusion of the intestine [86, p. 303].

Furthermore, Mathieu described a method for distinguishing fluid within the stomach from that emanating from the intestines:

> I noted that there was false ascites only in the left decubitus position. In contrast, in the right lateral decubitus position, dullness due to fluid within the stomach follows a convex line moving inferiorly, stopping slightly below the umbilicus. Below was the intestinal sound. Thus, it may be unclear whether there is an intestinal obstruction or gastric dilatation caused by pyloric stenosis. In those cases, the characteristic dullness corresponds to fluid within the stomach, and radiographic examination eliminates all doubts [86, p. 306].

Thus, Mathieu sign refers to dullness on percussion following a convex line from the stomach to slightly below the umbilicus in pyloric stenosis.

4.2.19 Butters Sign

We were unable to identify any historical information on George Butters. In the May 1915 issue of *Nürnberger medizinische Gesellschaft und Poliklinik* (Nuremberg Medical Society and Polyclinic), Wilhelm Voit in *Münchener medizinische Wochenschrift* used the term Butters cancer while reporting the case of a 39-year-old man with cancer involving the hepatic flexure of the colon. Initially, it was thought that the patient had a duodenal ulcer (Table 4.1). However,

> [o]ccult blood remained after 14 days. With the most precise daily palpation, subtle, shiftable resistance under the right costal arch in the parasternal line was concerning. Occult blood persists; neither macroscopic blood nor mucus is present in the stool. (…) Since the palpable resistance and occult blood persisted, the diagnosis of flexural carcinoma was made. Operative resection confirmed the diagnosis of a walnut-size carcinoma. (…) This case confirms the observation that constant occult blood in the feces, despite the strictest ulcer diet, almost always speaks for carcinoma [87, p. 1119].

Thus, Butter sign refers to shiftable resistance under the right costal arch in a parasternal line occurring in carcinoma of the hepatic flexure.

4.2.20 Kloiber Sign

Hans Kloiber (1883–1950) was born in Grüntegernbach, Landkreis Erding, Germany, and served as an assistant at the surgical university clinic in Frankfurt am Main [88, 89]. He was appointed assistant radiologist, followed by a senior radiologist at the radiographic institute of Baden-Baden Hospital from 1921 to 1946 [88, 89]. Kloiber described a radiographic finding in acute and chronic small bowel obstruction (Table 4.1):

> A chance observation in front of the X-ray screen caused me to refrain from giving a contrast agent. X-ray of a patient before taking the barium meal shows a strong clearing of the abdomen. I found several gas pockets with liquid levels to be the cause. Based on this observation, the diagnosis of ileus was made, and the operation confirmed my assumption.

The liquid levels are caused by fluid accumulating in the intestine due to congestion and gas formed from fermentation processes. If such a patient is placed upright, gas and liquid separate from one another by a horizontal line. One only needs to perform a fluoroscopy or, even better, an X-ray while standing, and then it is easy to detect the liquid level with the gas bubbles. Sometimes there are many and other times, a few gas bubbles, depending on the location of the disease and the duration of the incarceration. From this, a tentative diagnosis is made. A few liquid levels near the stomach indicate a high-seated intestinal obstruction, whereas numerous fluid levels in the small pelvis indicate a deep-seated intestinal obstruction [90, p. 1065]. (…) Since then, I have used this symptom systematically for X-ray diagnosis. The usefulness of the procedure was tested on a large body of definite cases of ileus, and the experience was made that in ileus, this sign was present in a more or less pronounced manner. Then dubious cases were also examined, and it was found that it was always possible to determine that if there were liquid levels with gas bubbles, it was actually ileus. The X-ray diagnosis was confirmed without exception by the subsequent operation. (…) Finally, I consider the fluid level with gas bubbles to be a pathognomonic sign and, therefore, a decisive sign for the diagnosis of ileus [90, p. 1066].

Thus, Kloiber sign refers to air-fluid levels detected in the upright X-ray in bowel obstruction.

4.2.21 Hedri Sign

For biographic information regarding Hedri see Chap. 8—Spleen Signs. Hedri described an intraoperative method for determining the viability of the colon (Table 4.1):

In intestinal resection, the epiploic appendices provide reliable and rapid information. It is easy to excise an epiploic appendage of a suspected bowel and see if its stump bleeds from the artery. If this is the case, you can leave that part of the intestine or combine the ends of the intestine. In the opposite case, we absolutely have to remove the bowel or continue with the resection. Ligation of the epiploic appendices is easy to perform and has no disadvantages. Therefore, these are reliable indicators of the nutritional status of the large intestines. In the most careful perusal of the literature pertaining to this, I found nothing of such an observation, which prompted me to bring this to your attention [91, p. 353].

There are several signs attributed to Hedri. The current one refers to determining the viability of a segment of bowel by excising an epiploic appendage to see whether the stump bleeds. The other Hedri sign is used to identify a rupture of the spleen or liver (see Chap. 8—Spleen Signs).

4.2.22 Gold Sign

Ernst Gold (1891–1967) was born in Vienna, Austria, and received his medical degree from the University of Vienna [92]. He served as a faculty member and associate professor in surgery at the University of Vienna [92, 93]. Gold had his venia legendi (authorization to teach) revoked and was expunged from the University of Vienna during National Socialism, immigrating to the United States [92, 94].

Gold described a finding at the surgical clinic of the University of Vienna under Prof. Anot Eiselsberg (1860–1939) on rectal examination in 14 of 16 patients with small bowel obstruction (Table 4.1):

> The nature of our sign of ileum is seen by following the individual findings recorded in the case histories. In most cases of small bowel obstruction, the bowel can be palpated from the cul-de-sac. Even though under normal conditions, the small intestine is a constant component of the contents of the small pelvis, it is usually not accessible for direct palpation from the pouch of Douglas. In order to palpate the small intestines during the rectal examination, certain changes must have taken place above the areas of the narrowed intestinal lumen. These changes involve an increase and abnormal composition of the intestinal contents that liquefy and accumulate, leading to widening of the intestinal loops and early hypertrophy of the muscular intestinal wall resulting from intestinal obstruction. An abnormal loop formation of the prestenotic position of the small bowel is also found early [95, p. 96].

Gold concluded that this phenomenon is prevented in cases of large bowel obstruction at the level of the cecum, which "lies like a lid in front of the entrance to the small pelvis, so that later when the congestion involves the small intestines, they can no longer sink down." He also described, in some cases early in the disease course, a "cushion-like protrusion" or bulge extending into the Douglas pouch [95, p. 97]. He found that unlike peritoneal effusions due to various causes, it was possible to displace the bulge with the examining finger in cases of small bowel obstruction.

Thus, Gold sign refers to bulging, inward displacement, and reduction of the rectal wall at the level of the pouch of Douglas in cases of small bowel obstruction.

4.2.23 Fleischner Sign

Felix George Fleischner (1893–1969) was born in Vienna, Austria, and received his medical degree from the University of Vienna Medical School in 1919 [96, 97]. He was an intern at Karolinen Children's Hospital and First Medical Clinic of the University and a resident and assistant at Wilhelminen Hospital from 1921 to 1929 [96]. He served under the auspices of Guido Holzknecht (1872–1931) at the Central Roentgen Institute from 1929 to 1930 and was an associate professor in radiology at the University of Vienna in 1931 [96]. He was chief of the roentgen department of the Vienna C.S. Child's Hospital [96, 97].

His venia legendi (authorization to teach) was revoked from the University of Vienna during National Socialism in 1938. He emigrated to the United States, where he was appointed to the radiology department at the Massachusetts Hospital and was a private practitioner in Greenfield, Massachusetts, from 1940 to 1942 [96–98]. Fleischner was appointed radiologist and eventually chief of the radiology department at Beth Israel Hospital from 1942 to 1960, with faculty appointments at Harvard (ascending to the rank of clinical professor of radiology in 1952) and Tufts

College of Medicine (assistant professor in 1945) [96–98]. He was appointed consultant in radiology at Peter Bent Brigham Hospital, Massachusetts General Hospital and Veterans Affairs Hospital in Boston, and Wet Roxbury, Massachusetts [96].

The Fleischner Society was named in his honor and founded in 1969, dedicated "to the development of roentgenology of the chest as a discipline in its own right" [99]. His name is eponymously associated with the dense horizontal line of atelectasis and healed infarction, located in the lower lobes 1–3 cm above the dome of the diaphragm (Fleischner lines) and a pulmonary sign (Fleischner sign) involving a prominence of the central pulmonary artery, caused by pulmonary embolism or thrombosis of this vessel [97].

Fleischner reported the results of over a hundred cases and described a novel radiographic finding in patients with ileocecal tuberculosis (Table 4.1):

> The diagnosis of ileocecal tuberculosis has not been emphasized. Upon reviewing the literature, insufficiency of the valve is understood and discussed as the consequence of a liquid enema in the lower loop of the small intestines. The recently described findings of rigid walls of the ileum suggest that insufficiency occurs even with oral contrast. I observed this in all such cases. The mouth of the ileocecal valve is seen as being patent. One has to rotate the patient or apply pressure to bring the area into view to avoid the overlying cecal shadow. Therefore, I am providing evidence for the insufficiency of the ileocecal valve by attaching great diagnostic importance to the detection of the openness of the valve as confirmed by its gross anatomical changes [100, p. 385–386].

Thus, incompetence of the ileocecal valve is caused by an ulcerative and fibrotic process that transforms the bowel into a rigid thick-walled tube with a narrowed lumen at the distal ileum.

4.2.24 Hintze Sign

There is limited historical information on Arthur Hintze (1881–1946). Hintze served as director of the Roentgen and Radium Institute of the Surgical University Clinic in Berlin from 1917 to 1935 [101, 102]. During this time, he was an associate professor in surgery and radiology [102, 103]. He was appointed deputy director at the General Institute against Tumorous Diseases beginning in 1935 [101, 102].

Hintze described the radiographic feature first mentioned by von Wahl on physical examination at the Roentgen Congress in 1919 (Table 4.1):

> [I]t consists in the detection of a severely distended, immobile bowel loop fixed in the abdomen. (…) [t]he gas-inflated loop is specific for obstruction of an intestinal loop and its circulation. The small intestinal loop is abundantly filled with gas and liquid. This von Wahl's symptom, which I made visible on X-ray, fulfills its task, in the most perfect way, of clarifying the diagnosis of ileum. It is immediately clear whether it is a small-intestinal loop with the typical Kerckring folds or a large-intestinal loop, which at most shows haustral marking. (…) The strength of the gas filling and the narrowness of the wall contour allow a conclusion to be drawn as to the nearness of the risk of perforation. If the wall contour is wide despite the abundant gas filling as has only been observed in sigmoid volvulus, this suggests that the disease is intermittent and is preceded by a series of attacks of bowel torsion with

spontaneous reversal. Finally in these cases the immediate cause for the disease of the ileum can be seen from the X-ray. In volvulus, one can see the constriction furrows at the twisted base of the loop and one can draw a conclusion as to whether the volvulus is of the left-hand or right-hand form based on whether the shorter leg of the sling and point of torsion are on the right or left side [103, p. 1547–1548].

Thus, Hintze sign refers to the presence of gas and liquid-filled distended loop of strangulated small bowel.

4.2.25 Burgess Sign

Arthur Henry Burgess (1874–1948) was born in Manchester, UK, and received his Master of Science in 1895 and Bachelor of Medicine and Bachelor of Surgery degrees from the Manchester Medical School in 1896 [104–107]. He was elected fellow of the Royal College of Surgery in 1899, house surgeon to Manchester Children's Hospital, Pendlebury, in 1897, and Resident Surgical Office (RSO) to the Manchester Royal Infirmary (MRI) in 1900 [104, 107]. His other appointments included visiting surgeon at the Manchester Union Hospital, Crumpsall, and a surgical officer at Christie Cancer Hospital [106]. At MRI, he was appointed honorary assistant surgeon in 1905, full surgeon in 1910, and consulting surgeon in 1934 [106]. During World War I, from 1914 to 1918, he was in charge of the Officer's Ward at the Second Western General Hospital, as consulting surgeon to the Mesopotamian Expeditionary Force, and later as consulting surgeon and chief of the surgical division in a General Hospital [104, 106, 107]. At the Victoria University of Manchester, he was a lecturer in surgery in 1907 and a professor of clinical surgery from 1921 to 1934 [104, 106, 107].

Burgess was elected president of the British Medical Association in 1929 [104, 106, 107]. He was an honorary doctor of Manitoba University in 1930, president of the Manchester Surgical Society in 1922, the Manchester Medical Society from 1925 to 1926, and the Association of Surgeons in 1933, and vice-president of the Royal College of Surgeons from 1934 to 1936 [104, 106, 107].

His character as described by Prof. Geoffrey Jefferson, prior house surgeon of Arthur Burgess:

> Burgess's work was completely sincere; there never was a less evasive man in his or anything else. Industry, sobriety, thoroughness, honesty, are the works that best express him—indeed he could not always restrain his irritation over the claims made by those whose sense of artistry caused them to advance statement that were more "required" than exact, who indulged thus in scientific romanticism. (…) Burgess excelled in another important way—namely, his encouragement of the younger surgeons, not of one pupil alone but of several [107, p. 1007].

Burgess described a palpatory finding in patients with acute intestinal obstruction (Table 4.1):

Whenever the outline of dilated coils was seen, with the peristaltic wave passing along, one might be absolutely certain that it was a case of obstruction which had been in existence for at least several weeks. Sometimes, even when peristalsis was not visible, it was palpable. By keeping the hand over the abdomen the coil underneath could be felt alternately, hardening and softening. That condition of palpable peristalsis, again indicated obstruction of some considerable standing [108, p. 556].

Thus, Burgess sign refers to palpable hardening and softening of the coil of the bowel occurring in intestinal obstruction.

4.2.26 Fèvre Sign

Marcel Paul Luis Edmond Fèvre (1897–1978) was born in Arras, Pas-de-Calais, France, and after completing an extern and internship trained under the tutelage of Louis Ombrédanne (1871–1956), pediatric and plastic surgeon, and Marcel Lance (1874–1960), a pediatric orthopedic surgeon at Hôpital des Enfants Malades (Hospital for Sick Children), Paris [109, 110], he also completed an internship with Victor Veau (1871–1949), a pediatric surgeon. Fèvre was appointed hospital surgeon in 1933, associate professor in 1939, at the pediatric surgical clinic of the Faculty of Medicine, Paris, in 1940, Hôpital St. Louis in 1942, and surgeon to the Hôpital des Enfants Malades in 1949. He was knighted Grand Officer of the Legion of Honor and was a member of the French Academy of Medicine [109, 110].

Fèvre described three signs of intussusception, which include, based on their order of appearance, painful crises, vomiting, and bloody anal discharge (Table 4.1):

The pain is intense, excruciatingly painful, and colicky. (…) There is a sense of painful pressure when examining the child during the crisis. The first colic attack begins in a previously healthy child whereby suddenly he/she begins to cry, clenches their fists, flexes their thighs, and waves their arms and legs—the abdomen contracts, preventing deep palpation. Then symptoms resolve, and the child is calm, chatters smiles, and plays. Suddenly the pain reappears with the same characters, a quarter of an hour to an hour, sometimes later after the previous crisis. The intermittency of these paroxysmal crises remains the major characteristic that should suggest intussusception. The first vomiting generally accompanies or follows the first painful attack. This vomiting may reoccur during subsequent seizures. (…) Vomiting is less frequent than painful crises: as a rule, a child with intussusception vomits what he/she consumes. However, the child often refuses the breast or any other food. Vomiting becomes less and soon disappears. Beware of this period of interruption because, when vomiting resumes, it occurs late, and is often bilious. The bloody anal discharge appears after a few hours and affirms the dreaded intussusception. These bloody emissions can assume different appearances including: traces of brownish blood staining the nappies; bloody serous fluids; bloody mucus; sometimes brownish melaena; exceptional hemorrhage of red blood; and, quite often, actual stool but colored dark brown with blood mixed in it. In short, the character that dominates these bloody emissions is their polymorphism. However, we often notice that the quantity of blood is not enormous. The smell of these stools is variable, often bland; a sickening and unpleasant odor indicates that the small intestine is involved in the intussusception [111, p. 176–177].

Thus, Fèvre sign refers to the clinical features of intussusception.

4.2.27 *Kantor Sign*

John Leonard Kantor (1890–1947) was born in Moscow, Russia, and immigrated to the United States that same year [112]. He received his medical and doctoral degrees from the College of Physicians and Surgeons Medical School of Columbia University (currently Columbia University Vagelos College of Physicians and Surgeons), New York, in 1912. Kantor completed an internship at Mt. Sinai Hospital and was a clinical assistant in gastroenterology at the Mt. Sinai Dispensary Clinic [113]. He served during World War I and II in the United States Army Medical Corps [112]. He was chief of the Vanderbilt Gastroenterology Clinic at Columbia Presbyterian Hospital from 1919 to 1932, associate professor in medicine in 1924, and associate clinical professor of medicine since 1939 at Columbia University College of Physicians and Surgeons [112]. Kantor also held appointments at Montefiore Hospital in New York City (gastroenterologist and associate roentgen-ologist), Beth David Hospital, Sharon Hospital in Connecticut, Will Roger Hospital in Saranac Lake, New York, and National Jewish Hospital [114].

Kantor described the roentgenographic appearance of the ileum in six patients with Crohn disease (Table 4.1). The most dramatic finding consisted of the following:

> [s]tring sign, a name borrowed from A.W. Crane. This is a thin, slightly irregular shadow suggesting a cotton string in appearance and extending more or less continuously from the region of the last visualized loop of ileum through the entire extent of the filling defect and extending at the ileocecal valve. It represents the attenuated barium filling of the greatly contracted intestinal lumen [115, p. 2018].

He recognized that the "string sign" may be found in other diseases, including tuberculosis, syphilis, and sarcomas involving the terminal ileum. Thus, Kantor sign refers to the thin string-like radiographic shadow due to a radiographic filling defect as occurring in regional ileitis or Chron disease.

4.2.28 *Dennis Sign*

Clarence Dennis (1909–2005) was born in St. Paul, Minnesota, USA, and received his medical degree from the Johns Hopkins School of Medicine in 1935 [116, 117]. He completed an internship and residency at the University of Minnesota and a Ph.D. degree in 1940 under the aegis of Owen Harding Wangensteen (1898–1981) [116, 118]. He was a member of the faculty of surgery at the University of Minnesota and ascended to the rank of full professor of surgery and administrative head of surgery at Minneapolis General Hospital [117, 119].

He was appointed chair in the Department of Surgery at State University of New York (SUNY) Downstate Medical Center, Brooklyn, from 1951 to 1972 and also served as a surgeon-in-chief at Kings County Hospital Center [116, 118–121]. He was appointed to direct the Division of Technological Applications, previously named the Medical Device Application Branch, at the National Heart and Lung Institute in Bethesda, Maryland, from 1972 to 1974 [121]. He joined the surgical faculty at the SUNY in Stony Brook and the Veterans Administration Hospital in Northport, NY, from 1975 to 1988 [116–118, 120]. Dennis moved to St. Paul and was later appointed director of the University of Minnesota's Cancer Detection Center from 1991 to 1996 [116, 118, 120, 121].

He is best recognized as the co-inventor of the multiple-screen blood pump oxygenator used in heart-lung machines [121]. His name is eponymously associated with Dennis clamp, used in abdominal surgery [121]. He is the recipient of several honors and awards, including the Modern Medicine Distinguished Achievement Award in 1973, the John H. Gibbon Award by the American Society Extracorporeal Technician in 1974, and the Laufman-Greatbach Prize by the Association for the Advancement of Medical Instrumentation for his pioneering work in cardiovascular surgery and devices in 1984. He also received an honorary doctorate from SUNY, Brooklyn, in 1988 [116, 117]. He was a member of the American College of Surgeons and the Nations Society for Medical Research, to name a few [116].

In a tribute to Dennis and his character, Gus Tanaka, an intern at SUNY Downstate, recalled:

> After Tanaka was diagnosed with a tuberculous pulmonary effusion, a week after being selected for the internship, rather than advising him to seek another career path, as Tanaka feared, "the kindly Dr. Dennis came to my bedside and assured me that I would not be dropped from the program", and outlined a program that would assure Tanaka a better chance of getting a decent night's rest [121, p. 802].

Dennis and Toon described auscultatory findings in patients with small bowel obstruction (Table 4.1):

> Borborygmus. Arrival of more gas and fluid with each cramp causes splashing; the pitch of the sound heard with a stethoscope rises as the bowel wall becomes more tightly stretched until the characteristic tinkle is heard. Cramps simultaneous with borborygmi at 3 to 10 minute-intervals are almost pathognomonic of small bowel obstruction [122, p. 62].

Thus, Dennis sign refers to cramps occurring with borborygmi every 3 to 10 minutes in small bowel obstruction.

4.2.29 Hunt Sign

Claude J. Hunt (1890–?) was born in Warren County, Kentucky, and received his medical degree from the School of Medicine at Kansas University [123]. He completed an internship at the Kansas City General Hospital and was a house surgeon at Wesley Hospital, Kansas City, Missouri [123]. He was a surgical assistant with W.J. Frick, a Kansas City surgeon. He completed postgraduate studies at Washington University School of Medicine, St. Louis, Harvard Medical School, Boston, and overseas at the University of Montpelier, France, and the University of Vienna, Austria [123]. He served as a lieutenant at Oswego Kansas City-based hospital in France during World War I [124].

He was Chief of the Hunt Surgical Service; chief of surgery at Research Hospital, Kansas City; surgeon at the Research Clinic, Kansas City General Hospital, Menorah Hospital, and St. Mary's Hospital; and faculty at the University of Kansas Medical School, Kansas City, Missouri [124].

He was elected president of the Jackson County Missouri State Medical Society, American Goiter Association, and Missouri State Surgical Society and was chairman of the Southern Medical Association Surgical Section [123, 125–127]. He was also an honorary member of the St. Paul Surgical Society, Philadelphia Proctological Society, and Rocky Mountain Radiological Society [123].

Hunt described the radiographic finding in intestinal obstruction and strangulation (Table 4.1):

> In simple obstruction the proximal bowel distends, coil by coil, and gradually assumes a transverse relationship to the long axis of the body, and the valvulae conniventes can be seen when the obstructed bowel assumes this characteristic stepladder pattern. (…) On the contrary, if the distended loop of bowel assumes no definite pattern, is found distended in an irregular manner and is darker than in previous type and if the valvulae conniventes are not seen or are poorly visible it may be said that the obstruction is one of a strangulated type [128, p. 463].

Thus, Hunt described the X-ray appearance of the bowel in simple obstruction and during the early stages of intestinal strangulation. In obstruction without strangulation, there are air-fluid levels, while in strangulated obstruction, the distended loop assumes no specific pattern, and the valvulae conniventes are either scarcely or not seen.

4.2.30 Kinsella Sign

Victor John Kinsella (1900–1983) was born in Sydney, New South Wales, Australia, and received his medical training at Sydney University, qualifying in 1922 [129]. He was a resident medical officer at Prince Alfred Hospital, Sydney, followed by an appointment as a medical superintendent at Lewisham Hospital, Sydney [129]. He was an assistant to Sir Hugh Berchmans Devine (1878–1959) in 1926 and completed postgraduate surgical training in 1929 at the General Hospital in Vienna under the auspices of Hans Finsterer (1877–1955) [129].

Kinsella was an honorary surgeon at Hornsby Hospital, Sydney, Australia, from 1931 to 1934, followed by an appointment with the same title at St. Vincent's Hospital. He earned a fellowship in the Royal College of Surgeons in 1930 and a medical degree from the University of Sidney in 1950 [129].

Kinsella described in his book titled *The Mechanism of Abdominal Pain* (Table 4.1):

> Morely states that if the pain arises from the jejunum it is felt above the umbilicus. But Chester Jones also Miller, Abbott and Karr, distended a small balloon at various levels of the gastro-intestinal tract and found that the pain from all parts of the small intestine was situated in the umbilical area. Occasionally it is passed through to the back. In one case only did it deviate appreciably from the midline and pass to the right iliac fossa [130, p. 188].

According to Bailey, Kinsella described an observation found in acute small bowel obstruction:

> Pain in the back, usually low in the lumbar region, occurs occasionally. Such pain is caused by tension on the mesentery occasioned by extreme increase of intraluminar pressure, the pain usually being associated with strangulated obstruction [131, p. 508].

Thus, Kinsella sign refers to lower back pain in patients with acute small bowel obstruction.

4.2.31 Patel Sign

Manubhai Dahyabhai Patel (1914–1973) was born in Nar town, Kaira district of Gujarat, India, and received his medical degree from Grant Medical College Bombay. He served at the Shree Sayaji General Hospital in Baroda, India [132].

We could not locate Manubhai Dahyabhai Patel's paper where he described the sign. Hamilton Bailey recommended that the bell of the stethoscope be firmly applied just below and to the right of the umbilicus and held in this position for up to 5 min. He reported on the auscultatory finding described by Patel (Table 4.1) (Fig. 4.1):

> [i]n paralytic ileus the clinician must expect to hear, no the hissing, turbulent, rumbling sounds associated with the colic of intestinal obstruction, but an ominous silence, not as profound as to warrant its frequent description of "death-like", but a hush, broken only the "lub, dub" of the patient's heart-beat transmitted, presumably, to the abdomen via the over-distended intestinal coils (M.D. Patel), broken also by succession splashes if the patient moves, and, in all but the last stages of paralytic ileus, broken, too by very occasional, weak tinkles [132, p. 240].

Thus, Patel sign refers to the auscultation of the heartbeat in the abdomen in patients with paralytic ileus.

4.2.32 Piulachs Sign

Pedro Piulachs Oliva (1908–1976) was born in Barcelona, Spain, and received his medical degree in Barcelona in 1931. He was awarded the Medicode Guardia Prize in 1932 [133–135]. He practiced at the medical facilities of Santiago de Compostela in 1940; Zaragoza, and Barcelona in 1943, the latter as professor of surgical pathology at the Faculty of Medicine from 1943 to 1976. He was appointed dean of the Faculty of Medicine of the Autonomous University of Barcelona [133].

Piulachs served as president of the Spanish Association of Surgeons, the Mediterranean Surgery Society, the Sarria Association of Biologists, the Catalan Society of Surgery from 1956 to 1961, and the National Association of Surgery [133]. He was a member of the Royal Academies of Barcelona and Madrid and the recipient of the Commendation of Civil Order of Alfonso X of Castile in 1966 [133, 135].

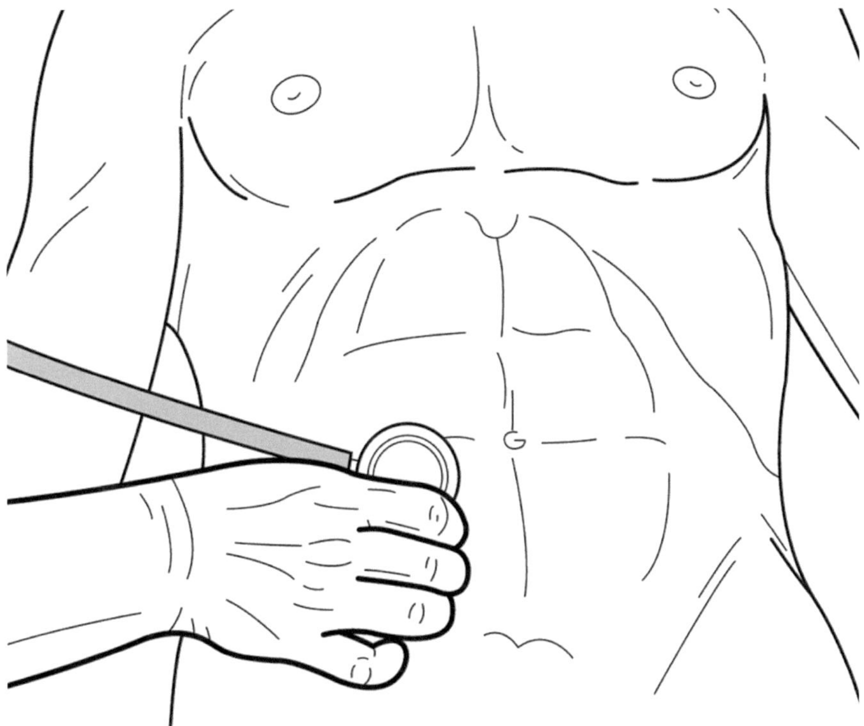

Fig. 4.1 Patel sign (by Ryan Yale)

In addition to his contributions to the sciences, Piulachs was a humanist, philosopher, and poet who wrote under the pen name Jorge Montiel [133, 134]. For the quality of his contributions, he was awarded the City of Barcelona Prize for Catalan poetry in 1970 and Virgil Prize by the Catalan Society of Surgery [133].

As to a description of his character:

> He systematized a series of surgical interventions and founded the Spanish School of Surgery. His scientific personality placed Spanish medical science on par with the most advanced countries. He always stood out for his great common sense, clarity, and exceptional work in teaching [136, p. 15]. (…) He was a humble and simple man in treatment but acquired an enormous stature on the chair's podium or in the triune of the lecturer. With a sharp, brilliant mentality and words and a tendency for irony and humor, both in private conversation and public discourse, he possessed extraordinary clarity that made it easy to understand complex concepts [135, p. 31].

A sign or test (Piulachs flank pinch) and syndrome (Piulachs–Hederich syndrome) have been eponymously named in honor of Piulachs. We were unable to locate Piulachs's paper on the flank pitch sign [137]. A description of this sign of appendicitis is found in Chap. 5—Appendicitis: Somatic and Visceral Nerve Reflexes Signs: Mechanisms and Pathophysiologic Approach in Acute and Chronic Disease.

Piulachs and Hederich described two cases in which there was acute dilation of the colon caused by dolicomegacolon (abnormal, elongated, redundant colon)—the latter is part of a visceral syndrome due to episodic hypersympathonia:

> [w]e have observed a type of dynamic occlusion which appears suddenly with enormous meteorism, without gas emission or evacuation of feces. (…) [t]ype of acute paralytic dynamic occlusion described as a complication of dolicomegacolon. We consider this complication a homolog in the colon of the dilation of the stomach that complicates the megastomach; that is why we designate it with the name of acute dilation of the colon [138, p. 1702]. In this condition, there is no evidence of mechanical occlusion or vascular injury. Patients present with intermittent diffuse abdominal pain with dilation of the colon: In acute colon dilation, meteorism is considerable; it is usually atonic without peristalsis and predominately supraumbilical. By radiological examination in volvulus, the enormous dilated loop is observed, which does not admit the opaque enema. In contrast, in acute dilation, a global colon dilation is observed [138, p. 1703].

When a probe is inserted into the colon, gas without liquid is expelled, causing deflation of the abdomen and immediate symptomatic relief. Thus Piulachs sign refers to acute colon dilation occurring in patients with a congenital deformity marked by being elongated and redundant (dolicomegacolon). This finding presumably represents the condition referred to as acute intestinal pseudo-obstruction.

Table 4.1 Small and large bowel signs

Name	Year	Description of sign	Significance
Dance [7]	1826	The cecum and the colon are displaced to the left side of the abdomen and are now located at the sigmoid flexure. The absence of the ascending colon and cecum causes a depression on the right side of the abdomen. A longitudinal enlarged voluminous mass is present on the left side of the abdomen	Intussusception
Cruveilhier [12]	1849	There are two characteristic signs of strangulation caused by intussusception: swelling and hematochezia	Intussusception
Blatin [14]	1877	The abdomen is distended without fluctuation. Percussion caused the abdomen to move and tremble, similar to a gelatinous mass	Intestinal obstruction
Cherchevsky [16]	1883	The episodes occurred unexpectedly. From disease onset, the volume or stool's diameter was noticeably smaller. Usually, the stool frequency increases four or five days before the spell. Instead of just one a day, there were two or even three bowel movements, with the feces usually molded into the shape of a sausage. The feces thinned out even more and eventually broke off into distinct, rounded pieces ranging from the size of a walnut to that of a hazelnut—this form degenerated into ribbons somewhat thicker toward the middle and flattened toward the edges. Later the evacuations were only the thickness of a pencil, after which they became quite liquid and were expelled in the form of a very thin jet. Simultaneously with this final form, there was a painful sensation under the costal margins and the pains described above, signifying the beginning of the attack. These gradually changes in the form and consistency of the stools preceded the severe crises. Simultaneously with the onset of pain under the false ribs, the patient's face becomes pale and slightly cyanotic, breathing accelerated to 26-28 bpm; the transverse diameter of the heart slightly exceeds the left parasternal line; the heartbeat slowed with the pulse decreasing from 70 to 60. The upper part of the abdomen is distended. Percussion makes a sonorous and tympanic noise heard with a metallic undertone. At the onset of the attack, the bloating, in most cases, is circumscribed, sometimes occurring in the epigastrium, while at other times, at the right or left colon flexures	Irritable bowel syndrome (mixed variant)
Wahl [23]	1886	The darker color, increased gaseous dilation, and congestion of the portion of the intestine above the obstruction lead to the point of constriction	Strangulating bowel obstruction

(continued)

Table 4.1 (continued)

Name	Year	Description of sign	Significance
Hirschsprung [28]	1888	Dilation and thickening of the walls, especially the muscularis, of the large intestines with a normal-appearing rectum. The mucosa in dilated segments has considerable erosions and ulcerations, which vary significantly in size and depth. The finger could easily be inserted into the rectum which was often full of feces on exploration	Dilation and hypertrophy of the distal colon
Gangolphe [34]	1893	Constriction of the intestinal loop results in a sero-bloody liquid in the peritoneal cavity and intestines. The quantity of fluid is proportional to the extent of the trapped intestinal loop and the intensity of the constriction	Strangulated bowel obstruction
Schlange [37]	1894	With intestinal obstruction, the efferent portion of the intestine is always empty and collapses, while the afferent portion is dilated. In the absence of peritonitis, peristaltic movements occur in the dilated intestine. The movements are strongest where obstruction develops slowly (e.g., a slowly growing mass with strictures) because here, the muscularis of the proximal intestine has time to hypertrophy	Intestinal obstruction
Mya [43]	1894	On inspection, two furrows are observed from top to bottom and from right to left. One is located 1 cm below the umbilicus in the midline, the other 6 cm above it. These two sulci circumscribe an enormous intestinal loop. Above the superior sulcus, there is a second tubular protrusion directed transversally. The median loop measured between the two grooves is 11 cm. The upper loop measures 6 cm	Dilation and hypertrophy of the distal colon
Gersuny [47]	1896	The intestinal mucosa adheres to the viscous collection of feces, forming a mass when the finger is pressed intensively and detaches itself again when the pressure is released	Dilation and hypertrophy of the distal colon
Bayer [50]	1898	The patient's abdomen shifts to the left in the upper and right in the lower half, forming an S-shaped bead. An oblique bulge runs diagonally from the top left to the bottom right, bending to the left again in the right hypogastrium and extending to the bottom right in the cecal region. It is stretched to the point of bursting and was hemispherically round, "like a bent knee." The saddle-shaped indentation was found on the left at the border between the epigastrium and hypogastrium. The largest protrusion usually occurs with pronounced colon meteorism, which conforms to the same protrusion in the opposite abdominal region	Sigmoid volvulus

Bouveret [55]	1899	Observe the patient's abdomen as he/she complains of colic. A strong, globular swelling lifts the abdominal wall in the right iliac fossa, epigastrium, and umbilicus. In contrast, the hypochondrium and left iliac fossa remain soft and depressible and maintain their normal configuration. During the painful crisis, an oblique line may be found extending from the middle of the right femoral arch to the left costal margin, dividing the abdomen into two parts: the right colon, with strong peristaltic contractions, and the left colon, without these strong peristaltic contractions. Later, if the obstruction is complete, it may also involve the small intestine. At that time, the sign no longer has the same value. However, generalized abdominal peristalsis starts and sometimes remains localized to the right side	Transverse colon obstruction
Anschütz[a] [60]	1902	Local gaseous dilation is observed in patients with cecal obstruction and a closed ileocecal valve	Colon obstruction
Nothnagel [66]	1905	(1) Ileal succession splash: In intestinal stenosis, there is frequently a feeling of fluctuation on palpation, and occasionally a distinct succussion sounds heard proximal to the stenosis (2) Early in distal colonic obstruction, only the large intestine is distended, with dilation present at the flanks: In stenosis of the sigmoid flexure complicated by gaseous dilation from stasis, the upper and lateral aspects of the abdomen are usually distended. The distension of the lateral aspect of the abdomen is generally called flank meteorism. Flank gaseous distension may be unilateral when the bowel distension is limited to certain colon sections. This may occur even when stenosis is in the sigmoid flexure, for only a short segment of the bowel above the stricture may be distended (3) Percussion sound is located over the same site as the ileus: In cases of bowel stenosis, no definite and reliable information is gained by percussion. There is only one point of diagnostic importance: when local gaseous distension is limited to a circumscribed area of the bowel, which can be identified by percussion. Whenever this condition is found, efforts should be directed toward identifying other signs of bowel constriction in this area. Localized tympanites is of value only in the diagnosis of narrowing of the bowel when combined with other symptoms	Bowel obstruction
Lane [74]	1910	A new band forms beneath the last few inches of the mesentery of the small intestines. This band is initially part of the undersurface of the mesentery. Later it forms a ligament distinct from the mesentery. The ligament contracts and deforms the ileum, producing a kink or obstruction, particularly in the erect posture. Because of this kink, the small intestines dilate, potentially extending up to the pylorus	Small bowel obstruction

(continued)

Table 4.1 (continued)

Name	Year	Description of sign	Significance
Stierlin [77]	1911	An infiltrative, indurated, and ulcerative processes of the cecum and ascending colon radiographically identified after 5 to 6 hours by the absence of a physiological shadow in this colon section. Cecal tuberculosis is, therefore, the absence of the cecum and ascending colon shadows between the lower ileum and transverse colon. Radiographically, ulcerations and infiltrates are seen in the remainder of the colon by a gap corresponding to the diseased section	Cecal tuberculosis
Cole [82]	1914	A deformity of the cap or sphincter is present and caused by the surrounding induration and cicatricial contraction of an ulcer crater. The induration within an ulcer projects into the cap's lumen, causing a displacement of contrast. It may be so small as to present only a constant dent on the side of the cap, or it may be extensive as to distort the lumen of the cap. Alternatively, the process may involve one-half of the cap without distorting the other half	Duodenal ulcers
Mathieu [86]	1914	(1) Intestinal fluid and stasis accumulate proximal to an area of stenosis are demonstrated by extensive clapotage (splashing sound) and percussion dullness (2) Method for distinguishing fluid within the stomach from the intestines: It may be difficult to distinguish intestinal obstruction from gastric dilatation due to pyloric stenosis. The stomach is dull, only in the left decubitus position. In contrast, in the right lateral decubitus position, dullness caused by fluid within the stomach follows a convex line at the bottom, stopping slightly below the umbilicus. Intestinal sounds are present below this area	Intestinal obstruction
Butters [87]	1915	Subtle, shiftable palpable resistance under the right costal arch in the parasternal line and occult blood suggests right (hepatic) flexural carcinoma	Colon cancer at the right flexure
Kloiber [90]	1919	Gas and liquid are found on a standing fluoroscopy or X-ray separated by a horizontal line. The number of air-fluid levels varies depending on the location of the disease and the duration of the incarceration. Several air-fluid levels near the stomach suggest a more proximal obstruction, while numerous fluid levels in the pelvis indicate more distal small bowel obstruction	Small bowel obstruction
Hedri [91]	1920	Excision of an epiploic appendage at its base causes arterial bleeding	Colon viability
Gold [95]	1924	Palpation of the small intestines during the rectal examination requires an increase and abnormal composition of the intestinal contents that liquefy and accumulate, proximal to the small bowel obstruction, leading to widening of the intestinal loops and early hypertrophy of the muscular intestinal wall, and an abnormal loop of the prestenotic portion of the small bowel	Small bowel obstruction

Fleischner [100]	1928	The opening of the ileocecal valve is patent. Rotate the patient or apply pressure to bring the area into view in order to avoid an overlying cecal shadow	Insufficiency of the ileocecal valve
Hintze [103]	1928	Small intestinal loops show the typical Kerckring folds (valvular conniventes) and large intestinal loops shows haustral marking	Bowel obstruction
Burgess [108]	1929	Obstruction present for at least several weeks is signified by observing an outline of dilated coils of the intestines seen with the peristaltic wave. Sometimes, even when peristalsis was not visible, it was palpable. By keeping the hand over the abdomen, the coil underneath could be felt alternately, hardening and softening	Intestinal obstruction
Fèvre [111]	1930	The pain is intense, excruciatingly, and colicky. One senses that the child is experiencing painful pressure on examination during the crisis. The first colic attack begins suddenly. The child cries, clenches his hands and thighs and waves his arms and legs—the abdomen contracts, preventing deep palpation. Then symptoms resolve, and the child is now calm, chatters, smiles, and plays. Suddenly the pain reappears a quarter of an hour, an hour, sometimes later after the previous crisis with the same character. The intermittency of these paroxysmal crises is the primary characteristic suggesting intussusception. Initial vomiting generally accompanies or follows the first painful attack. This vomiting may reoccur during subsequent episodes. Vomiting is less frequent than painful crises: as a rule, a child with intussusception vomits what he/she eats. However, the child often refuses to eat. Vomiting occurs less frequently and then resolves. Beware of this period of interruption because, when vomiting resumes, it occurs later and is often bilious. The bloody emission from the anus appears after a few hours and affirms intussusception. These bloody emissions contain traces of brownish blood staining the nappies, bloody serous fluids, bloody mucus, sometimes brownish melaena, hemorrhage of red blood, and, quite often, actual stool, but colored brown, dark with blood mixed with it. In short, the character that dominates these bloody emissions is their different forms. However, often the quantity of blood is not enormous. The smell of these stools is variable, often bland; sickening and unpleasant odors indicate the small intestine's participation in the intussusception	Intussusception
Kantor [115]	1934	The "string sign" is a thin, slightly irregular shadow extending continuously from the region of the last visualized loop of ileum through the entire extent of the filling defect to the ileocecal valve	Ileal stenosis

(continued)

Table 4.1 (continued)

Name	Year	Description of sign	Significance
Dennis [122]	1946	The arrival of more gas and fluid with each cramp causes splashing. The pitch of the sound auscultated with a stethoscope rises as the bowel wall becomes more tightly stretched until the characteristic tinkle is heard. Cramps occur simultaneously with borborygmi at 3- to 10-min intervals	Small bowel obstruction
Hunt [128]	1948	In simple obstruction the proximal bowel distends, coil by coil, and gradually assumes a transverse relationship to the long axis of the body. The valvulae conniventes can be seen. The obstructed bowel assumes this characteristic stepladder pattern. In strangulated type of obstruction the distended loop of bowl assumes no definite pattern, is found distended in an irregular manner, is darker than in previously, and if the valvulae conniventes are not seen or are poorly visible	Intestinal obstruction and strangulation
Kinsella [130]	1948	Pain from all parts of the small intestine is usually situated in the umbilical area, and occasionally referred to the back in the lower lumbar region	Small bowel obstruction
Patel [132]	1973	The bell of the stethoscope is firmly applied just below and to the right of the umbilicus and held in this position for up to 5 min. In paralytic ileus, the abdomen is silent. Only the "lub, dub" of the patient's heartbeat transmitted, presumably, to the abdomen via the overdistended intestinal coils broken by succession splashes if the patient moves	Paralytic ileus
Piulachs [138]	[n.a.]	Acute paralytic dynamic occlusion appears suddenly with enormous meteorism, without gas emission or evacuation of feces as a complication of dolicomegacolon. Patients present with intermittent diffuse abdominal pain with dilation of the colon. In acute dilation of the colon, meteorism is considerable; it is usually atonic without peristalsis and predominately located supraumbilical	Acute colon dilation

[a] Denotes an individual who supported anti-semitism, racial acts, or committed crimes against humanity

4.3 Conclusion

Signs of the small and large intestines were identified through observation, palpation, and auscultation. Many of these signs are unknown and not recognized by those whose discovery was first published. They provide the reader with a more in-depth appreciation of the physical examination skills employed by these physicians as a method of diagnosis.

References

1. Skinner HA. The origin of medical terms. Baltimore: The Williams & Wilkins; 1949.
2. Celsus AC. The fourth book of Aurelius Cornelius Celsus. In: Lee A, editor. On medicine: chapter 1 – of the internal parts of the human body. London: E. Cox; 1831. p. 239–45.
3. Gurlt E, Hirsch A. Dance, Jean-Baptiste-Hippolyte. In: Biographisches Lexikon der hervorragenden Ärzte aller Zeiten und Völker, vol. 6. Wien: Urban & Schwarzenberg; 1888. p. 670.
4. [No Author]. Jean-Baptiste Hippolyte Dance (1797–1832). Progrès Méd. 1936;13:17–9.
5. Dechambre A. Dance, Jean-Baptiste-Hippolyte. In: Dictionnaire Encyclopédique des Sciences Médicales, tome 25. Paris: G. Masson; 1880. p. 385–6.
6. Delmas V. Dance, Jean Baptiste Hippolyte. Comité des travaux historiques et scientifiques. 2011. http://cths.fr/an/savant.php?id=105491. Accessed 20 Nov 2022.
7. Dance JBH. Mémoire sur les invaginations morbides des intestins. In: Répertoire Général d'Anatomie et de Physiologie Pathologiques, et de Clinique Chirurgicale, vol. 1. Paris: Chez Boiste; 1826. p. 195–214.
8. Vayre P. Jean Cruveilhier (1791–1874), chirurgien promoteur de la preuve par les faits à la médecine fondée sur la preuve. E-mémoires l'Acad Natl Chirurg. 2008;7:1–12. https://e-memoire.academie-chirurgie.fr/ememoires/005_2008_7_2_001x012.pdf. Accessed 12 Nov 2022.
9. Després A. Nécrologie: Cruveilhier. In: La Revue Scientifique de la France et de l'Étranger, vol. 2. Paris: Germer Baillière; 1872. p. 908.
10. Cruveilhier, Jean (1791–1874). Correspondance familiale. 2013. http://correspondancefamiliale.ehess.fr/index.php?4489. Accessed 12 Nov 2022.
11. [No Author]. Jean Cruveilhier (1791–1874), pathological anatomist. JAMA. 1966;195:683–4.
12. Cruveilhier J. Quatrième classe: des déplacements par invagination. In: Traité d'Anatomie Pathologique Générale, vol. 1. Paris: J.-B. Baillière; 1849. p. 513–88.
13. Blatin H, Nivet V. Tratado de las Enfermedades de las Mujeres. Cadiz: Sociedad de la Revista Médica; 1845.
14. Blatin H. Masse d'hydatides (?) rendues par l'anus, frémissement hydatique. In: Davaine C, editor. Traité des Entozoaires et des Maladies Vermineuses de l'Homme et des Animaux Domestiques. Paris: J.-B. Baillière et fils; 1877. p. 524–5.
15. Rolleston HD. Hydatid cysts. In: Diseases of the liver, gall-bladder and bile ducts. London: MacMillan and Co.; 1912. p. 391–425.
16. Cherchevsky M. Contributions à la pathologie des névroses intestinales. Rev Méd. 1883;3:876–900.
17. Cherchevsky M. Sur un nouveau signe de sclérose de la crosse de l'aorte. Sem Méd. 1898;18:409–10.
18. Ottow R. Von Wahl, Eduard Georg. In: Album Dorpato-Livonorum. Dorpat: Druck von H. Laakmanns Buch-und Steindruckerei; 1908. p. 160.
19. Kröger C. Von Wahl, Eduard Georg. In: Birkenruher-Album, 1825–1892. St. Petersburg: Buch- und Steindruckerei; 1910. p. 261–2.

20. Hasselblatt Arnold, Otto Gustav. Album academicum der Kaiserlichen Universität Dorpat. Münchener Digitalisierungszentrum. https://daten.digitale-sammlungen.de/~db/bsb00000433/images/index.html?id=00000433&fip=eayayztsewqeayaxssdasyztsqrseayaxs&no=165&seite=433. Accessed 18 Nov 2022.

21. Pagel J. Wahl, Eduard von. In: Biographisches Lexikon, hervorragender Ärzte des neunzehnten Jahrhunderts. Berlin: Urban und Schwarzenberg; 1901. p. 1802–3.

22. Edward Georg von Wahl. Austria forum. https://austria-forum.org/af/AustriaWiki/Eduard_Georg_von_Wahl. Accessed 17 Nov 2022.

23. Wahl E. Zur Casuistik der Laparotomien und Enterostomien bei Darmocclusion. St Pet med Wochenschr. 1886;11:183–4.

24. Rovsing T. Harald Hirschsprung: født 14. December 1830, død 11. April 1916. Hospitalstidende. 1916;59:389–92.

25. Borgbjærg A. Harald Hirschsprung. Dansk Biografisk Leksikon. 2011. https://biografiskleksikon.lex.dk/Harald_Hirschsprung. Accessed 20 Nov 2022.

26. Monrad S. Professor Harald Hirschsprung. Ugeskr Laeger. 1916;78:606–8.

27. Hirschsprung H. Fälle von Darminvagination bei Kindern, behandelt im Königin Louisen Kinderhospital in Kopenhagen während der Jahre 1871–1904. Mitt Grenzgeb Med Chir. 1905;14:555–74.

28. Hirschsprung H. Stuhlträgheit Neugeborener in Folge von dilatation und hypertrophie des colons. Jahrb Kinderh. 1888;27:1–7.

29. [No Author]. Michel Gangolphe (1858–1919). Lyon Méd. 1919;128:477–85.

30. Molin H. Discours prononcé aux funérailles de Michel Gangolphe. Lyon Méd. 1919;129:577–81.

31. Molin H. Michel Gangolphe, 1858–1919. Lyon Chir. 1920;17:1–12.

32. [No Author]. Le Dr. Michel Gangolphe. In: Polybiblion. Paris: Bureaux du Polybiblion; 1919. p. 304.

33. Nové-Josserand G. Mort du docteur Gangolphe. Lyon Méd. 1919;128:612–3.

34. Gangolphe M. Nouveau signe de l'occlusion intestinale par étranglement. Rev Chir. 1893;13:403–4.

35. Schlange, Friedrich Ernst Hans. Biographisches Lexikon hervorragender Ärzte. http://www.zeno.org/Pagel-1901/A/Schlange,+Friedrich+Ernst+Hans. Accessed 10 Oct 2022.

36. [No Author]. Tagung der Deutschen Gesellschaft für Chirurgie. Arch klin Chir. 1923;1:49.

37. Schlange H. Über den Ileus. Samm klin Vortr. 1894;35:63–86.

38. [No Author]. Professor Giuseppe Mya. Br Med J. 1911;1:471–2.

39. [No Author]. La morte del Prof. Giuseppe Mya. Rass Clin Ter. 1911;10:56–8.

40. Picchi L. Il Presidente pronuncia il seguente discorso in commemorazione del prof. Giuseppe Mya. Sperimentale. 1911;65:93–100.

41. Belfani S. Commemorazione del Socio fondatore prof. Giuseppe Mya. Biochim Terapia Sperimentale. 1911;3:47–8.

42. Collective. Dizionario Biografico degli Italiani, vol. 77. Roma: Istituto dell'Enciclopedia Italiana; 2012.

43. Mya G. Due osservazioni di dilatazione ed ipertrofia congenita del colon (megacolon congenito). Sperimentale. 1894;48:215–20.

44. Robert Gersuny. Wien Geschichte Wiki. 2021. https://www.geschichtewiki.wien.gv.at/Robert_Gersuny. Accessed 18 Nov 2022.

45. Collective. Gersuny, Robert (1844–1924). In: Österreichisches Biographisches Lexikon, 1815–1950, vol. 1. Wien: Verlag der Österreichischen Akademie der Wissenschaften; 1957. p. 431.

46. Sturm H. Biographisches Lexikon zur Geschichte der böhmischen Länder, vol. 1. München: Oldenbourg Verlag; 1979.

47. Gersuny R. Ueber ein Symptom bei Kothtumoren. Wien klin Wochenschr. 1896;9:889–92.

48. Carl Bayer. Literarische Landkarte der deutschmährischen Autoren. https://limam.upol.cz/Authors/Detail/110. Accessed 18 Nov 2022.

49. Kreuter A. Bayer, Carl. In: Deutschsprachige Neurologen und Psychiater: ein biographisch-bibliographisches Lexikon von den Vorläufern bis zur Mitte des 20. Jahrhunderts, vol. 1. München: K.G. Saur; 2013. p. 78.

50. Bayer C. Characteristischer Meteorismus bei Volvulus des S romanum. Arch klin Chir. 1898;57:233–42.

51. Pallasse E. Lettre de Lyon: Léon Bouveret – César Tournier. Le Progrès Méd. 1929;18:787–90.

52. Français H. Nécrologie: Léon Bouveret (1850–1929). Paris Méd. 1929;72:313.

53. François M. Bouveret, Léon. Comité des travaux historiques et scientifiques. 2020. https://cths.fr/an/savant.php?id=111465. Accessed 18 Nov 2022.

54. Léon Bouveret, 1850–1929. Portraits de Médecins. https://www.medarus.org/Medecins/MedecinsTextes/bouveret_leon.htm. Accessed 20 Nov 2022.

55. Bouveret L. La symphyse gastro-colique. Rev Méd. 1899;19:323–36.

56. Vierhaus R. Anschütz, Willy. In: Deutsche Biographische Enzyklopädie, vol. 1. München: K.G. Saur; 2005. p. 184.

57. Alfred Wilhelm Anschütz. Kiel Directory of Scholars. https://cau.gelehrtenverzeichnis.de/person/7f8006b2-ccad-69ce-5dfc-4d4c607e7a6d?lang=en. Accessed 4 Nov 2022.

58. Alfred Wilhelm Anschütz (1870–1954). Ehrenbürger innen von Kiel. https://www.kiel.de/de/kiel_zukunft/stadtgeschichte/_ehrenbuerger/alfred_wilhelm_anschuetz.php. Accessed 4 Nov 2022.

59. Anschütz, Willy. Deutsche Gesellschaft für Chirurgie. https://www.dgch.de/index.php?id=86&L=0PD. Accessed 4 Nov 2022.

60. Anschütz W. Ueber den Verlauf des Ileus bei Darmcarcinom und dem localen Meteorismus des Cöcum bei tiefsitzendem Dickdarmverschluss. Arch klin Chir. 1902;68:195–221.

61. [No Author]. Obituary: Hermann Nothnagel, MD. Br Med J. 1905;2:215.

62. [No Author]. Hermann Nothnagel (1841–1905). Nature. 1941;148:388.

63. Leyden EV. Hermann Nothnagel. Ztschr klin Med. 1905;57:1–7.

64. Mannaberg J. Hermann Nothnagel. Münch med Wochenschr. 1905;52:1687–9.

65. Wechsberg F. Hermann Nothnagel. Wien klin Rundschau. 1905;19:505–8.

66. Nothnagel H. Nothnagel's encyclopedia of practical medicine, vol. 11: diseases of the intestines and peritoneum. Rolleston HD, editor. (trans: A. Stengel). Philadelphia: W.B. Saunders & Company; 1905.

67. Lane, Sir William Arbuthnot (1856–1943). Plarr's Lives of the Fellows. Royal College of Surgeons of England. https://livesonline.rcseng.ac.uk/client/en_GB/lives/search/detailnonmodal/ent:$002f$002fSD_ASSET$002f0$002fSD_ASSET:376515/one?qu=%22rcs%3A+E004 332%22&rt=false%7C%7C%7CIDENTIFIER%7C%7C%7CResource+Identifier. Accessed 7 Nov 2022.

68. Jones AR. Sir William Arbuthnot Lane. J Bone Jt Surg. 1952;34:478–82.

69. [No Author]. Obituary: Sir W. Arbuthnot Lane, Bt, CB, FRCS, consulting surgeon, Guy's Hospital. Br Med J. 1943;1:115–6.

70. [No Author]. Classic articles in colonic and rectal surgery: Sir William Arbuthnot Lane, 1856–1943. Dis Colon Rectum. 1985;28:750–7.

71. [No Author]. Sir William Arbuthnot Lane, Bart, CB MS, FRCS. Postgrad Med J. 1943;19:29.

72. [No Author]. Sir W. Arbuthnot Lane's resignation from the British Medical Association. Can J Med Surg. 1925;58:177–8.

73. [No Author]. Society reports: report of special clinic at the New York Polyclinic Hospital. Am Pract. 1913;47:654–60.

74. Lane WA. Chronic intestinal stasis. Surg Gynecol Obstet. 1910;11:495–500.

75. Sauerbruch F. Eduard Stierlin. Münch med Wochenschr. 1919;66:1445.

76. Lüdin M. Prof. Dr. med. Eduard Stierlin. Schweiz med Wochenschr. 1920;50:115.

77. Stierlin E. Die Radiographie in der Diagnostik der Ileocoecal: Tuberkulose und andere Krankheiten des Dickdarms. Münch med Wochenschr. 1911;58:1231–5.

78. Andresen AF. Lewis Gregory Cole, 1874–1954. Gastroenterology. 1955;28:867–71.

79. Orndoff BH. Lewis Gregory Cole, MD, 1874–1954. Radiology. 1955;64:597–9.

80. Linton O. Lewis Gregory Cole. J Am Coll Radiol. 2007;4:195–6.
81. [No Author]. Announcement and book reviews: Lewis Gregory Cole, MD – Friedenwald medalist. Radiology. 1946;46:81.
82. Cole LG. The diagnosis of post-pyloric (duodenal) ulcer by means of serial radiography. Lancet. 1914;183:1239–44.
83. Lereboullet P. Nécrologie: Albert Mathieu. Paris Méd. 1917;25–26:273–4.
84. Bougier L. Albert Mathieu. In: Hygiène Scolaire. Paris: Masson et Cie; 1916. p. 145–58.
85. Ségal A. Le docteur Albert Mathieu, les Maladies de l'Appareil Digestif et de la Nutrition et le monde médical de son temps. Hegel. 2011;4:21–7.
86. Mathieu A. Note sur la valeur séméiologique du clapotage abdominal et de la fausse ascite pour le diagnostic de l'occlusion intestinale. Arch Mal Appar Dig. 1914;8:301–6.
87. Voit W. Demonstration eines resezierten (Dr. Butters) Carcinoma flexurae coli dext. Münch Med Wochenschr. 1915;62:1119.
88. Kütterer G, Kloiber H. In: Lebensdaten verdienter Persönlichkeiten in den ersten Jahrzehnten der Röntgenologie. Norderstedt: Books on Demand GmbH; 2015. p. 299.
89. Weber B. Nachruf: Hans Kloiber. Fortschr Geb Rontgenstr. 1951;74:105.
90. Kloiber H. Die Röntgendiagnose des Ileus ohne Kontrastmittel (Mit Demonstration von Röntgenbildern). Münch med Wochenschr. 1919;66:1065–6.
91. Hedri A. Ein sicheres Zeichen für die Lebensfähigkeit des Dickdarmes. Zentralbl Chir. 1920;47:352–3.
92. Blumesberger S, Doppelhofer M, Mauthie G. Gold, Ernest. In: Handbuch österreichischer Autorinnen und Autoren jüdischer Herkunft 18. bis 20. Jahrhundert, vol. 1. München: K.G. Saur; 2002. p. 429.
93. Ernst Gold. Gedenkbuch für die Opfer des Nationalsozialismus an der Universität Wien 1938. Universität Wien. https://gedenkbuch.univie.ac.at/page/1/person/ernst-gold. Accessed 5 Nov 2022.
94. Ernst Gold (1891–1967): Vertrieben 1938. Van Swieten Blog. Universitätsbibliothek Medizinische Universität Wien. https://ub.meduniwien.ac.at/blog/?p=1184. Accessed 5 Nov 2022.
95. Gold E. Über ein differentialdiagnostisch verwertbares Zeichen bei Ileus. Mitt Grenzgeb Inn Med Chir. 1924;38:78–101.
96. Fleischner, Felix. Social Networks and Archival Context. https://snaccooperative.org/ark:/99166/w6sc1kr1. Accessed 19 Nov 2022.
97. Maizlin ZV, Cooperberg PL, Clement JJ, Vos PM, Coblentz CL. People behind exclusive eponyms of radiologic signs: part I. Can Assoc Radiol J. 2009;60:201–12.
98. Koren N. Fleischner, Felix George. In: Jewish Physicians: a Biographical Index. Jerusalem: Israel Universities Press; 1973. p. 174.
99. [No Author]. Announcements and books received. Radiology. 1970;97:694.
100. Fleischner F. Die Darmtuberkulose im Röntgenbild. In: Holfelder H, Holthusen H, Jungling O, Martius H, editors. Ergebnisse der medizinischen Strahlenforschung, vol. 3. Leipzig: Verlag von Georg Thieme; 1928. p. 359–423.
101. Eckart WU. Prof. Arthur Hintze (1881–1946). In: 100 Jahre organisierte Krebsforschung. Stuttgart: Georg Thieme Verlag; 2000. p. 52.
102. Fischer W, Hierholzer K, Hubenstorf M, Walther PT, Winau R. Exodus von Wissenschaften aus Berlin: Fragestellungen, Ergebnisse, Desiderate – Entwicklungen vor und nach 1933. Berlin: Walter de Gruyter; 1994.
103. Hintze A. Allgemeine topische und Ursachendiagnosen des Ileus durch die Röntgenuntersuchung. Med Klin. 1928;40:1547–8.
104. [No Author]. Arthur Henry Burgess (1874–1948). Br J Surg. 1948;36:104–5.
105. Arthur Burgess. Medical manuscripts collection. Archives hub. https://archiveshub.jisc.ac.uk/search/archives/3d4fc2b0-f608-3873-8169-4182500c73d5?component=6344feb6-b5c1-3938-95fa-d096b7f739b4. Accessed 12 Oct 2022.
106. Burgess, Arthur Henry (1874–1948). Plarr's lives of the fellows. Royal College of Surgeons of England. https://livesonline.rcseng.ac.uk/client/en_GB/lives/search/detailnonmodal/ent:$002f$002fSD_ASSET$002f0$002fSD_ASSET:376102/one?qu=LIVES_OCCUPATIO

N%3D%22Urological+surgeon%22&qf=LIVES_HONOURS%09Titles%2FQualifications %09FACS+1931%09FACS+1931. Accessed 20 Nov 2022.

107. [No Author]. Prof. A.H. Burgess, MSc, FRCS, LLD. Br Med J. 1948;1:1007.

108. Burgess AH. Acute intestinal obstruction. CMAJ. 1929;20:556.

109. Jacotot H, Léger L, Hennet S. Fèvre, Marcel Paul Louis Edmond. Comité des travaux historiques et scientifique. 5 Apr 2020. https://cths.fr/an/savant.php?id=3566. Accessed 20 Nov 2022.

110. Léger L. Éloge de Marcel Fèvre (1897–1978). Bull Acad Nat Méd. 1978;162:359–65.

111. Fèvre M. Signes, diagnostic précoce, indication du traitement dans l'invagination intestinale aiguë du nourrisson. Sem Hôp Paris. 1930;6:176–80.

112. Adler C, Szold H. Kantor, John Leonard. In: American Jewish year book, vol. 50. Philadelphia: Jewish Publication Society of America; 1949. p. 518.

113. [No Author]. John Leonard Kantor. In: Columbia University in the City of New York: Catalogue of Officers and Graduates, vol. 16. New York: Columbia University; 1916. p. 1908.

114. Mackin J. Kantor, John Leonard (1890–1947). In: Notable New Yorkers of Manhattan's Upper West Side: Bloomingdale-Morningside heights. New York: Fordham University Press; 2020. p. 41.

115. Kantor JL. Regional (terminal) ileitis: its roentgen diagnosis. JAMA. 1934;103:2016–21.

116. Clarence Dennis. The Clarence Dennis Papers. National Library of Medicine: Profiles in Science. https://profiles.nlm.nih.gov/spotlight/bx. Accessed 20 Nov 2022.

117. Blood O. Dr. Clarence Dennis and the development of a heart-lung machine for open heart operations. Downstate Health Sciences University. https://www.downstate.edu/about/our-history/_documents/exhibits/denis.pdf. Accessed 20 Nov 2022.

118. Clarence Dennis, 96. The Washington Post. 17 July 2005. https://www.washingtonpost.com/ archive/local/2005/07/17/clarence-dennis-96/eba05d36-3606-4f1e-8a3e-ff1bf04439c3/. Accessed 20 Nov 2022.

119. Altman LK. Clarence Dennis, builder of machine crucial to heart surgery, dies at 96. The New York Times. 20 July 2005. https://www.nytimes.com/2005/07/20/obituaries/clarence-dennis-builder-of-machine-crucial-to-heart-surgery-dies.html. Accessed 20 Nov 2022.

120. Nelson VJ. Clarence Dennis, 96; physician was pioneer in open-heart surgery. Los Angeles Times. 19 July 2005. https://www.latimes.com/archives/la-xpm-2005-jul-19-me-dennis19-story.html. Accessed 20 Nov 2022.

121. Oransky I. Obituary: Clarence Dennis. Lancet. 2005;366:802.

122. Dennis C, Toon R. Small bowel obstruction. Bull Univ Minn Hosp. 1946;18:62–72.

123. [No Author]. Claude J. Hunt, MD. J Fla Med Assoc. 1955;41:745.

124. [No Author]. War work: Hunt, Claude J. The war record of the University of Kansas, vol. 19. Lawrence: Department of Journalism Press; 1918. p. 26.

125. [No Author]. Dr. Claude J. Hunt, President. J Missouri Med Assoc. 1925;22:199.

126. [No Author]. Missouri: Claude J. Hunt. South Med J. 1958;51:1075.

127. [No Author]. American Goiter Association: President, Claude J. Hunt. In: McDonough's Illinois Medical Directory. Chicago: McDonough & Company; 1952. p. 43.

128. Hunt CJ. Early diagnosis and Roentgen manifestations of obstruction of small bowel. Arch Surg. 1948;57:460–9.

129. Kinsella, Victor John (1900–1983). Plarr's Lives of the Fellows. Royal College of Surgeons of England. https://livesonline.rcseng.ac.uk/client/en_GB/lives/search/detailnonmodal/ ent:$002f$002fSD_ASSET$002f0$002fSD_ASSET:379575/one?qu=%22rcs%3A+E00739 2%22&rt=false%7C%7C%7CIDENTIFIER%7C%7C%7CResource+Identifier. Accessed 4 Nov 2022.

130. Kinsella VJ. The mechanism of abdominal pain. Sydney: Australasian Medical Publishing; 1948.

131. Bailey H. Demonstration of physical signs in clinical surgery. 13th ed. Bristol: John Wright & Sons; 1960.

132. [No Author]. Dr. M.D. Patel. J Indian Med Assoc. 1973;61:240.

133. Tenia 67 años: ha muerto el doctor Piulachs. Diario de Barcelona. 26 March 1976. https:// www.galeriametges.cat/Upload/Documents/9/98.pdf. Accessed 21 Nov 2022.

134. [No Author]. Ha fallecido el catedratico Don Pedro Piulach Oliva. La Vanguardia, 26 March 1976. p. 23.
135. Marfa FVB. Obito de Pedro Piulachs Oliva: Día de luto para la medicina mundial. El Correo Catalán, 26 March 1976. p. 31.
136. Sarró M. Recuerdo entrañable del professor Piulachs. La Vanguardia, 17 Sep 1989. p. 15.
137. Llibre Commemoratiu I Volum – 150è Aniversari. Acadèmia de Ciències Mèdiques i de la Salut de Catalunya i de Balears. https://institucional.academia.cat/docs/llibres-historia/llibre_150_aniversari.pdf. Accessed 5 Nov 2022.
138. Piulachs P, Hederich H. La dilatación a aguda del colon, complicación del dolicomegacolon. Día Méd. 1949;21:1702–5.

Chapter 5
Appendicitis: Somatic and Visceral Nerve Reflexes Signs: Mechanisms and Pathophysiologic Approach in Acute and Chronic Disease

5.1 Introduction

5.1.1 Somatic and Visceral Reflexes

Physicians identified and reported on various clinical techniques during the nineteenth and twentieth centuries to diagnose appendicitis, eponymously named signs, to honor their accomplishments. These signs provide further support for the bedside diagnosis of acute and chronic appendicitis and supplement other imagining techniques. Different patterns and locations of abdominal pain in appendicitis are explained by whether the splanchnic (viscerosensory and visceromotor) and/or cerebrospinal (somatosensory and somatomotor) nerve pathways are activated. Activation occurs spontaneously or is expressed through superficial (somatic) or deep (visceral) palpation [1].

In acute appendicitis early in the disease course, Pacinian mechanoreceptors and splanchnic afferent nerve fibers within the appendix respond to stretch (distension). The pain fibers travel with splanchnic sympathetic nerves through the superior mesenteric, gastric, and hepatic plexuses to the dorsal root ganglion. In general, visceral efferent pain fibers, in general, travel along the same spinal cord segments as their afferent nerve counterparts. Visceral pain is perceived in the midline (epigastric and periumbilical regions) and is fixed regardless of the position of the appendix, reflecting its embryologic nerve origin. This pain is generally deep-seated, poorly localized, bilaterally distributed, and more widespread, and it extends to involve the T8–T10 dermatomes (viscerosensory reflex) [1]. What is not widely appreciated is that in some cases, when visceral pain is abrupt and severe due to rapid distension of the appendix, there is a "spill-over" phenomenon at peak pain intensity, causing a direct stimulation of efferent neurons (cerebrospinal nerve pathway) from splanchnic afferent nerves due to their anatomical juxtaposition in the dorsal root of the spinal cord [1]. Thus, abrupt and severe visceral appendiceal pain is perceived

S. H. Yale et al., *Gastrointestinal Eponymic Signs*, https://doi.org/10.1007/978-3-031-33673-7_5

within the cerebral cortex as well as causing activation of alpha-motor neurons and efferent nerve pathways in intercostal nerves that innervate abdominal muscle causing involuntary abdominal spasm (guarding) in the absence of inflammatory involvement of the parietal peritoneum. This pain and muscle spasm is located at the right T10–T11 dermatomes (viscerosensory and visceromotor segmental reflex).

In contrast, inflammation that extends to involve the parietal peritoneum of the abdominal wall in acute appendicitis activates the cerebrospinal nerve pathway. This pathway is stimulated by movement, cough, superficial palpation, and removal of palpatory hand or other maneuvers at a site(s) of tenderness at the parietal peritoneum on the abdominal wall. It involves afferent pain signals transmitted through intercostal nerves to the dorsal root ganglion and cortical pathways, and efferent pathways stimulating alpha-motor neurons in the anterior rami with the signal transmitted to the same intercostal nerves on the anterior abdominal wall causing abdominal muscle spasms and guarding (somatomotor segmental reflex). These somatic segmental reflexes localize the pain and spasms to the same area at the inflamed peritoneum, usually at the T10–T12 dermatomes. In general, there is a point on this dermatomal segment involving the anterior abdominal wall, representing the site of greatest pain first recognized by Charles McBurney (1845–1913) in 1889 and colloquially known as McBurney point. The point is between an inch and a half and 2 in. to the right anterior superior iliac spine on a straight line drawn from that process to the umbilicus. What is not widely recognized by many clinicians is that this point represents the location on the anterior abdominal wall where the parietal peritoneum is reflexively irritated by appendiceal inflammation and not the location of the appendix. Hence, in cases where the appendix is retrocecally located in the pelvis or involving the posterior abdominal wall, pain is less likely to be found at McBurney point. Nevertheless, when there is superficial palpatory tenderness at McBurney point, a clinician can be reasonably sure that the disease represents acute appendicitis.

The sequence of events leading to activation of reflexes during the acute and chronic stages of appendicitis can be summarized as follows: In early acute appendicitis, the disease is confined to the appendix or periappendiceal region, a viscerosensory reflex is present, causing a centralized visceral pain perceived at the T8–T10 dermatomes. In some cases, when the disease is of rapid onset and severe, there may be a "spill-over" effect into somatic segments (visceromotor and/or viscerosensory segmental reflexes) at the right T10–T11 dermatome. In the later stages of acute appendicitis, the parietal peritoneum may be involved caused by perforation and extension of the inflammatory process to the anterior abdominal wall, such that somatic (somatosensory and somatomotor segmental reflexes) segmental pain pathways at the right T10–T12 dermatome or other regions of the abdominal wall are now involved. In chronic appendicitis, the disease is again primarily confined to the appendix. As such, only visceral pain pathways are involved, which can be centralized or located in the right lower quadrant, similar to what occurs in acute appendicitis.

Understanding how these maneuvers are performed and the disease is expressed assists clinicians with the means to determine the presence or absence of appendicitis, knowledge of the pathophysiologic process, and the location of the pain. Teaching the pathophysiologic process while the sign is being taught and performed provides the learner with a more fundamental and in-depth appreciation of the physical examination's role in enumerating the disease process and establishing a diagnosis.

This chapter reviews the abdominal signs of acute and chronic appendicitis involved in the activation of somatic and visceral pathways and their accompanying symptoms. In the subsequent chapter discussed are other signs named in the absence of activation of nerve pathways. We present the signs as originally described to avoid misrepresenting that enumerated by the primary authors. The signs are grouped using a pathophysiologic approach and listed chronologically based on the year they were first reported.

5.2 Historical Background

The disease acute appendicitis has been contentious since its presumed original description by Jean François Fernel (1497–1558) in 1554 [2]. For over three centuries, there has been the absence of a unified consensus among physicians regarding the source, diagnostic features, and treatment of this disease. It was Reginald Heber Fitz (1843–1913) who, in 1886, established a comprehensive description of the disease in his landmark presentation and publication in 257 patients, titled *Perforating Inflammation of the Vermiform Appendix: With Special Reference to its Early Diagnosis and Treatment* [3]. Fitz was the first to coin the term "appendicitis" and distinguish it from inflammatory processes involving the cecum or pericecal regions (typhlitis, perityphlitis, perityphlitis abscess). Fitz stated that "the term appendicitis was preferred to typhlitis, as avoiding the possibility of a misunderstanding, and as localizing the disease in its usual place of origin." [3, p. 13]. He further established, elaborated on, and described the clinical features, diagnosis, course, macroscopic pathological features, and treatment of this disease. We provide excerpts from his time-honored description of appendicitis and appendiceal perforation, given its significance and clarity of presentation to the history of appendicitis:

It was found that the disease occurred most frequently among previously healthy youths and young adults, especially males; that a fecal concretion or foreign body was present as a local cause in more than three-fifths of the cases. Attacks of indigestion and acts of violence, especially when indirect, were exciting causes in one-fifth of the cases. The action of these causes was favored by a constipated habit, or by congenital or acquired irregularities in the position and attachment of the appendix. The first characteristic symptom of a perforating appendicitis was found to be a sudden, severe, abdominal pain. This occurred in 84% of the cases and usually in the right iliac fossa, where tenderness could always be found, even when the pain was referred to some other locality. (…) Fever was the next characteristic symptom and occurred in the course of 24 hours. Finally came the swelling which made its appearance in the course of three days. The chief source of danger from the appendicular peritonitis arose from its becoming generalized. Such a result followed most frequently between the second and fourth days. (…) If it became evident that general peritonitis was imminent at the end of 24 hours after the sudden intense pain the appendix should be exposed and removed. (…) More favorable results in the future were to follow the earliest possible opening of the swelling. This in most instances was at the outset, a sac formed by circumscribed peritonitis. It was usually present on the third day of the disease, dating from the pain, its first marked characteristic symptom [3, p. 13].

Hence, his work was immeasurable in providing the first unified conceptualization of the disease and its prompt surgical treatment, thus challenging prevailing thinking about the disease up to that time.

5.3   Somatic Segmental Nerve Pathway Signs

There are various maneuvers, as elucidated through signs, in which somatic pain caused by irritation of the parietal peritoneum is elicited by patient movement, cough, superficial palpation, and other techniques, including pinching, twisting, or releasing the depressed palpatory hand on the anterior abdomen wall (somatosensory segmental reflex). Other signs require the contraction of the abdominal muscles (somatomotor segmental reflex). In addition to the eponymously named signs included in this review, two recent maneuvers are worth mentioning. Tzortzopoulou et al. described the jumping up (j-up) test in children with suspected acute appendicitis, which involves asking the patient to "jump and try to reach both rising hands a toy hanging down from the ceiling of the examination room" [4, p. 1]. Pain in this study was assessed by comparing the child's facial expression to the Bier pain scale. In another study, Eid and Al-Kaisy asked patients with suspected acute appendicitis whether they experienced increased abdominal pain while traveling over a "speed (traffic control) bump" or "Holly hump" [5]. Both studies reported high sensitivity (87%, 90.5%) with lower specificity (70%, 40%) for the J-up and speed bump, respectively [4, 5]. It should be noted that neither of these studies assessed the location of the pain. The high sensitivity suggests that this test and sign correctly identify patients with peritonitis. The lower specificity is consistent with other conditions occurring intra-abdominally that causes peritonitis.

5.4   Eponymous Signs

5.4.1   McBurney Sign (Point)

Charles Heber McBurney (1845–1913) was born in Roxbury, Massachusetts, USA, and received his medical degree from the College of Physicians and Surgeons (renamed Columbia University in 1912, and Columbia University Roy and Diana Vagelos College of Physicians and Surgeons in 2017), New York in 1870 [6, 7]. He completed his internship at Bellevue Hospital in New York City and received his postgraduate training in Vienna, Paris, and London [7]. He returned in 1873 to the

College of Physicians and Surgeons with an appointment as an assistant demonstrator in anatomy. He was appointed assistant surgeon at Bellevue in 1880 and surgeon-in-chief at Roosevelt Hospital, New York City, in 1888. From 1889 to 1894, he was appointed professor of surgery, followed by a position as professor of clinical surgery until 1907, after which he was bestowed the title of professor emeritus of surgery at the College of Physicians and Surgeons [7]. McBurney was a fellow of the American Medical Society, an honorary fellow of the Royal College of Surgeons, Edinburgh, in 1905, and a member of the New York Academy of Medicine and Surgical Society of Paris, among others [8].

In addition to the eponym "McBurney point/sign," he is also recognized for his contribution to the use of rubber gloves during surgery asepsis, pyloric stenosis, a method for reducing dislocation of the humerus as a complication of a fracture at or near the surgical neck, extraction of a common bile duct stone through an incision in the duodenum and ampulla, inguinal hernia repair, and the operative incision in patients with acute appendicitis (McBurney incision) [9–14]. This technique involves splitting rather than cutting the external and internal oblique muscle bundles, aponeurosis, and transversalis muscle to expose the appendix in patients with non-perforated appendicitis [12].

Regarding his character:

> As a teacher and lecturer, McBurney was simple, clear, and eminently practical. (…) In his relations with the house staff of the hospital he was always absolute master. (…) To his patients he was gentle, self-sacrificing, sparing himself not at all. His manner was always charming, and I have never seen a sweeter smile on any human face than he did show. He inspired absolute confidence in those under his care. His winning manner, absolute devotion to duty, and superior intelligence aroused in those who worked with him professionally the highest admiration, affection, and esteem [15, p. 979].

At the New York Surgical Society in 1889, he presented the sign describing the location of appendiceal pain at the right lower abdominal quadrant: "The seat of greatest pain, determined by the pressure of one finger, has been very exactly between an inch and half and two inches from the anterior spinous process of the ilium on a straight line drawn from that process to the umbilicus." [16, p. 678] (Table 5.1) (Fig. 5.1).

It is of interest that Ludwig Traube (1818–1876) described in 1871 the case of a 32-year-old man, "It began initially with moderate pain, which first appeared in the lower half of the abdomen between the middle of the anterior superior spine and umbilicus that continued to increase in intensity until it became more severe by late noon yesterday" [17, p. 55]. Two days later, he wrote that the "Abdomen is very distended, tense, and sensitive to pressure everywhere but especially to the right at the point mentioned above the iliac spine and umbilicus" [17, p. 56].

The most common finding in patients with acute appendicitis is local tenderness which initially may be masked by more generalized pain. The point of maximum tenderness at McBurney point is fixed. It thus represents not the position of the appendix but the site on the anterior abdominal wall where the T10 and T12 sensory afferent nerves are most commonly irritated by parietal peritoneal appendiceal

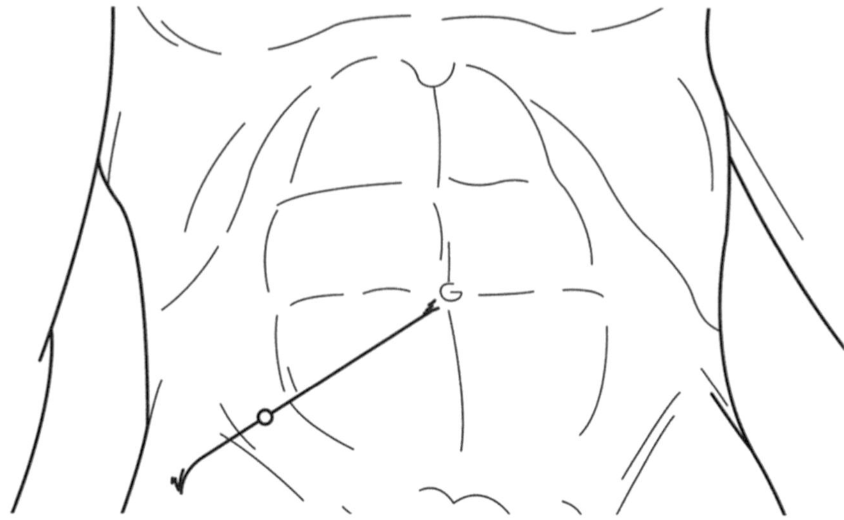

Fig. 5.1 McBurney sign (by Ryan Yale)

inflammation. This finding may be absent in patients with a thickened abdominal wall or omental fat or whose appendix is located retrocecally in the pelvis or the fossa on the posterior abdominal wall [18]. Other sites of cutaneous tenderness on the anterior abdominal wall may also be involved, as described by Cope, Lanz, Clado, and Gray [18]. In general, pain over McBurney point provides surgeons reasonable confidence that the appendix is more likely to be involved [18]. Hence, even today, surgeons routinely search for this physical sign in patients presenting with acute or subacute abdominal pain.

During the initial clinical examination in patients with acute appendicitis, Soda et al. reported a sensitivity of 83% and specificity of 45% at McBurney point. The positive predictive value was 76%, and the negative predictive value was 56% [19]. A meta-analysis reported a positive likelihood ratio of 1.29 (range of 1.06–1.57) and a negative likelihood ratio of 0.25 (range 0.12–0.53) for McBurney point in acute appendicitis [20]. Results from these studies should be interpreted with caution and examined based on their clinical context.

5.4.2   Perman Sign

Emil Samuel Perman (1856–1946) was born in Östersund, Sweden, and received his medical licensure in 1887 and medical degree in 1889 from the Karolinska Institute, Solna, Sweden [21, 22]. He served as an assistant surgeon at Sabbatsberg Hospital in Stockholm from 1886 to 1891, associate professor of surgery at Karolinska Institute from 1891 to 1896, and chief physician at Crown Princess

Lovisa's Care Institution for Sick Children in Stockholm from 1892 to 1899 [21, 22]. Perman was appointed chief physician in the surgical department of Sabbatsberg Hospital, Stockholm, from 1899 to 1919 [22]. He described two methods for diagnosing acute appendicitis in 1904:

> A symptom, the significance which was first pointed out by Dieulafoy (abdominal guarding), which is of great importance and one that I have always found to be accurate when present, involves muscle tension over the cecal tract and adjacent portion of the abdomen when touched or lightly pressed. If this symptom is found, you can be almost certain that there are already many changes in and around the appendix-free or limited gangrene or perforation with incipient purulent peritonitis. Additionally, I found another symptom: pain localized to the ileocecal area when pressure is applied to the left side of the abdomen [23, p. 806].

These findings are consistent with the activation of somatomotor segmental reflexes with superficial palpation in the right lower abdominal quadrant. A somatosensory or viscerosensory segmental nerve reflex occurs when pressure is applied to the left side of the abdomen (see Sect. 5.6.6) (Table 5.1). We are unaware of any study that evaluated the sensitivity or specificity of this sign.

5.4.3 Blumberg-Shchetkin Sign

5.4.3.1 Moritz Blumberg

Jacob Moritz Blumberg (1873–1955) was born in Posen, province of Silesia, Prussia (currently Poland), and received his medical degree from the University of Breslau, Wroclaw (now University of Wroclaw, Poland) in 1897 [24]. During World War I, he served in the German army and was instrumental in devising a rapid method for delousing the Russian prisoners of war and hence successfully contained and prevented a typhus epidemic on the eastern front. This accomplishment was later described as "one of the greatest achievements in military medical history" [24]. He left Berlin during World War II and practiced in London, England, with his son Ernst Friedrich Blumberg (1908–1973), who also specialized in surgery, gynecology, and radiology [24].

In addition to the sign which bears his name, Moritz Blumberg's other notable surgical accomplishments included redesigning the rubber surgical glove (Blumberg glove), designing an instrument to facilitate suturing of the perineum, describing the buttonhole incision, and developing a procedure for temporary sterility in women [24]. His character was described as a "sympathetic, yet firm personality having inspired immediate confidence in those who sought his advice" [24].

Blumberg described in 1907 a method for determining whether the parietal peritoneum is irritated by an inflamed appendix (Fig. 5.2):

> Very different results occur when pressure is applied compared to when the palpating hand is raised. In my opinion, it is always necessary to consider these two movements separately based on the type of pain they induce. For example, first, apply pressure on the area of the

abdomen to be examined and ask the patient whether it is painful. After listening to the response, suddenly lift the palpating hand and ask the patient whether it was painful when the hand was removed and which of the two types of pain was greatest. (…) I noted an extremely violent pain, causing the patient to momentarily grimace, when the palpating hand was suddenly lifted. During an acute episode the patient stated with certainty that the pain was greatest when the hand was suddenly lifted compared to when it was pressed. In cases of less severe inflammation involving the peritoneum, the pain when the hand was suddenly lifted was similar to when the hand was pressed. As the healing process progressed, the pain was less when the hand was lifted and finally remained only vaguely present, presumably caused by adhesion, when the hand was lifted. The pain completely disappeared when chronic disease was present [25, p. 1177]. (…) The method can be applied accurately since it is not a matter of assessing the extent of the pain but comparing the intensity of the two pains. This information is reliably conveyed by the patient [25, p. 1178].

Blumberg recognized the peritoneal origin of the pain and that it was present in cases of acute appendicitis and other inflammatory processes involving the peritoneum [25]. He concluded that this finding suggests a serious underlying intra-abdominal process if it occurs suddenly after disease onset. At the same time, its gradual decrease in intensity provides reassurance of the resolving underlying peritoneal process [25] (Table 5.1).

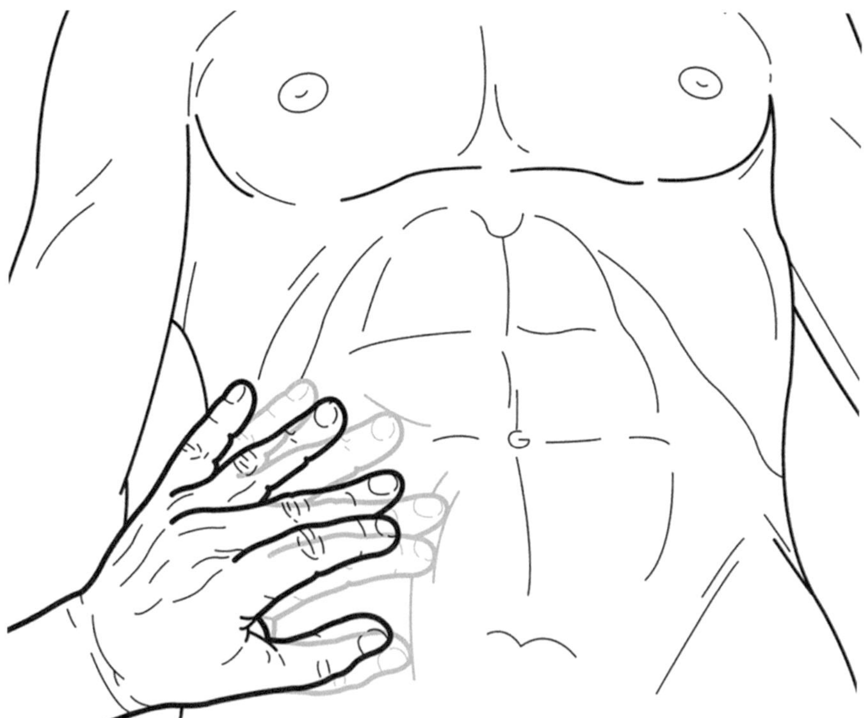

Fig. 5.2 Blumberg (Shchetkin) sign (by Ryan Yale)

5.4.3.2 Dmitri Shchetkin

Dmitri Sergeevich Shchetkin (1851–1923) was born in Ryazan, Russia, and received his medical degree from St. Petersburg Medical and Surgical Academy in 1877 [26]. He was an intern during the Russo-Turkish war (1877–1878) and completed a one-year internship at the Clinical Military Hospital in St. Petersburg, where the focus of his studies was directed toward obstetrics and gynecological surgery [26, 27]. Here he successfully passed the doctorate in medicine certification examination and doctoral dissertation, delivered at the St. Petersburg Medical and Surgical Academy, titled "On Conditions Predisposing to the Development of Venous Thrombosis after Ovariectomy." [26]. Shchetkin served as vice-president of the Ryazan Medical Society from 1884 to 1888, a senior (chief) physician at the Ryazan Provincial Zemstvo Hospital from 1888 to 1902, and a senior physician at the Penza Provincial Zemstvo Hospital from 1902 to 1917 [26, 27].

Shchetkin and other gynecologists and surgeons practicing at Ryazan, Russian Empire in the late 1880s, and Penza Provincial Zemstvo I Hospital, the Soviet Union in 1902, were reportedly performing this sign before Blumberg's 1907 publication [26–29]. Shchetkin reported at the Penza Medical Society in 1908 the following sign found in patients with peritonitis:

> The symptom is that if you put your hand over the patient's abdomen and lightly press, pain in the abdomen is usually not felt. The patient feels severe pain soon after the examiner lifts his hand from the abdominal wall. The symptom is particularly characteristic in cases of local peritonitis because it accurately indicates the location of the disease on the peritoneum. It also serves as a valuable sign for general peritonitis. In addition to this, it is an important finding in the differential diagnosis of peritonitis and abdominal wall pain simulating peritonitis [27, p. 51].

In his paper "On the abdominal tremor," Shchetkin described another palpatory finding in patients with intestinal adhesions; a vibratory sensation transmitted to the abdominal wall while talking in patients with intra-abdominal adhesions extending between the intestines and the abdominal wall [28].

Several studies have evaluated the Blumberg-Shchetkin sign in patients with acute appendicitis. Andersson (2004) reported a positive and negative likelihood ratio of 1.99 and 0.39, respectively [20]. In a study of 100 patients presenting with right iliac fossa pain, Golledge et al. (1996) reported a sensitivity and specificity of 82% and 89%, respectively, with a positive predictive value of 86% [30]. Additionally, in a large case series, a sensitivity ranging from 40 to 95%, specificity 20 to 89%, and positive and negative likelihood ratios of 2.1 and 0.5 were found [31]. Recall that the sign demonstrates the presence of rebound tenderness caused by irritation of the parietal peritoneum. Thus, a moderately high suspicion of the disease suggests that the patient is likely to have peritonitis if the test is positive. Conversely, the low likelihood ratio is consistent with a lower risk of peritonitis in a patient with a negative test.

5.4.4 *Illoway Sign*

Henry Illoway (Illovy) (1847–1932) was born in Kolin, Bohemia, and received his medical degree from Miami Medical College of Cincinnati, Ohio, in 1869 [32–37]. He completed his residency training at Cincinnati Hospital from 1869 to 1870 and was a private practitioner and later a visiting physician at the Jewish Hospital, Cincinnati [32, 33, 35, 37].

Illoway was appointed professor of diseases of children at Cincinnati College of Medicine and Surgery in 1888 [35, 37]. He studied in Berlin under the tutelage of Ismar Isidor Boas (1858–1938) and Emanuel Mendel (1839–1907) and in Vienna with Leopold (Löb) Oser (1839–1910). He then returned to the USA to treat gastrointestinal diseases and serve the poor in New York City beginning in 1894 [34, 35, 37]. He was a fellow of the New York Academy of Medicine and a member of the New York County Medical Society, Society of Medical Jurisprudence, and German Medical Society, among others [33, 36].

Illoway described a maneuver for diagnosing appendicitis (Table 5.1) (Fig. 5.3):

> The patient is placed at full length upon the operating table or chair for the purposes of examination. This is made in the usual way, and when all the data have been obtained, I tell him or her: (a) to flex the leg upon the thigh and the thigh upon the trunk. I now ask if the movement, or rather the upward pressure thus made, causes any pain or soreness in the lower portion of the right half of the abdomen, i.e., the appendicular region. If the answer is "no" or "very little," either I myself, flex (b) the thigh more closely, more forcibly upon the trunk or direct the patient to do so. Again, I inquire, does it cause pain or soreness, or does it increase the pain or soreness? I now have the patient, (c) extend the leg to full length with a quick and rather sudden movement, and ask whether this has caused any pain or soreness. If neither of these movements has caused any appreciable pain or soreness, I direct the patient to execute the same movements with the left leg, and to compare the sensation produced, as to whether it is any different from that caused by the right leg, or whether it is the same on both sides. (…) It is the pain or even soreness produced both on flexion and extension—and I lay the greater stress on the extension—that I regard as a positive and unfailing sign of the presence of appendicitis [38, p. 252–253].

Pain felt on the right iliac fossa suggests inflammatory involvement of the more proximal portion of the psoas muscle or an area adjacent to the psoas muscle (iliopsoas). We are unaware of any study that evaluated the sensitivity or specificity of this sign.

5.4.5 *Caden Sign*

James Albert Corscaden (1881–1964) was born in Providence, Rhode Island, USA, and received his medical degree from the College of Physicians and Surgeons (renamed Columbia University in 1912), New York, in 1906 [39]. He completed an internship at Presbyterian Hospital, New York, in 1907 and was a private practitioner at the time of the publication with Ellsworth Eliot, Jr. (1864–1945) of their manuscript titled "Intussusception with Special Reference to Adults" in 1911 [39, 40].

Ellsworth Eliot, Jr. was a surgeon, and Corscaden served as an assistant surgeon in the outpatient department at Presbyterian Hospital [40]. Corscaden was appointed

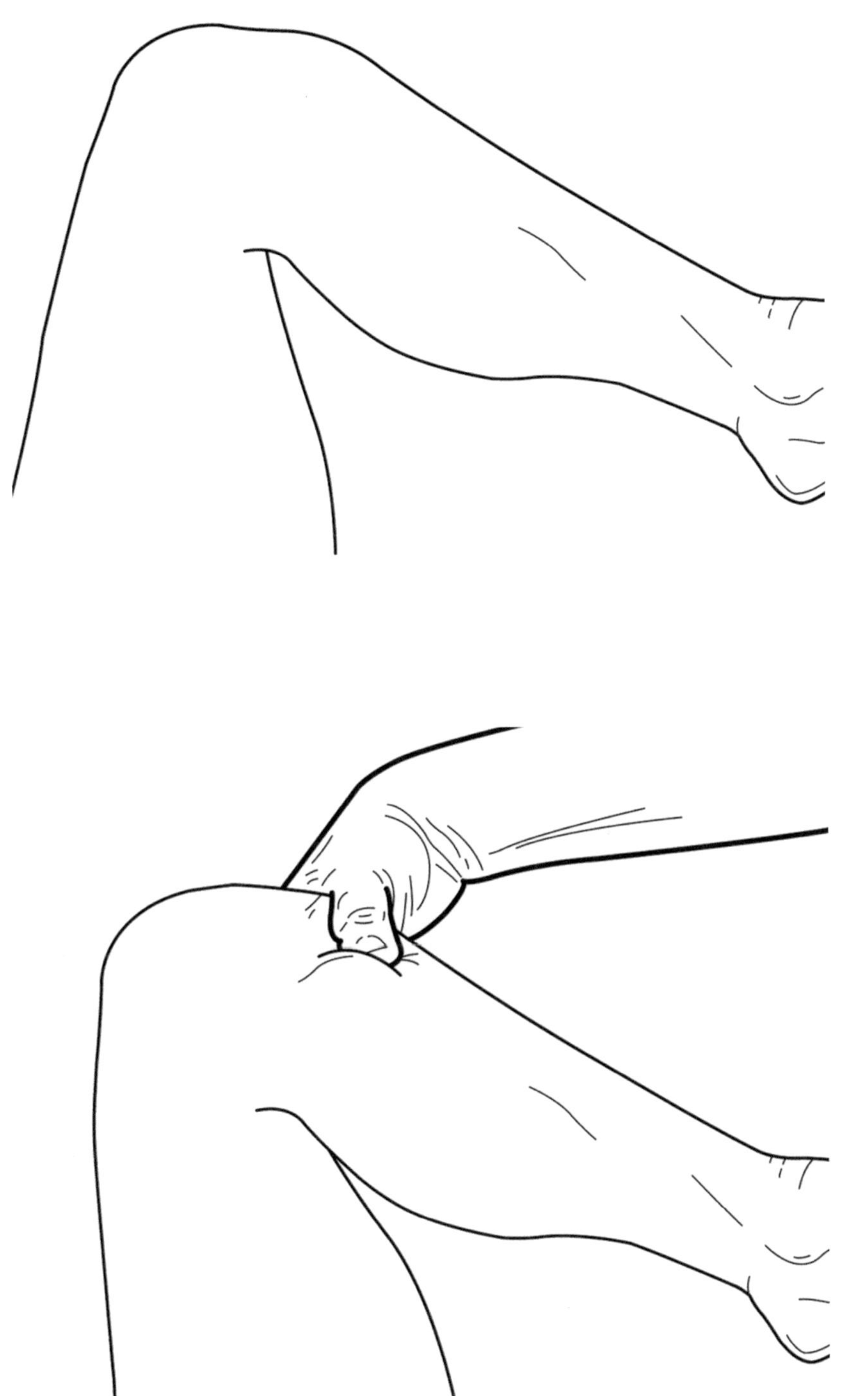

Fig. 5.3   Illoway sign (by Ryan Yale)

to the College of Physicians and Surgeons faculty in 1938. He held an appointment in the Department of Obstetrics and Clinical Gynecology at the College of Physicians and Surgeons, where he remained throughout his career [39].

Eliot and Corscaden described the findings that distinguish acute appendicitis from intussusception:

> A correct diagnosis is usually possible by noting that the tumor associated with appendicitis is almost invariably fixed and enjoys little if any respiratory movement. Moreover, the associated muscular rigidity is of great importance. In appendicitis it is almost always most marked in the lower right quadrant, while in intussusception the symptom, if present, is generally more marked on one side or the other of the umbilicus, while the intervening abdomen between this area and either inguinal region is either less rigid or entirely free from any rigidity whatever [40, p. 184].

Thus, Caden or Corscaden sign refers to muscular rigidity in the lower right abdominal quadrant (somatomotor and/or visceromotor reflex) (Table 5.1). It is unclear why any attribution for this sign was not credited to Eliot. We are unaware of any study that evaluated the sensitivity or specificity of this sign.

5.4.6 Chutro Sign

Pedro (Piedro) Chutro (Cortajerena) (1880–1937) was born in Chascomús, province of Buenos Aires, Argentina, and received his medical degree at the Faculty of Medicine, University of Buenos Aires in 1904 [41]. His doctoral thesis was titled "Fracturas de la Extremidad Inferior del Húmero en los Niños" (Fractures of the Lower Extremities of the Humerus in Children) [42, 43]. During his medical training, he worked in the Children's Surgical Service at the Hospital de Clinicas under the aegis of Alejandro Posada (1870–1902) and Marcelino Herrera Vegas (1870–1958) [43]. He continued his studies in Vienna, Berlin, and Paris and, upon his return, served as head of the surgical service in 1908 and a substitute professor of operative medicine at Teodoro Álvarez Hospital in 1909 and the surgical clinic in 1914 [41, 43].

During World War I, he was appointed first assistant at Lycée Buffon Hospital, Paris, in 1915, rising to the rank of commander of the surgery services [41, 43, 44]. Here he successfully treated osteomyelitis and bone sinuses caused by wounds. For his work, he received the Distinguished Service Medal from the USA and the Knight of the Legion of Honor from France [43, 45]. Upon his return to Buenos Aires, Chutro served as full professor of the surgical clinic at Durand Hospital, followed by an appointment as titular professor and chair of clinical surgery at Ramos Mejía Hospital in 1919 [41, 44].

Among his other accomplishments, he was a founding member of the Society of Surgery of Buenos Aires in 1911, a member of the Academy of Medicine in Paris and the National Society of Surgery from 1916, and a foreign correspondent for the division of surgery in the National Academy of Medicine from 1920 to 1937 [44]. He identified the method of adding sodium citrate to blood to prevent its coagulation in 1914 [46].

A description of his character by Domingo Prat:

> As a physician, he was rigid, stern, and a zealous guardian of the precious health of the sick, which society entrusted to his care. He believed in the need for a harmonious existence and

respect for the pain of his fellow men. He prevented it not because that took away the brilliance of his operations, but because of his love for his neighbor and his deep respect for the hospitalized patient. This part of his personality constituted a model of discipline and order, which morally and technically constituted an exemplary role model for early physicians. For this reason, his surgical clinic service stood out for its exemplary operation and discipline. This great teacher, who just disappeared from the surgical stage from Río de la Plata, constitutes an extraordinary and irreplaceable loss for Argentine surgery and Río de la Plata [47, p. 114, 116].

Pedro Chutro described a finding observed in patients with acute appendicitis:

For a long time, I have been struck by the frequent occurrence of the deviation of the abdominal midline to the right. This type of appendicular sign can be easily observed because the pigmentation almost always follows the tracing of the midline. The deviation follows a curved shape, with a more or less pronounced arch, convex to the right and whose most protruding point is at the level of the navel. The explanation of this phenomenon is straightforward; pathophysiology teaches us that when the peritoneum is inflamed, the broad muscle, especially the transversus, goes into permanent contraction and moves the linea alba to the right, with the skin accompanying the muscle plane. The navel plays an important role. Frequently it is difficult to confirm the tracing of the midline. When extending a thread from the xiphoid process to the middle of the pubic symphysis, it is observed that the entire navel is placed to the right of said line as if it had moved laterally [48, p. 4]. (…) This sign is important concerning the disease's progress since the navel's return to its usual place and shape does not follow the disappearance of other symptoms; it returns slowly [48, p. 5].

Chutro found that inflammation of the parietal peritoneum causes abdominal wall contraction (somatomotor reflex) and deviation of the umbilicus to the right (Table 5.1). We are unaware of any study that evaluated the sensitivity or specificity of this sign.

5.4.7 ten Horn Sign

Carel Hendrik Leo Herman ten Horn (1884–1964) was born in Veendam, Groningen, The Netherlands. He served as a voluntary assistant, followed by a first assistant in the surgical clinic at the University of Amsterdam from 1908 to 1914 [49]. He was the director of the surgical and urological departments at the Den Helder Naval Hospital, The Netherlands, from 1914 to 1915. His academic appointments included a professor by special appointment (extraordinary professor) in 1916, a full professor from 1916 to 1918, and a director of the Department of Surgery of the Faculty of Medicine and Health Sciences, Ghent University, Belgium, from 1917 to 1918 [49].

He described the method and expected findings in patients with acute appendicitis after applying traction on the right spermatic cord (Fig. 5.4):

During the examination, one must avoid any unnecessary pressure on the testis. Grasp the spermatic cord between the thumb and index finger above the testis. Gentle pulling of the spermatic cord produces a displacement of the parietal peritoneum near the inner inguinal ring. It is well known that the slightest pull is painful when the peritoneum is inflamed [50, p. 1537].

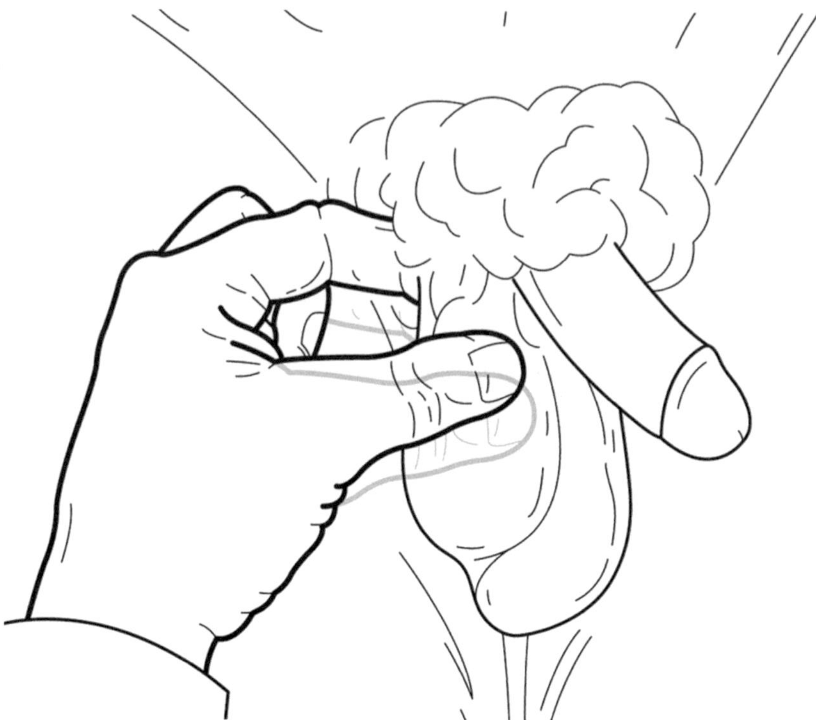

Fig. 5.4 ten Horn sign (by Ryan Yale)

ten Horn found that twelve patients with acute appendicitis reported pain in the right iliac fossa after downward traction on the right spermatic cord. In some cases, he also noted that traction on the left spermatic cord was also painful. In these cases, abundant serofibrinous exudate was found intraoperatively within the abdominal activity [50]. Thus, traction of the right spermatic is believed to cause pain in the right iliac fossa due to the apposition of the gonadal vessel and connective tissue against the inflamed parietal peritoneum in cases of perforated appendicitis (Table 5.1). We are unaware of any studies that assessed the sensitivity and specificity of this sign.

5.4.8   Lanz Sign

Otto Lanz (1865–1935) was born in Steffisburg, Thun district, Canton of Bern, Switzerland, studied medicine at the Universities of Geneva, Bern, Basle, and Leipzig, and received his medical degree from the University of Bern in 1891 [51]. He became an associate professor in surgery in 1893 and a surgical assistant at the University Clinic under Theodor Kocher (1841–1917) from 1890 to 1897 [51]. Lanz was a private practitioner in Lindenhofspital, Switzerland, and a full professor of surgery at the University of Amsterdam in 1902 [51]. He was an avid art collector who possessed a collection of paintings from the fourteenth through the sixteenth centuries. Part of the collection was displaced at the Rijksmuseum in Amsterdam in

1935, forcefully acquired in 1941, and later returned after the war [51]. In addition to the sign of appendicitis, which bears his name, Lanz also contributed to asepsis, thyroid surgery, and mesh split-skin graft [51, 52].

As to a description of his character:

> If he sometimes outwardly seemed a little stern, anyone who had once felt the warm look in his eyes knew that he was facing a sympathetic, understanding man and, at that moment, regarded him more as a fatherly friend than a scholar. And how many consulted him for other than physical suffering. His concern for the patients entrusted to him knew no bounds. When a patient was in danger of life, he did not depart from the sickbed, accustomed to every means that might still help, and many a person owes their life to his faithful care where everything seemed already lost [52, p. 1368].

Lanz described a finding involving the inguinal canal in patients with appendicitis (Fig. 5.5):

> Based on dozens of cases of acute appendicitis examined, I have the impression that the cremaster reflex on the right side is usually weakened or absent. In addition, in acute cases, I have often found that the right spermatic cord is thickened probably as a result of collateral edema, and exquisitely sensitive to pressure when it is rolled back and forth with the fingers when examined at the exit from the anterior inguinal ring, at the medial attachment of the Poupart ligament, just lateral to the pubic tubercle. For years I have also repeatedly taken the opportunity to use the muscular defense to follow a finger inserted into the inguinal canal. At the same time, one occasionally feels a degree of tension in the anterior canal wall, which is quite striking compared to the left side. One can easily and painlessly insert the fingertip or entire index finger into the inguinal canal on the left. The intensely stretched inferior border of the inferior oblique and transversus muscle on the right side prevents penetration of the finger into the inguinal canal. Trying to perform the same maneuver on the right side is painful, while it is not painful on the left side. The patients complain of pain on coughing when the finger is inserted [53, p. 1705–1706].

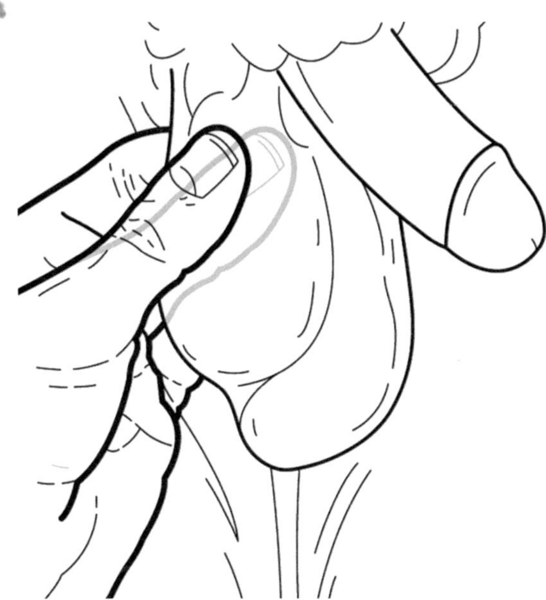

Fig. 5.5 Lanz sign (by Ryan Yale)

Lanz described the absent or diminished right cremasteric reflex, thickened and tender right spermatic cord, and tension involving the right anterior wall of the inguinal canal in males with acute appendicitis (Table 5.1). We are unaware of any studies that assessed this sign's sensitivity and specificity.

5.4.9   Morris Sign

Robert Tuttle Morris (1857–1945) was born in Seymour, Connecticut, USA, and received his medical degree from the College of Physicians and Surgeons (renamed Columbia University in 1912), New York, in 1882 [54, 55]. He was an assistant house surgeon at Bellevue Hospital from 1882 to 1884 and subsequently traveled abroad to Europe for additional training in surgery [54]. He was on staff as an instructor in surgery at the faculty of Post Graduate Medical School, New York, in 1889 and chair and attending surgeon from 1898 to 1917 [55]. Morris was an associate editor of the *New England Medical Monthly* and *Journal of the Linnean Society of Natural History* [54]. He was elected president of the American Therapeutic Association in 1916 [55].

As to his character:

> Doctor Morris was always an interesting and impressive figure in the surgical clinic. His chief purpose was to arouse the attention of his students, to stimulate them to think. His case presentations were rarely logical expositions but rather entertaining and dramatic, interlarded with an abundance of surgical aphorisms. He used irony to arouse attention and had a sly and subtle wit. Sarcasm was not in his speech and he was always a worthy opponent in medical debate. Doctor Morris possessed in a singular degree serenity, urbanity, dignity, and restless curiosity of mind. He was a fluent lecturer on widely diverse subjects; his spirit and his mind were attuned to the rapid evolution not only of medicine but also the cognate sciences [55, p. 958].

Morris described two findings to assist in the diagnosis of chronic appendicitis. The first involved a point of tenderness on the anterior abdominal wall:

> [t]he greatest degree of tenderness on pressure is at the point a half inch to the right of the navel, close to the spinal column, and corresponding to the right sympathetic lumbar ganglion [56, p. 2036].

This point of tenderness was absent in acute cases of appendicitis, and if it occurs in pelvic irritations or infection, it is present bilaterally (Table 5.1). The other finding was referred to as the "cider barrel sign" a term used to describe the percussion sound on the right side of the abdomen in patients with chronic appendicitis.

5.4.10   Cope Signs

Sir Vincent Zachary Cope (1881–1974) was born in Hull, Kingston-upon-Hull, England, and conferred his medical degree with honors from St. Mary's Hospital Medical School, London [57]. He remained at St. Mary's Hospital throughout his career, practicing surgery and maintaining a zest and passion for medical history [57, 58]. He joined the medical corps in 1914 and served in World War I from 1916 to 1919 [57]. His first book,

Surgical Aspects of Dysentery Including Liver-Abscess, published in 1920, described his and his colleagues' experiences with the surgical management of dysentery during the war [57]. He authored the time-honored book, *The Early Diagnosis of the Acute Abdomen* in 1921, with revisions extending to the fourteenth edition [58, 59].

In the Royal College of Surgeons, he was a court of examiners and council member and chairman of the committee to the Ministry of Health, responsible for surveying hospital facilities, workforce, and training from 1949 to 1952 [57, 58]. He compiled under the direction of an Inter-Services Editorial Board the volumes *Medicine and Pathology* in 1952 and *Surgery* in 1953 of the History of the Second World War [58]. In recognition of these works, he was bestowed knighthood in 1953 [58]. Cope wrote other historical books, essays, and biographies that are too numerous to enumerate in this brief biographical sketch. Many societies recognized and honored his distinguished career, including the Royal College of Surgeons, the Medical Society of London, and the Royal Society of Medicine [58]. In the words of William Richard Lefanu (1904–1995):

> In private life he was the most equable, modest, and friendly of men. (…) He often said that the good surgeon must feel for his patients, but never let this sympathy disturb his judgment or treatment; he had the strength to obey this counsel of perfection in his own case [58, p. 308].

Three signs have been named for Cope, with two, psoas and obturator, used to diagnose appendicitis. The third, a misnomer, is incorrectly named in the literature in patients with cholecystitis. O'Reilly and Krauthamer coined the term "Cope sign" to describe their finding of two patients with acute cholecystitis and bradycardia [60]. Cope, however, in his paper "A sign of gall-bladder disease," reported:

> For six months before my recent illness, I occasionally had attacks of profuse sweating and increased pulse rate that woke me from sleep, but usually passed off within half an hour. They were not accompanied by any pain. A physician found my heart normal. (…) I do not know whether the nocturnal bout of sweating and rise in pulse rate had any connexon with the presence of gall stones, but it may be significance that since the operation a year ago I have not had a similar attack [61, p. 147–148].

Cope's symptoms of increased heart rate caused by biliary colic and chronic calculous cholecystitis were consistent with the activation of alpha-adrenergic sympathetic pathways [62]. The phenomenon that O'Reilly and Krauthamer (1971) reported was a cardio-biliary reflex, a group of disorders involving afferent and efferent nerve pathways that inappropriately lead to vasodilation, bradycardia, hypotension, and syncope [60]. The afferent pathway for this reflex originates in the gallbladder, is vagally mediated, and activated in response to mechanical stimulation resulting in bradyarrhythmia (e.g., atrioventricular block, high grade, or complete heart block) and other symptoms secondary to heightened parasympathetic tone [63].

Cope described two maneuvers in the diagnosis of acute appendicitis. The first was reported in 1921 and referred to as the iliopsoas rigidity (psoas extension test) (Table 5.1) (Fig. 5.6):

> It is well known that if there is an inflamed focus in relation to the psoas muscle the corresponding thigh is often flexed by the patient to relieve the pain. A lesser degree of such contraction (and irritation) can be determined often by making the patient lie on the opposite side and extending the thigh on the affected side to the full extent. Pain will be caused by the maneuver if the psoas is rigid from either reflex or direct irritation [59, p. 42].

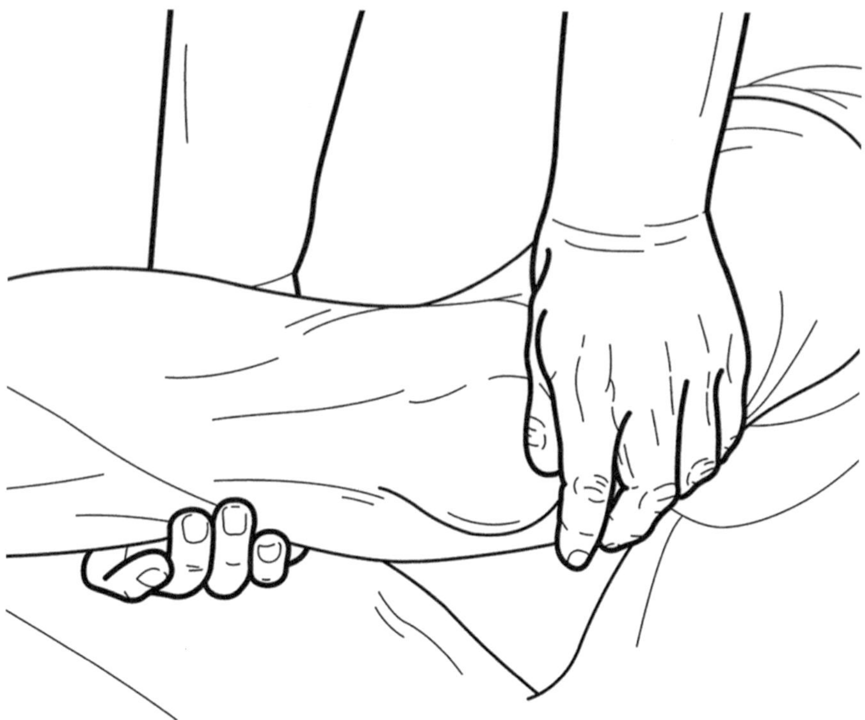

Fig. 5.6 Cope (Iliopsoas) sign (by Ryan Yale)

A variation of this test that departs from Cope's original description includes having the patient supine and flexing the thigh against the examiner's hand placed above the knee. In severe cases, the inflammation may cause a fixed flexion deformity of the hip [64]. This maneuver is most likely positive in cases of retrocecal appendicitis in which the inflamed appendix is juxtapositioned against the psoas muscle, a primary or secondary psoas abscess arising from the psoas, a paraspinal condition, or a disorder involving the ureter or bladder [65]. A negative test is more likely to be found if the anterior abdominal wall is rigid or the inflammation is subacute [65–67]. The sensitivity of the psoas sign ranges from 13 to 42%, specificity of 79–97%, and a positive likelihood ratio of 2.0 for detecting appendicitis [63, 64]. Andersson reported a positive likelihood ratio of 2.31 (1.36–3.91) and a negative likelihood ratio of 0.85 (0.76–0.95) for the psoas sign in acute appendicitis [20]. Thus, a positive psoas sign increases the probability of having appendicitis, while a negative test result only modestly decreases the likelihood of disease.

Vasilii (Vasily) Parmenovich Obraztsov's (1849–1920) name has been associated with the psoas test. We were unable to verify his description of the test and the year it was reported [68, 69]. In a study on 19,346 patients with acute appendicitis, Obraztsov sign was identified in 62.1% of those with acute appendicitis and in 3.7% of patients in which the appendix was in a retrocecal position [70]. A sliding palpatory technique for deep abdominal palpation has been attributed to Obraztsov-Strazhesko [71].

Cope, in 1919, described another method to diagnose acute appendicitis in cases where appendiceal or other causes of pelvic inflammation are located below the pelvic brim adjacent to the lateral wall (Table 5.1) (Fig. 5.7):

> The right thigh is slightly flexed (so as to relax the psoas muscle) by the surgeon, who stands on the right of the patient; the limb is then fully rotated at the hip, first internally and then externally, so as to put the obturator internus through a full range of movement. The sign is positive if the patient complains of hypogastric pain when the limb is moved in this manner [72, p. 537].

According to Cope, the obturator test is more likely to be positive under the following circumstances:

> Since the fascia covering the obturator internus is fairly dense, the test is not positive unless the inflammation is considerable; and, with a positive result, one always expects the appendix to be adherent to, or even an abscess to be contiguous to, the fascia. I have found this sign of assistance not only in cases of appendicitis, but also in other pelvic conditions such as rupture ectopic gestation, and I have no doubt that it will often prove of value in doubtful cases [72, p. 537].

Examples of conditions that irritate the obturator internus muscle include inflammatory fluid in the pelvis, abscess, or perforated appendix. This test has been found to have a low sensitivity (8%) and high specificity (94%) in diagnosing appendicitis [67]. It should be recognized that Cope only described the location of the pain for

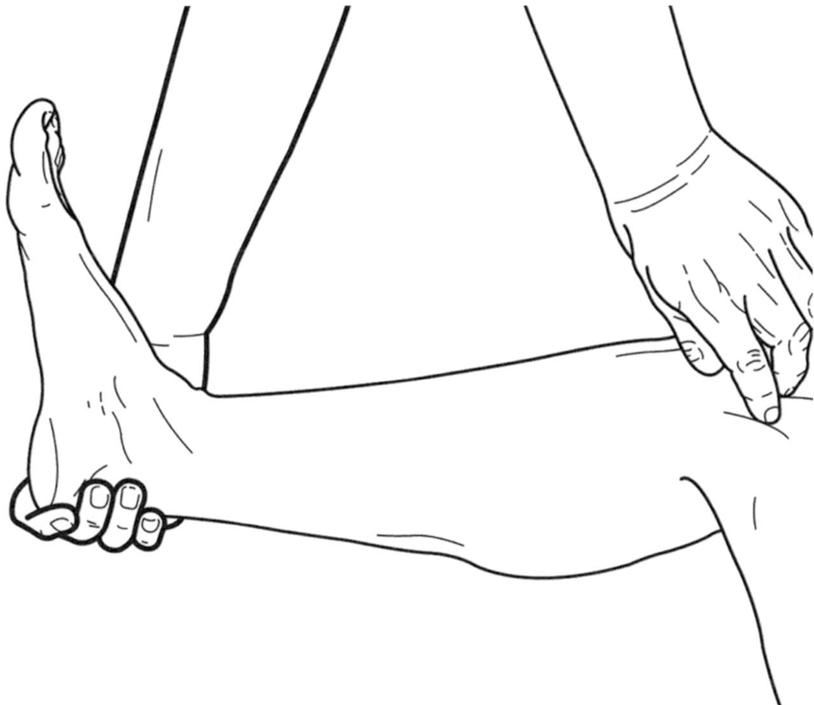

Fig. 5.7 Cope (Obturator) sign (by Ryan Yale)

the obturator and not the psoas sign. The psoas and obturator internus muscles are retroperitoneally located. Unlike the obturator internus, which is innervated by the L5-S2 nerves, the psoas muscle is located within the lower abdomen and pelvis, originates from the vertebral bodies of T12 and L1–L3, inserts in the less trochanter of the femur, and is innervated by L1–L4 nerves. Thus, depending on the location of the inflammatory process along the course of the right psoas muscle, pain may be perceived in the lower back, right lower quadrant, inguinal and hypogastric regions, hip, thigh, or knee. Inflammation of the obturator internus or other structures within the pelvis innervated by lumbosacral nerves causes pain to be perceived within the hypogastrium (suprapubic region).

Interestingly, Cope described the clinical symptoms of testicular pain occurring in acute appendicitis in the absence of signs elicited on physical examination. The pain may be present early in the course of the disease, occur in the right, left, or both testicles, and last up to two days. He postulated that the pathophysiologic mechanism involved the activation of sympathetic fibers arising from T10 spinal cord segment-nerves fibers also innervating the appendix. This mechanism represents a viscerosensory reflex of referred pain [73]. Furthermore, he also recognized the finding of testicular contraction on the right side in patients with acute appendicitis which he believed to be caused by irritation of the genito-crural (genitofemoral nerve) [73].

5.4.11 Gregory Sign

We were unable to identify any historical information on Arthur Gregory. At the time of the publication of his sign in 1922, he served as chief physician of the surgical department of the Vologda Military Hospital, Russia [74].

Gregory described a method for diagnosing acute, subacute, and chronic appendicitis. His discussion of the sign occurring in chronic appendicitis is found under visceral segmental reflexes. The somatic nerve reflex sign involves:

> Percussion midway between the umbilicus and anterior superior iliac spine causes tremor of the small intestines which is transmitted unimpeded (muscle contraction is absent) to the diseased appendix causing pain at McBurney's point. In acute and subacute appendicitis, the symptoms are clearly pronounced; even slight percussion causes an intense pain sensation at McBurney's point [74].

Gregory also found another somatic and visceral nerve reflex sign:

> In some cases, where the appendix is located medially due to adhesions in the areas of the small intestine, percussion between the umbilicus and the anterior superior iliac spine causes pain not only at McBurney's point but also at umbilicus and epigastrium. With the appendix in a pelvic position, pain during percussion was felt in the suprapubic region [74, p. 398].

Thus, Gregory sign refers to pain occurring at McBurney pain upon percussion of the abdomen between the umbilicus and anterior superior iliac spine or directly at McBurney point in acute and subacute appendicitis (somatosensory nerve reflex)

(Table 5.1). The referred nature of the pain at the umbilicus and epigastrium occurs in cases where the appendix is located medially and is consistent with a viscerosensory nerve reflex. Likewise, pain in the hypogastrium is consistent with somatosensory nerve reflex caused by irritation of nerves within the pelvis.

5.4.12   Sattler Sign

There is limited historical information on Eugen Sattler. He was a senior surgeon in the surgical university Clinic and St. Stefan Hospital in Pressburg (Budapest) until 1925 and in the surgical department of the polyclinic for war invalids, widows, and orphans in Budapest in 1926 [75–78].

Sattler presented a lecture at the September 15th, 1923, Congress of the Society of Hungarian Surgeons, where he described a maneuver for isolating the iliopsoas muscle as a method for distinguishing appendicitis from right adnexitis:

> We achieve this when the upper body is in a sitting position, and the legs are in a horizontal position with the axis of the upper body. In this position, the origin and insertion of the sartorius and tensor fasciae latae move closer to each other, causing their musculature to be completely relaxed. The patient sitting on a straight bed with the legs outstretched is asked to lift the right leg. In doing so, the patient flexes the hip joint, triggering isolated iliopsoas action. To accurately perform the examination, the legs must be extended so that the auxiliary muscles do not become active. Most patients tend to bend the upper body backward in order to support the painful iliopsoas activity with the accessory muscles. Therefore, an assistant must support the patient's back with his hand. The patient holds his hands beside his body but does not lean on them. When asked to do so, the patient tries to raise his leg. In healthy people, this occurs only under a slight angle; in weak or ill patients, of course, at an even smaller angle. Now I take hold of the patient's right leg and bend it further, asking him to point my finger to the painful spot in his abdomen. The point which I call the "appendix point" so designated is the boundary point of the right lateral third, on a straight line connecting the two anterior superior iliac spines (the point determined by Lanz). This point is almost the same in all cases, regardless of the position of the four known locations the processus vermiformis occupies. In some cases, there may be an insignificant change in the position of this point, a little up or down [79, p. 349–350].

He postulated that this maneuver causes the appendix to be compressed between the psoas muscle and the abdominal wall. Sattler also described the location of adnexal tenderness, which he named the adnexal point:

> During further investigations, I noticed that female patients described another spot as the painful point in adnexitis. With the help of the same examination method, the female patients with diseases in the adnexa described a painful spot, which I called the "adnexal point," as a painful point. I could paraphrase this point so that it corresponds to the lower point of an isosceles triangle, the two sides of which are the length of the outer third of the area of a straight line connecting the two anterior superior iliac spines. The proximal limb falls in this line, and the base of the triangle is half the length of the limb [79, p. 350].

Thus, Sattler sign refers to pain located at Lanz point occurring upon flexion of the extended leg onto the abdomen. The mechanism is more likely to be accounted for by inflammation involving the iliopsoas muscle rather than compression of the appendix between the psoas muscle and abdominal wall (Table 5.1).

5.4.13 Gray Sign

Sir Henry McIlree Williamson Gray (1870–1938) was born in Aberdeen, Scotland, and received his medical degree from the University of Aberdeen Medical School, graduating with honors in 1895. In Aberdeen, he was a private surgical practitioner from 1896 to 1903 [80]. He served as a surgeon during the South African (Boer) War and was invalided home with the rank of Major [81, 82]. During World War I, he obtained the rank of colonel in the Army Medical Service in 1914, consulting surgeon to the British Extraordinary Force in Rouen, France, and from 1917 as a consulting surgeon to the British Third Army [81, 82]. Gray was awarded the Order of the Bath Companion in 1916 and St. Michael and St. George Companion in 1918 [80]. He was appointed consultant of the Special Military Surgery in England until 1919. In that same year, Major (Temp. Lieut. Col.) Gray of the Royal Army Medical Corps (Territorial Force) was annotated Knights Commander of the Military Division of the said Most Excellent Order [83].

Gray served as consultant surgeon to the Royal Hospital for Sick Children beginning in 1923 and was appointed surgeon-in-chief at the Royal Victoria Hospital and as faculty at McGill University, Montreal, Quebec, Canada [81, 82]. The appointment of Gray at McGill University was contentious as he was not appropriately vetted and consequently usurped through the university teaching hospital appointment protocol committee chaired by Principal Sir Arthur Currie (1875–1933) [80].

In recognition of his appointment to the Royal Victoria Hospital and McGill University and commemorating his contributions while at Aberdeen, the following was said about Gray:

> The profession in the North of Scotland and indeed, throughout Great Britain will receive with very mixed feelings the announcement that Sir Henry W. Gray, KBE, CB, surgeon to the Aberdeen Royal Infirmary, has accepted the appointment of chief of the surgical staff of the Royal Victoria Hospital, Montreal. On the one hand they will congratulate Canada on having obtained his services, and Sir Henry Gray himself on the wide scope which the great McGill Medical School and the splendidly appointed Victoria Hospital will offer him; but on the other they will regret that Scotland and Aberdeen should lose a teacher of such well-deserved popularity and a surgeon of so much originality and skill [84, p. 730].

Gray resigned from his position at the Royal Victoria Hospital two years later and became a private practitioner and head of a private hospital in Montreal, Canada [80, 81].

Gray described a method for diagnosing submesenteric appendicitis:

> If one presses with the point of a finger somewhere about 11/2″ below and to the left of the umbilicus one can frequently elicit tenderness there. Occasionally, at the tender spot, there seems to be a small aperture in the rectus sheath. It is possible that this tender spot corresponds to the point of emergence of the terminal branch of the 11th dorsal nerve. The amount of pressure required to produce the feeling of tenderness is estimated. The pressure is relaxed and then with the back of the hand diffuse pressure is made and sustained over the appendix region, which is usually also tender. Then the same amount of pressure is exerted at the same spot as before on the left side, with the point of a finger of the other hand. If the sign is positive the tenderness there is not now appreciated by the patient or is lessened considerably in degree. This sign, when positive, is evidence of the presence of

either a submesenteric appendix or a Lane's terminal ileal membrane. If the presence of a retrocecal or retrocolic appendix has been already established, then this sign indicates a Lane's membrane only [85, p. 36–37].

Thus, Gray sign refers to pain occurring by pressure exerted 11/2 in. below and to the right of the umbilicus in acute appendicitis. We are unaware of any study that evaluated the sensitivity or specificity of this sign.

5.4.14 Przewalsky Sign

We could not identify any historical information on B. Przewalsky (B. Przewalski). He served as chair in the department of the I. Military Hospital Kharkov in Ukraine (Southern Russia) when he published his paper "Diagnostik der Appendicitis chronica" (Diagnostics of Chronic Appendicitis) [86].

Przewalsky identified a finding in patients with chronic appendicitis (Fig. 5.8):

> The patient lies supine on a table with the legs positioned a hand width apart. The leg to be examined lies within the heel of the examiner's hand, a few inches above the table. The examiner begins to count the seconds when his hands are removed. (…) Healthy people can maintain both legs stretched above the table for about two minutes. The extended right leg cannot remain elevated for more than 15 seconds if the right iliacus muscle is atrophic and if there is lymphadenopathy surrounding the right iliac artery [86, p. 1079].

Przewalsky identified on palpation enlarged lymph nodes surrounding the right circumflex iliac artery and atr ophy of the right iliacus muscle laterally from the external iliac artery resulting from the inflammatory process in adult patients with chronic appendicitis. These findings accounted for the functional weakness in flexion of the right leg [86, p. 1078]. We are unaware of any study that evaluated the sensitivity or specificity of this sign. Przewalsky described another finding involving air within the rectal ampulla in patients with acute appendicitis (see Chap. 6).

5.4.15 Gray (Shoulder) Sign

Irving Gray (1892–1953) was born in New York City, USA, received his medical training at New York University and in the Medical College of Bellevue Hospital, and received his medical degree from the latter in 1913 [87, 88]. He was an intern at the Jewish Hospital, Brooklyn, New York City, from 1913 to 1915, was the recipient of the Glover C. Arnold Surgical Prize in 1914 and entered general practice in 1915 [87, 89].

He was an associate in medicine and chief of the gastro-enterologic clinic at the Jewish Hospital, Brooklyn, and a gastroenterologist at the Brooklyn State Hospital [90]. He was also a staff physician at the Seaview Hospital, Staten Island, New York; consulting physician in Cumberland; Rockaway Beach Hospital; Long Beach

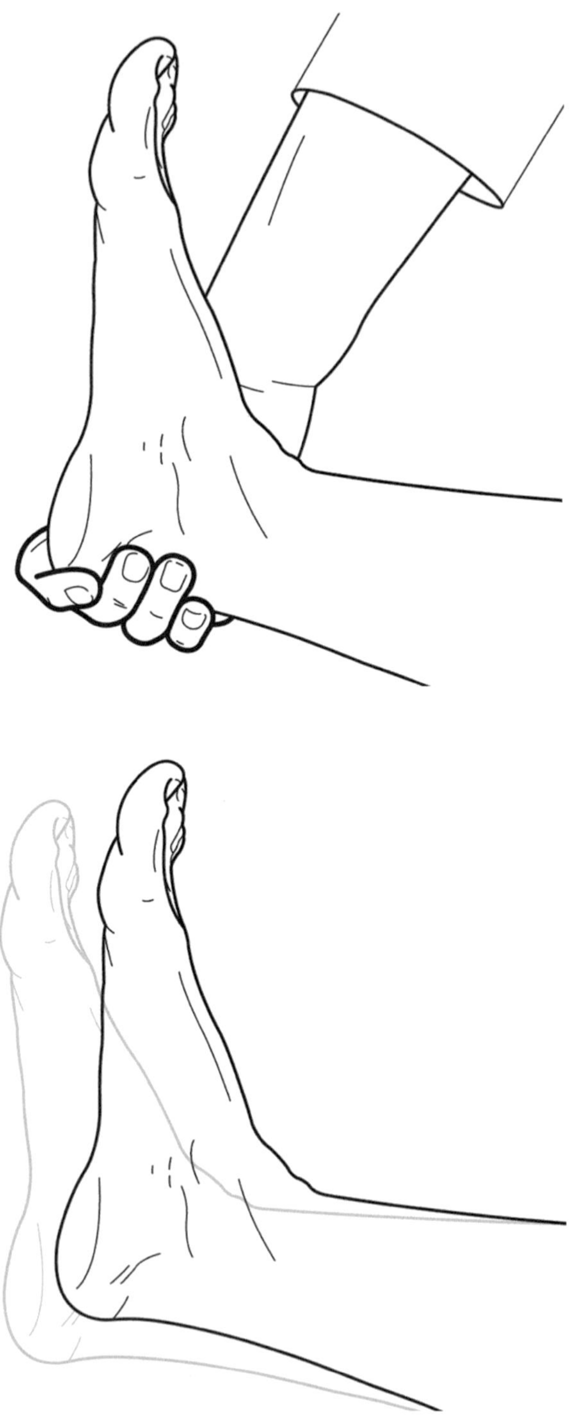

Fig. 5.8 Przewalsky sign (by Ryan Yale)

Hospital, St. Joseph's Hospital, Rockaway Beach and Post-Graduate Hospital, Manhattan, New York City. Gray served as a lieutenant in the medical corps of the United States Navy during World War I [87, 88, 90]. He was a member of the Medical Society of the State of New York, the Kings County Medical Society, American Medical Association, and the New York Heart Association [87, 91].

Gray reported on three cases by which pain in the left shoulder occurring in patients with chronic appendicitis was caused reflexively through the phrenic nerve. The pathogenesis involved:

> [a]n associated pylorospasm with increased gastric tension and upward pressure on the left diaphragm which proved to be the cause of the phrenic shoulder pain [92, p. 899]. In its origin the phrenic nerve is in communication with the descending branches of the cervical plexus. These branches become cutaneous near the clavicle. Thus we see how pain in the left shoulder region may occur when the left phrenic nerve is irritated as a result of reflex pylorus spasm in chronic appendicitis [92, p. 895].

Thus, Gray sign refers to pain in the left shoulder in patients with acute appendicitis. The pathogenesis is presumably caused by peritonitis and diaphragmatic irritation secondary to appendiceal perforation (Table 5.1).

5.4.16 Iliescu Sign

We were unable to identify any historical information on Michail (Mihail) O. Iliescu. At the time of the publication of his sign, he was an assistant surgeon in the department of the Colentian Hospital, Bucharest [93].

Iliescu described a palpatory finding in patients with acute and chronic appendicitis (Table 5.1):

> I found pain on pressure at the right phrenic point, located in the neck between the two heads of the sternocleidomastoid muscles. (…) [t]o find it, one must look for it precisely in the middle of the "phrenic triangle," formed laterally by the two heads of the sternomastoid and inferiorly by the internal segment of the clavicle. Perhaps the phrenic nerve cannot be directly compressed, and only the terminal branches of the superficial cervical plexus is compressed. The phrenic originates from the fourth, fifth, sixth, and sometimes from the third cervical nerves. Even though the pain was relatively superficial and cutaneous in some cases that does not necessarily mean that the phrenic does not externalize the painful point of the appendix in the neck. During my initial research, I believed that only the right phrenic was positive, but now I must say that the two phrenic points are sensitive to pressure. However, the right is incomparably more sensitive compared to the left. The patient is able to distinguish this difference [93, p. 315–316].

The sign was present in all of his 105 cases of acute and latent appendicitis, resolved after an appendectomy, and was absent in patients with salpingo-oophoritis and pelvic peritonitis [93]. The sign resolved when ice was applied and reoccurred when the disease flared. He postulated that the finding was caused by ascending right lymphangitis involving the phrenic nerve [93]. We are unaware of any study that evaluated the sensitivity or specificity of this sign.

5.4.17 Chapman Sign

Charles Leopold Granville Chapman (1876–1951) was born in Hessle, Yorkshire, England, studied medicine at Guy's Hospital, and was appointed member of the Royal College of Surgeons, licentiate of the Royal College of Physicians in 1897, and a fellow of the Royal College of Surgeons, England, in 1909 [94, 95]. He practiced surgery in Grimsby, England, and in 1919 was appointed to the Grimsby and District Hospital. He was a member of the Royal College of Obstetricians and Gynecologists in 1934 and chairman of the Grimsby Division of the British Medical Association from 1933 to 1934 [94, 95]. A description of his character as articulated in his obituary:

> He was one of the best of that excellent type, the general-practitioner specialist. He maintained a high standard of surgery in the local hospital. (…) Doctors scattered throughout the country will look back with gratitude and pleasure upon the warm hospitality which was always afforded to them at his home in Grimsby [95, p. 590].

Chapman described a method for diagnosing acute appendicitis and other conditions which cause an acute abdomen with peritonitis:

> The "rising test" consists in the patient putting both hands down by the side of the thighs and then raising himself in bed by means of the abdominal muscles. This produces pain immediately, and the patient fails to raise himself or complains of pain in doing so. This test will prove positive when there is little or no tenderness in the abdomen. In my hands it has frequently proved the presence of acute abdomen, and is often the decisive factor in doing an immediate operation [96, p. 786].

Thus, Chapman sign refers to pain occurring when the patient is asked to sit up from a supine position (Table 5.1). We are unaware of any study that evaluated the sensitivity or specificity of this sign.

5.4.18 Sumner Sign

There is limited historical information on Franklin W. Sumner. He practiced surgery at Dorset County Hospital, Dorchester, Dorset, England, and was elected fellow of the Royal College of Surgeons, Edinburgh [97]. He described a sign in acute appendicitis:

> The patient lies on his back, limp, his arms by his sides, breathing freely with his mouth wide open, his tongue protruded, and his glottis open (making no noise on respiration). The warmed hand of the surgeon is than placed on the lower abdomen, the metacarpophalangeal joints resting on the pubes and the fingers kept rigid, together extended, and pointing first to the right clavicle when examining the right side and to the left clavicle when examining the left side; by a gentle movement of the metacarpophalangeal joints, wrist, and elbow, and without any deep pressure of the phalanges, the muscle tone of the two sides is several times compared, when it will be found that there is a definite increase of tone on the right side as compared with the left [97, p. 106–107].

Thus Sumner sign refers to the presence of increased abdominal muscle tone in patients with peritonitis secondary to acute appendicitis (Table 5.1). We are unaware of any study that evaluated the sensitivity or specificity of this sign.

5.4.19 *Brittain Sign*

We were unable to identify any historical information on R. Brittain, an intern at the Richmond Memorial Hospital, Virginia, USA, who observed in July 1928 a finding in a patient with gangrenous appendicitis [98]. George Paul LaRoque (1876–1934) named the sign in honor of Dr. Brittain, who was the first to observe the finding and to describe the examination technique which required that (Table 5.1):

> The patient should be quietly at rest, the bedclothes pulled well down, a careful inspection made before the examining hand is applied and the patient's mind diverted from the test. Careful palpation of the left side and upper abdomen is made before the right lower quadrant is touched. Then, upon a gentle touch of the lower right quadrant, especially at the McBurney area, as soon as the finger is applied the testicle is seen to retract upwards. As long as the finger is held in contact the testicle remains in this position. As soon as it is removed the testicle will drop back to its original position. It has been observed in some cases that, with the hand remaining gently on the abdominal wall, the testicle may drop back to its original position and then upon removal of the finger will again retract (rebound retraction) [98, p. 193–194].

LaRoque, who was a professor of clinical surgery at the Medical College of Virginia and surgeon to Memorial, St. Philip, Dooley, Sheltering Arms and Retreat for the Sick Hospital, Richmond, Virginia, reported that "We have now observed in nearly 500 cases of gangrenous appendicitis and have failed to observe it in more than 300 other acute abdominal affections, such as intestinal obstruction, gallbladder and ulcer diseases, kidney and ureteral obstruction, and nonsurgical affection, such as functional colicky pains, following dietetic indiscretions and the taking of purgative medicine" [98, p. 192]. LaRoque believed that this sign is pathognomonic for gangrenous appendicitis. He postulated that activation of the motor nerve reflex arc causes contraction of the cremasteric portion of the internal oblique muscle [98].

Thus, Brittain found that in male patients with gangrenous appendicitis, pressure over the right lower abdominal quadrant caused contraction of the cremaster muscle, drawing the testis into the upper portion of the scrotum. When the pressure is released, the testis resumes its normal position (Table 5.1). Summer wrote that "I agree with LaRoque and Brittain that this sign is pathognomonic of a gangrenous appendix in a high percentage of cases" [99, p. 476]. We are unaware of any studies that evaluated the sensitivity or specificity of this sign. The pathogenesis, although not stated, may be secondary to irritation of the genital branch of the genitofemoral nerve found in the right lower quadrant.

5.4.20 *Fotheringham Sign*

Wenceslao Tejerina Fotheringham (1901–1985) was born in Rio Cuarto, Cordoba, Argentina [100, 101]. He was appointed physician to Albeto Baraldi Service at Centennial Hospital [101]. Fotheringham was a full professor of surgical pathology and associate professor of clinical surgery at the Rosario School of Medicine in 1940 [102]. The following year he was appointed head of the surgery service at the Italiano Rosario Hospital [101].

He served on the executive committee of the Fifth National Congress of Medicine in Rosario in 1934, appointed to the Official University Education Advisory Council [101]. He was an honorary professor at the Universities of Montevideo and Santiago de Chile. Fotheringham was a founding member of the Rosario Society of Surgery, serving as its president from 1938 to 1939 and 1954 to 1955. He was elected president of the Argentine Association of Surgery at the 21st Argentine Congress of Surgery [101].

Fotheringham reported a sign found in patients with acute appendicitis (Table 5.1):

> We observed an acute finding involving the peritoneum in right iliac fossa, Apply full downward pressure in the left iliac fossa and abruptly withdraw the hand, as if to investigate Rovsing's sign. The patient experiences an intense pain that radiates from the right fossa to the navel or epigastric region, sometimes traversing the midline to the left side. When the patient is asked where the pain is most severe, he sometimes points to the periumbilical region. In some cases, the sudden decompression of the left iliac fossa is accompanied by such intense pain that the confused and disoriented patient cannot accurately determine the source of pain. Repeating the maneuver once or twice more requires the patient's full attention to specify the radiation of pain [102, p. 65–66].

Fotheringham believed that the radiation of the pain to the periumbilical region when palpating and releasing the hand in the left lower quadrant is specific for acute peritonitis. He acknowledged that this sign had been previously described but differed from the one he described (Table 5.1):

> Before concluding, I want to clarify that Jacob described a similar sign in acute appendicitis, a sign known by his name that consists of pain in the right iliac fossa caused by sudden decompression on the left. Mondor stated that it is not just one more sign of peritonitis of the iliac fossa since Jacob did not mention the umbilical or epigastric radiation of this provoked pain that we judge to be of genuine diagnostic interest [102, p. 67].

We are unaware of any study that evaluated the sensitivity or specificity of this sign.

5.4.21   Mastin Sign

Edward Vernon Mastin (1891–1962) was born in Mobile, Alabama, USA, and received his medical degree from the University of Pennsylvania in 1916 and a Master of Sciences in 1922. He completed an internship at the Polyclinic Hospital from 1916 to 1917 and a surgical fellowship at the Mayo Clinic Rochester, Minnesota, from 1917 to 1922 [103–106]. During World War I, he served with distinction in the Medical Corps of the U.S. Army and was discharged with the rank of captain [103].

Mastin received his Master of Science degree in surgery at the University of Minnesota in 1922 [103, 104]. He was appointed visiting surgeon at St. Louis City Hospital and instructor in anatomy at Washington University, St. Louis, in 1926 [103]. He was an assistant professor of surgery at St. Louis University School of Medicine, chief of surgery at St. Luke's Jewish and St. Louis City Hospitals, assistant surgeon at St. Mary's and Firmin Desloge Hospitals, and consulting surgeon at the Missouri Pacific and Frisco Employees' Hospitals and Beaumont Medical

Building in St. Louis [103, 105, 106]. At the time of the publication of the sign, which bears his name, he was a surgeon in the surgical department at St. Louis University School of Medicine, St. Louis, Missouri [107]. He was a member of several medical organizations, including the St. Louis Medical Society and Surgical Societies and Southern Medical Association (president in 1945) [103, 104].

Mastin reported two cases who presented with right clavicular and shoulder pain associated with nausea and vomiting. Palpatory pressure over the area of the acutely inflamed appendix exacerbated the pain, which was relieved after an appendectomy. Mastin postulated that:

> Relief of pain in the upper chest and shoulder region following appendectomy indicates that the pain was caused by inflammation of the appendix, consequently it was referred pain. Since the areas to which the pain was referred is supplied by the third, fourth and fifth cervical nerves, the afferent impulses arising at the site of inflammation must have entered the spinal cord in the corresponding cervical segments. The only nerve connected with this segment of the spinal cord, which includes afferent fibers that reach the abdomen, is the phrenic. Consequently these must be regarded as cases in which the pain was referred via the phrenic nerve [107, p. 776].

Thus, Mastin sign refers right clavicular and shoulder pain in patients with acute appendicitis with peritonitis (Table 5.1). We are unaware of any study that evaluated the sensitivity or specificity of this sign.

5.4.22 Richet - Netter Sign

5.4.22.1 Charles Richet

Charles Robert Richet (1850–1935) was born in Paris, France, and received his medical degree from the Faculty of Medicine, University of Paris, in 1876. He was appointed associate professor of physiology in the Faculty of Medicine, Paris, in 1877 and chair of physiology from 1887 to 1927 [108–110]. With the French physiologist Paul Portier (1866–1962), he identified the immunologic phenomenon coining the term "anaphylaxis" in 1902 and was awarded the Nobel Prize for this work in 1913 [108, 109].

Richet was the recipient of the Grand Cross of the Legion of Honor, a member of the French Academy of Medicine in 1898 and the French Academy of Sciences in 1914 [108, 110]. He was editor of *Revue Scientifique* from 1878 to 1902 and co-editor of *Journal de Physiologie et de Pathologie Générale* beginning in 1917 [109]. He was editor of the 9-volume set of *Dictionnaire de Physiologie* from 1895 to 1912 [109, 110].

Richet was also a philosopher, poet, novelist, playwright, statistician, and engineer [108, 110]. His view of eugenics and his position as president of the French Eugenic Society, as expressed in his 1919 book *La Sélection Humaine* marred his accomplishments and is contrary to the principles of an eponym being an honorific term [111].

5.4.22.2 Henry Netter

We were unable to identify any historical information on Henry Netter. Richet and Netter identified the right thigh adductor muscle contracture in 40 of 50 patients with acute or chronic appendicitis:

> The patient is supine with the mouth open, thighs semi-flexed, heels flat on the bed, knees adducted, and muscles completely relaxed. The hand or fingers are placed on the medial surface of each knee. At the same time, pressure is directed outward to abduct the knees such that their external surface is in contact with the bed as the mechanism to assess for limitation of abduction. This maneuver must be performed by exerting soft, constant, and equal pressure bilaterally without jerks [112, p. 317]. The finding was independent of the position, anatomical variations, or severity of appendicitis and occurred early and late in the disease. They postulated that this condition was caused by a reflex mechanism involving the eleventh intercostal nerve. The authors noted that in most cases, there is only a slight contracture or simple hypertonia, with abduction being less on the right side than the left side. They recommend repeating the maneuver several times to appreciate the sensation of resistance during abduction [112, p. 318].

According to the authors, the sign was present in 40 of 100 children and adults with acute appendicitis, including a case of appendicular abscess [112]. Thus, Richet - Netter sign refers to the presence of hypertonia or contracture on abduction of the right thigh (Table 5.1).

5.4.23   Ben-Asher Sign

Solomon Ben-Asher (1894–1949) was born in Russia, immigrated to the USA, and resided in New Jersey throughout most of his childhood and adult life. He received his medical degree from the University and Bellevue Hospital Medical College (renamed New York Grossman School of Medicine in 2019) in 1923 [113]. He served as a cardiologist at Bellevue Hospital and a visiting physician at Greenville Hospital, New Jersey. During World War I, he served in the Army with the Chemical Warfare Branch in Washington, D.C. He was a member of the International and American Gastroenterological Associations, an associate fellow of the American College of Physicians, and a fellow of the American College of Chest Physicians [113]. As described by Irving Willner, MD, Governor of the College of Chest Physicians, New Jersey, "He was known as an inspiring and tireless worker by his friends and patients" [113].

Ben-Asher described the "cough sign" as a method to diagnose acute appendicitis:

> For many years, I have utilized the cough sign in the examination of acute abdominal cases and have found it of great value in the differential diagnosis, and almost pathognomonic of acute appendicitis. In eliciting the sign, the examiner places the tip of his fingers under the left costal margin in the region of the spleen. The patient is then asked to take a deep breath, exhale completely, and then cough. When positive, the patient will pin to the area of the suspected appendicitis as the site of severe pain [114, p. 369].

Ben-Asher did not describe the location of the pain in acute appendicitis (Table 5.1). In his study of 400 cases of patients with acute abdominal pain admitted to Greenville Hospital, New Jersey, Ben-Asher identified 198 cases of uncomplicated appendicitis and 202 cases of non-appendiceal disease. The cough sign was identified in 71% of patients with acute appendicitis and 24% with non-appendiceal disease [114].

5.4.24 Markle Sign

George Bushar Markle (1921–1999) was born in Hazleton, Pennsylvania, USA, and received his medical degree from the University of Pennsylvania Medical School, Philadelphia, Pennsylvania, in 1946 [115]. He completed an internship at Geisinger Medical Center in Danville, Pennsylvania, and a surgical fellowship at the Mayo Clinic in Rochester, Minnesota, in 1952 [115]. He served as a surgeon in World War II and was Chief of Surgery stationed during the Korean War at Fort Monroe Army Hospital, Virginia, from 1952 to 1954. He was a diplomate of the American Board of Surgery and practiced surgery at Carlsbad Regional Medical Center, New Mexico, from 1954 to 1994 [115].

Markle described the heel-drop jarring test, which is performed as follows (Table 5.1) (Fig. 5.9):

> The patient is asked to stand knees straight, with or without shoes. The clinician stands on his toes for a few seconds and, relaxing suddenly, comes down with his full weight upon his heels with a definite thump. The unsuspecting patient does likewise and may be quite surprised to feel a definite pain wherever there is inflammation in the abdomen. Not only can he tell you usually quite positively, if there is pain, but also can tell just where the pain is most severe [116, p. 721].

Markle studied 43 patients with confirmed appendicitis and found rebound tenderness in 86% and a positive heel-drop jarring test in 93%. In those patients with a positive sign, 92% were able to identify the location of their underlying disease [116]. In another similar study (1985) by Markle, a positive heel-drop jarring test was found in 74% of 190 patients with acute appendicitis, of which 71% were able to identify the underlying source of inflammation [117]. Ahn et al. (2016) found a sensitivity and specificity of 69% and 65%, respectively, for the heel-drop jarring test and a sensitivity and specificity of 59% and 63% for rebound tenderness [118]. Compared to other factors assessed in this study, the heel-drop jarring test had the highest odds ratio of 3.4 [118]. A sensitivity and specificity of 85% and 30% positive heel-drop jarring test and odds ratio of 2.5 were reported by Menteş et al. (2010) [119]. Combining other factors (white blood cell count $\geq 11.9/mm^3$ and right lower quadrant abdominal pain) with a positive heel-drop jarring test resulted in an odds ratio of 9.75 with a positive predictive value of 96% in diagnosing acute appendicitis [119]. The lower specificity identified in these studies may reflect the presence of diseases involving the abdominal wall [118, 119]. Overall, the heel-drop jarring test is useful for diagnosing acute appendicitis. Importantly, its utility is further improved when combined with other findings in acute appendicitis.

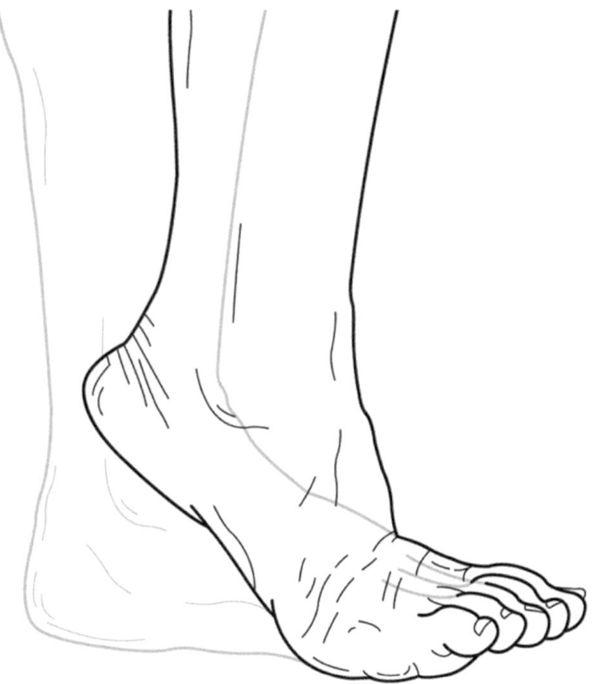

Fig. 5.9 Markle sign (by Ryan Yale)

5.4.25 *Dunphy Sign*

John Englebert Dunphy (1908–1981) was born in Northampton, Massachusetts, USA, and received his medical degree from Harvard Medical School in 1933. He was trained in surgery at Peter Bent Brigham Hospital (currently Brigham and Women's Hospital) in Massachusetts and completed a fellowship at the Lahey Clinic, Burlington, Massachusetts; Massachusetts General Hospital, Boston (George Gorham Peters Traveling Fellow); and Harvard Medical School, Boston (Arthur Cabot Research Fellow). He joined the faculty in the surgery department at Harvard Medical School, practicing in the Newton-Wellesley area in 1939 [120, 121].

During World War II, Dunphy served as captain and commanding officer of the surgical service of the Fifth General Hospital of the United States Army at Belfast and Southern England [122]. He was chief of surgery in 1943, rising to the rank of lieutenant colonel. For his meritorious service, he received the bronze star and Commander of the Ordre de la Santé Publique (The Order of Public Health) from the French government for his service to public health and protection. After the war, he returned to his prior position at Harvard and Brigham Hospital as a part-time senior associate professor [120].

Dunphy was appointed professor of surgery at Harvard Medical School and was the first director of the Fifth Surgical Service at the Boston City Hospital in 1955, where he was instrumental in establishing the Sears Surgical Laboratories. He was appointed the Kenneth H.A. MacKenzie professor of surgery and chairman of the Department of Surgery at the University of Oregon in 1959 [122]. He left Oregon and was appointed professor and chairman of the Department of Surgery at the University of California, San Francisco, in 1964. It was here that he established the trauma center and trauma research program. He also served as associate chief of staff of education at the Veterans Hospital in San Francisco from 1975 to 1979 [121].

Dunphy received many awards and accolades, including ten honorary degrees and six honorary fellowships in the Royal Colleges. He was one of the few surgeons who served as president of three surgical organizations—the American Surgical Association, the Society of University Surgeons, and the American College of Surgeons [120, 122]. A summary of Dunphy's accomplishments and character as in the words of Geoffrey Nunes, "Let us remember and honor J. Englebert Dunphy—a skilled surgeon, an organization man, a jovial party man, a caring physician, a curious biologist, an enthusiast teacher, and profound humanist who left a legacy that consists not only of surgical teaching but also of a body of philosophy about patient care" [122, p. 470]. In a tribute to Dunphy, Thomas K. Hunt wrote:

> His last written works were in support of the hospice concept and included a classic paper, "On caring for the patient with cancer". As he often did, he meant the word "caring" to have two meanings—one professional, and one very personal. He truly cared for his patients. Every resident who "cared" in a normally professional sense for one of Dunphy's patients learned how much Dunphy "cared" in the personal sense; and residents and colleagues alike who became zealously professional were made to recognize quickly how important it was "to care" in a personal sense as well [120].

Dunphy described a method for determining the presence of peritoneal inflammation in his book *Physical Examination of the Surgical Patient* (Table 5.1):

> The patient should first be asked to cough. In the presence of acute peritoneal inflammation this usually elicits a sharp twinge of pain localized to the involved area. It is extremely valuable to elicit the "cough tenderness" and have the patient point with one finger to the exact area of pain. This localizes the area of inflammation before the examiner so much as touches the patient. He can thus avoid palpating this area until the remainder of the abdominal examination is completed [123, p. 137].

Golledge et al. (1996), in a prospective study of 100 consecutive patients presenting with right lower quadrant abdominal pain, found 44 cases of histologically confirmed acute appendicitis and 14 with a normal appendix [30]. The cough test was found to have a sensitivity of 82%, a specificity of 56%, a positive predictive value of 56%, and diagnostic accuracy of 64% [30]. In a study of 866 patients with acute appendicitis, a sensitivity of 95.1% and specificity of 80% were found for Dunphy sign [124]. Dixon et al. (1991) reported an odds ratio of 1.42 for abdominal pain aggravated by coughing among 395 patients with histologically confirmed acute appendicitis [125]. Although helpful in diagnosing peritonitis, these findings suggest that Dunphy sign lacks sufficient specificity to confirm the diagnosis of acute appendicitis. Therefore, a negative sign should not exclude the diagnosis of acute appendicitis.

5.4.26   *Piulachs Sign*

Historical information on Pedro Piulachs Oliva (1908–1976) is found in the small and large bowel chapter. A sign or test (Piulachs flank pinch) and syndrome (Piulachs-Hederich) have been eponymously named in honor of Piulachs. We were unable to locate Piulachs's paper on the flank pitch sign. Accordingly, "Pain caused by compression of the right flank in the case of appendicitis. The maneuver is performed by placing the thumb on iliac spine and remaining fingers in the direction of the lumbar fossa" [126, p. 237]. The right flank is then squeezed. A positive test caused pain and abdominal guarding impeding hand closure. The same procedure should be performed on the left flank.

Table 5.1 Somatic reflex signs in appendicitis

Name	Year	Description of sign	Method	Pathophysiologic mechanism
McBurney [16]	1889	The site of greatest pain is identified by applying pressure in the right lower abdominal quadrant using one finger at a point located 1 1/2–2 in. along a straight line extending from the anterior spinous process of the ilium to the umbilicus	Palpation	Somatosensory
Perman [23]	1904	1. Muscle tension at the cecum and adjacent abdominal region when touched or lightly pressed 2. Pain localized to the ileocecal area when pressure is applied to the left side of the abdomen	Palpation	Somatomotor/somatosensory
Blumberg-Shchetkin [25, 27]	1907 1908	Apply pressure to the abdominal area where the patient complains of discomfort. Suddenly lift the palpating hand, and ask the patient whether he/she experienced pain when removing the hand. Ask the patient whether the pain worsens when the hand is depressed or removed	Palpation	Somatosensory

(continued)

Table 5.1 (continued)

Name	Year	Description of sign	Method	Pathophysiologic mechanism
Illoway [38]	1908	The patient is supine on a table or sitting on a chair. Ask the patient to flex the leg upon the thigh and the thigh upon the trunk. Then ask if the movement, or rather the upward pressure causes any pain or soreness in the lower portion of the right half of the abdomen, i.e., the appendicular region. If the answer is "no" or "very little," either further forcibly flex the thigh upon the trunk or ask the patient to do so. Again, inquire, does it cause pain or soreness, or does it increase the pain or soreness? Now ask the patient to fully extend the leg with a quick and rather sudden movement and inquire whether this caused any pain or soreness. If neither of these movements caused appreciable pain or soreness, ask the patient to execute the same movements with the left leg and compare the sensation produced to determine whether it is any different from that caused by the right leg or whether it is the same on both sides. If pain or soreness is present on flexion and extension—Place the more significant importance on extension—Regard it as a positive sign of appendicitis	Palpation	Somatosensory
Caden [40]	1911	Muscular rigidity is prominent in the lower right quadrant	Palpation	Somatomotor
Chutro [48]	1912	The abdominal midline frequently deviates to the right with the pigmentation almost always follows the tracing of the midline. The deviation follows a curved shape, with a more or less pronounced arch, convex to the right with most protruding point located at the umbilicus. Frequently it is difficult to confirm the tracing of the midline. When extending a thread from the xiphoid process to the middle of the pubic symphysis, the entire navel is placed to the right of the line as if it had moved laterally	Observation	Somatomotor (superficial reflex)

ten Horn [50]	1914	Grasp the spermatic cord between the thumb and index finger above the testes, avoiding unnecessary pressure on the testis. Gently pull the spermatic cord	Palpation	Somatosensory
Lanz [53]	1914	The right cremaster reflex is usually weakened or absent. In acute cases, when the spermatic cord is rolled back and forth as it exits the anterior inguinal ring at the medial attachment of Poupart ligament just lateral to the pubic tubercle, it is thick and exquisitely sensitive to pressure. When inserting a finger into the inguinal canal, a greater tension in the right anterior canal wall is felt compared to the left side, where one can easily and painlessly insert the fingertip or the entire index finger into the inguinal canal. The intensely stretched inferior border of the inferior oblique and transversus muscle on the right side prevents the penetration of the finger into the inguinal canal. When attempting to perform the same maneuver on the right side, it is painful, and not painful on the left side. The patient complains of pain in coughing after the finger is inserted into the inguinal canal	Palpation	Somatosensory/somatomotor
Morris [56]	1917	The greatest tenderness on pressure is at the point ½ inches to the right of the navel, close to the spinal column	Palpation	Somatosensory
Cope [72]	1919	Obturator test. The examiner slightly flexes the right thigh and then internally and externally rotates the right hip. Pain is located in the hypogastrium	Maneuver	Somatosensory
Cope [59]	1921	Iliopsoas extension. The patient lies on the left side. The examiner extends the right thigh. The location of the pain was not specified	Maneuver	Somatosensory

(continued)

Table 5.1 (continued)

Name	Year	Description of sign	Method	Pathophysiologic mechanism
Gregory [74]	1922	Percussion midway between the umbilicus and anterior superior iliac spine causes tremors of the small intestines which is transmitted unimpeded (muscle contraction is absent) to the diseased appendix, causing pain at McBurney's point. This symptom occurring in acute and subacute appendicitis is pronounced—Slight percussion causes an intense pain sensation at McBurney's point. Direct percussion at McBurney's point is also usually painful in acute and subacute appendicitis	Percussion	Somatosensory (acute, subacute)/ viscerosensory (chronic appendicitis)
Sattler [79]	1924	The patient is placed in a sitting position with the legs horizontal position to the axis of the upper body. Ask the patient to lift the right leg. In doing so, the patient flexes the hip joint, triggering isolated iliopsoas action. To accurately perform the examination, extend the legs so that the auxiliary muscles do not become active. An assistant must support the patient's back with his hand. The patient holds his hands beside his body but does not lean on them. When asked to do so, the patient tries to raise his leg. In healthy people, this occurs only under a slight angle; in weak or ill patients, of course, at an even smaller angle. Now, take hold of the patient's right leg and bend it further, asking him to point using the examiner's finger to the painful spot in his abdomen. The point, which I call the "appendix point" so designated, is the boundary point of the right lateral third, on a straight line connecting the two anterior superior iliac spines (the point determined by Lanz)	Maneuver	Somatosensory

Gray [85]	1925	Pressure is applied to the abdominal wall using the finger pointed 11/2 inches below and to the right of the umbilicus. This tender spot may have a small opening in the rectus sheath. The amount of pressure required to produce tenderness is estimated. The pressure is relaxed, and then using the dorsum of the hand, diffuse pressure is made and sustained over the appendix region. The same amount of pressure is exerted at the exact location on the left side using the point of a finger on the left hand.	Palpation	Somatosensory
Przewalsky [86]	1925	The patient lies supine on a table with the legs positioned a hand width apart. The leg to be examined lies within the heel of the examiner's hand, a few inches above the table. The examiner begins to count the seconds when his hands are removed. (…) healthy people can maintain both legs stretched above the table for about 2 minutes. The extended right leg cannot remain elevated for more than 15 seconds if the right iliacus muscle is atrophic and if there is lymphadenopathy surrounding the right iliac artery	Maneuver	Somatomotor
Gray (shoulder) [92]	1925	Pain in the left shoulder	Observation	Somatosensory (chronic appendicitis)
Iliescu [93]	1926	Pain on pressure occurs at the right phrenic point, located in the neck between the two heads of the sternocleidomastoid muscles. The pain occurs in the middle of the "phrenic triangle," which is formed laterally by the two heads of the sternomastoid and inferiorly by the internal segment of the clavicle. The right phrenic point is more sensitive compared to the left	Palpation	Somatosensory
Chapman [96]	1927	The patient places their hands down by the side of the thighs and is asked to raise himself/herself in bed using only their abdominal muscles	Passive	Somatosensory

(continued)

Table 5.1 (continued)

Name	Year	Description of sign	Method	Pathophysiologic mechanism
Sumner [97]	1930	The patient lies quietly on his/her back with the arms lying by their side, breathing freely with their mouth wide open, tongue protruding, and glottis open. The examiner places his/her warm hand on the lower abdomen with the metacarpophalangeal joints resting on the pubis. The fingers are rigid, adducted, extended, and pointing first to the right clavicle when examining the right side and to the left clavicle when examining the left side. Compare the muscle tone of the two sides by gently moving the metacarpophalangeal joints, wrist, and elbow without any deep finger pressure	Palpation	Somatomotor
Brittain [98]	1931	Carefully palpate the left side of the abdomen. Superficially palpate the right lower quadrant at McBurney point. When the finger is applied to this area, the testicle retracts upwards. The testicle drops back to its original position as soon as the finger is removed. In some cases, while the hand remaining gently on the abdominal wall, the testicle may drop back to its original position. Upon removing the hand, the testicle retracts (rebound retraction)	Palpation	Somatomotor
Fotheringham [102]	1934	Apply full downward pressure in the left iliac fossa and abruptly withdraw the hand. The patient experiences intense pain that radiates from the right fossa to the navel or epigastric region, sometimes traversing the midline to the left side. Ask the patient where the pain is most severe, and he/she sometimes points to the periumbilical region. In some cases, the sudden decompression of the left iliac fossa causes such intense pain that the patient cannot accurately determine the source of pain. Repeat the maneuver several times to clarify the location of the pain's radiation	Palpation	Somatosensory

Mastin [107]	1936	Relief of pain in the upper chest and shoulder region following appendectomy indicates that the pain is due to inflammation of the appendix; consequently, it represents referred pain	Observation	Somatosensory
Richet-Netter [112]	1937	The patient is supine with the mouth open, thighs semi-flexed, heels flat on the bed, knees adducted, and muscles completely relaxed. Place the hand or fingers on the medial surface of each knee. At the same time, apply pressure outward to abduct the knees such that their external surface is in contact with the bed as the mechanism to assess for limitation of abduction. Perform this maneuver by exerting soft, constant, and equal pressure bilaterally without jerks. In most cases, there is only a slight contracture or simple hypertonia, with abduction being less on the right side than the left side. Repeat the maneuver several times to appreciate the sensation of resistance during abduction	Palpation	Somatomotor
Ben-Asher [114]	1943	The examiner places the tip of his/her fingers under the left costal margin. Ask the patient to take a deep breath, exhale, and cough	Palpation and cough	Somatosensory
Markle [116]	1973	Ask the patient to stand with the knees straight, with or without shoes, and observe the examiner. The clinician stands on his/her toes for a few seconds and relaxes suddenly, coming down with his/her full weight upon their heels with a definite thump. The patient now completes the same maneuver. Ask the patient if they experienced pain and, if so, its location	Observation	Somatosensory
Dunphy [123]	1975	Ask the patient to cough	Cough	Somatosensory
Piulachs [126]	[n.a.]	Place the thumb on the right iliac spine and remaining fingers in the direction of the lumbar fossa. Squeeze the flank	Palpation	Somatosensory/somatomotor

5.5 Visceral Segmental Nerve Pathway Signs

The activation of visceral nerve pathways occurs in early acute or chronic appendicitis when the disease remains primarily confined to the appendix. As previously noted, in some cases, when the appendiceal inflammatory infiltrates is rapid and severe in onset, visceral afferent nerve fibers in the dorsal root ganglion may "spillover" to involve somatic efferent nerves (cerebrospinal pathways), leading to abdominal wall pain and spasms (guarding) at spinal cord segments T10–T11 (viscerosensory and visceromotor reflexes). Furthermore, it is important that physicians distinguish pain found on superficial versus deep palpation and recognize that both superficial and deep pain may be present in the case of peritonitis secondary to appendiceal perforation, which may be clinically indistinguishable. A carefully performed physical examination may assist in sorting out and sorting through these findings.

5.6 Eponymous Sign

5.6.1 Meltzer Sign

Samuel James Meltzer (1851–1920) was born in Ponevyezh, Courland, Russia (currently Lithuania), and received a doctor of medicine degree at the University of Berlin, Germany, in 1882 [127, 128]. He immigrated to New York City in 1883 to practice medicine and later conducted research at the Welch Laboratory at Bellevue and the Curtis and Prudden Laboratories at the College of Physicians and Surgeons (currently Vagelos College of Physicians and Surgeons). He was appointed head of the Department of Physiology and Pharmacology in 1907 [128].

Meltzer was elected president of the American Physiological Society, Society for Experimental Biology and Medicine, American Gastro-Physiological Society, American Society for the Advancement of Clinical Research, Association of American Physicians, American Association for Thoracic Society (1918), and Society of Clinical Investigation [129]. Noteworthy, he founded the societies of Experimental Biology of Medicine and the American Society of Clinical Investigation. He served as chair of the Department of Experimental Physiology and Pharmacology at the Rockefeller Institute of Medical Research, New York, from 1903 to 1919 [128, 129]. His contributions to medical sciences were unparalleled, spanning multiple scientific disciplines. He pioneered an artificial respiration technique as a means to provide anesthesia during surgery in 1912, recognized asthma as an allergic disease, promoted the use of face masks to prevent infectious diseases, recommended the use of oxygen in heart disease, established the use of a nasogastric tube for prolonged gastric feeding, recommended the use of the abdomen for dialysis, developed an assay for adrenalin, and identified the relationship between a strained pancreatic emulsion and its ability to lower glucose levels [128, 130].

A brief reflection and insight into Meltzer's character and intellect as described by Howell:

> He was not content to simply catalogue his observations and publish them as isolated facts which somehow would find their place in the growing structure of science. They were for him the subject of much reflection. He regarded them as revelation of the processes of the body which he must try to interpret, and his genuinely scientific mind was constantly seeking to formulate general theories to fit or to embrace the facts that were disclosed by his experiments. Nothing seemed to give him greater pleasure than to discuss these theoretical possibilities with his fellow workers, and from many conversations of this kind which it was my good fortune to enjoy I got always the impression of a mind constantly on the alert to understand and interpret his results and full of a certain eager expectancy of discoveries of importance. His theories and generalizations in turn supplied him with the interest and energy to devise new work, so that throughout his long career there was never any lack of problems to be attacked nor any diminution in enthusiasm for research [130, p. 6].

Meltzer described a method for distinguishing appendicitis from circumscribed rheumatic myositis in 1902 (Table 5.2):

> After pressing firmly over the tender spot until a distinct pain is elicited, I relax the pressure to such a degree as to leave just a minimum of pain, and then induce the patient to flex the thigh gradually to a strong degree. If the pain is due to a tissue lying between the abdominal wall and iliopsoas, it becomes immediately intensified, in fact the patient refuses soon to continue the contraction. When the pain is due to a rheumatic myositis, the contraction of the iliopsoas exerts practically no effect upon it [131, p. 102].

Meltzer did not define the location of the pain with this maneuver. Pain is likely caused by tenderness upon palpation by the examiner's finger on the inflamed appendix. We are unaware of any study that assessed the sensitivity or specificity of this sign.

5.6.2 Sherren Sign

James Sherren (1872–1945) was born in Weymouth, Dorset, England, and received his medical training from the London Hospital Medical College, qualifying as a fellow of the Royal College of Surgeons, England, in 1900 [132]. He was appointed demonstrator of anatomy and surgical tutor to the London Hospital Medical College, followed by appointments at the London Hospital as a surgical registrar in 1901 and assistant surgeon in 1902 [132, 133]. Sherren was elected a member of the Royal Medical and Chirurgical Society (merged with other societies to become the Royal Society of Medicine in 1903) and the Clinical Society of London in 1906 (merged with the Royal Society of Medicine in 1907) [134, 135]. During World War I, as colonel of the Army Medical Services, he served as consulting surgeon to the War Office and Yarrow Military Hospital, Broadstairs, and surgeon to the King George Military Hospital and King Edward VII's Hospital for Officers. He was awarded the

Commander of the Order of the British Empire medal for his services in 1919 [132, 133].

At the University of London, he served as an examiner for surgery and was a member of the Senate. In 1926, he resigned to serve as a naval medical officer. On his return, he resumed surgical practice at the Cornelia and East Dorset Hospital, Poole, England [132]. Regarding his character and unique characteristics in the words of Mr. H. Souttar:

> The passing of James Sherren closes a unique career and removes a figure memorable in the story of the London Hospital. (…) He was a great surgeon and a great teacher, but it will always be a real man that we shall remember him. (…) [t]hose of us who know him realized that in his life there were three great loves—the sea, music, and his work [132, p. 670].

Within the Royal College of Surgeons, he served as an examiner in anatomy for the primary fellowship, a member of the Court of Examiners, and from 1917 to 1926 was a member of the Council, acting as a vice-president from 1925 to 1927 [133].

He identified a method for delineating cutaneous hyperalgesia in cases of acute appendicitis (Table 5.2) (Fig. 5.10):

> Cutaneous hyperalgesia is tested by gently pinching or stroking the skin, beginning if possible, in an area which is not tender and working towards the suspected tender area and so marking out its boundaries. Care is necessary in order to avoid bringing out any deep tenderness which may be present. The skin only must be stimulated and all pressure on deeper structures avoided. In appendicitis cutaneous hyperalgesia varies from a complete band extending on the right side from the middle line below the umbilicus in front to the lumbar spines behind, down to a small circular spot a little above the middle point between the umbilicus and the anterior superior spine. This band corresponds to the eleventh dorsal area of head. Very often the tenderness extends somewhat into the tenth dorsal area also and occasionally, but not often, into the twelfth dorsal area, sending a tongue shaped process over the gluteal region. The width of the band is in an adult about three inches [136, p. 817].

Sherren also reported on a cutaneous area more commonly found in patients with acute appendicitis:

> The usual area is on the right side of the abdomen and of a triangular shape. So often is this triangular area present that I am in the habit of describing it in my notes as the "appendix triangle" of cutaneous tenderness. This triangle is situated to the right iliac regions. Its lower boundary reaches almost to Poupart's ligament. Its inner almost to the middle line, and its apex is a little outside the anterior superior spine, sometimes extending to the mid-axillary line [136, p. 817].

Sherren described the area(s) of cutaneous hyperalgesia, which he attributed to the degree of distension of the appendix. Thus, this finding represents a viscerosensory reflex. We are unaware of any study that evaluated the sensitivity or specificity of this sign.

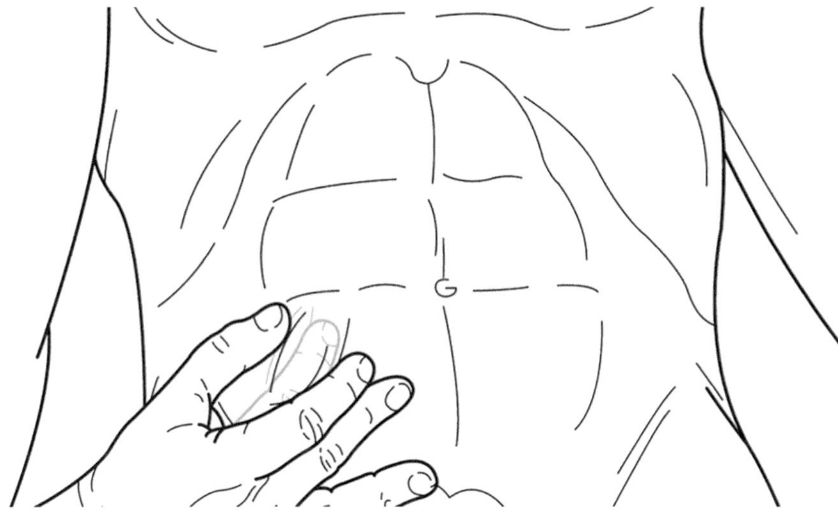

Fig. 5.10 Sherren sign (by Ryan Yale)

5.6.3 Mackenzie Sign

Sir James Mackenzie (1853–1925) was born in the town of Scone in highland Perthshire, Scotland, and received his bachelor of medicine and master of surgery degrees from Edinburgh University in 1878 [137–140]. He was appointed resident physician at Edinburgh Royal Infirmary, followed by further medical training in Vienna [139, 140]. He was involved in general medical practice with William Briggs and John Brown in Burley, Lancashire, in 1879 [138, 140]. Mackenzie received his medical degree in 1882. He moved to London as a general practitioner in 1907, was appointed to the Mount Vernon Hospital for Diseases of the Chest in 1909, and at the London Hospital as a lecturer on cardiac research in 1910. He led the cardiac department at the London Hospital in 1913 and was a cardiac consulting physician until 1918 [136–140]. During World War I, from 1914 to 1918, Mackenzie was instrumental in establishing a military heart hospital in Colchester in 1917 [141, 142]. He moved to St. Andrews, Scotland as a private practitioner and founded the Institute for Clinical Research [137, 139, 141]. The institute aimed to elucidate the significance of symptoms early in the disease course to prevent common diseases [138]. In addition to understanding cardiac arrhythmia and murmurs, Mackenzie's work sought to assess the impact of signs and symptoms on the disease state and prognosis.

He published his first book, *The Study of the Pulse*, in 1902 and *Diseases of the Heart* in 1907. He was knighted and elected fellow of the Royal Society in 1915 and was an honoring consulting physician to the King in Scotland in 1920 [138–140]. The Sir James Mackenzie Cardiological Society was named in his honor in 1926 and was the antecedent to the American College of Cardiology [142].

As to a description of his character:

> From all accounts it appears that Mackenzie was, to use the simplest language, both a great and good man. Few physicians have ever given so much of themselves to their patients, and it is certain that none have done so while at the same time carrying out first-rate research. His richness in humility and gentleness made him deeply loved not only by his patients but by all his colleagues [137, p. 483].

The sensory nerves from appendicitis arise from the right eleventh and twelfth dorsal and first and second lumbar spinal cord segments. Mackenzie recognized that:

> Not only may the disturbance of these nerve cells be recognized by the presence of pain, but their excessive irritability can be demonstrated by the presence of hyperanesthesia in the tissues forming the external body wall. (…) It is more readily demonstrated, however, in the erector spinae and muscles of the abdomen, and particularly in those over the right iliac fossa. The slightest pressure here is often felt as pain. One can readily demonstrate that the tenderness is not due to the inflamed peritoneum by slightly raising a portion of muscle away from the peritoneum before applying pressure, or, in cases where the pain and tenderness is widespread, by finding this tenderness in the muscles of the lumbar region, where pressure can be applied without the possibility of involving the peritoneum [143, p. 67].

Thus, Mackenzie sign refers to the superficial cutaneous hyperesthesia involving the right erector muscles and muscles in the right iliac fossa in patients with appendicitis (Table 5.2).

5.6.4 Sicard Sign

Jean-Marie-Athanase Sicard (1872–1929) was born in Marseille, France, studied medicine in Marseille and hospitals in Paris, and received his medical degree in 1899 [144]. He completed an internship in neurology and a doctoral thesis on the cerebrospinal fluid in patients with neurosyphilis under the aegis of George-Fernand-Isidore Widal (1862–1929) in 1901. Sicard was appointed chief of the clinic in 1901, Doctor of the Paris Hospital in 1903, and associate professor in 1907 [144]. During World War I, he served as an attendant, followed by the head of the neurological center for the Marseille region in Toulon, France. He was appointed chief of services from 1910 to 1929 and professor of medical pathology at the Necker Hospital, Paris, in 1923 [144]. Among his other contributions, he introduced injecting a sclerosing solution for varicose veins and alcohol for treating trigeminal neuralgia and described a technique for managing peripheral nerve injuries, amputation stumps, and causalgia (currently named complex regional pain syndrome). He and his student Jacques Forestier (1890–1978) introduced Lipiodol® as a radiopaque contrast agent in diagnostic radiology [144]. Regarding his character:

> From the life and work of Jean Sicard, we draw another lesson. Research and purpose, research for purpose. I would say that these were the two driving forces of this great physician. But research must not lose sight of its objective, which is to contribute to the relief of the sick. Sicard knew that medicine has a lot to lose by moving too far away from the sick and that research should not be locked in the secrecy of faculties or in the sanctuary of the laboratory [145, p. 61].

He described the absence of the superficial abdominal reflex in patients with acute appendicitis:

> Suddenly under the influence of a unilateral excitation, we see the abdominal wall contract into a depression often localized to the corresponding side. It is necessary that the touch is fast and elicited, for example, by the nail gliding superficially over the skin. If the contact causes a painful pinching or pinprick of the skin, the abdominal muscles become immobilized, and the reflex is ineffective. A rim located at the epigastric cutaneous region under the false ribs corresponds to the superior third of the abdominal muscle contraction, the para-umbilical region contraction is located at the middle third, and contraction of the lower third occurs near the hypogastric region. By the way, each of these three reflexes is elicited by moving the finger from a central medial to a lateral position over the muscle. Here, the right abdominal reflex and its para-umbilical type (hypogastric) must be involved since these are the ones affected in most moderately affected cases of appendicitis. At the same time, the left side continues to react normally. In four cases successfully treated, I noted the unilateral absence of the right abdominal reflex during the acute episode and that the reflex quickly returned to normal during convalescence. In a more recent observation in a case of peritonitis, the reflex was absent bilaterally. (…) [i]n two cases of appendicitis, the unilateral sign existed concurrently with pain, exquisite hyperesthesia, and abdominal muscle contraction [146, p. 19].

Thus, Sicard sign refers to the absence of the right superficial abdominal nerve reflexes in patients with appendicitis (Table 5.2). The superficial abdominal reflex involves spinal cord segments T6–T12, whereby the upper abdomen involves the T6–T8, midabdominal T8–T10, and lower abdomen (T10–T12) nerves. The absence of a superficial abdominal reflex in acute appendicitis may reflect activation of visceromotor reflexes or ongoing inflammation of the parietal peritoneum causing persistent pain and reflex spasm of the abdominal wall in the right lower quadrant (somatomotor reflex). We are unaware of any study that evaluated this sign's sensitivity of specificity.

5.6.5 *Berthomier-Michelson Sign*

5.6.5.1 André-Auguste Berthomier

André-Auguste Berthomier (1848–1914) was born in Allier, Langy, France, and served as an interne of the Lyon Hospital from 1842 to 1846. He was appointed adjunct surgeon in the Moulin Hospital in 1848 [147]. During the time of the publication of his book titled, *Mécanisme des Fractures du Coude chez les Enfants, leur Traitement par l'Extension* (Mechanism of Elbow Fractures in Children, Their Treatment by Extension), he was a doctor of medicine at the Faculty of Paris and Laureate of the School of Medicine for which he served from the period of 1869 to 1871 [147, 148]. Berthomier was a physician at the Secondary School in Seine, Yzeures, in 1888; chief of surgery at the General Hospital in 1891 and Moulin Hospital in 1898—the latter for which he was later recognized as an honorary surgeon [148]. His son, named André Berthomier—also a physician, wrote his thesis at the Paris School of Medicine in 1906 titled, *Les Courants de Haute Fréquence dans les Dermatoses (Dites Autrefois) Diathésiques (Prurit, Eczéma, Psoriasis, Acné)* (High Frequency Currents in Dermatoses, Formerly Called-Diathetic: Pruritus,

Eczema, Psoriasis, Acne). He was honored as a recipient of the Legion of Honor (Chevalier) on July 11, 1908 [147, 148].

Berthomier, at the 19th French Congress of Surgery in 1906, described a finding that he believed to be pathognomonic for chronic appendicitis (Table 5.2):

> The symptoms consist of the very marked differences in the pain intensity caused by the pressure on the cecal-appendicular region based on whether the patient is supine or in the left lateral decubitus position. The characteristic difference is often the only symptom to recognize chronic appendicitis. Several times I found that exploration of McBurney point in the supine position left suspicion for the presence of chronic appendix. In contrast, exploration in the lateral decubitus confirmed my impression [149, p. 167].

From his description, it is unclear the intensity of the palpatory pressure exerted in the right lower abdominal quadrant at McBurney point. Furthermore, he did not expressly state the location of the pain. Based on what is known regarding superficial and deep pain, and the nature and course of chronic appendicitis, it is inferred that Berthomier was applying firm and deep pressure at the right lower quadrant abdomen. Berthomier described his experience with this maneuver:

> I also studied the same symptom in 57 cases treated with either a right salpingectomy or right salpingectomy with subtotal hysterectomy. On examination, I found the opposite result, mainly; acute pain was present in the supine position and either absent or less intense in the left lateral position. In no case was there a diseased appendix or cecum. In 10 other cases where the bimanual examination indicated salpingitis, pressure in the left lateral decubitus position produced an overt exacerbation of pain. In these cases, the appendix was adherent to the ovary and the fallopian tube [149, p. 169].

It is believed that the left lateral recumbent position causes the omentum, intestines, mesentery, fallopian tube, and other non-retroperitoneal structures to be displaced to the left, enhancing the accessibility of the appendix, a fixed structure to direct palpation.

Some authors refer to this as the Berthomier-Michelson sign. There is a 1911 manuscript published by F.G. Michelson, titled "Zur Frage von der primären chronischen Appendizitis und ihrer differentiellen Diagnose" (On the Question of Primary Chronic Appendicitis and Its Differential Diagnosis). However, this paper postdates Berthomier's description in 1906 [150].

5.6.6 Rovsing Sign

Niels Thorkild Rovsing (1862–1927) was born in Flensburg, Germany, and received his medical degree from the University of Copenhagen in 1885 [151, 152]. He earned his doctorate in 1889 based on research conducted at the Frederik Hospital Clinical-Surgical Laboratory, Denmark, titled, *On the Etiology, Pathogenesis, and Treatment of Cystitis*. He was appointed reserve surgeon for Oscar Thorvald Bloch (1847–1926) from 1889 to 1892, a surgeon at Queen Louis's Children Hospital, Denmark from 1892 to 1902, and chief surgeon at the Red Cross Hospital, Platanvej, Copenhagen, Denmark, from 1896 to 1900 [151, 153]. Concurrently, he started in collaboration with Eilert Adam Tscherning (1851–1919) and Leopold Meyer (1852–1918), a private clinic in Lundsgade followed by another in Vendersgade, Copenhagen, where he practiced until 1899. In 1899, Rovsing received a teaching appointment as a professor of operative surgery in Rosenvænget, Copenhagen. However, he was compelled to establish a private surgical clinic to care for his patients because he was not allowed access to hospital beds [152, 153].

Rovsing was a senior surgeon at the Kongelig Frederiks (King Frederick) Hospital in Copenhagen in 1904 [151, 152]. He supported the construction of the Rigshospitalet (State Hospital), Copenhagen, a more modern hospital for its time established in 1910 to replace the Kongelig Frederiks Hospital, as its primary goal was to improve the delivery of surgical care. His chief work was in cystitis, tuberculosis of the urinary tract, and diseases involving the gallbladder and gallstones [151]. He served as a co-editor for the *Hospitalstidende* journal in 1892 and editor-in-chief in 1908 [148]. Rovsing was a founding member, in collaboration with Eilert Adam Tscherning (1851–1919) of the Danish Medical Society in 1908, and an honorary member of the Edinburgh Medico-Chirurgical Society and the Association of Surgeons of Great Britain and Ireland [151, 152]. Among his other accomplishments, he was a consistory member in 1911, honorary doctor of surgery in 1914, and rector from 1919 to 1920 at the University of Copenhagen. He was appointed Minister of Education of Denmark in 1920 [153]. A tribute to Rovsing as described in his obituary:

> The death of Professor Rovsing has robbed the Danish medical profession of a striking and forceful personality. It is always difficult to say how much anyone's success in life depends on character and personality and how much on intellect. But in Rovsing's case there can be no doubt that, both in force of character and weight of intellect, he was a head and shoulders above his fellows [151].

Rovsing described in his 1907 paper titled "Indirektes Hervorrufen des typischen Schmerzes an McBurney's Punkt: Ein Beitrag zur Diagnostik der Appendizitis und Typhlitis" (Indirect Method of Evoking Typical Pain at McBurney's Point: A Contribution to the Diagnosis of Appendicitis and Typhlitis), a method for diagnosing appendicitis and typhlitis (Fig. 5.11):

> I wondered whether I could elicit the typical pain in the right iliac fossa by applying pressure at the left iliac fossa. This involves compressing the descending colon by pushing the fingers of my right hand onto the fingers of the left hand placed flat against the abdomen in the left iliac fossa. Using this method, the hands slide upward toward the left colonic flexure [154, p. 1258].

Rovsing described a proposed mechanism for the pathogenesis of this maneuver (Table 5.2):

> I thought that the pain at McBurney's point was due to the increased pressure and tension caused by gas within the transverse colon. The cecum and appendix are known to be strongly influenced by increased pressure and resistance caused by strictures within the rectum and at the sigmoid flexure and ileocecal valve, which prevents gas from escaping into the small intestines. Within the cecum, the opening to the appendix is the only place where intestinal gas is forced. I believe that in cases of appendicitis or cecal inflammation, increased tension by compression of the intestines produces pain at the point of the inflammation. I did not expect that this maneuver would be such a fine, safe and valuable diagnostic aid as it turned out when it was used in over 100 cases [154, p. 1257].

Physicians often inaccurately perform this maneuver, applying only downward pressure with one or both hands in the left lower quadrant or applying deep and even pressure in the left lower quadrant and then suddenly release the hand(s) [155, 156] (see Sect. 5.4.20). This reflects the incorrect translation of this sign in the English literature [156]. Traube described palpatory pressure in the left lower quadrant in 1871 and Perman in 1904. However, Rovsing sign is unique in that it involves palpatory downward pressure and compression in coordination with a sliding movement toward the left colonic flexure. Thus, a positive Rovsing sign refers to the presence of right lower quadrant abdominal pain caused by the retrograde movement of intestinal gas causing increased tension at the cecum and inflamed appendix in a patient with a competent ileocecal valve. Others have postulated that the pain is caused by impingement of the inflamed appendix due to rightward displacement of the ileum or shifting and friction of the inflamed appendix against the parietal peritoneum [157].

Davey found the sign to be positive in 5 of 303 cases of acute appendicitis [156]. After performing this maneuver, he could not identify any evidence through manometric or barium enema studies of gas in the cecal region [157]. These findings support the contention that the mechanism is due to inflammation of the parietal peritoneum over the iliopsoas muscle. If that is the case, then the maneuver represents a somatosensory, not a viscerosensory reflex.

A positive likelihood ratio ranging from 1.5 to 4.23 with a sensitivity ranging from 19% to 75% and a specificity of 58% to 93% has been reported for this sign [157]. These findings suggest that this sign may be helpful in diagnosing acute appendicitis, albeit limited, which may reflect the inconsistency in technique, the extent of the disease (confined to the appendix or involving the parietal peritoneum) when performing this maneuver, or incompetent ileocecal valve.

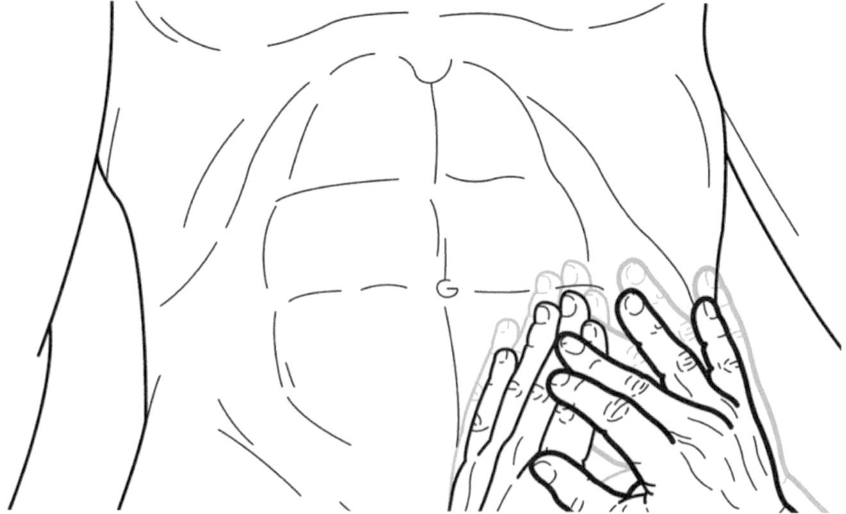

Fig. 5.11 Rovsing sign (by Ryan Yale)

5.6.7 *Chase Sign*

Ira Carleton Chase (1868–1933) was born in Oberlin, Ohio, USA, and received his A.M. degree from Oberlin College, Ohio in 1898 [158, 159]. He was initially appointed professor of physics and chemistry at the old Fort Worth University, Texas, in 1893 and chair of chemistry and toxicology in 1894 [158, 159]. He later pursued a medical career and received his medical degree from the New York and Bellevue Hospital Medical College in 1899. After graduation, he worked in group practice in Fort Worth, Texas, and was appointed professor of anatomy in the medical department in 1901 and chair in 1910 at Fort Worth University. He was dean of the Fort Worth Medical College and associate professor of surgery in 1913 [158, 159].

Chase was associate editor of the *Oberlin Review* from 1890 to 1891, co-editor of the *Texas Medical Gazette*, and first editor-in-chief of the *Texas State Journal of Medicine* from 1905 to 1910 [158]. He was active in the Texas Medical Association serving as general secretary at Denison, Texas, from 1902 to 1903. He was also the Texas delegate to the American Medical Association and served as a judicial council member [158]. Chase was a fellow of the American College of Surgeons in 1915. He authored the textbooks *The Chemical Examination of Gastric Contents* in 1891 and *A Laboratory Manual of Medical Chemistry* in 1897 [158, 159].

As to a description of his character:

> C.S. Laymen who have come to know Doctor Chase of Fort Worth have been impressed not only by his unusual abilities in his profession but equally well by his personal character his elevated purpose, and all the qualities that make the physician a real leader in the slow evolution of humanity to a higher and better civilization [160, p. 144].

Chase described a palpatory method which he referred to as the "cecal distension test" for diagnosing acute appendicitis (Table 5.2):

> The patient is best placed on a hard, low bed or table. The knee should be flexed and two pillows placed under the head and shoulders, giving a dorsal semirecumbent position, rendering the abdomen flaccid for the most satisfactory abdominal compression. The surgeon stands on the patient's left, facing the feet. The palmar surfaces of the fingers on the right hand are placed under the patient's left inguinal region and the fingers of the left hand used to reinforce the right. Deep pressure is then made backward, slowly drawing the fingers deeply and forcibly upward under the left costal arch. This procedure is intended to compress the lower portion of the descending colon and force its gaseous content into the transverse, and thence to the ascending colon. The pressure being maintained with the fingers of the left hand, the right hand is then removed and placed over the upper portion of the descending colon, or better and forcibly depressed. A gaseous compression wave will travel across the transverse and down the ascending colon and on arriving at the cecum will produce cecal distention, yielding a typical sharp pain in the right iliac fossa, if inflammation of the cecum or appendix be present [161, p. 610].

Chase postulated that the maneuver:

> [i]f carefully carried out will demonstrate conclusively, I believe, the presence or absence of active inflammation in the cecum or appendix by the typical colicky pains usually following in the right iliac region [161, p. 610].

He found that the test was helpful in patients with rigidity or tenderness in the right lower quadrant precluding direct palpation in this region. Chase acknowledged the paper published by Rovsing, entitled "Indirektes Hervorrufen des typischen Schmerzes an McBurney's Punkt" (Indirect Production of Typical Pain at McBurney's Point) in *Zentralblatt für Chirurgie* on November 5, 1907, prior to completion of this paper presented to the North Texas Medical Association in December 1907 [161].

5.6.8 Bastedo Sign

Walter Arthur Bastedo (1873–1952) was born in Newmarket, Ontario, Canada, and received his doctorate in pharmacy from the New York College of Pharmacy and medical degree from Columbia University College of Physicians and Surgeon (currently Columbia University Vagelos College of Physicians and Surgeons), New York, in 1899 [162, 163]. Throughout his career, he was affiliated with St. Mary's, St. Vincent's, and Staten Island (consulting physician), City Hospital (attending physician from 1913 to 1919), and St. Luke's Hospital, New York [164, 165]. He was appointed attending staff at St. Luke's Hospital, ascending to the attending and consultant physician rank from 1899 to 1927 [162, 165].

He was an instructor in pharmacology at Cornell University Medical School, New York, from 1899 to 1901, an instructor in materia medica and pharmacology, an assistant in applied therapeutics, an associate in pharmacology, and an assistant professor of clinical medicine at Columbia University College of Physicians and Surgeons [162, 163, 166]. At Columbia University's Vanderbilt Clinic, he served as chief of the clinic in gastroenterology from 1902 to 1908 [167].

Bastedo was a member of the New York Board of Health advisory council from 1911 to 1919. He was chairman of the section of pharmacy and therapeutics of the American Medical Association from 1918 to 1919 and president and chairman of the board of trustees on revisions to the *United States Pharmacopoeia* from 1919 to 1920 [161]. Bastedo served as councilor of the gastroenterologist association in 1919 and officer of the New York Association for Medical Education in 1921 [167–169]. He received the honorary degree of Doctor of Science from Columbia University in 1929 and an honorary degree of Master of Science from Philadelphia College of Pharmacy and Science in 1934 [163].

Bastedo read before the Medical Society of the County of Richmond, Virginia, a method of dilating the colon to differentiate chronic appendicitis from other causes of right lower quadrant abdominal pain. The method involves insufflating air into the colon using an atomizer bulb and a soft rubber rectal tube. He reported in patients with chronic appendicitis (Table 5.2):

> In the routine examination of digestive patients by colon dilation, I noted, some three years ago, that acute pain or tenderness in the region of McBurney's point on dilatation of the colon regularly meant appendicitis. I have now many cases in which the finding has proven

by operation, and in every case operated upon in which the sign was positive a disease appendix has been found. (…) In no operation cases with the sign negative was appendicitis found [170, p. 110].

In 37 patients undergoing laparotomy for abdominal pain, this sign was positive in 23 patients with chronic appendicitis [171, p. 398]. Hertz in his 1913 paper on Bastedo sign reported:

> In my own experience, I have only obtained a positive Bastedo's sign in appendicitis, the appendix having always been found diseased at the subsequent operation, with the possible exception of one case, which is still too recent to form a judgment as to whether the removal of an apparently normal appendix will cause the symptoms to disappear [172, p. 187].

Although not a practical maneuver, Bastedo sign used a nonpalpatory technique to introduce air into the proximal colonic segment. He did not describe the location of the pain induced by this maneuver. Thus, it represented another method similar to that proposed by Rovsing, Owen, and Chase, causing air to move into the ascending colon and appendix. We are unaware of any study that evaluated the sensitivity or specificity of this sign.

5.6.9 Caden Sign

Historical information about Eliot and Corscaden is found under the somatic segmental nerve pathway signs section. The sign eponymously named for Caden reported that the abdominal rigidity in appendicitis as distinguished from intussusception "[i]is almost always most marked in the lower right quadrant, while in intussusception the symptom, if present, is generally more marked on one side or the other of the umbilicus, while the intervening abdomen between this area and either inguinal region is either less rigid or entirely free from any rigidity whatever" [40, p. 184]. We were unable to determine whether this pain represented a somatomotor or visceromotor reflex and thus included this in both sections.

5.6.10 Aaron Sign

Charles Dettie Aaron (1866–1951) was born in Lockport, New York, USA, and received his medical degree in 1891 from the University of Buffalo, New York [173, 174]. He served as house surgeon at Harper Hospital, Detroit, Michigan, from 1891 to 1893 and as city physician in Detroit from 1893 to 1895 [173, 175]. He traveled to Europe to further advance his medical training at the University of Berlin and the Universities of Giessen, Vienna, Wurzburg, Heidelberg, Paris, and London from 1896 to 1902 [174, 175]. At the Detroit College of Medicine and Surgery (currently Wayne State University School of Medicine), he served as a lecturer in materia medica and therapeutics in 1898 and professor of gastroenterology and dietetics from 1905 to 1938. Among his many accolades, he was the recipient of the honorary degree of Doctor of Science from the University of Heidelberg, Germany, in 1910 [173, 174]. He served as a member of the American College of Physicians council, president of the Northern Tri-State Medical Association and Detroit Academy of Medicine, and the first vice-president of the American Therapeutic Society [174]. It is important to recognize that Aaron was the primary founder of the American Gastroenterological Association and served as its secretary-treasurer from 1897 to 1910 [175]. He authored two books, *Diseases of the Stomach* in 1911 and *Diseases of Digestive Organs* in 1915 [176]. Aaron identified in patients with chronic appendicitis (Table 5.2):

> Continuous firm pressure with the ends of the first three fingers over McBurney's point induced a referred distress or pain in the epigastrium or precordial region. (…) Since then, in many cases of chronic appendicitis with digestive symptoms, I have been able to induce a referred pain or distress in the epigastrium, left hypochondrium, umbilical, left inguinal or precordial region by a continuous firm pressure over the appendix [177, p. 350].

Aaron postulated that chronic appendiceal inflammation causes connective tissue proliferation and scar formation that impinges on the surrounding nerve fibers containing afferent pathways to the superior mesenteric, gastric, and hepatic sympathetic plexuses [177]. Chronic firm pressure in the right lower quadrant stimulates these nerve endings resulting in reflex activation of afferent nerve pathways and visceral nerve reflexes. This finding is plausible as viscerosensory midline abdominal pain may be present during recurrent acute episodes of chronic appendicitis. We are unaware of any study that evaluated the sensitivity or specificity of this sign.

5.6.11   Bassler Sign

Anthony Bassler (1874–1959) received his medical degree from Bellevue Hospital Medical College, New York, in 1889. Along with Dr. Lewis Brinton (1861–1929), he was co-editor of the *American Journal of Gastroenterology* in 1911, which combined with the journal, *Proctologist* and renamed the *Proctologist and Gastroenterologists* journal in 1916. That same year, Bassler was appointed consulting gastroenterologist at Christ's Hospital in New Jersey and 2 years later Professor of Gastroenterology at Fordham University Medical School and New York Polyclinic Medical School and Hospital [178, 179].

Bassler was one of the incorporators of the New York Society for the Advancement of Gastroenterology in 1932, which changed its name to the National Society for the Advancement of Gastroenterology in 1934, and finally, the American College of Gastroenterology in 1943. He served as its president from 1936 to 1948 [180, 181]. He also served as the first chairman of the section of gastroenterology of the American Medical Association and was the American president of the International Society of Gastroenterology and Hepatic Insufficiency. He was a fellow of the National Society for the Advancement of Gastroenterology and an honorary member of the Belgian Gastroenterological Society [182]. Bassler was decorated with the Legion of Honor of France and received an honorary Legum Doctor (LL.D.) degree from Hahnemann Medical College in Philadelphia [182].

Several honorary tributes were published in the *American Journal of Gastroenterology* commemorating Anthony Bassler. As articulated by Louis L Perkel, MD, FACG:

> Dr. Anthony Bassler will long be remembered as one of the pioneers in the establishment of gastroenterology as a recognized specialty. Those of us who had the privilege of knowing him since we began practicing our specialty will never forget his kindness and helpfulness. He was truly an inspiration to his younger colleagues. His passing is not only a personal blow to his myriad of friends, but also an irreparable loss to the College as well as to the medical profession [183, p. 761].

Bassler described in 1913 a maneuver for diagnosing chronic appendicitis:

> [n]ote the position of the right edge of the rectus muscle on the umbilical-spine line maintaining the site with the finger. Having the patient rise to a sitting position helps in palpating the rectus edge. Standing at the right and facing the patient (for right-handed individuals) the thumb is placed vertical on the abdomen, the tip of the thumb pointing to the ensiform, when it is slowly pressed backward into the abdomen, not inward, outward, up or down. When the thumb has been sunk about half-way down to the back of the abdominal cavity, it is swung to the right of the patient at a right angle to the downward pressure line. This pinches the appendix against the iliacus muscle and unyielding structures under and at the side of it, and usually elicits pain or tenderness [184, p. 207–208].

Bassler believed that this method of examining the appendix was helpful in cases where percussion was ineffective in identifying the cecum. He did not describe the location of the pain (Table 5.2). We are unaware of any study that evaluated the sensitivity or specificity of this sign.

5.6.12 Reder Sign

Francis Reder (1864–1936) was born in New Athens, Illinois, USA, and received his medical degree from St. Louis Medical College (Washington University Medical School) in 1884 [185, 186]. He completed an internship at St. Louis City Hospital and Female Hospitals and received further postgraduate medical training at the German Hospital, New York, under the aegis of G.A. Gerster (1874–1974) [185]. Reder was appointed house surgeon at this hospital from 1886 to 1888 [186]. He traveled abroad for additional studies and training at the universities of Berlin in 1888, Munich, Vienna, and Paris in 1891 and 1901 [185, 186].

Reder was president of the St. Louis Surgical Society in 1929 and a member of several societies, including the American College of Surgeons and the St. Louis Surgical Society [185]. He was elected an honorary member of the St. Louis Medical Society in 1935 [185, 187]. Reder was a private practitioner and general surgeon for the Burlington Railway System and chief of the clinic for diseases of the rectum at Washington University, St. Louis, Missouri [186].

As to insights into his character as articulated by Fred W. Bailey:

> Honored at home and abroad, loved and respected by all who knew him, he possessed the admirable attributes of professional dignity, ability and congenial personality. To him the world was a stage, and his profession the plot, in which he labored daily, administering to the needs of his fellow men [185, p. 150].

Reder described a method for distinguishing chronic appendicitis with adhesions from chronic appendicitis without adhesions:

> The "point" in the rectum, however, has invariably given a positive reaction in the presence of a chronically diseased appendix. The part of the rectum concerned in this examination is the first portion. It commences at the sacro-iliac synchondrosis, usually the left side, is entirely covered with peritoneum and has a mesorectum, which gives that portion of the bowel a certain amount of mobility. (…) Within the lumen of the bowel at the junction with the sigmoid, about 31/2 or 4 inches above the margin of the anus, there exist aggregations of circular fibres that form a valve. This valve is constant, is known as the valve of O'Beirne, and varies but little in its distinctive circular characteristics. It serves as a landmark, and is an important factor in the examination [188, p. 16].

During the examination, the patient is positioned supine with legs flexed, and a finger is inserted into the rectum until O'Beirne's valve is reached. He identified a point in the first portion of the rectum as a method for diagnosing chronic appendicitis. The examination is performed as follows:

> In making the examination to reach the "point" the patient is comfortably placed on the examining table upon his back, with both legs flexed. The index-finger, well lubricated, is introduced into the rectum, and a search made for O'Beirne's valve. It is absolutely necessary that the valve be located. (…) The valve having been located, the finger is hooked into it and gentle traction made upon the structure to test the mobility of that portion of the rectum. The tip of the finger is allowed to rest within the lumen of the valve and the patient asked if he experiences any pain. Should there be any pain, it is generally referred to the sphincter area of the rectum. By allowing the finger to rest for a short time this pain will subside. It is desirable that the patient be entirely free from pain while the examining finger is in this position. After being assured of the total absence of pain by the patient, the tip of the finger is gently pushed upward toward the right iliac fossa, when, in the event of an appendix lesion, the finger will touch a point beyond the valve that will cause great pain. As a control maneuver a similar "point" may be touched by sweeping the examining finger toward the left inguinal fossa, usually with negative result [188, p. 16–17].

Thus, Reder sign refers to the presence of appendiceal inflammation detected through palpation of O'Beirne valve on digital rectal examination (Table 5.2). We are unaware of any study which evaluated the sensitivity or specificity of this sign.

5.6.13 Owen Sign

Edmund Blackett Owen (1847–1915) was born in Finchingfield, England, received his medical training at St. Mary's Hospital, London, diploma for membership in the Royal College of Surgeons in 1868, and fellowship in the Royal College of Surgeons in 1872 [189]. He was appointed demonstrator of anatomy from 1868 until 1875 [189]. At St. Mary's Hospital, Owen had multiple appointments, including as a lecturer in anatomy from 1876 to 1888 and surgical lecturer until 1896. He also served on staff, first as an assistant surgeon in 1877, full surgeon in 1883, and consulting Surgeon in 1898 at the Hospital for Sick Children, London. He was a surgeon to outpatients in 1871, full surgeon in 1882 until his retirement in 1902, whereby he was named consulting surgeon [189].

Among his other appointments, in the Royal College of Surgeons, he served as a member of the council from 1897 to 1913, vice-president for two terms (1905–1906 and 1906–1907), a member of the board of examiners in anatomy and physiology in 1883, fellowship board and examiner in anatomy for the second examination of the conjoint board in 1884, and court of examiners from 1888 to 1899 [189, 190]. He also served as an examiner in surgery at the Universities of Durham, London, and Cambridge [189].

Owen was an active member of the British Medical Association, serving as secretary in the section of surgery at the annual Liverpool meeting in 1883, vice-president at the annual meeting in Cardiff, Wales, in 1885, vice-president of the section of surgery, and president of the section of surgery at the annual meeting in Swansea, Wales, in 1903 [189]. In 1900, he was appointed to the office of chairman of the constitution committee, chairman of the colonial committee in 1902, and chairman of the council from 1907 to 1910 [189, 190].

Among his many other accolades, he was honorary associate and Knight of the Grace of the Order of St. John of Jerusalem, orator of the medical society in 1897, and president of the Harveian Society, to name a few [189]. During World War I, he served as surgeon-in-chief of the St. John Ambulance Brigade and British Red Cross. Owen received the Cross of the Legion of Honor in 1903 for his services at the French Hospital beginning in 1901 [191].

A description of his character as enumerated by Francis Richardson Cross:

> In the passing of Edmund Owen, the profession of surgery has lost one of its leaders, respected for his uprightness and high sense of duty, and honored for the active part he has taken in medical ethics, and in the progress and improvement of surgical practice and in its teaching. (…) Owen was always in good spirits, courteous, and amusing, but not at the expense of others. I never remember him saying an unkind word of any colleague, and he showed no unfair bias against the opinions he did not agree with. If he could not speak well or kindly of men or matters, he did not discuss them. He was a hard worker. He wrote and spoke forcibly and well. Perhaps by nature somewhat impulsive, he carefully considered his subject with ability, shrewdness and common sense, and, having formed his opinion, he was fearless and honest in expressing his views, which were usually sound and accurate [189, p. 202–203].

Owen described a method for diagnosing acute appendicitis (Table 5.2):

> If in the case of appendicitis, when the colon contains much gas, firm pressure is made with the hand over the descending colon, the gas is forcibly driven towards the caecum, and the inflamed tissues being disturbed, the patient may complain of pain in the right iliac fossa. This would scarcely happen in the case of ovaritis or other pelvic diseases, so it may prove useful as a diagnostic measure in obscure cases of appendicitis. Again, it may be that a person with appendicitis tolerates a considerable amount of pressure with the hand over the right iliac fossa, and if the steady pressure is maintained long enough to drive some of the gas out of the blind end of the large intestine, and the hand is then suddenly taken off, the quick return of gas into the caecum so disturbs the inflamed appendix that the patient calls out with pain [192, p. 49–50].

It should be recognized that Niels Thorkild Rovsing had previously described a similar maneuver in 1907 [154], seven years before Owen. We are unaware of any study that evaluated the sensitivity or specificity of this sign.

5.6.14 Wachenheim Sign

Frederick L. Wachenheim (1870–1913) was born in New York City, USA, and received his medical degree from Columbia University College of Medicine and Surgeons (currently Columbia University Vagelos College of Physicians and Surgeons), New York City [193]. He served at Sydenham Hospital and the polyclinic at Mount Sinai Hospital and was chief of the clinic children's department, Mount Sinai Hospital Dispensary, New York [194, 195].

He was a member of the Academy of Medicine, the American Medical Association, and the committee of the prevention of tuberculosis from the Charity Organization Society of the City of New York [191, 192]. He authored *The Climatic Treatment of Children* in 1907 [195].

Wachenheim described a method for diagnosing acute appendicitis in cooperative children:

> High palpation of the right iliac fossa, per rectum, elicits tenderness and pain in the McBurney region when appendicitis is present, never under normal conditions. To determine this point to our satisfaction, it is necessary to observe certain precautions. In the first place, we must gain the confidence of the little patient, assuring him that that the procedure will not be distressing. Secondly, we must introduce the examining finger quite painlessly; this can always be done if we exercise patience; the ordinary rectal examination is far too often conducted brutally, causing the patient considerable pain and alarm. It is evident that no clear statement can be obtained from a child whose sphincter has been violently dilated. With free lubrication and slow dilatation, this procedure can be rendered absolutely painless, even at the age of six or seven years. The valuable diagnostic point in the fact that the patient complains of no discomfort, until the introduced finger reaches the right iliac fossa, when the child complains of a sharp pain in the neighborhood of McBurney's point. To assure ourselves that the pain is in no relation to the mere rectal examination, we must ask the child to point out the site of the pain; if due to a rough introduction of the finger, the patient will invariably point to the anus, if appendicular, it will always be correctly localized, provided the intelligence of the child is adequate, as I have usually found it to be after the age of eight years, and often much earlier [196, p. 198].

A similar maneuver was described by Reder [188], although Wachenheim did not specifically require digital palpation of O′ Beirne valve (Table 5.2).

5.6.15 Blaisdell Sign

Silas Canada Blaisdell (1856–1929) was born in Winterport, Maine, USA, and received his medical degree from New York University Medical College in 1882 [197, 198]. After graduation, he was a private practitioner in Brooklyn, NY, and lecturer in applied and comparative anatomy at New York University Medical College, a lecturer in regional anatomy in the dental school at the New York College of Dentistry, and a surgeon-in-chief of Eastern District Hospital, Brooklyn, NY. He was a member of the Kings County Medical Society, Brooklyn, NY, and Brooklyn Medical and Surgical Society, to name a few [197, 198].

Blaisdell reported a test used in the diagnosis of appendicitis (Table 5.2):

> *[t]he pain is increased when the patient is turned to the left and diminished when he is turned back on his right side.* The pain is not so intense when the patient is on his back as on the left side. (…) In making the test the abdomen must not be allowed to touch the bed thereby allowing the viscera no support when it pulls to the left and drags along the sensitive appendix thereby causing additional pain [199, p. 285–286].

He believes this finding had not been previously reported, although Berthomier described a similar palpatory maneuver in 1906 [149]. This patient presumably had mesenteric adenitis as the appendix is a fixed (retroperitoneal) structure and does not shift when the patient is moved to the left lateral decubitus position.

5.6.16   Baldwin Sign

James Fairchild Baldwin (1850–1936) was born in Orangeville, New York, USA, and received his medical degree from Jefferson Medical College, Philadelphia, Pennsylvania, in 1874 and Master of Arts degree from Oberlin College, Oberlin, Ohio, in 1875 [200]. He was appointed professor of physiology and anatomy at the Starling Medical College, Columbus, Ohio, from 1875 to 1882 [201–203]. Baldwin was a founding member of the Columbus Medical College in 1876 (merged with Starling Medical College in 1892). He was the first editor-in-chief, along with John Waterman Hamilton (1823–1898), from 1876 to 1894 and independently from 1894 to 1898 of the *Ohio Medical Recorder* (named *Ohio Medical Journal* in 1881 and *Columbus Medical Journal* in 1882), which was supported by the Central Ohio Medical Society [201–203].

Baldwin was also a founding member of the Ohio Medical University in 1892 (united with Starling Medical College to become Starling Ohio Medical College in 1907 and subsequently Ohio State University College of Medicine in 1914), where he was professor of gynecology and chancellor from 1890 to 1899 [202–204]. He served as president of the Central Ohio Medical Society in 1889 and was a member of this society throughout his career [203–207]. He founded Grant Hospital in Columbus, Ohio, in 1900 and served as chief of staff [202]. He was president of the Ohio State Medical Association from 1919 to 1920 and the American Association of Obstetricians, Gynecologists, and Abdominal Surgeons in 1923 [202].

Baldwin, in a discussion of a case of a patient with retrocecal appendicitis, described the maneuver and mechanism involved in eliciting this test:

> In the vast majority of cases, when you have such a condition, you can by pressure elicit tenderness such as the doctor described; then tell the patient to keep the knee stiff and lift

> the right leg: as the psoas muscle contracts under your fingers, the tenderness become much
> more marked, and the leg drop with an expression of pain from the patient. The appendix
> rests on the psoas muscle, and when brought up under the fingers get pinched. I have made
> the diagnosis in this way over and over again, and have never failed to find a retrocecal
> appendix [208, p. 254].

Thus, extending the right thigh and knee onto the pelvis causes discomfort because the psoas muscle and fingers compress the inflamed retrocecal appendix (Table 5.2). Baldwin did not define the location of the pain. This sign is similar to the one reported by Meltzer in 1902 [131].

5.6.17 Rosenstein Sign

Paul Rosenstein (1875–1964) was born in Graudenz, German Empire (currently Grudziadz, Poland) and received his doctorate in 1898 [209]. He served as a junior physician at the Institute of Pathology in Königsberg, Prussia, and at the Gynecological and Surgical Hospital in Berlin, Germany [209, 210]. At the Hasenheide Hospital in Berlin, he served as director of the surgical department in 1909 and adjunct professor of urology and chair of the surgical department. He was director of the surgical polyclinic of the Jewish Community Hospital, Berlin, in 1917 [209, 210]. Rosenstein served as president of the Berlin Urological Society until 1933. During National Socialism, he and other Jewish physicians were forced from their positions and banned from practicing medicine [209, 210].

Rosenstein described a maneuver as a method for differentiating acute or chronic cecal or appendiceal pain from other causes of abdominal pain. The bedside test is performed as follows:

> The patient is placed on his/her left side with the anterior superior spines of the ilium per-
> pendicular to the surface. Pressure is applied to the right side, three fingerbreadths inside
> and slightly below the right anterior superior spine. If the cecum or appendix is inflamed,
> the patient experiences intense pain [211, p. 644].

Rosenstein did not define the location of the pain. Pyotr Porfiryevich Sitkovsky (1922) reported in his paper titled, "About one of the clinical signs in inflammation of the appendix," the same maneuver described by Rosenstein two years earlier [212]. Rosenstein postulated that the inflammatory hyperemia and increased cecal or appendiceal volume exert increased traction and pressure on the mesentery as it falls to the midline when the patient assumes the left lateral decubitus position. He also recognized that the inflammatory processes within the mesentery or mesenteriolum might also contribute to the pain. Sitkovsky believed the pain was due to increased mesenteric traction caused by the inflamed appendix and activation of interceptors within the mesentery [212] (Table 5.2).

The finding by Rosenstein and Sitkovsky is presumably caused by shifting of the mesentery, which allows unimpeded access to the inflamed appendix when the patient is placed in the left lateral decubitus position.

5.6.18 *Kocher Sign*

Emil Theodor Kocher (1841–1917) was born in Bern, Switzerland, and received his medical degree from the University of Bern in 1866 [213]. He completed his postgraduate studies in Zurich, Berlin, Paris, London, and Vienna. He habilitated in surgery at the University of Bern and was appointed surgical assistant in the clinic to George Albert Lücke (1829–1894). Kocher was a general practitioner and lecturer in Berlin and was later appointed full professor and director of the surgical clinic at the University of Bern in 1872, a position he maintained throughout his career [213–216].

His name is best recognized in connection with the treatment and management of goiter, although he contributed substantially to other fields of medicine and surgery [213, 217]. He also devised new surgical instruments and novel surgical techniques for which his name is eponymously ascribed [218]. He was awarded the Nobel Prize for his extensive work on the pathology, physiology, and surgical management of the thyroid gland in 1909 [219].

As a description of his character as articulated by Albert Kocher:

> He was highly respected and loved by his students, as he knew better than anyone else how to impart his unyielding rigor to everything that concerned the sick and thus combine friendly collegiality with his students. His impeccable example and the fine, distinguished way in which he imparted his knowledge to his students, modestly concealing his superiority, spurred everyone on to the highest degree [216, p. 7].

Among his numerous accolades, he was an honorary fellow of the Royal College of Surgeons and an honorary member of the Royal Society of Sciences, Uppsala; Swiss Natural Research Society; honorary member of the American Surgical Society; president of the German Society of Surgeons, Berlin; and elected chairman of the First International Congress of Surgeons, Brussels [215, 220].

Albert Vogel, a resident in Kocher's surgical clinic, published Theodor Kocher's (1814–1917) work titled "Die Behandlung der Appendizitis an der chirurgischen Klinik der Universität Bern" (The Treatment of Appendicitis at the Surgical Clinic of the University of Bern) in 1921 was based on a presentation delivered by Kocher at the inaugural meeting of the Swiss Society of Surgery on 8 March 1913. The publication was delayed for one year due to the onset of World War I. The name Kocher has been paired with Volkovich and is sometimes referred to as the Kocher-Volkovich sign, which describes initial pain in the epigastrium, followed by pain in the right lower quadrant [221–223]. Kocher reported:

> In our opinion, initial vomiting, and localization of pain in the epigastrium followed by the diffuse spread and gradual fixation in the classical place, McBurney point, occurs because of general peritoneal inflammation. This inflammation should not be confused with the serous type of peritonitis which develops later if the appendix becomes gangrenous or perforates. We can explain the diffuse pain, particularly at the umbilical and epigastric regions, because the appendix is not painful in the first stages of the disease, with the pulling on the peritoneum being the source of pain. Local pain develops if infiltration of the mesentery occurs [223, p. 2–3].

As currently known, pain initially located in the epigastric and periumbilical regions represents a viscerosensory nerve reflex. In contrast, pain in the right lower quadrant is caused by viscerosomatic (visceromotor and viscerosensory) and somatic (somatosensory and somatomotor) segmental reflexes, the latter secondary to inflammation of the parietal peritoneum. Thus, Kocher described the classic presentation and sequence of events of acute appendicitis (Table 5.2).

5.6.19 Sloan Sign

Leroy Hendrick Sloan (1892–1961) was born in Aurora, Illinois, and received his medical degree from Rush Medical College, Chicago, Illinois, in 1917 [224]. He completed an internship at Cook County Hospital in Chicago, Illinois, and furthered his postgraduate training in Vienna and London. He returned to Chicago and ascended to the chief of medical service at Illinois Central Hospital, a position he held from 1921 to 1957 [224]. Other appointments in Chicago included attending physician at Cook County Hospital, associate professor of Medicine at Rush Medical College, and clinical professor of medicine at the University of Illinois College of Medicine, Chicago [224].

Among his other accomplishments, he served as president of the American College of Physicians and was chairman of the Joint Commission for Accreditation of Hospitals [224]. His character as described by Ford K. Hick:

> He had the gift of favorably affecting the lives of almost everyone with whom he came in contact. He was a counselor, confidant, and sponsor to many physicians. Any physician, student or patient who really knew Dr. Sloan has some anecdote to recite expressing his individuality and capacity for helping other people [224, p. 601].

He described a maneuver for detecting appendicitis in patients with a heavy muscular abdomen (Fig. 5.12):

> The patient, keeping the knee straight, raises the right heel from the bed while the examiner places his left hand over the right lower quadrant of the abdomen and applies pressure to it with the fingers of the right hand. The psoas muscle is thus put on tension while the appendix is compressed between it and the left hand of the examiner [18, p. 142].

Sloan did not define the location of the pain (Table 5.2). The sign is similar to that described by Meltzer in 1902 [131]. We are unaware of any study that evaluated the sensitivity or specificity of this sign.

5.6.20 Gregory Sign

Historical information on Arthur Gregory is found under the section somatic segmental nerve pathway signs. Gregory percussed midway between the umbilicus and anterior superior iliac spine and found that:

> In chronic appendicitis it is often necessary to use stronger percussion, sometimes with two fingers, and to press in the abdominal walls with the fingers of the left hand, in order to maintain the symptom. Some patients report that they do not feel any pain, but rather a slight shaking or a light blow at McBurney's point. Direct percussion at McBurney's point is also usually painful in acute and subacute appendicitis, but often completely painless in

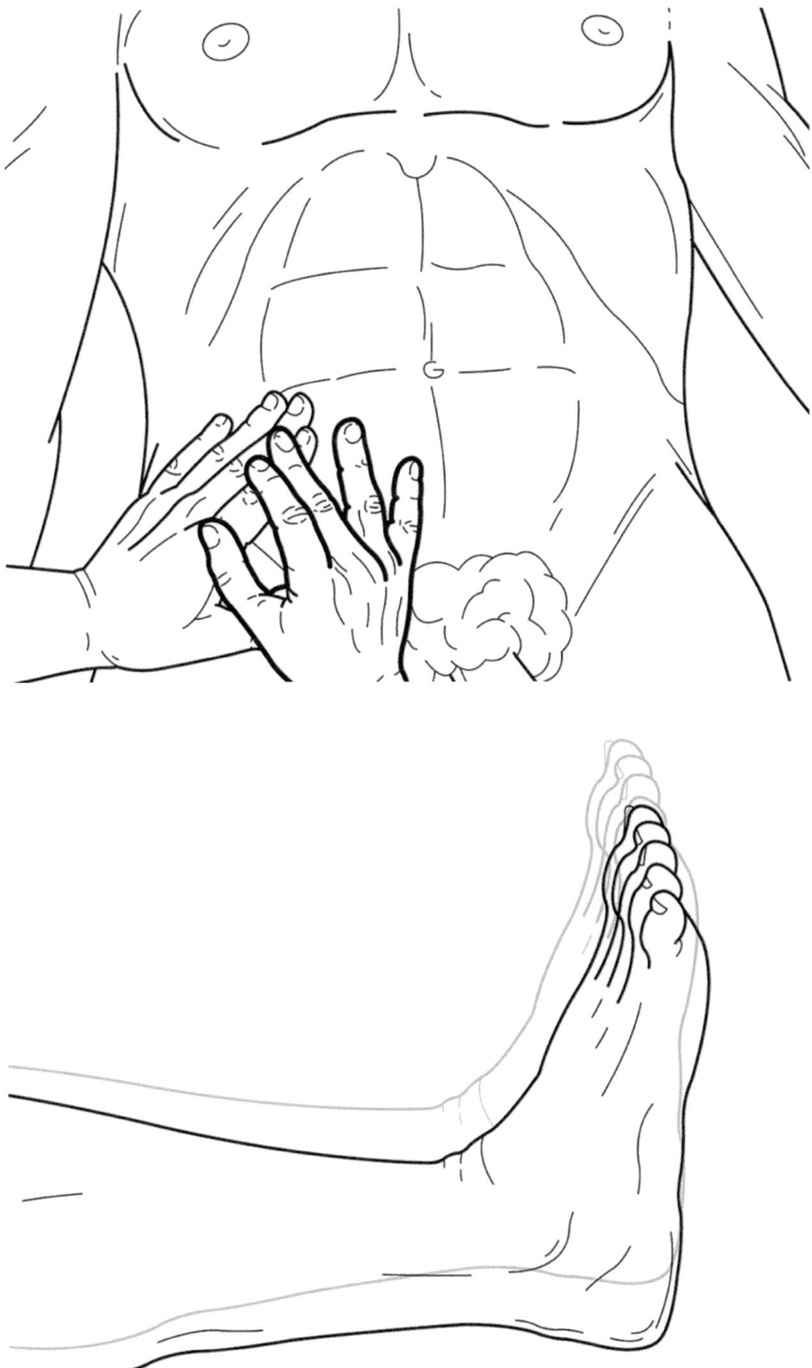

Fig. 5.12 Sloan sign (by Ryan Yale)

chronic appendicitis. It is possible that muscular contraction so reduces the transmission of the shock to the diseased appendix that there is no sensation of pain at all. With percussion on the left side, the vibration is transmitted unimpeded to the diseased appendix. It has often been found that in chronic appendicitis symptoms disappears after palpation of the appendix, only to return after a few minutes. It is possible that the intense sensation of pain on palpation numbs the sensation of pain for a time [74, p. 398].

Thus, Gregory recognized that in chronic appendicitis, no pain is found when percussing over McBurney point. Pain is elicited when firm percussion and deep palpation are applied activating viscerosensory segmental reflexes.

5.6.21 Soresi Sign

Angelo Luigi Maria Soresi (1877–1951) was born in Piacenza, Italy, received medical training in Naples and Rome, and graduated in 1903 [225]. He immigrated to the USA, where he was a professor of surgery at Homeopathic Medical College, Flower Hospital, and was later appointed chief surgeon at Green Point Hospital, Brooklyn, New York. During World War I, he served as captain of the surgical department at the Military Hospital, Green Cross (site of the elementary school of Torino) [225]. Among his accomplishments, he is credited for administering combined spinal epidural anesthesia in 1937 and the surgical management of hiatal hernias [226, 227].

Soresi described a maneuver for diagnosing appendicitis (Table 5.2):

> The patient flexes the thighs. The hand is applied to the region of the hepatic flexure of the colon. While the patient breathes as deeply as possible, the hand is pressed very gently under the costal margin. The patient is told to cough, and is then asked whether any pain is felt; the answer may be yes or no. When it is "yes," the patient, on being asked whether the pain is felt, without hesitation will indicate McBurney's point when a true appendicitis is present. (…) The sign is elicited through gently pressure on the appendiceal region by the gas contained in the intestine, when the patient coughs, while the hand of the surgeon compresses the colon, and by the pressure of the contracting abdominal muscles [228, p. 1766].

We are unaware of any studies which assessed the sensitivity or specificity of this sign.

5.6.22 Tresidder Sign

Lieutenant Colonel Alfred Geddes Tresidder (1881–1970) received his medical training at the London Hospital, qualifying in 1906 [229]. He graduated M.B., B.S. in 1907 and was a member of the Indian Medical Service, a military medical service in British-ruled India, in 1908. Tresidder received his medical degree in 1911 [229]. He was appointed to the London Hospital as an ear, nose, and throat (ENT) surgeon and received his Master of Science degree in 1931 [229]. After World War I, he was a civil surgeon to the Bombay presidency, India, held the position as major civil surgeon to Nasik, Hyderabad, Sindh, and Poona, and provided medical care to Lord Lloyd (1879–1941), Governor of Bombay. Tresidder was appointed Companion, Order of the Indian Empire in 1927 [229]. In approximately 1931, he was appointed surgeon to the Blackheath and Charlton Hospitals in South East London and joined the Emergency Medical Service in 1939. He held a commission as an ENT surgeon in the Royal Army Medical Corps, serving at Woolwich, Netley, and Bath [229]. From 1946 to 1957, he served as a consulting ENT surgeon at St. Helier's Hospital and senior clinical assistant to the Central London, Throat, Nose, and Ear Hospital. Tresidder remained active after retirement as a locum for ENT surgeon and at the Post Office for the Treasury Medical Service. He rose to the military rank of lieutenant-colonel [229].

Tresidder observed a finding in a 17-year-old male with an acute episode of chronic appendicitis: "[t]he patient was lying on his abdomen and on being questioned he explained that he found that this was the most comfortable position on which he could lie [230, p. 376]." The appendix was found to be located retrocecally and adherent to the posterior wall of the cecum. Tresidder postulated that "Presumably the adoption of this position would allow the cecum to fall forward and away from the inflamed retro-caecal appendix, and in doing so relieve to some extent the pressure on the organ" [230, p. 376]. We are unaware of any studies which assessed the sensitivity or specificity of this sign (Table 5.2).

5.6.23 *Livingston sign*

Edward Meakin Livingston (1895–1969) was born in Sparta, Wisconsin, USA, and received his medical degree from New York University in 1919 [231–233]. He was an instructor in surgery in 1921, an assistant clinical professor of surgery, an assistant visiting surgeon third division, and subsequently, an associate visiting surgeon at Bellevue Hospital, New York [234]. He published with George T. Pack (1898–1969) the books *End-Results in the Treatment of Gastric Cancer: An Analytical Study and Statistical Survey of Sixty Years of Surgical Treatment* in 1939 and *Treatment of Cancer and Allied Diseases* in 1940 [235, 236]. During their later writing, he was an assisting attending surgeon at Memorial Hospital in New York. With Edward Milton Foote, he coauthored the sixth edition of *Principles and Practice of Minor Surgery: A Textbook for Students and Practitioners* in 1929 (formerly named *A Textbook of Minor Surgery* by Edward Milton Foote) [237].

In the preface of his book *A Clinical Study of the Abdominal Cavity and Peritoneum* in 1932, he stated:

> So increased, however, has my estimate become of the diagnostic possibilities in the careful bedside examination of the patient, that I already feel amply repaid for any expenditure of time and effort. And if the reading of this volume there be those who derive even a small degree of the pleasure which I have had in its preparation my payment shall have multiplied [234, p. viii–ix].

Livingston described a triangular shape zone of cutaneous tenderness as "the most important single sign or symptom of acute appendicitis" [238, p. 630]. Based on clinical observation, the area of skin tenderness was maximum at the center of the triangle and does not extend beyond its borders. The appendix skin triangle consists of the following:

> A line from the umbilicus to the highest point on the right iliac crest forms the upper side;
> a line carried from this point to the right pubic spine forms its lower side, while a line from
> the right pubic spine to the umbilicus closes the triangle [238, p. 635].

Livingston acknowledged that other areas of cutaneous tenderness on the anterior abdominal wall might occur in patients with appendicitis. However, a positive skin test for the diagnosis of appendicitis is most likely when an area of hyperesthesia, bordered by a triangular area with maximal tenderness in its center, is located in an area in the right lower quadrant of the anterior abdominal wall. Sherren described a similar triangular area of cutaneous hyperesthesia in the right lower quadrant in patients with acute appendicitis [136].

Livingston emphasized that this bedside "pinch test" or "traction method" of sensory testing should involve a vigorous twisting or pulling motion of the skin and subcutaneous tissues between the thumb and forefinger. Areas of noninvolved pain should be tested for comparison, while heat or cold may be used to further assist in defining the border of hyperesthesia or show a sensory change in the involved area. In an observational study of 428 patients, acute appendicitis was confirmed in 367, and 317 (86%) were found preoperatively to have cutaneous hyperesthesia limited to the appendiceal triangle [238] (Table 5.2).

5.6.24   Klein Sign

Limited historical information was identified for William Klein (1881–1970). He was a member of the Department of Surgery at Morrisania City Hospitals and Bronx Hospital, Bronx, New York, in 1938 [239]. Klein described a method for distinguishing acute appendicitis from acute mesenteric adenitis and other diseases involving the cecum:

> Tenderness is found over a small area to the right of the umbilicus, but much higher than McBurney's point. The tender area may extend even above the umbilicus on the right side. The left side at the same time is free from tenderness. The patient is then turned on the left side and allowed to remain in this position for thirty seconds or more. Palpation in this position finds the tender area previously noted on the right side now shifted to the left of the umbilicus and absent on the right side. The patient is turned on the right side and allowed to rest for a short period, and palpation then reveals absence of tenderness on the left side and more marked tenderness on the right. In this position the tenderness in the area in question is more extensive than when the patient was resting on his back [239, p. 578–579].

Klein accounted for the pathogenesis of this finding:

> The shifting tenderness is easily explained if one remembers the anatomic outline of the mesentery. When the patient is turned on either side the mesentery of the small intestines will gravitate to the extreme dependent part of the abdomen. The cecum and appendix have little mobility and cannot be shifted to the left with a change of the body position. This one sign, when present, has always differentiated mesenteric adenitis from acute appendicitis [239, p. 579].

This sign is similar to that described by Berthomier-Michelson in 1906 and 1911, respectively, Blaisdell in 1916, and Rosenstein in 1920. We are unaware of any study that evaluated this sign's sensitivity or specificity (Table 5.2).

5.6.25   *Altschüler Sign*

Emil Altschüler (1879–1942) was born in Speyer in Rheiland-Pfalz, Germany, and studied medicine in Heidelberg, Berlin, and Strasbourg [240]. He served as an assistant physician at the Hygienic-Bacteriological Institute and Institute for Fighting Typhoid from 1902 to 1904 and in 1904 as an assistant physician at Freimaurer Hospital, Hamburg. Altschüler was an assistant and senior physician at the University Surgical Clinic, Strasburg, and received his doctorate in 1909 [240]. In Frankfurt am Main, he rose to chief surgeon at the Jewish Community Hospital. During World War II, Altschüler immigrated to Israel and was appointed chief physician in the surgical department at Bikur Cholim Hospital, Jerusalem [240].

Altschüler described a finding in 1938 in patients with acute and chronic retrocecal appendicitis:

> The third, fourth, and little finger of the left hand are laid on the outer border of the ileum and the left index-finger on the inner border. If the index-finger is very gradually moved over the soft parts from the anterior superior spine downwards, every case of retrocoecal appendicitis shows a definite, often very painful sensitivity, usually restricted to a small area. In severe cases there is also very definite localized muscle spasm in the same place, sometimes higher, sometimes lower. The abdomen is usually not sensitive to pressure and the usual points of tenderness are absent [241, p. 892].

Thus, the sign refers to pain and muscle spasm located over the right pelvic margin in acute and chronic retrocecal appendicitis (Table 5.2). We are unaware of any study that evaluated this sign's sensitivity of specificity.

5.6.26   *Alders Sign*

Nicholas Alders (1904–1995) was born in Budapest, Hungary, and received his medical degree from the University of Vienna in 1928 [242]. He practiced obstetrics and gynecology in Vienna but was forced to flee to London, England, during World War II. After qualifying in 1941, he served initially as a surgeon in the emergency medical services and registrar in gynecological and obstetrics at the Royal Victoria and West Hants Hospital, Bournemouth, England, and at the East Dorset Group of Hospital, Southwest Metropolitan Regional Hospital Board, England, in 1954 [242–244]. He was appointed a fellow of the Royal College of Surgeons, Edinburgh, in 1945; a member of the Royal College of Obstetricians and Gynecologists in 1951; and a fellow of the International College of Surgeons, Bournemouth, 1953 [242, 245]. Alders described a maneuver for differentiating uterine from extrauterine (e.g., appendiceal) complications (Table 5.2):

> With the patient lying straight on her back, the examining fingers find the area of maximum tenderness to pressure on the abdominal wall. While the fingers remain in contact with that area without altering the intensity of pressure, they are exerting to elicit pain, the patient is made to turn over on the opposite side so that the plane of the anterior abdominal wall is approximately vertical. The pain produced by the pressure of the fingers will be less or will have entirely disappeared if the lesion is uterine and has fallen away from the examining fingers—"shifting tenderness" [246, p. 1194–1195].

Alders did not specifically state the location of the pain on palpation of the abdomen. Based on the principle of viscerosensory segmental reflex, it is postulated that the pain is located along the T10–T11 dermatome. According to Alders, the pain caused by uterine conditions, including hemorrhage or leiomyoma, becomes less intense or disappears when the patient turns to the opposite side. If the pain is extrauterine in origin, as in the case of appendicitis, ovarian torsion, or diverticulitis, it remains unchanged when the patient moves to the left decubitus position. This finding occurs because these are retroperitoneal structures and thus fixed in position. Findings from this maneuver are not helpful when there is an enlarged palpable uterus or where the uterus is fixed due to the adhesions to the abdominal wall. Studies evaluating Alders sign are limited. One study by Chen et al. (1999) found Alders sign was present in approximately 36% (5 of 14) of pregnant patients with acute appendicitis [247].

5.6.27   Bryan Sign

Williams McIver Bryan, Jr. (1917–2007) was born in Savannah, Georgia, and received his medical degree from the Medical College of South Carolina in 1944 [248]. At the University of Tennessee College of Medicine, he received his Master of Science degree and served as the Fred Adair Teaching Fellow in the Department of Obstetrics and Gynecology [248]. He was chief in the obstetrics and gynecology department at Columbia General Hospital, South Carolina (currently Prisma Health Richland Hospital). Bryan also served as a consultant at Baptist Medical Center (currently Prisma Health Baptist), Richland Memorial (currently Prisma Health Richland), and Providence Hospitals, Columbia [248].

Among his other accolades, he served as president of the South Central Obstetrical and Gynecological Society, diplomate and Life Fellow of the American College of Obstetricians and Gynecologists, and a fellow of the American College of Physicians [248]. He was also a member of the board of directors for the American Red Cross United Fund and the committee for Maternal Welfare for the State of South Carolina [248].

In his discussion of appendicitis during a presentation at the 17th Annual Meeting of the South Atlantic Association of Obstetricians and Gynecologists, Bryan reported a method for diagnosing appendicitis during pregnancy and the puerperium that involved applying "Pressure on the pregnant uterus from the left side will often elicit pain in the right lower or middle quadrants" [249, p. 1205]. The presence of pain in this location suggests activation of the viscerosensory segmental pain reflex caused by compression of the gravid uterus on the inflamed appendix. Kurtz et al. reported the presence of Bryan sign in 31 of 37 (83.8%) followed by rebound tenderness in 24 of 35 (68.6%) cases of appendicitis occurring during pregnancy [250] (Table 5.2).

5.6.28   Arapov Sign

Dmitry Alekseyevich Arapov (1897–1984) was born in Moscow, Russia, and received his medical degree from the Medical Faculty of the Second Moscow State University in 1929. He served at the Nikolai Vasilyevich Sklifosovsky First Aid

Research Institute in Moscow under the aegis of Sergei Yudin (1891–1954), chairman of the surgical department [251]. He was appointed deputy chief surgeon of the military medical directorate of the ministry of defense and chief surgeon of the USSR Navy from 1953 to 1970 [251].

His most highly recognized works were related to gas gangrene caused by axillary fragments lodged in a wound and the use of nitrous oxide to prevent shock. Arapov was appointed corresponding member of the USSR Academy of Medical Science in 1953, an honored scientist of the Russian Soviet Federative Socialist Republic in 1959, an honorary member of the All-Russian, Moscow, Kazakh, and Tajik Surgical Societies, and a member of the International Society of Surgeons. He received many honors and awards, including the Order of the Red Banner, the Red Star, and the Badge of Honor and Medal [251].

Arapov et al. described a physical finding in patients with acute appendicitis (Table 5.2):

> Irritation of the peritoneum is determined according to this rule: The hand is used to apply superficial pressure over the anterior abdominal wall at a distance from the right iliac fossa. Pain after deep and sharp pressure at the right ileal fossa confirms that the appendix, not the peritoneum, is involved. The absence of irritation of the pelvic peritoneum, as determined by rectal and vaginal examination, provides additional information [252, p. 25].

Arapov did not delineate the location of the pain. We are unaware of any study that evaluated this sign's sensitivity of specificity.

5.6.29 Marek Sign

Vitezslav Marek is currently a member of the Department of Surgical Oncology, St. Elizabeth Hospital, Medical School of Comenius University, Bratislava, Slovak Republic [253]. Marek et al. (2021), in their paper titled "Acute appendicitis: clinical anatomy of the new palpation sign," introduced a novel viscerosomatic palpatory sign used in the diagnosis of acute appendicitis [253]. The authors' method is unique, and the technique was modified slightly for infants and children. Patients are placed in the left recumbent position with knees flexed, which displaces the mesentery slightly to the left, providing better palpatory access to the appendix, while flexion of the knees and thighs relaxes the anterior abdominal wall. In infants and children, the technique involves applying firm pressure on the anterior abdominal wall in the lumbar region using the thumb directed posteriorly while simultaneously palpatory pressure is applied in the right hypogastrium region using the second, third, and fourth fingers of the same hand. A bimanual method in adults involves applying the same technique with the thumb, but in this case, the fingers of the left and right hand are used to apply pressure in the right hypogastrium. According to Marek et al., "If a deep palpation induces abdominal contracture, preventing the palpation of the iliac artery pulsations, the sign is considered positive, indicating a high probability of AA and the need for a surgical revision" [253, p. 219].

The authors state that the sign can be used during the early and later stages of appendicitis and involves the activation of visceromotor segmental reflexes. It is recognized that these segmental reflexes become clinically indistinguishable in cases of acute appendicitis with perforation causing secondary inflammation of the parietal peritoneum. In cases of inflammation of the parietal peritoneum, abdominal wall contraction occurs during superficial palpation (somatomotor segmental reflex). Thus, conditions other than acute appendicitis, which causes peritonitis and impedes palpation of the iliac artery pulsation, will cause a false-positive Marek sign. We are unaware of any study that evaluated this sign's sensitivity or specificity (Table 5.2).

5.6.30 Ott Sign

We were unable to verify the author's identify or source text for Ott sign. According to Donnell B. Cobb, Ott sign:

> [i]s obtained by having the patient turn on the left side, thus producing a painful dragging sensation on the right lower quadrant as the cecum and inflamed appendix tend to sag toward the left and pull against the mesentery [254, p. 476].

Robertson and Robertson (1947) referred to Ott sign (Table 5.2):

> When the patient is on his left side there is a feeling of distress and of a painful dragging sensation as if a heavy body in the abdomen had fallen to the left, sometimes referred to as the "mesenteric pull" [255, p. 19].

Thus, Ott sign refers to the dragging sensation in the right lower quadrant when the patient is placed in the left lateral decubitus position.

5.6.31 Baron Sign

We were unable to identify the text source and biographical information of the Baron sign. According to Robertson and Robertson (1947), Baron found in chronic appendicitis that the (Fig. 5.13):

> [r]ight psoas muscle was frequently sensitive to pressure. The patient must be recumbent, relaxed and told to breathe deeply. The examiner's second third and fourth fingers of the right hand are placed on Poupart's ligament and pressure is made in the direction of the psoas muscle. The patient is told then to elevate the leg of the same side with knee extended, forming an angle at the hip of about 45 degrees. In this position the palpating fingers readily detect the psoas muscle thus made tense. Similar palpation should be made on both sides for purposes of comparison; even in the healthy individual the tensed muscle may be sensitive, but when the appendix is involved, the tenderness is more marked on the right side. However, the psoas, in being covered by the peritoneum, is also painful in the presence of sacrospinal and gluteal muscle myalgias-in arthroses of the lumbar region of the spine, the lumbosacral and ileosacral joints and sometimes in sciatica [255, p. 22] (Table 5.2).

Thus, Baron sign refers to the viscerosensory reflex elicited through palpation and extension of the leg.

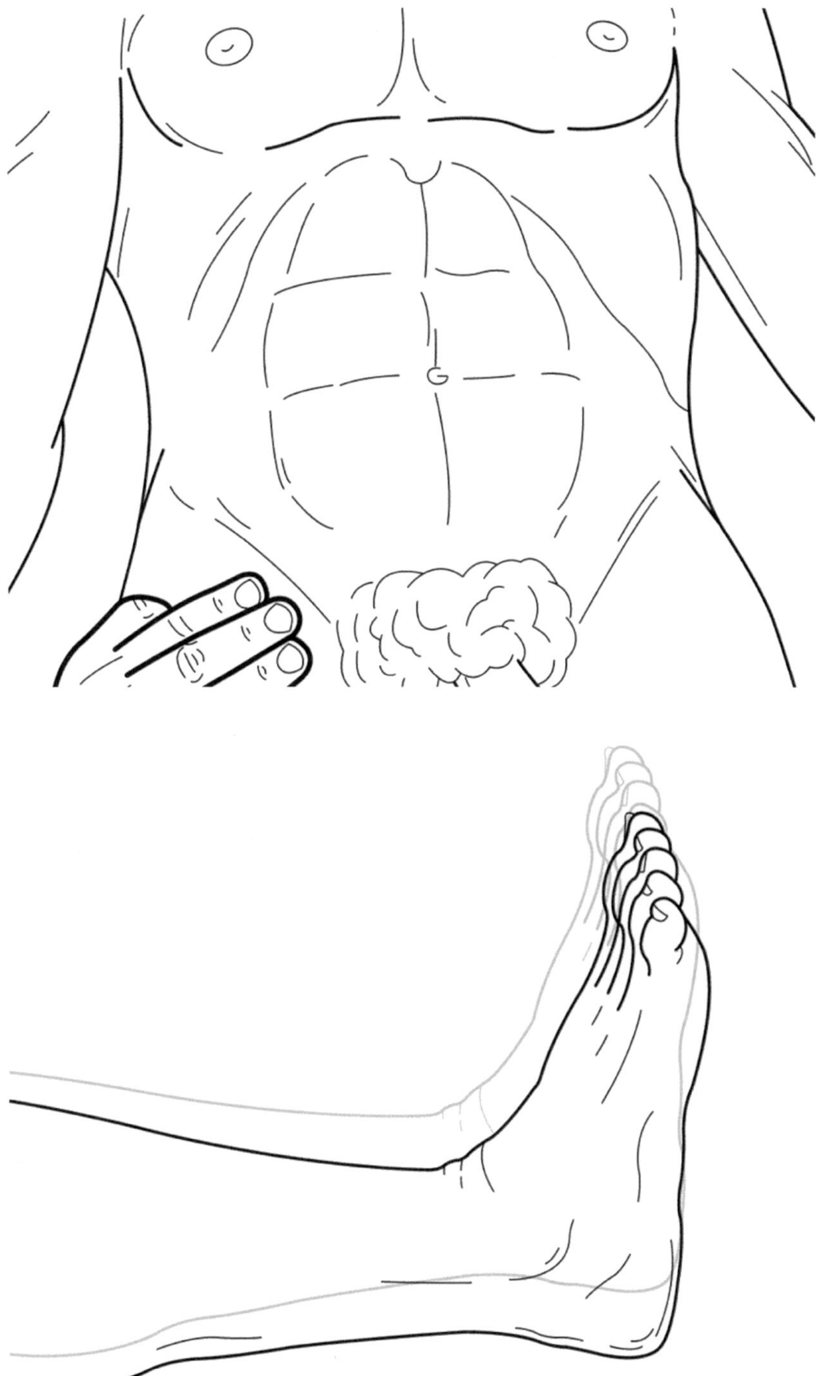

Fig. 5.13 Baron sign (by Ryan Yale)

5.6.32   *Donnelly Sign*

There is a paucity of information on Daniel Joseph Donnelly. He was a private practitioner in gynecology, appointed instructor in materia medica in 1918, and was an associate professor of medicine at Temple University, Philadelphia [256–258]. He served as secretary and treasurer of the Samaritan Hospital Medical Society, Philadelphia, in 1917 [259].

We were unable to identify the source text for Donnelly sign. Robertson and Robertson wrote in their book *Diagnostic Signs, Reflexes and Syndromes*, published in 1947 (Table 5.2):

> Dr. Daniel Donnelly of Philadelphia has described a sign indicative of retrocecal appendicitis. When the right leg is in full extension and abducted, it causes the psoas muscle to be brought into prominence. Pressure then made over the right inferior quadrant and especially in and just below McBurney's region elicits pain in proportion to the degree of inflammation in the appendix and its surroundings [255, p. 24].

This description suggests the activation of viscerosensory nerve pathways as the mechanism of abdominal pain.

Table 5.2 Visceral reflex signs in appendicitis

Name	Year	Description of the sign	Method	Pathophysiologic mechanism
Meltzer [131]	1902	Apply firm pressure over the tender spot on the anterior abdominal wall. When pain occurs, release the pressure so that the patient experiences only minimal discomfort. Now, ask the patient to flex the thigh	Palpation	Viscerosensory
Sherren [136]	1903	1. In a location distant from the tender area, gently pinch or stroke the skin. While moving inward toward the tender area, repeat this process and determine its boundary. Cutaneous hyperalgesia is found either as a wide band extending to the right side from the midline below the umbilicus in front to the lumbar spine or as a small circular area slightly above the midpoint on a line drawn between the umbilicus and anterior superior spine. Occasionally, the tenderness extends to the gluteal region as a tongue-shaped band three inches in width. 2. Triangular area or "appendix triangle" of cutaneous tenderness in the right iliac regions. Its lower boundary reaches almost to Poupart ligament. Its inner almost extends to the middle line, and its apex is slightly outside the anterior superior spine, sometimes extending to the mid-axillary line	Palpation	Viscerosensory
Mackenzie [143]	1903	Excessive irritability of the nerve cell is responsible for the pain and hyperesthesia in the tissues occurring on the abdominal wall. It is more readily demonstrated in the erector spinae and muscles of the abdomen, particularly those over the right iliac fossa. Pain occurs when slight pressure is applied to this region. One can readily demonstrate that the tenderness is not due to the inflamed peritoneum by slightly raising a portion of muscle away from the peritoneum before applying pressure or, in cases where the pain and tenderness are widespread, by finding this tenderness in the muscles of the lumbar region	Palpation	Viscerosensory
Sicard [146]	1905	A depression of the abdominal wall occurs on the same side where a superficial touch is applied. The reflexes are divided into an epigastric, paraumbilical, and hypogastric zone and elicited by moving the finger from a central medial to a lateral position. The paraumbilical and hypogastric reflexes are involved in appendicitis	Palpation	Visceromotor

(continued)

Table 5.2 (continued)

Name	Year	Description of the sign	Method	Pathophysiologic mechanism
Berthomier-Michelson [149, 150]	1906 1911	A marked difference in pain intensity is found at the cecal-appendicular regions depending upon whether the patient is positioned in the supine or left lateral decubitus position. Palpation of McBurney point in the supine position showed no evidence of chronic appendicitis, while palpation in the lateral decubitus confirms the diagnosis	Palpation	Viscerosensory (chronic appendicitis)
Rovsing [154]	1907	Compress the descending colon by pushing the fingers of the right hand onto the fingers of the left hand placed flat against the abdomen in the left iliac fossa. Using this method, the hands slide upward toward the left colonic flexure	Palpation	Viscerosensory
Chase [161]	1908	Place the patient on a hard, low bed or table. Flex the knee and place two pillows under the head and shoulders, giving a dorsal semi-recumbent position. Stand on the patient's left side, facing the feet. Place the palmar surfaces of the fingers of the right hand under the patient's left inguinal region and the fingers of the left hand to reinforce the right hand. Deep pressure is applied gradually backward, drawing the fingers deeply and forcibly upward under the left costal arch. The intent of this maneuver is to compress the lower portion of the descending colon and force its gaseous content into the transverse and thence to the ascending colon. Maintain pressure with the fingers of the left-hand hand. Remove the right hand, place it over the upper portion of the descending colon, and apply more forcibly depression. A gaseous compression wave will travel across the transverse and down the ascending colon and, on arriving at the cecum, produces cecal distention, yielding a typical sharp pain in the right iliac fossa if inflammation of the cecum or appendix is present	Palpation	Viscerosensory
Bastedo [170]	1910	Insufflate air into the colon. Pain or tenderness in the region of McBurney point on dilatation of the colon is consistent with appendicitis	Instilling air in colon	Viscerosensory
Caden [40]	1911	Muscular rigidity is prominent in the lower right quadrant	Palpation	Visceromotor
Aaron [177]	1913	Continuous firm pressure applied with the first three fingertips over McBurney point induces referred pain in the epigastrium or precordial region	Palpation	Viscerosensory (chronic appendicitis)

Bassler [184]	1913	Identify the right edge of the rectus muscle with the finger, located on a line extending from the umbilicus to the anterior superior iliac spine. Ask the patient to rise to a sitting position. Stand to the right and face the patient (for right-handed individuals). The thumb is placed vertically on the abdomen at the point identified by the finger. Position the tip of the thumb pointing to the ensiform and slowly press backward (not inward, outward, up, or down) into the abdomen. With the thumb depressed about halfway down to the back of the abdominal cavity, swing it to the patient's right at a right angle to the downward pressure line. This maneuver causes the appendix to become pinched against the iliacus muscle and other fixed structures located inferiorly and laterally	Palpation	Viscerosensory (chronic appendicitis)
Reder [188]	1913	The patient is positioned supine with their legs flexed. Insert a finger into the rectum reaching for O'Beirne's valve. The tip of the finger is allowed to rest within the lumen of the valve, and the patient asked if he experiences any pain. The answer is usually no. pain, if present, is generally referred to the sphincter area of the rectum. This pain will subside after allowing the finger to rest for a short time. (…) after being assured of the total absence of pain by the patient, the tip of the finger is gently pushed upward toward the right iliac fossa. The finger will touch a point beyond the valve that will cause significant pain in the case of appendicitis. Sweeping the examining finger toward the left inguinal fossa is a control point. The location of the pain was not specified	Palpation	Viscerosensory (chronic appendicitis)
Owen [192]	1914	Applying firm pressure with the hand over the descending colon causes gas within the colon to be driven forcibly toward the cecum, and the patient will complain of pain in the right iliac fossa. Steady pressure is maintained long enough to move some of the gas out of the blind end of the large intestine. Then, suddenly remove the hand. In that case, the rapid return of gas into the caecum disturbs the inflamed appendix so that the patient again complains of pain	Palpation	Viscerosensory

(continued)

Table 5.2 (continued)

Name	Year	Description of the sign	Method	Pathophysiologic mechanism
Wachenheim [196]	1916	To identify this point, gain the child's confidence, assuring them that the procedure will not be distressing. Introduce the examining finger with lubrication and slow dilation relatively painlessly into the rectum. The patient does not complain of discomfort until the introduced finger reaches the right iliac fossa. Here, the child complains of sharp pain in the neighborhood of McBurney's point. The child is asked to identify the site of the pain. If it is due to the rough introduction of the finger, the patient will invariably point to the anus. If appendicular, it is generally correctly localized, particularly in children eight years and older. The location of the pain was not specified	Palpation	Viscerosensory
Blaisdell [199]	1916	*Pain increases in intensity when the patient turns to the left and diminishes when they turn back to their right side.* When performing the test, the abdomen must not touch the bed to avoid supporting the viscera. The absence of support to the viscera pulls it to the left and drags it along the sensitive appendix causing additional pain. The location of the pain was not specified	Observation	Viscerosensory
Baldwin [208]	1916	The examiner asks the patient to extend their knee and lift the right leg. The leg drops, and the patient complains of pain. The location of the pain was not specified	Passive	Viscerosensory
Rosenstein [211]	1920	Place the patient in the left lateral decubitus position. Apply pressure to the right side, three fingerbreadths inside and slightly below the right anterior superior spine. The location of the pain was not specified	Palpatory	Viscerosensory
Kocher [223]	1921	The initial vomiting and localization of pain is in the epigastrium, followed by diffuse spread, and the gradual fixation at McBurney point occurs because of general peritoneal inflammation	Observation	Viscerosensory
Sloan [18, 223]	1922	The patient keeps their knee straight and raises the right heel from the bed while the examiner places his left hand over the right lower quadrant of the abdomen and applies pressure to it with the fingers of the right hand. The location of the pain was not specified.	Palpatory	Viscerosensory

	Year	Description	Method	Type
Gregory [74]	1922	Direct percussion at McBurney's point is often painless in chronic appendicitis. It has often been found that in chronic appendicitis, symptoms disappear after palpation of the appendix, only to return after a few minutes	Palpatory	Viscerosensory
Soresi [228]	1924	The examiner applies the hand to the region of the hepatic flexure of the colon. While the patient breathes as deeply as possible, the hand is pressed gently under the costal margin. The patient is told to cough and asked whether they felt any pain. If the answer is "yes," the patient, on being asked where the pain is felt, without hesitation, will indicate McBurney point when appendicitis is present	Palpation	Viscerosensory
Tresidder [230]	1925	The patient lies on their abdomen and, on being questioned, explains that they found this was the most comfortable position from which they could lie. The location of the pain was not specified	Observation	Viscerosensory
Livingston [234]	1932	A noninvolved area of the skin is picked up between the thumb and forefinger and pulled directly away from the abdomen. Traction is maintained outward until the patient reports discomfort. The initial degree of traction represents the intensity standard for that particular patient. The **pinch test** applies vigorous twisting pinches on all parts of the abdominal skin. An identical stimulus applied to an inflammatory area causes an immediate defensive response by the patient (winces, cries out, or reaches for the examining hand). Testing with heat and cold are further refinements that may aid in determining the limits of hyperesthesia or demonstrate the complete sensory change within the involved zone	Palpation	Viscerosensory
Klein [239]	1938	Tenderness is located over a small area to the right of the umbilicus but higher than McBurney point. The tender area may extend even above the umbilicus on the right side. The left side is nontender. The patient is turned to the left lateral decubitus position and remains for ≥30 seconds. Palpation identifies that the tender area previously identified on the right side is absent and has now shifted to the left of the umbilicus. The patient is now turned on their right side and allowed to rest for a short period. Palpation in this position reveals absent left and more marked tenderness on the right. Furthermore, the tender area is more extensive in this position than when the patient rests on their back	Palpation	Viscerosensory

(continued)

Table 5.2 (continued)

Name	Year	Description of the sign	Method	Pathophysiologic mechanism
Altschüler [241]	1938	Place the third through fifth fingers of the left hand on the outer border of the ileum and the left index finger on the inner border. The index finger is gradually moved downward over the soft parts from the anterior superior spine. A circumscribed area of abdominal tenderness is present. In severe cases, there is a localized muscle spasm in the exact location, or sometimes in a higher or lower position, at the right pelvic margin. The abdomen wall is usually not sensitive to pressure, and the usual points of tenderness are absent	Palpatory	Viscerosensory/ visceromotor (acute and chronic retrocecal appendicitis)
Alders [246]	1951	With the pregnant woman lying straight on her back, the examiner's fingers identify an area of maximum tenderness and applies pressure to the abdominal wall. Ask the patient to turn toward the left decubitus position while maintaining contact with the area of tenderness without altering the pressure exerted to elicit pain	Palpation	Viscerosensory
Bryan [249]	1955	Pressure on the pregnant uterus from the left side causes pain in the right lower or middle quadrants	Palpation	Viscerosensory
Arapov [252]	1968	With the fingers over the anterior abdominal wall, shallow pressure is applied first at a site distant from the right iliac fossa. Pain after deep and sharp pressure at the right ileal fossa confirms that the appendix, not the peritoneum, is involved. The rectal and vaginal examination confirms whether the pelvic peritoneum is also inflamed	Palpatory	Viscerosensory
Marek [253]	2021	The patient is placed in the left recumbent position with the knees and thighs flexed. In infants and children, firm pressure is applied to the anterior abdominal wall in the lumbar region using the thumb directed posteriorly, while palpatory pressure is applied in the right hypogastrium region using the second, third, and fourth fingers of the same hand. A bimanual method in adults involves applying the same technique with the thumb, but in this case, the fingers of the left and right-hand push in the right hypogastrium	Palpatory	Visceromotor

Ott [254, 255]	[n.a.]	When the patient is on their left side, there is a feeling of distress and a painful dragging sensation as if a heavy body in the abdomen had fallen to the left, sometimes referred to as the "mesenteric pull." The location of the pain was not specified	Observation	Viscerosensory
Baron [255]	[n.a.]	The patient is recumbent, relaxed, and told to breathe deeply. The examiner places the second, third, and fourth fingers of their right hand on Poupart's ligament, and pressure is applied downward toward the psoas muscle. Ask the patient to elevate the leg on the same side with the knee extended, forming an angle at the hip of about 45 degrees. In this position, the palpating fingers readily detect the psoas muscle, thus made tense. For purposes of comparison, apply similar palpation on both sides. Tenderness is more marked on the right side when the appendix is involved	Palpation	Viscerosensory/ visceromotor
Donnelly [255]	[n.a.]	The right leg is placed in full extension and abducted. Apply pressure over the right inferior quadrant below (McBurney's region). Pain elicited is proportional to the degree of inflammation in the appendix and its surroundings. The location of the pain was not reported	Palpation	Somatosensory

5.7 Conclusion

Despite advanced imaging techniques, history and physical examination remain the cornerstone in diagnosing acute and chronic appendicitis. There is an overlap in the performance of some clinical signs and activation of the same nerve pathway. Gaps remain in our knowledge regarding the reliability and validity of these signs in the clinical diagnosis of appendicitis. These limitations involve not performing the sign as initially described, lack of description or standardization of the maneuver, and failure to correlate the location of the appendix and the extent of the disease with the clinical examination. A further variation of these signs also depends on whether the appendix is located in its most common retrocecal or retro-appendiceal position. Clinicians performing these maneuvers must be aware of how they should be appropriately conducted, their limitations, pain location, and the significance of a positive test result. Knowledge of the fundamental anatomical aspects of the appendix, the site of the pain, and the location of the inflammatory process allows clinicians to correlate pathophysiologic principles to the mechanism involved in a positive test. These signs must be rigorously studied using a standardized methodology to further clarify and elucidate their role and utility in clinical practice.

References

1. Sherman R. Abdominal pain. In: Walker HK, Hall WD, Hurst JW, editors. Clinical methods: the history, physical, and laboratory examinations. 3rd ed. Boston: Butterworth; 1990. p. 443–7.
2. Fernelii I. Universa Medicina. Parisiis: Apud Andream Wechelum; 1554.
3. Fitz RH. Perforating inflammation of the vermiform appendix: with special reference to its early diagnosis and treatment. Philadelphia: Wm. J. Dornan; 1886.
4. Tzortzopoulou AK, Giamarelou P, Tsolia M, Spyridis N, Vakaki M, Passalides A, et al. The jumping up (J-up) test: making the diagnosis of acute appendicitis easier in children. Glob Pediatr Health. 2019;6:1–7.
5. Eid MM, Al-Kaisy M. The utility of the speed bump sign for diagnosing acute appendicitis. Am J Emerg Med. 2020;38:1551–3.
6. Sylvester CH, Rocheleau WF. McBurney, Charles. In: The new practical reference library, vol. 3. Chicago: The Dixon-Hanson Company; 1908. p. 451.
7. [No author]. Charles McBurney (1845–1913): point, sign, and incision. JAMA. 1966;197:1098–9.
8. [No author]. Death: Charles McBurney, MD. JAMA. 1913;61:1826–7.
9. McBurney C. Removal of biliary calculi from the common duct by the duodenal route. Ann Surg. 1898;28:481–6.
10. McBurney C. The use of rubber gloves in operative surgery. Ann Surg. 1898;28:108–19.
11. McBurney C. Dislocation of the humerus complicated by fracture at or near the surgical neck, with a new method of reduction. Ann Surg. 1894;19:399–415.
12. McBurney C. The incision made in the abdominal wall in cases of appendicitis, with a description of a new method of operating. Ann Surg. 1894;20:38–43.
13. McBurney C. Operations for pyloric stenosis. Ann Surg. 1886;3:372–80.
14. McBurney C. Surgery: on a method of operation for the radical cure of inguinal hernia. In: Braithwaite J, editor. The retrospect of practical medicine and surgery. New York: W.A. Townsend; 1890. p. 184.

15. Johnson AB. Charles McBurney, MA, MD. NY Med J. 1913;998:978–9.
16. McBurney C. Experience with early operative interference in cases of disease of the vermiform appendix. NY Med J. 1889;50:676–84.
17. Traube L. Entzündung des Bindegewebes und des Peritonäum in der Umgegend des Coecum mit Fäcal - Obstruction des Colon. In: Gesammelte Beiträge zur Pathologie und Physiologie. Berlin: Verlag von August Hirschwald; 1871. p. 55–6.
18. Boyce FF. The clinical picture and diagnosis of appendicitis. In: Acute appendicitis and its complications. New York: Oxford University Press; 1949. p. 113–54.
19. Soda K, Nemoto K, Yoshizawa S, Hibiki T, Shizuya K, Konishi F. Detection of pinpoint tenderness on the appendix under ultrasonography is useful to confirm acute appendicitis. Arch Surg. 2001;136:1136–40.
20. Andersson REB. Meta-analysis of the clinical and laboratory diagnosis of appendicitis. Br J Surg. 2004;91:28–37.
21. Levertin A. Svenskt porträttgalleri XIII. Läkarekåren ed. Stockholm: H.W. Tullbergs; 1889.
22. Hofberg H. Svenskt Biografiskt Handlexikon: Alfabetiskt Ordnade Lefnadsteckningar. Stockholm: Albert Bonniers Förlag; 1906.
23. Perman ES. Om indikationerna för operation vid appendicit samt redogörelse for å Sabbatsbergs sjukhus opererade fall. Hygiea. 1904;66:797–847.
24. [No author]. Moritz Blumberg. Br Med J. 1955;2:440–1.
25. Blumberg JM. Ein neues diagnostisches Symptom bei Appendicitis. Münch med Wochenschr. 1907;54:1177–8.
26. Kasatkin VM. Vydaiushchiĭsia deiatel' zemskoĭ meditsiny D.S. Shchetkin [A prominent man in Zemstvo medicine, D.S. Shchetkin]. Klin Med (Mosk). 1987;65:126–7.
27. Kasatkin VM. O peritoneal'nom simptome Shchetkina-Bliumberga [The Shchetkin-Blumberg peritoneal symptom]. Feldsher Akush. 1989;54:51–2.
28. Yudin AC. Achievements in surgery. Inform Bull Embassy Union Soviet Socialist Republic. 1945;5:8.
29. [No author]. 1939–1945 World War. Information Bulletin. The Embassy. 1946;5:66–131.
30. Golledge J, Toms AP, Franklin IJ, Scriven MW, Galland RB. Assessment of peritonism in appendicitis. Ann R Coll Surg Engl. 1996;78:11–4.
31. McGee SR. Abdominal pain and tenderness. In: Evidence-based physical diagnosis. 2nd ed. St. Louis: Saunders Elsevier; 2007. p. 572–87.
32. Rechcigl M. Henry Illoway. (1847–1932). In: American men and women in medicine, applied sciences and engineering with roots in Czechoslovakia practitioners—educators—specialists—researchers. Bloomington: AuthorHouse; 2021.
33. Collective. Henry Illoway. In: Distinguished Successful Americans of our Day. Chicago: Successful Americans; 1911. p. 304.
34. Landman I. Illoway, Henry. In: The universal Jewish encyclopedia: an authoritative and popular presentation of Jews and Judaism since the earliest times, vol. 5. New York: Universal Jewish Encyclopedia; 1939. p. 539.
35. Collective. Illoway, Henry. The National Cyclopedia of American biography, vol. 16. New York: James T. White; 1918. p. 417.
36. [No author]. Death of fellows of the academy. Bull NY Acad Med. 1932;8:105.
37. Mauthe G, Doppelhofer M, Blumesberger S. Illoway, Henry. In: Doppelhofer SBM, Mauthe G, editors. Handbuch österreichischer Autorinnen und Autoren jüdischer Herkunft: 18. bis 20. Jahrhundert, vol. 1. Wien: K.G. Saur; 2011. p. 587.
38. Illoway H. A pathognomonic symptom (or sign) of appendicitis not hitherto described. Arch Diagn. 1908;1:250–4.
39. Corscaden JA. Columbia University Irving Medical Center. Augustus C. Long Health Sciences Library. https://www.library-archives.cumc.columbia.edu/obit/james-corscaden. Accessed 28 Mar 2022.
40. Eliot E, Corscaden JA. Intussusception with special reference to adults. Ann Surg. 1911;53:169–222.
41. [No author]. Pedro Chutro. Aregentines Today. 1920;2:957–8.

42. Chutro P. Fracturas de la Extremidad Inferior del Húmero en los Niños. Buenos Aires: J. Peuser; 1904.
43. Buzzy A. Piedro Chutro, Figure o Argentine Surgery ALMA culturalmedicina. http://www.almarevista.com/revista/sin-categoria/eduardo-braun-menendez/. Accessed 22 Mar 2022.
44. Pedro C. Committee for historical and scientific work. https://cths.fr/an/savant.php?id=3240#. Accessed 22 Mar 2022.
45. Frédet P. Medical conditions in south American. Bull Pan Am Un. 1921;52:48–58.
46. Ureña PH. Historia cultural y literaria dela América hispánica. 2nd ed. Madrid: Editorial Verbum; 2008.
47. Prat D. Profesor Pedro Chutro. Rev Cir Urug. 1937;8:114–6.
48. Chutro P. El Ombligo de los Appendiculares. Buenos Aires: Imprenta de Coni Hermanos; 1912.
49. ten Horn C. Ugentmemorialis. Universiteit Gent ten Horn, Carel 1885-1964. http://www.ugentmemorialis.be/cataolg/000005248. Accessed 11 Aug 2022.
50. ten Horn C. Zur Diagnose der Appendicitis. Berl klin Wochenschr. 1914;3:1537–8.
51. Boschung U. Otto Lanz. Histroisches Lexikon der Schweiz HLS. https://hls-dhs-dss.ch/de/articles/014461/2008-09-09/. Accessed 21 Aug 2022.
52. Van Cappellen D. In memoriam Prof. Dr Otto Lanz Ned Tjdschr Geneeskd. 1935;79:1366–8.
53. Lanz O. Untersuchung auf Genitalsymptome zur Unterstützung der Diagnose bei Appendizitis. Zentralbl Chir. 1914;41:1705–7.
54. Collective. Morris, Robert Tuttle. In: The National Cyclopedia of American Biography, vol. 1. New York: James T. White; 1893. p. 393.
55. Chas GH. Robert Tuttle Morris, 1857–1945. Ann Surg. 1946;123:957–9.
56. Morris RT. Appendicitis and the gynecologist. JAMA. 1917;69:2036–7.
57. Burke MRP. The dexterous hand: Zachary Cope, surgeon and author, 1881–1974. Surg News R Aust Coll Surg. 2016;17:40–2.
58. [No author]. Obituary: Vincent Zachary Cope, Kt, MD, MS, FRCS. Med Hist. 1975;19:307–8.
59. Cope Z. Method of diagnosis: The examination of the patient—determination of iliopsoas rigidity. In: The early diagnosis of the acute abdomen. London: Henry Frowde and Hodder & Stoughton; 1921. p. 42.
60. O'Reilly MV, Krauthamer MJ. Cope's sign and reflex bradycardia in two patients with cholecystitis. Br Med J. 1971;2:146.
61. Cope Z. A sign of gall-bladder disease. Br Med J. 1970;3:147–8.
62. Vacca G, Battaglia A, Grossini E, Papillo B. Tachycardia and pressor responses to distention of the gallbladder in the anesthetized pig. Med Sci Res. 1994;22:697–9.
63. Kusumoto FM, Schoenfeld MH, Barrett C, Edgerton JR, Ellenbogen KA, Gold MR, et al. 2018 ACC/AHA/HRS guideline on the evaluation and management of patients with bradycardia and cardiac conduction delay. Circulation. 2019;140:e382–482.
64. Cope Z. Method of diagnosis: the examination of the patient—determination of iliopsoas rigidity. In: Siren W, editor. Cope's early diagnosis of the acute abdomen. 17th ed. Oxford: Oxford University Press; 1987. p. 36.
65. Prabhu S. Clinical signs and syndromes in surgery. Bangalore: Jaypee Brothers Medical Publisher; 2011.
66. Izbicki JR, Knoefel WT, Wilker DK, Mandelkow HK, Müller K, Siebeck M, et al. Accurate diagnosis of acute appendicitis: a retrospective and prospective analysis of 686 patients. Eur J Surg. 1992;158:227–31.
67. Berry J Jr, Malt RA. Appendicitis near its centenary. Ann Surg. 1984;200:567–75.
68. Kovalyova ON, Ashcheulova TV. Propedeutics to internal medicine, part 1: diagnostics. 2nd ed. Vinnytsia: Nova Knyha Publishers; 2011.
69. Augustin G. Acute abdomen during pregnancy. Cham: Springer; 2014.
70. Butsenko VN, Antoniuk SM. Znachimost' otdel'nykh simptomov ostrogo appenditsita [Significance of the separate symptoms in acute appendicitis]. Klin Khir. 1992;2:33–5.
71. Natalskyaya NY, Moseichuk KA. Remembering the great: Vasily Parmenovich Obraztsov. Tabrichesky Med Biol Bull. 2019;22:101–3.

72. Cope VZ. The thigh-rotation or obturator test: a new sign in some inflammatory conditions. Br J Surg. 1919;7:537.

73. Cope VZ. Genito-urinary symptoms in acute appendicitis. Proc R Soc Med. 1921–22;15:1–3.

74. Gregory A. Ueber ein neues diagnostisches Symptom bei Appendizitis. Zentralbl Chir. 1922;49:397–8.

75. Sattler E. Synoviale Sehnenscheidenentzündungen als Gewerbs - erkrankung an Händen und Füßen. Arch klin Chir. 1923:259–70.

76. Sattler E. Über die Amputationen. Ztschr Orthop Chir. 1926;47:268–75.

77. Sattler E. Ueber Rivanol - Behandlung. Ztschr Immunitätsforsch Exper Therap. 1925;45:81–5.

78. Sattler E. Die Aethernarkose Fortsch Ther. 1926;2:11–5.

79. Sattler E. Differential-diagnostische Möglichkeit zwischen akuter Appendicitis und Adnexitis mit Hilfe einer neuen Untersuchungsmethode. Dtsch Z Chir. 1924;187:347–52.

80. Hanaway J, Cruess R, Darragh J. McGill Medicine, 1885–1936, vol. 2. Montreal: McGill-Queen's University Press; 2006.

81. [No author]. Obituaries: Sir Henry McIlree Williamson Gray. CMAJ. 1938;39:612.

82. [No author]. Colonel Sir Henry McIlree Williamson Gray. Scotland's War Aberdeenshire's War. http://www.scotlandswar.co.uk/gray_hmw.html. Accessed 20 Jun 2022.

83. [No author]. Major Temp. Lieut. Col. Henry McIllree Williamson Gray, CB, CMG, MB, FRCS. JRAMC. 1919;33:115.

84. [No author]. Sir Henry Gray. Br Med J. 1923;1:730.

85. Gray SH. Physical factors in the production of appendicitis: points in diagnosis, their influence on surgical treatment. Ill Med J. 1925;48:33–8.

86. Przewalsky B. Diagnostik der Appendicitis chronica. Zentralb Chir. 1925;52:1078–9.

87. Hazelton HI. Long Island - Burroughs and counties: the boroughs of Brooklyn and Queens, counties of Nassau and Suffolk, Long Island, New York, 1609–1924, vol. 6. New York: Lewis Historical Publishing; 1925.

88. [No author]. Supreme court appellate division third department. New York: NY State; 1931.

89. [No author]. The Glover C. Arnold surgical prize: Irving Gray. In: New York University Catalogue. New York: University of the City of New York; 1914. p. 464.

90. [No author]. Irving Gray, MD. Med Clin N. 1925;9:547.

91. [No author]. Irving Gray, MD, Brooklyn, NY. Bull Am Heart Assoc. 1935;1:x.

92. Gray I. Left shoulder pain of phrenic origin: a reflex symptom in chronic appendicitis. Am J Med Sci. 1925;170:894–9.

93. Iliescu M. Nouvelles contributions à l'étude du signe du phrénique droit dans l'appendicite. Bull Acad Méd (Paris). 1926;96:315–7.

94. [No author]. Calendar of the Royal College of Surgeons of England. London: Taylor & Francis; 1899.

95. [No author]. Obituary: C.L. Granville Chapman. Br Med J. 1951;1:590.

96. Chapman CLG. The "rising test" for acute abdomen. Br Med J. 1927;2:786.

97. Sumner FW. An important sign in acute appendicitis. Br Med J. 1930;1:106–7.

98. LaRoque GP. Brittain's pathognomonic sign of gangrenous appendicitis. Am J Med Sci. 1931;182:191–5.

99. Summer JE. Prognosis in surgery of the abdomen: the acute appendix. Nebr Med J. 1932;17:473–7.

100. Fotheringham WT. Geneaología Familiar. https://genealogiafamiliar.net/getperson.php?personID=I95398&tree=BVCZ. Accessed 5 Sept 2022.

101. Fotheringham WT. La Voz de la Biblioteca. https://www.facebook.com/lavozdelabiblio/photos/02-de-junio-de-1901nace-wenceslao-tejerina-fotheringhamnaci%C3%B3-el-02-de-junio-de-1/2374847309418607. Accessed 5 Sept 2022.

102. Fotheringham WT. A propósito del valor diagnóstico de un signpo de appendicitis. Rev Méd Rosario. 1934;24:65–8.

103. Walters HE. In Memoria: Edward Vernon Mastin. Trans South Surg Assoc. 1958;71:332–3.

104. [No author]. Dr. Edward Vernon Mastin, President of the southern medical association. South Med J. 1945;38:559.

105. Collective. Mastin, Edward Vernon. In: Dictionary of medical specialist certified by American boards. Los Angeles, CA: The University of California; 1953. p. 1691.
106. [No author]. Edward Vernon Mastin, MD. Bull Washington Univ St Louis. 1926;24:22.
107. Mastin EV. Shoulder and clavicular pain in appendicitis. Ann Surg. 1936;103:773–80.
108. Binet L. Charles Richet (1850–1935). Revue des deux Mondes. 1950;15:417–28.
109. Richet C. Biographical. The Nobel Prize. https://www.nobelprize.org/prizes/medicine/1913/richet/biographical/. Accessed 20 Aug 2022.
110. [No author]. Prof. Charles Richet. Nature. 1935;136:1017–8.
111. Richet CR. La sélection humaine. Paris: Libraire Félix Alcan; 1919.
112. Richet C, Netter H. Un nouveau signe d'appendicite: la contracture des adducteurs du côté droit. Paris Méd. 1937;43:317–8.
113. Willner I. Obituary: Solomon Ben Asher (1894–1949). ACCP. 1949;16:508.
114. Ben-Asher S. The value of the cough sign in acute appendicitis. Am J Dig Dis. 1943;10:368–70.
115. [No author]. Obituaries: Dr. George Bushar Markle, IV native of Hazleton, dies. Hazleton Standard-Speaker; 1999. p. 2.
116. Markle GB. A simple test for intraperitoneal inflammation. Am J Surg. 1973;125:721–2.
117. Markle GB. Heel-drop jarring test for appendicitis. Arch Surg. 1985;120:243.
118. Ahn S, Lee H, Choi W, Ahn R, Hong JS, Sohn CH, et al. Clinical importance of the heel drop test and a new clinical score for adult appendicitis. PloS One. 2016;11:e0164574.
119. Menteş Ö, Eryilmaz M, Coşkun K, Harlak A, Özer T, Kozak O. The importance of heel drop physical examination sign in diagnosis of acute appendicitis. Eur J Surg Sci. 2010;1:77–82.
120. Hunt TK. University of California: In Memoriam, 1996, John Englebert Dunphy, surgery. San Francisco, University of California; 2011. http://texts.cdlib.org/view?docId=hb767nb3z6&chunk.id=div00029&brand=calisphere&doc.view=entire_text. Accessed 28 Jun 2022.
121. [No author]. United Press International. Dr. J. Englebert Dunphy, an internationally known surgeon. https://www.upi.com/Archives/1981/12/25/Dr-J-Englebert-Dunphy-an-internationally-known-surgeon-at/6739378104400/. Accessed 28 Jun 2022.
122. Nunes GC. The legacy of J. Englebert Dunphy. Am J Surg. 1995;169:466–70.
123. Dunphy JE, Botsford TW. Examination of the abdomen: the appraisal of abnormal findings. In: Physical examination of the surgical patient: an introduction to clinical surgery. Philadelphia: W.N. Saunders; 1975. p. 136–46.
124. Irdris SA, Shalayel MH, Awad TO, Idris TA, Ali AQ, Mohammed SA. The sensitivity and specificity of the conventional symptoms and signs in making a diagnosis of acute appendicitis. Sudan J Med Sci. 2009;4:55–61.
125. Dixon JM, Elton RA, Rainey JB, Macleod DA. Rectal examination in patients with pain in the right lower quadrant of the abdomen. Br Med J. 1991;302:386–8.
126. Acadèmia de Ciències Mèdiques I de La Salut de Catalunya I de Balears. Llibre Commemoratiu 1 Volum 150 èAniversari. https://institucional.academia.cat/docs/llibres-historia/llibre_150_aniversari.pdf. Accessed 5 Aug 2022.
127. [No author]. Dr. Samuel J. Meltzer, physiologist, dies. New York Times. 1920. p. 15.
128. Meltzer A. Samuel James Meltzer, MD, March 22, 1851–November 7, 1920. Proc Soc Exp Biol Med. 1987;184:370–4.
129. Brainard ER. History of the American Society for Clinical Investigation, 1909–1959. J Clin Invest. 1959;38:1784–837.
130. Howell WH. Biographical memoir: Samuel James Meltzer, 1851–1920. Washington, DC: National Academy of Sciences; 1926.
131. Meltzer SJ. On the contraction of the iliopsoas muscle as an aid in the diagnosis of the content of the iliac fossa. NY Med J. 1902;76:100–3.
132. [No author]. Obituary: James Sherren, CBE, FRCS. Br Med J. 1945;2:670.
133. [No author]. Sherren, James (1872–1945). Plarr's lives of the fellows. Royal College of Surgeons of England. https://livesonline.rcseng.ac.uk/client/en_GB/lives/search/detailnonmodal/ent:$002f$002fSDASSET$002f0$002fSD_ASSET:376771/one?qu=%22rcs%3A+E004588%22&rt=false%7C%7C%7CIDENTIFIER%7C%7C%7CResource+Identifier. Accessed 22 Jul 2022.

134. [No author]. Resident fellows: Sherren, James. Med-Chir T. 1904;87:xlix.

135. [No author]. List of members: Sherren, James. Tr Clin Soc. 1906;39:xxxix.

136. Sherren J. On the occurrence and significance of cutaneous hyperalgesia in appendicitis. Lancet. 1903;162:816–21.

137. Stevenson I. Sir James Mackenzie, 1853–1925. Am Heart J. 1953;46:479–84.

138. Brown GH. Sir James Mackenzie. The Royal College of Physicians. https://history.rcplondon.ac.uk/inspiring-physicians/sir-james-mackenzie. Accessed 10 Jun 2022.

139. [No author]. Obituary: Sir James Mackenzie FRS. Nature. 1925;115:271.

140. [No author]. Sir James Mackenzie (1853–1925), beloved clinician. JAMA. 1966;196:591–2.

141. Wade EG. Sir James Mackenzie, 1853–1925, MF, FRCP, FRS. In: Elwood WJ, Tuxford AF, editors. Some Manchester doctors: a biographical collection to mark the 150th anniversary of the Manchester medical society, 1834–1984. Manchester: Manchester University Press; 1984. p. 101–7.

142. Klingfield P, Hollman A. The sir James Mackenzie Cardiological society and the American College of Cardiology. Am J Cardiol. 1996;78:808–13.

143. Mackenzie J. The nature of the symptoms in appendicitis. Br Med J. 1903;2:66–8.

144. Palmerini A. Enciclopedia Italiana di Scienze, Lettere ed Arti. Roma: Istituto della Enciclopedia Italiana; 1936.

145. Haas C. Jean-Athanase Sicard et la Société médicale des hôpitaux de Paris. Hist Sci Méd. 1988;22:61–3.

146. Sicard JA. Le réflexe cutané abdominal au cours de la fièvre typhoïde et de l'appendicite chez l'enfant. Presse méd. 1905;13:19–20.

147. Berthomier AA. Résumé les services [original handwritten resume]. Paris: French Academy of Surgery; [n.a.].

148. Berthomier AA. Mécanisme des fractures du coude chez les enfants, leur traitement par l'extension. Paris: V. Adrien Delahaye et Cie; 1875.

149. Berthomier AA. De l'examen dans le décubitus latéral gauche pour le diagnostic difficile de l'appendicite. In: Dix-neuvième Congrès de Chirurgie. Paris: Association Française de Chirurgie; 1906. p. 167–9.

150. Michelson FG. Zur Frage von der primären chronischen Appendizitis und ihrer differentiellen Diagnose. Russk Vrach St Peterb. 1911;31:1243–7.

151. [No author]. Niels Thorkild Rovsing. Br Med J. 1927;1:265.

152. Hognason K, Swan KG. Niels Thorkild Rovsing: the surgeon behind the sign. Am Surg. 2014;80:1201–6.

153. Aagaard OC. Thorkild Rovsing. Danish Biographical Lexicon. https://biografiskleksikon.lex.dk/Thorkild_Rovsing. Accessed 28 Jun 2022.

154. Rovsing T. Indirektes Hervorrufen des typischen Schmerzes an McBurney's Punkt: Ein Beitrag zur Diagnostik der Appendizitis und Typhlitis. Zentralbl Chir. 1907;34:1257–9.

155. Wagner JM, McKinney WP, Carpenter JL. Does this patient have appendicitis? In: Simel DL, Rennie D, editors. The rational clinical examination: evidence-based clinical diagnosis. New York: McGraw Hill; 2009. p. 53–9.

156. Prosenz J, Hirtler L. Rovsing sign revisited: effects of an erroneous translation on medical teaching and research. J Surg Educ. 2014;71:738–42.

157. Davey WW. Rovsing's sign. Br Med J. 1956;2:28–30.

158. [No author]. Dr. Ira Carleton Chase, the fifty-third president of the State Medical Association of Texas. Tex State J Med. 1920;16:35–6.

159. Moulton CW. Chase, Ira Carleton. In: The Doctor's Who's Who. New York: Saalfield Publishing; 1906. p. 51.

160. Paddock BB. Ira Carleton Chase AM, MD, FACS. In: History of Texas: Fort Worth and Texas Northwest Edition. Chicago: Lewis Publishing; 1922. p. 144–5.

161. Chase IC. A new test for the differential diagnosis of appendicitis. JAMA. 1908;50:610–1.

162. [No author]. Obituaries: Dr. Walter Arthur Bastedo. Ann Intern Med. 1953;38:174.

163. [No author]. Deaths: Walter Arthur Bastedo. JAMA. 1952;150:233–4.

164. Matthews B. Columbia University Quarterly, vol. 6. New York: Columbia University Press; 1912.
165. [No author]. News items. Columbia Alumni News. 1915;7:541.
166. [No author]. Catalogue and General Announcement, 1907–1908: Catalogue of the Officers and Students of Columbia College; Columbia University in the City of New York, vol. 1908. New York: Columbia University. p. 13.
167. [No author]. New York Association for Medical Education Reorganizes. Med Rec. 1921;99:488.
168. [No author]. Medical news. JAMA. 1919;73:435.
169. Andresen AF. Dr. Walter Arthur Bastedo, 1873–1952. Gastroenterology. 1953;25:91–2.
170. Bastedo WA. Artificial dilation of stomach and colon as aids abdominal diagnosis; with a helpful sign in chronic appendicitis. Med Surg Rep St Luke's Hosp. 1910;2:104–11.
171. Bischoff CW. Zur Differentialdiagnose der Appendicitis chronica. Monatsschr Geburtshilfe Gynakol. 1914;40:398–404.
172. Hertz AF. Bastedo's sign: a new symptom of chronic appendicitis. Proc R Soc Med. 1913;6:185–8.
173. Marcus JR, Daniels JM. The concise dictionary of American Jewish biography. Brooklyn, NY: Carlson Publishing; 1994.
174. [No author]. Dr. Charles D. Aaron. In: Michigan Jewish history: early Jewish physicians in Michigan. Michigan: Jewish Historical Society of Michigan; 1962. p. 8.
175. [No author]. C.D. Aaron dies at 91; noted doctor. Detroit, MI: Detroit Free Press; 1951. p. 32.
176. [No author]. The American literary yearbook: a biographical and bibliographical dictionary of living north American authors, vol. 1. Minnesota: Publisher Henning; 1919.
177. Aaron CD. A sign indicative of chronic appendicitis. JAMA. 1913;60:350–1.
178. [No author]. News items: The American journal of gastroenterology. NY Med J. 1911;94:1239.
179. [No author]. New note. Ill Med J. 1916;29:316.
180. ACG's History. American College of Gastroenterology. https://gi.org/about/acgs-history/. Accessed 7 Sep 2022.
181. The founding and the early years, 1932–1954. American College of Gastroenterology. https://s3.gi.org/members/annbook/chapter1.pdf. Accessed 7 Sep 2022.
182. [No author]. College news notes. Ann Intern Med. 1936;9:1272–3.
183. Weiss S. In memoriam: Anthony Bassler, MD, FACG. Am J Gastroenterol. 1959;32:757–70.
184. Bassler A. Pinching the appendix in the diagnosis of chronic appendicitis. Am J Med Sci. 1913;146:204–9.
185. Bailey FW. Francis Reder, 1864–1936. Ann Surg. 1939;110:149–50.
186. Goodwin EJ. Francis Reder, biographical sketch. In: A history of medicine in Missouri. St. Louis: W.L. Smith; 1905. p. 253–4.
187. Reder F. History presidents. St Louis Surgical Society. https://www.saintlouissurgicalsociety.org/history/presidents. Accessed 12 Jul 2022.
188. Reder F. A sign of diagnostic value in obscure cases of chronic appendicitis elicited by rectal palpation. Int Clin. 1913;23:13–7.
189. [No author]. Obituary: Edmund Owen. Br Med J. 1915;2:200–3.
190. Owen EB (1847–1915). Plarr's live of fellows. Royal College of Surgeons of England. 2015. https://livesonline.rcseng.ac.uk/client/en_GB/lives/search/detailnonmodal/ent:$002f$002fSD_ASSET$002f0$002fSD_ASSET:375057/one?qu=%22rcs%3A+E002874%22&rt=false%7C%7C%7CIDENTIFIER%7C%7C%7CResource+Identifier. Accessed 24 Jul 2022.
191. Baume A. The late Mr. Edmund Owen. Lancet. 1915;186:359.
192. Owen E. Appendicitis: a plea for immediate operation, vol. 181. Bristol: John Wright and Sons; 1914.
193. Spengler O. Dr. Frederick L. Wachenheim. In: Das deutsche Element der Stadt New York; biographisches Jahrbuch der Deutsch-Amerikaner New Yorks und Umgebung. New York: Spengler; 1913. p. 271.

194. Collective. The Charity Organization Society of the City of New York, vol. 19-21. New York: Committee on the Prevention of Tuberculosis; 1902-1903. p. 4.
195. Wachenheim FL. The climatic treatment of children. New York: Rebman Company; 1907.
196. Wachenheim FL. A contribution to the diagnosis of appendicitis in childhood. Arch Pediatr. 1916;32:197–9.
197. Chamberlain JL. Blaisdell, Silas Canada. In: Universities and Their Sons—New York University: its history, influence, equipment and characteristics, vol. 2. Boston: R. Herndon Company; 1903. p. 247.
198. Little GT. Silas Canada Blaisdell. In: Genealogical and family history of the state of Maine, vol. 4. New York: Lewis Historical Publishing; 1909. p. 2252–3.
199. Blaisdell SC. The turning test in appendicitis. Arch Diagn. 1916;9–10:285–6.
200. [No author]. James Fairchild Baldwin. In: General Catalogue of officers and students, 1857–1900. Michigan: Ellis Publishing; 1900. p. 103.
201. Columbus Medical College. https://library.osu.edu/site/mhcb/2011/02/21/columbus-medical-college/. Accessed 14 Aug 2022.
202. [No author]. In memoriam: James Fairchild Baldwin, MD. Ohio Med J. 1936;32:264.
203. Origins of the OSU College of Medicine. https://library.osu.edu/site/mhcb/2014/01/05/origins-of-the-osu-college-of-medicine/. Accessed 14 Aug 2022.
204. Stevenson RB. A history of the Columbus medical association: The first seventy-five years, 1869–1945. Columbus: Columbus Medical Association; 2021.
205. Curtis JM, George M. James Fairchild Baldwin, MD, 1850–1936. Ohio State Archaeol Hist Q. 1947;56:374–8.
206. Centennials and Timeline of Medical Education in Central Ohio. The Ohio State University. University Libraries Historical Reflection: The Medical Heritage Center Blog. https://library.osu.edu/site/mhcb/category/the-ohio-state-university-college-of-medicine/ Accessed 14 Aug 2022.
207. [No author]. Editorial articles. Columbus Med J. 1899;23:43.
208. Davis JDS. Value of pain, jaundice, and tumor mass in the differential diagnosis of diseases of the right upper quadrant of abdomen. Tr Am Ass Obst Gynec. 1916;29:246–57.
209. Killy W, Vierhaus R. Dictionary of German biography, vol. 8. München: K.G. Saur; 2005.
210. Moll FH, Krischel M, Rathert P, Fangerau H. Urologie und Nationalsozialismus: Paul Rosenstein, 1875–1964: zerrissene Biographie eines jüdischen Urologen. Urologe. 2011;50:1143–53.
211. Rosenstein P. Der Mesenterialdruckschmerz ein einfaches differentialdiagnostisches Merkmal der Blinddarmentzündung. Zentralbl Chir. 1920;26:644–5.
212. Sitkovksy P. [About one of the clinical signs in inflammation of the appendix]. Turkestansk Med Zurn. 1922;1:37.
213. [No author]. Professor Theodor Kocher. Br Med J. 1917;2:168–9.
214. [No author]. Professor Theodor Kocher. Boston M S J. 1918;178:29–31.
215. Widmer M. The passing of a great man—professor Dr. Theodore Kocher Albany M Ann; 1917. p. 471–3.
216. [No author]. Theodor Kocher. Separatabdruck aus der Beilage "Nekrologe" zu den Verhandlungen der Schweiz. Freiburg: Verhandlungen der Schweiz Naturf Gesellschaft; 1917.
217. Tröhler U. Emil Theodor Kocher (1841–1917). J R Soc Med. 2014;107:376–7.
218. Karoye OF, Baribote O. Emil Theodor Kocher and surgical eponyms: a story of diligence, hard work and excellence. Yenagoa Med J. 2021;3:3–7.
219. Kocher T. Biographical. Nobel Prize. https://www.nobelprize.org/prizes/medicine/1909/kocher/biographical/. Accessed 8 Aug 2022.
220. [No author]. Theodor Kocher (1841–1917). Nature. 1941;148:222.
221. [No author]. N.M. Volkovitch. JAMA. 1914;63:1146.
222. Sachdeva A, Futta AK. Advances in pediatrics. In: Mahaveer pediatric surgery. New Delhi: Jaypee Brothers Medical; 2012. p. 1432.

223. Vogel A. Die Behandlung der Appendizitis an der chirurgische Klinik der Universität Bern. Arch klin Chir. 1921;115:1–85.
224. Hick FK. LeRoy Hendrick Sloan, MD, 1892–1961. Med Clin N Am. 1962;46:601–2.
225. Torino JM. 1915: la scuola Giuseppe Parini è adattata a Ospedale militare della Croce Verde (prima parte). Bdtorino. http://www.bdtorino.eu/sito/stampa_immagini. php?id=28917&data=21%20Maggio%202018&pubblicazione=Articolo%20scritto%20 da%20Milo%20Julini. Accessed 30 Aug 2022.
226. Gazdić VS. A brief history of anaesthesia. Gazdić Scr Med. 2020;51:190–7.
227. Kappáz GT. Avaliacão da qualidade de vida e fatores associdos à satisfacão dos pacientes submetidos ao tratamento cirúgico da Doenca do Refluxo Gastroesofágico. Dissertacão apresentad à Faculdade de Medicina da Universidade de São Paulo para obtencão do título de Mestre em Ciências. São Paulo: Faculdade de Medicina da Universidade de São Paulo; 2013.
228. Soresi AL. A helpful sign in the diagnosis of appendicitis. JAMA. 1924;1:1766.
229. [No author]. Obituary notices: lieutenant-colonel a.G. Tresidder CIE, MD, MS, FRCS, IMS (Retd). Br Med J. 1970;3:289.
230. Tresidder AG. An interesting sign in retro-cæcal appendicitis. Ind M Gaz. 1925;60:376.
231. [No author]. Edward Meakin Livingston. In: New York University – report of officers 1920–1921, 1921–1922. New York: New York University; 1922. p. 370.
232. [No author]. Livingston, Edward Meakin. In: Alumni directory, 1849–1919. Wisconsin: University of Wisconsin; 1921. p. 202.
233. Livingston EM. Family Search. Updated 2019-12-10. https://ancestors.familysearch.org/en/ L2SP-S8C/edward-meakin-livingston-1895-1969. Accessed 2 Feb 2022.
234. Livingston EM. A clinical study of the abdominal cavity and peritoneum. New York: P.B. Hoeber; 1932.
235. Pack GT, Livingston EM. End-results in the treatment of gastric cancer: an analytical study and statistical survey of sixty years of surgical treatment, vol. 198. New York: P.B. Hoeber; 1939. p. 263.
236. Pack GT, Livingston EM. Treatment of cancer and allied diseases. New York: P.B. Hoeber; 1940.
237. Foote EM, Livingston EM. Principles and practice of minor surgery. 6th ed. New York: D. Appleton; 1929.
238. Livingston EM. The skin triangle of appendicitis: a discussion of its significance and its diagnostic value as observed in more than four hundred cases of acute appendicitis. Arch Surg. 1926;13:630–43.
239. Klein W. Nonspecific adenitis: a report of one hundred and forty cases. Arch Surg. 1938;36:571–85.
240. Altschüler E. Judische Pflege-geschichte. Jewish Nursing History. https://www. juedische-pflegegeschichte.de/recherche/?limiter=network&cmd=limitObject&dataI d=107868945880153&sid=e0f4d9434fd61f318ac4879c511ad9ae&id=131724555879435. Accessed 14 Sep 2022.
241. Altschüler E. A diagnostic sign for retrocaecal appendicitis. Lancet. 1938;231:891–2.
242. Fisher R. Nicholas Alders. Br Med J. 1995;311:1294.
243. Alders N. Cavernous haemangioma of the perineum. J Obst Gyn Br Empire. 1949;56:1038–40.
244. [No author]. Medical news: appointments. Br Med J. 1955;1:176.
245. [No author]. Mr. Nicholas Alders. In: Constitution and by-laws of the International College of Surgeons and the United States section. Chicago: International College of Surgeons; 1953. p. 43.
246. Alders N. A new sign for differentiating uterine from extrauterine complications of pregnancy and puerperium. Br Med J. 1951;2:1194–5.
247. Chen CF, Tan KH, Shin FC, Chen HI. Acute appendicitis during pregnancy. J Med Sci. 1999;19:252–62.

248. [No author]. Williams Bryan Jr. The Post and Courier. Legacy. https://www.legacy.com/us/obituaries/charleston/name/williams-bryan-obituary?n=williams-bryan&pid=97086959&fhid=5564. Accessed 21 Aug 2022.
249. Bryan WM Jr. Surgical emergencies in pregnancy and in the puerperium. Am J Obstet Gynecol. 1955;70:1204–13.
250. Kurtz GR, Davis RS, Sproul JD. Acute appendicitis in pregnancy and labor, a report of 41 cases. Obstet Gynecol. 1964;23:528–32.
251. Arapov DA. Biography. The Great Russian Encyclopedia. https://cityshin.ru/en/metal-processing/dmitrii-alekseevich-arapov-biografiya-dmitrii-alekseevich-arapov/. Accessed 14 Sep 2022.
252. Arapov DA, Simonian KS, Kaplan BS. Paradoksy ostrogo appenditsita [Paradoxes of acute appendicitis]. Vestn Khir Grek. 1968;101:22–6.
253. Marek V, Záhorec R, Durdík S. Acute appendicitis: clinical anatomy of the new palpation sign. Clin Anat. 2021;34:218–23.
254. Cobb DB. Appendicitis: the two P's and the highest mortality in the world. North Carolina Med J. 1940:472–8.
255. Robertson WME, Robertson HF. Diagnostic signs, reflexes and syndromes. Philadelphia: F.A. Davis Company; 1947.
256. [No author]. Daniel J. Donnelly. In: Samaritan hospital: twenty-second annual report from June 1, 1914 to June 1, 1915. Philadelphia: Temple University; 1916. p. 8.
257. [No author]. News. N Y Med Week. 1937;16:7.
258. [No author]. News items: the medical Department of the Temple University of Philadelphia. N Y Med J. 1908;88:802.
259. [No author]. State news items. Penn Med J. 1917;20:447.

Chapter 6
Miscellaneous Non-reflex Signs in Appendicitis

6.1 Introduction

In the late nineteenth century, physicians began recognizing the relationship between elevated white blood cells, serofibrinous exudate, and adhesions as markers of the inflammatory response. A variety of other findings detected in patients with appendicitis included detecting air within the colon or rectum, the texture of the abdominal muscles, and accentuation of the pulmonic component to the second heart sound. This chapter describes appendiceal signs whose pathogenesis is not based on the activation of cerebrospinal or visceral nerve pathways. The signs are reported chronologically from the date they were first reported.

6.2 Miscellaneous Eponymous Signs

6.2.1 Hayem–Sonnenburg Sign

6.2.1.1 Georges Hayem

Georges Hayem (1841–1933) was born in Paris, France, completed the boarding school competitive examination in 1863, and began his externship that same year [1]. He was appointed to the Hôpital des Enfants Malades (Hospital of the Sick Children), Paris, in 1864, followed by Lariboisière Hospital in the same city [2]. He was an assistant to Alfred Vulpian (1826–1887) and an intern at the Salpêtrière Hospital in 1865. Hayem was elected to the French Academy of Medicine, Paris, in 1866, received the Gold Medal in 1867, and served as its president in 1918 [3, 4]. He received his medical degree in 1868 with the thesis titled *Études sur les diverses formes d'encéphalite: anatomie et physiologie pathologiques* (Study of the Various Forms of Encephalitis: Pathological Anatomy and Physiology). Hayem completed

S. H. Yale et al., *Gastrointestinal Eponymic Signs*, https://doi.org/10.1007/978-3-031-33673-7_6

two aggregation theses titled *Des bronchites* (Bronchitis) in 1869 and *Des hémorragies intra-rachidiennes* (Intra-spinal Hemorrhage) in 1872. At the Faculty of Medicine in Paris, he was appointed assistant professor of the pathological laboratory, which he directed beginning in 1873 [5–7].

Hayem was appointed associate professor and hospital doctor in 1868 and served as a physician at the Central Hospital Office in 1872 and the Charity Hospital, Paris, in 1877 [1, 3, 4, 8]. He was named professor of clinical medicine at the Faculty of Paris and chair of therapeutics and materia medica at St. Antoine Hospital, Paris, in 1879 [3]. His contributions spanned multiple disciplines, including stomach disorders and blood pathology [4]. He is most highly recognized as being the French promoter of modern hematology, providing the first description of chronic hemolytic anemia, later named eponymously as Hayem-Widal or acquired type [9]. Hayem's books titled *Du sang et des ses altérations anatomiques* (Blood and Its Anatomical Alterations), published in 1889, and *Leçons cliniques sur les maladies du sang* (Clinical Lessons in Blood Diseases), published in 1900, were considered landmark works in the field of hematology during that time [9, 10]. He was a member of the French Academy of Medicine and was named Commander of the Legion of Honor in 1913 [11]. Hayem founded the journal *Revue des sciences médicales en France et à l'étranger* (Journal of Medical Sciences in France and Abroad) in 1873 and the French Society of Hematology, serving as its first president in 1931 [4]. The Leukemia Research Institute at Saint-Louis Hospital was also named in his honor in 1960 [8].

Hayem described the relationship between an elevated white blood cell count and unrecognized inflammation, suppuration, peritonitis, and appendicitis:

> The same year when I began to occupy myself continuously with the examination of the blood, a friend of mine asked me to determine the degree of anemia in a woman with puerperal mania. The patient's blood was frankly inflammatory. It formed lumps with liquid A (artificial serum used for diluting blood), and the number of white blood cells was very high. I, therefore, pronounced the existence of intense inflammation. In fact, the patient was suffering from suppurative pelvic-peritonitis. Since that time, other cases have been identified. It has been shown that examination of the blood often identifies ailments or complications that may go unnoticed in certain complex clinical cases. It is mainly in abdominal diseases of an obscure diagnosis that examining the blood can be beneficial. It can be used, for example, to distinguish hematocele from pelvic-peritonitis and to reveal the state of the peritoneum in diseases of the intestine or abdominal viscera, including constrictions and pseudo-constrictions, typhlitis and perityphlitis, perihepatitis, perinephritis, etc. [10, p. 1019–1020].

Leukocytosis is a well-recognized finding in patients with acute and chronic infectious and inflammatory processes (Table 6.1). This sign is a remarkable historical example of a universally well-known finding recognized in the late nineteenth century.

6.2.1.2   Eduard Sonnenburg

Eduard Hermann Sonnenburg (1848–1915) was born in Bremen, Germany, and received his medical degree in 1872. He served as an assistant at the surgical university clinic in Strasbourg under Georg Albert Lücke (1829–1894) from 1873 to 1880 (completed habilitation in 1876), followed by an appointment in Berlin as first assistant and head of the surgical university clinic with Bernhard Rudolf Konrad von Langenbeck (1810–1887) and as first assistant to Ernst von Bergmann (1836–1907) at the Royal Clinic until 1883 (completed habilitation in 1881) [12–14]. At Friedrich Wilhelm University, Sonnenburg was a private lecturer in 1881, appointed associate professor in 1883, and an honorary professor in 1908 [15]. He was appointed Geheimer Medizinalrat (Privy Medical Councilor) in 1899 [14]. Sonnenburg was director of the surgical department at the City Hospital of Berlin at Moabit from 1890 to 1915 [14, 16]. He served as editor of *Deutsche Zeitschrift für Chirurgie* (German Journal of Surgery) and was a founding member and first chairman of the Free Association of Surgeons of Berlin (currently Berlin Surgical Society) in 1886 [12, 13]. He served as consulting general physician of the Army Corps III at the onset of World War I and was appointed by the Ministry of Culture to direct the surgical clinic and lectures in Ziegelstrasse, Berlin, during August Karl Gustav Bier (1861–1949) temporary leave during the war [13]. Sonnenburg's lifework spanned multiple therapeutic areas, including burns, frostbite, surgical management involving the urinary bladder and prostate injuries, and perityphlitis [12–14]. In a description of his character:

> He was an international personality and enjoyed a worldwide reputation, especially in recognition of his operational accomplishments in the field of perityphlitis, which of course, only comprised a part of his significant achievements. The readers of our weekly, of whom he has been a loyal collaborator for many years, acknowledge the high value of his scientific work—work through which he did honor to Lücke's school and especially Langenbeck's in every respect. The distinguished and likable personality of Sonnenburg will never be forgotten in the broadest circles of our city among the Berlin specialists who made him the first chairman of the Society for Surgery and for whom he served with devotion and success as head of the surgical department of the Moabit Hospital [17, p. 591].

In his book titled *Pathologie und Therapie des Perityphlitis: Appendicitis Simplex und Appendicitis Perforativa* (Pathology and Therapy of Perityphlitis: Simple Appendicitis and Perforated Appendicitis), Sonnenburg wrote:

> With some experience, one can undoubtedly diagnose the condition of the appendix and peritoneum based on symptoms before the operation. However, as a rule, one finds pronounced gangrene with or without perforation in the vicinity of purulent progressive peritonitis. I made this claim years ago. Suppose the peritoneum has been severely infected by the spread of phlegmon, perforation, or gangrene. In that case, a serofibrinous exudate is located on the peritoneal surface near the focus. The exudate is clouded by the multiplication and disintegration of microbes and the resulting confluence of leukocytes, which present more rapidly and to a greater extent the more severe the infection. The more severe the infection, the greater the fibrin content so that delicate fibrinous adhesions are formed [18, p. 85].

Thus, Sonnenburg described the pathophysiologic process found intraperitoneally in patients with perforated appendicitis (Table 6.1).

6.2.2 *Roux Sign*

César Roux (1857–1934) was born in Mont-la-Ville, Switzerland, studied medicine at Geneva and Bern, and received his medical degree from the University of Bern, Switzerland, in 1880 [19, 20]. Notably, after graduation, he served as an assistant to Emil Theodor Kocher (1841–1917) at the Isle Hospital, Bern, from 1880 to 1883. He practiced as a private surgeon at Place de la Palud, Lausanne, Switzerland, from 1883 to 1887 and served as a professor of forensic medicine at the Faculty of Law from 1884 to 1888 [19, 20]. From 1887 to 1926, Roux served as chief surgeon at Cantonal Hospital in Lausanne and, from 1885 to 1889, was appointed extraordinary professor of forensic medicine at the Academy of Lausanne [19]. He was as director of the surgical clinic and the first professor of ordinary surgery and gynecology when the academia was renamed Lausanne University from 1890 to 1923 [20]. Roux received an honorary doctorate from the University of Paris and the Chicago School of Medicine and the titles—Commander of the Legion of honoris causa from the University of Berne in 1930, Commander of the Order of George I, Grand officer of the Order of the Crown of Italy, and Honorary President of the Swiss Society of Surgery [20]. He was an honorary member of the Bucharest Surgical Society of Medicine, Royal Academy of Medicine of Rome, American Society of Urology, Society of Medicine of the Canton of Bern, the Society of Medicine of Canton of Vaud, and the Military Academy of Medicine of St. Petersburg [20]. In addition to the sign that bears his name, he is best known for the surgical anastomotic operation Roux-en-Y, with the letter "Y" vaguely resembling the position of the intestines after bypass. He is also credited for performing the first successful operation to remove a pheochromocytoma in 1926 [21, 22].

Roux described a sign in his paper titled "Traitement chirurgical de la pérityphlite suppurée" (Surgical treatment of suppurative perityphlitis) for determining the presence of inflammatory infiltrate and pus in the abdomen caused by appendiceal perforation:

Early perforation and infiltration occur in the intestinal wall covered by the mesentery. The two mesentery layers are involved with the infiltrate, rapidly gaining access by the looser serosa layer on the inferior and anterior sides of the cecum and adjacent colon. The infiltrate causes thickening and somewhat rigidity of the intestinal wall. The wall is palpable and slightly dull to percussion. This sign, which we drew attention to at the Third French Congress of Surgery, has never failed us and proves that an abscess has formed and that pus, which is often undetected by the patient, his family, or his doctor, is present. Moreover, it is useless to wait until this infiltration extends further within the colon. The diagnosis is confirmed as soon as it appears on the cecum. It is easy to see, and one can imagine that the feeling of resistance offered by the cecal wall is similar in consistency to very soft cardboard soaked in hot water. This finding should not be confused with the presumed edge of the cecum infiltrated within the end of the muscular fibers of the external oblique or its fascia. (…) In a word, the surgeon should find the collected infiltrated pus in all cases of perforating appendicitis as soon as it involves the cecum. At this point, 48 hours at most has elapsed since the moment of perforation. It can be difficult to reach the abscess without opening the peritoneal cavity, which is isolated on all sides by adhesions [23, p. 211–212].

Furthermore, he described the method for detecting typhlitis or inflammation of the cecum and distinguishing it from perityphlitis (appendicitis):

> There are two findings, according to whether the disease originates in the cecum or the vermiform appendix. For the first, one has gone so far as to deny its existence (apart from the trauma, which ultimately in this region mimics any spontaneous inflammatory process). Nevertheless, we recognize the possibility of pericecal suppuration following a simple stercoral stasis. It is indeed here that the disease begins with stasis of feces, a foreign body, followed by irritation of the mucous membrane and muscle, and finally of the serosa. Stasis is followed by typhlitis or inflammation of the walls of the cecum. Perityphlitis (when the serosa is dull) forms plastic-like adhesions or suppuration nearby independent of a cecal perforation. It is possible and even probable that there is injury or ulceration of the mucosa. However, we cannot deny, a priori, the formation of pus around the caecum in the late period of a stercoral typhlitis. However, this form of suppurative perityphlitis is rare. In general, stercoral stasis soon gives way to a laxative or enema. (…) For a certain time after, there remains a substantial thickening of the cecal walls, and it is even possible to palpate this empty coecum, to move it back and forth. Only after weeks, the cecum resumes its normal state [23, p. 204].

Thus, Roux sign refers to palpable thickening, rigidity, and percussion dullness of the cecal wall in appendicitis (Table 6.1).

6.2.3 Mannaberg Sign

Julius Mannaberg (1860–1941) received his medical degree from the University of Vienna in 1884 and continued his training with Moritz Kaposi (1837–1902) at the Vienna General Hospital in 1887 and Hermann Nothnagel (1841–1905) at the I. Medical Clinic, Vienna, from 1887 to 1895. He completed his habilitation in 1895 [24, 25]. Mannaberg was promoted to the rank of first assistant in the I. Medical Clinic in 1894 [25]. During the summer months between 1890 and 1892, he received the Oppolzer Travel Scholarship, allowing him the opportunity to study malaria in Istria, Dalmatia, Croatia, Slavonia, and Austro-Hungarian monocracy. He worked in the Vienna Polyclinic as an internal medicine physician beginning in 1898, advancing to director, which he served from 1917 to 1930. He was appointed Associate Professor of Medicine at the University of Vienna in 1902 and elected to the Royal Society of Tropical Medicine in 1909 [26].

In his review of cases of acute appendicitis, Mannaberg identified the presence of "repetition of over-accentuation of the second pulmonary sound without any other explanation that could explain this symptom" [27, p. 209]. In his review of 88 patients seen at the Nothnagel Clinic from 1882 to 1892, this finding was identified in 10 (11%) of patients. In an additional 13 (85%) cases of acute appendicitis, the pulmonary sound was accentuated in 4 cases and, in 7 cases, considerably louder than the second heart sound [27, p. 210].

He accounted for the discrepancy of why this sign had not been previously recognized:

It will hardly seem strange that the symptom in question has not been found much more often than in the older case series. Despite all the accuracy and objectivity in describing the symptoms, the examiner's attention is always directed to the point where the disease is located. Therefore, it is understandable that we usually access the status of the heart in acute appendicitis in a somewhat superficial manner. Incidentally, to personally keep me as free as possible from any bias, I asked my esteemed colleague to judge the finding in most cases. I, therefore, hold myself entitled to the statement that in acute appendicitis accentuated of the pulmonary component of the second heart sound is found frequently. As far as I am aware, this finding has not been previously reported in the literature [27, p. 210].

Mannaberg was unable to explain the significance of this finding but recognized that "Further observation in a large number of cases of acute appendicitis and other pathological conditions of the abdomen may teach us, along with the other symptoms mentioned, the significance of this diagnostic finding" [27, p. 211]. We are unaware of any study that evaluated this sign's sensitivity of specificity (Table 6.1).

6.2.4   *Filatov Sign*

Nil Fedorovich (Fyodorovich) Filatov (1847–1902) was born in Mikhailovka, Saransk district, Penza province in Southern Russia, and received his medical training from the Faculty of Medicine at Moscow University in 1869 [28–30]. After returning to the Saransk district to work as a private practitioner he traveled to Vienna, Prague, Paris, Berlin, and Heidelberg to study diseases of children. Upon his return, he was appointed head to the Sofia Children's Hospital in 1875, received his medical degree in 1876 based on the thesis "On the Question of the Relationship of Bronchitis to Acute Catarrhal Pneumonia" and served as an associate professor in the Department of Obstetrics, Children's and Women's Diseases at Moscow University [28, 30]. He was appointed professor in the Department of Children's Diseases at Moscow University in 1891 and ordinary professor at Moscow University beginning in 1898. The Children's Clinical Hospital was named in his honor in 1922 [28–30]. He served as chairman of the Moscow Society of Pediatric Physicians. He is considered founder of the Russian Pediatric School [30].

Filatov described findings occurring early in patients with acute appendicitis:

> On the second or third day a circumscribed hardening in the form of an immovable tumor, very painful upon pressure, may be felt in the right iliac region at a point which exactly correspond to the caecum [31, p. 202].

Thus, Filatov described the inflammatory appendiceal swelling in the right lower quadrant in patients with acute appendicitis (Table 6.1). Pain in the right lower quadrant with palpation suggests activation of the viscerosensory reflex.

6.2.5   *Klemm Sign*

Paul Karl Otto Klemm (1861–1925) was born in Riga, Latvia, and received his medical degree in 1891. He was an assistant physician in Terbata, Latvia, assistant to the chair of the Department of Surgery at Riga City Hospital, and director of the Surgical Dispensary of the Red Cross from 1892 to 1895 [32]. Klemm was appointed chair and medical director of the surgical department in 1908. He was vice-president of the Riga Cross Society and a member of the Practical Doctors Society, for which he served as president and co-editor of *St. Petersburger medizinische Wochenschrift* (St. Petersburg Medical Weekly) [32]. Klemm's interests included the study of the acute and chronic forms of tetanus, particularly those involving the facial nerve (Klemm tetanus), osteomyelitis, hernias in children, abdominal shotgun injuries, aseptic suture materials, ligature of a fistula, and primary peritonitis [32].

Klemm, in 1906, described findings occurring in some patients with chronic appendicitis (Table 6.1):

> Another objective symptom that was detectable in most cases was the local gaseous dilation of the cecum, which persisted even after evacuation. I call this the air cushion symptom. On inspection, in thin patients with a scaphoid abdomen, one can perceive a protrusion in the right lower abdominal region. When palpating the abdomen, one can feel a mass of air the size of a man's fist. On intermittent light palpation, a squeaky, cooing sound is produced [33, p. 593].

Klemm believed that pain in the right iliac fossa at McBurney point and the large dilation of the cecum or "air-cushion" findings are two symptoms that are useful in distinguishing appendicitis from pseudo-appendicitis. He coined the term "anfalls-frei appendicitis" or "seizure-free appendicitis" in cases where intra-abdominal adhesion involves the cecum and colon with cecal dilation, presumably since they prevent movement of the cecum. Klemm attributed this condition to appendiceal inflammation but found in many cases that appendectomy did not resolve the patient's symptoms [34]. Hofmeister believed that these intra-abdominal bands or membranes over the colon and cecum were evidence of previous episodes of appendicitis or colitis [35].

6.2.6   *Kahn Sign*

Maurice Guttman Kahn (1873–1950) was born in Morrison, Illinois, and received his medical degree from Harvard University in 1898 [36]. He was surgeon to the Denver and Rio Grande RR and visiting physician to Children's Home and St. Vincent's Hospital Leadville, Colorado. Kahn founded the Cedars of Lebanon Hospital (previously called Kaspar Cohn Hospital) in Los Angeles, California, and was appointed chief of staff of surgery in 1913. He was professor of clinical surgery at Southern California University in 1928 [36].

Kahn identified the presence of bradycardia in six cases of gangrenous appendicitis:

> So it would appear from this given a case presenting other unmistakable signs of appendicitis, with a subnormal pulse, the tentative diagnosis of gangrene, with some reason, may be maintained [37, p. 2011].

Relative bradycardia may also be found in patients with peritonitis and sepsis secondary to acute appendicitis (Table 6.1).

6.2.7   *Dubard Sign*

There is limited historical information on Pierre-Marie-Maurice Dubard (1862–1941). He was born in Côte-d'Or, Bourgogne, France, served as professor at the School of Medicine in Dijon and was appointed chair of pathology and medicine clinics at the same school. He served as president of Côte d'Or Committee from 1926 to 1929 and from 1967 to 1971 [38–40].

Dubard reported on the association between gastric or duodenal ulcers and chronic appendicitis. In the first series of 36 patients who underwent a laparotomy for pyloric and subpyloric ulcers and strictures, an appendectomy was performed in 12 (33%) patients with chronic appendicitis. In the second series of 101 patients with juxta-pylori or a duodenal ulcer, 40 underwent gastroenterostomy, and in 18 (45%) cases, a concomitant appendectomy for chronic appendicitis was performed. The pneumogastric sign, or sensitivity upon pressure on the vagus nerve in the neck, was present in 17 of 18 patients. Dubard found that 80% of patients operated on with gastric ulcers had chronic pulmonary tuberculosis. Based on these findings Dubard concluded (Table 6.1):

> Since then, the meaning of the "pneumogastric sign" has been clarified: vagal neuritis, of pulmonary origin, causing localized ulcer and other chronic inflammatory disorders of the gastrointestinal tract in the organs innervated by this nerve. (…) The frequency of associated lesions of the gastrointestinal tract partly explains the post-operative failure of operations limited to a single organ (appendectomy, gastro-enterostomy). This observation implies as a corollary to the surgeon, the obligation to explore as complete as possible the digestive tract of the patient [41, p. 359–360].

Huchon in a thesis at Lyons proposed a pathogenesis for a simple gastric ulcer that assists in the diagnosis and prognosis. Dubard recognized the relationship between pulmonary tuberculosis and gastric ulcer and proposed that a:

> [c]hronic lesion of the lung causes irritation of the pulmonary terminals of the pneumogastric nerves resulting in a neuritis or neuralgia of this nerve. The neuritis in turn leads to trophic disturbance on the side of the stomach and consequently a gastric ulcer [42, p. 903].

Huchon called this association between pneumogastric neuritis and simple gastric ulcer Dubard sign [42]. In addition to tuberculosis, other conditions can cause a similar phenomenon, including aneurysms and cancer of the lung if the pneumogastric nerve is involved. Furthermore, Huchon found that in patients with a confirmed benign ulcer, pressure exerted at the neck always shows either one or both of these nerves sensitive to pressure which was absent in those with gastric cancer.

6.2.8   Williams Sign

Edward Johnston Williams (1872–1946) was born in Franklin Centre, Quebec, and received his medical degree from McGill University. He was appointed chief surgeon at Sherbrooke General Hospital, Quebec [43]. Williams was a major in the Canadian Army Medical Corps, commanded as chief surgeon at the No 1 Canadian Stationary Hospital at Lemnos and Salonika, Greece, the No 13 Canadian General Hospital, Hastings, Sussex, and the No 9 Canadian General Hospital in Shorncliffe, Folkestone, in 1918. He was the recipient of the Distinguished Service Order. He continued his surgical practice in Montreal after World War I [43].

Williams described the case of an 18-year-old male with bilateral inguinal pain. During herniorrhaphy, he found on the right side a:

> [m]ass was found to be a portion of the omentum. (…) After extensive dissection I separated from the cord a long appendix which extended down into the scrotum to the epididymis. This condition suggested to my mind the possibility of the appendix being dragged down into the scrotum with the testicles at the time of its descent form the abdominal cavity [44, p. 193].

Thus, Williams sign refers to the inflamed appendix herniating through the inguinal canal (Table 6.1).

6.2.9   Hönck Sign

There is limited historical information on Ernst Hönck. At the time of the publication of his sign, he was a physician practicing in Hamburg, Germany [45]. Hönck acknowledged Widmer's 1908 publication in *Münchener medizinische Wochenschrift* (Munich Medical Weekly) of a case of epityphlitis with peritonitis and the finding that the temperature of the right axilla was 0.3–1.5 higher compared to the left axilla:

> I have asserted in this study that at the onset of acute epityphitis the right sympathetic is irritated, and that in some cases after a time the irritation spreads to the left sympathetic. If this observation is correct, then in such cases the temperature of the left axilla would be higher than that of the right. This is indeed the case. In fact, in two recent cases I have found the left axilla warmer than the right; namely in one case of an unoperated acute epityphlitis, and the other occurring three weeks after operating on an acutely inflamed appendix. Both women had spontaneous left abdominal pain at the time and the difference in both was only 0.2°. (…) I venture to say beforehand that in some cases one will find a one-sided increases in temperature. In other cases a temperature difference will only be found at the trunk, and uncommonly, one will find that a crossing of the temperature differences takes place in such

a way that one finds the higher temperatures at the trunk on the right and a lower temperature on the left lower extremities and vice versa. Similar crossing might take place at the head. I am assuming that the sympathetic irritation is so strong that it becomes noticeable in the form of a rise in temperature in distant parts of the body. This, however, may of course will not always be the case [45, p. 1511].

We are unaware of the sensitivity or specificity of this sign (Table 6.1).

6.2.10   Widmer Sign

There is limited historical information on Charles Widmer. He served as a physician at the Lerchsche Hospital, Zofingen, in Switzerland [46, 47]. He reported in an 18-year-old female with acute appendicitis:

> [w]e became aware of a peculiar behavior of the temperature. The right axilla showed significantly higher values than the corresponding one on the left and this difference remained until the pulse and temperature curve returned to normal. (…) In addition to these objectively determined temperature differences on both sides, there was also a pronounced subjective feeling of heat on the right side of the trunk, from the surgical wound upward toward the neck [47, p. 620].

Widmer described his experience with measuring the temperatures in the axilla in perityphlitis:

> Years ago we had several opportunities measure temperature differences in both axillae in favor of the right side in perityphlitis. Given the relative unreliability of measuring the axillae in general, we paid no further attention to the matter, especially since the criterion of fever in appendicitis has long ceased to be the main one [47, p. 620].

We are unaware of the sensitivity or specificity of this sign (Table 6.1).

6.2.11   Przewalsky Sign

We were only able to identify limited biographical information on Bernard Przewalsky (Przewalski) (1880–?) (see Chap. 5). At the time of the publication of this sign, he was practicing medicine in Kharkov in Southern Russia [48]. Przewalsky reported the following novel finding:

> I would now like to draw the attention of the specialists to a symptom which, in my opinion, is suitable for securing the early diagnosis of acute septic peritonitis, namely, air (or gas) within the ampullae of the rectum without any sign of infiltration or partial protrusion of its walls into the rectal cavity. Such inflation of the rectum in acute appendicitis is a sign in the differential diagnostic which clearly distinguishes it from the symptoms of rectal involvement in the case of inflammatory processes involving the parametrium. I observed this symptom consistently in ill patients [48, p. 845].

We are unaware of any study that evaluated this sign's sensitivity or specificity (Table 6.1).

6.2.12   *Volkovich Sign*

Nikolai Markianovich Volkovich (1858–1928) was born in Horodnya, Chernigov Province, Ukraine. He received his medical degree with distinction from the Faculty of Medicine, Kyiv University, in 1882 and completed his surgical training at Professor Borngaunt's Hospital Surgical Clinic in Kyiv [49, 50]. He was appointed head of the surgical department at Alexandrine Hospital, Kyiv, in 1893, professor and head of the surgical clinic at Kyiv University Hospital in 1903, and from 1911 to 1922, led the department of surgery. During World War I, Volkovich was a surgeon at the University Hospital and consultant to the Southwest Guard of the Red Cross [49].

Volkovich was appointed chairman of the Eighth Congress of Russian Surgeons, founder of the Academy of Sciences in Ukraine, and organized and served as chairman of the Surgical Society of Kyiv [49]. He was chair of medical research at the Kyiv branch of the Main Board for Sciences at the Museum and Artistic Research Establishment in 1922. He was elected a full member of the Academy of Science of the Ukrainian Soviet Socialist Republic (SSR) in 1928 and an honorary member of the Society of Russian Surgeons, the Russian Surgical Society of Pirogov, and the Saratov Surgical Society [49]. In the words of Volkovich:

> The art of surgery is not only about performing technically difficult procedures. I mean the art that gives the doctor the right to be an expert clinician. By this, it is meant the art of recognizing the disease and the foresight about its course, the ability to intervene or patiently follow its course, and finally modify it accordingly if the intervention does not follow the expected outcome [51, p. 157].

A description of his character:

> N.M. Volkovich was not only an outstanding scientist and a brilliant surgeon but also an excellent teacher. His lectures on clinical surgery were clear and straightforward, deep in content and engaging in form, and full of examples from personal experience. Students admired his sensible visual teaching method [51, p. 157].

Volkovich's contribution to medicine and surgery cannot be overstated. His scientific works included rhinoscleroma, surgical management of the gallbladder and biliary duct diseases, appendicitis, bone tuberculosis, tuberculous peritonitis, obliterating endarteritis, and trauma, including bone injuries [49, 51–53]. In 1898, he described in his paper titled "On the question sectioning the abdominal integument during abdominal incision," a method that involves bluntly dissecting without obliquely incising the abdominal wall as an essential technique in the surgical management of appendicitis [50, 51]. It should be recognized that this technique was previously described and reported by McBurney in 1894. Volkovich described a method for diagnosing recurrent or chronic appendicitis (Table 6.1):

> I designated this feature as a "muscular symptom of chronic appendicitis" compared to the muscular sign that characterizes acute appendicitis. (…) In acute appendicitis, the abdominal muscles have an increased abdominal wall tone and tension that protrudes sharply on the right side. In cases of chronic appendicitis, or during intervals between attacks of appendicitis, there is a weakening of the abdominal wall and a noticeable softness and decrease in volume on the right side compared to the left side. This phenomenon is determined by comparing the feeling elicited by palpating both sides of the abdomen. First, determine the state of the iliac region as felt by palpation. Second, palpate at the hypochondrium and lumbar regions where

the broad abdominal muscle (oblique and transversalis), has not yet merged into the tendon fibers, appears to be the most firm. In these regions, one can assess their condition by grasping the soft tissues above the iliac crest between the fingers. The skin and soft tissue on the right side of the abdomen are more depressible, thinner, and easily grasped between the fingers. The reduction in the muscle volume on the right side is carefully determined visually by gazing horizontally with the patient in the supine position. The right iliac region appears more depressed compared to the left side. Additionally, when examining the patient posteriorly, the muscles in the right lumbar region appear less prominent and with a greater depression than in the hypochondrium. I also noted that the muscles on the affected side of the abdomen appear more fibrous, less elastic, softer, and with decreased volume. In other words, for the most part, the known manifestations of muscle atrophy are seen [54, p. 601–604].

Albert Vogel, a resident in Kocher's surgical clinic, published Theodor Kocher's (1814–1917) work titled "Die Behandlung der Appendizitis an der chirurgischen Klinik der Universität Bern" (The treatment of appendicitis at the surgical clinic of the University of Bern) in 1921. It was based on a presentation delivered by Kocher at the inaugural meeting of the Swiss Society of Surgery on 8 March 1913. The publication was delayed for 1 year due to the onset of World War I. The name Kocher has been paired with Volkovich and is sometimes referred to as the Kocher-Volkovich sign, which describes initial pain in the epigastrium, followed by pain in the right lower quadrant [55–57]. Information about Kocher sign is found in Chap. 5. We were unable to identify Volkovich's original paper within the literature where this finding was reported.

6.2.13　Morris Sign

Biographical information regarding Robert Tuttle Morris (1857–1945) is found in Chap. 5 under the somatic segmental nerve pathway. Morris described two findings in chronic appendicitis. The first was a palpatory tender point located a half inch to the right of the umbilicus [58]. The second phenomenon was:

> [p]ersistant distension of the ascending colon with gas. (…) The distention of the ascending colon with gas, which belongs particularly to chronic appendicitis, I call the "cider barrel sign." If we percuss the left side of the abdomen in a case of chronic appendicitis, we shall obtain a normal resonance note suggesting percussion of the cider barrel in October. If we percuss the right side of the abdomen, we obtain a percussion note suggesting that of the cider barrel in January [58, p. 2036–2037].

Morris sign refers to the tympanic percussion sound in the ascending colon caused by air in patients with chronic appendicitis (Table 6.1). We are unaware of any study which assessed the sensitivity or specificity of this sign.

6.2.14　Lockwood Sign

Charles Barrett Lockwood (1856–1914) was born in Stockton-on-Tees, England, and was a Member and Fellow of the Royal College of Surgeons in 1878 and 1881, respectively [59]. At St. Bartholomew's Hospital, London, he was a demonstrator in anatomy, teaching and conducting research in the anatomical department. Throughout his career, he maintained a strong interest in morphological anatomy and its practical application to surgery [60]. He served as house surgeon to the Dean Street Lock Hospital in 1878, an assistant resident anesthetist in 1879, house surgeon to Alfred Willett (1837–1913) in 1880, and surgeon to the Great Northern Central Hospital from 1882 to 1892 [61, 62]. He was appointed assistant surgeon in 1892, full surgeon in 1903, and consulting surgeon in 1912 to St. Bartholomew Hospital [59]. Lockwood maintained a keen interest in morphological anatomy and its practical application in surgery [61].

From 1886 to 1889, he was a Hunterian professor of comparative anatomy and physiology. From 1894 to 1895, he served as an elected member of the Royal College of Surgeons, England, and on the Council of the College in 1908 [62]. He founded the Anatomical Society of the British Anatomist in 1887, serving as its President in 1902. He also served as President of the Medical Society of Long and the Harveian Society of London. His character as described by one of his colleagues:

> In the wards of the hospital, he was beloved by his house surgeons and by his dressers. The patients seemed instinctively to know that they had a great man to deal with. His powers of observation were so keen that no malingerer ever escaped undetected. No point in the history of the case was considered too trivial, and no clinical fact was eliminated except after the most scrupulous scientific and pathological investigation [59, p. 903]. (…) He remained as keen on his work, as unsparing of himself, and as great a teacher. He was more than ever beloved by those who worked under him [59, p. 904].

Dr. Christopher Addison further wrote:

> But those who were permitted to enjoy the priceless privilege of his friendship knew well how affectionate and generous his nature was. He showed men how to help themselves and stimulated them to do it. He drew out those who made their best endeavors, pointed out the way, and so gave them an education of the best and most enduring kind. It is a joy to render homage to such a master—a bright example of the best in British surgery, and one whose influence on the lives of those he taught is growing always and reaching out to others, bringing thereby to him that ceaseless and unconscious tribute which is the lasting treasure of greatness [59, p. 904].

G.H. Colt [63] described the maneuver as performed by Charles Barrett Lockwood as a method to identify patients with chronic appendicitis (Fig. 6.1):

> The patient lies on his back with his head raised on a pillow and his knees drawn up, so that the superficial abdominal muscles are relaxed. The surgeon sits down near his right side and palpates the right iliac region near McBurney's spot with the three inner fingers of his left hand. If he feels a trickle of flatulence passing his fingers, and if this can be often repeated after waiting a half to one minute or a little longer, the patient has either a chronically inflamed appendix or adhesions near it [63, p. 942].

According to Colt, the "trickle of gas" was a small, fine crepitation with a higher note. Colt described his experience with the sign:

> During the last ten years I have tested this sign in over 600 cases verified by operation; it has, in fact, been the determining sign. It has been positive in every case but one. Two positives have been noted in cases which were not appendicular, but these had calcified glands in the ileocolic angle. Negatively the sign is of constant value in excluding appendicular adhesions of the appendix which is apparently normal on section. When the appendicular trouble is lying towards the pelvis the sign is felt lower down and nearer the middle line [63, p. 942].

We are unaware of any study that evaluated this sign's sensitivity or specificity (Table 6.1).

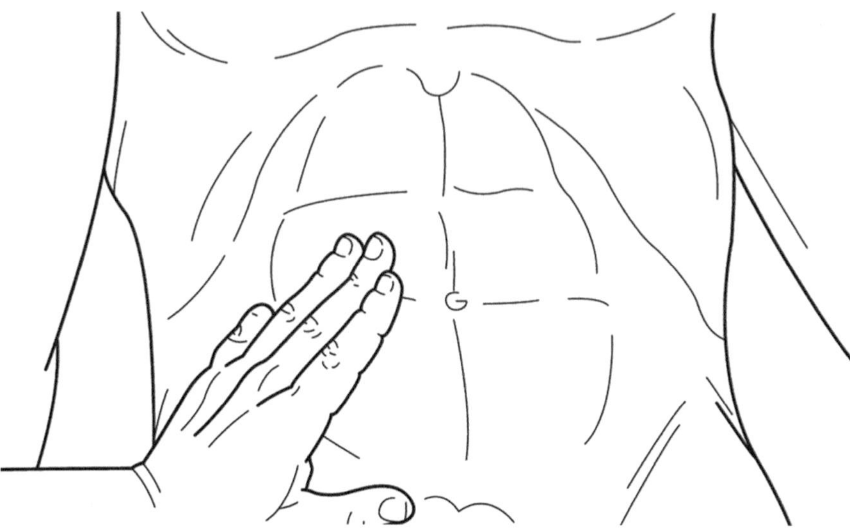

Fig. 6.1 Lockwood sign (by Ryan Yale)

6.2.15 Dott Sign

Norman McOmish Dott (1897–1973) was born in Colinton, Edinburgh, and received his Bachelor of Medicine and Bachelor of Surgery degrees from Edinburgh University Medical School in 1919 [64–67]. He served as a resident house surgeon at the Royal Infirmary from 1919 to 1920, followed by a lectureship and laboratory research in the physiology department at Edinburgh University under the aegis of Sir Edward Sharpey-Schafer (1850–1935) [64, 67]. Dott held appointments as an assistant surgeon at the Deaconess and Chalmer Hospitals, Edinburgh [64, 65].

He was the recipient of the Rockefeller Surgical Fellowship, where he served as a junior associate research fellow at the Peter Bent Brigham Hospital in Boston, Massachusetts, under the aegis of Harvey William Cushing (1869–1939) from 1923 to 1924, later returning to the Royal Hospital for Sick Children as a pediatric surgeon in ordinary in 1925 [64–67]. Dott established neurologic surgery as a subspecialty in 1931; was appointed lecturer in surgical neurology in the Royal Infirmary of Edinburgh in 1932; and later worked in the I. Department of Surgical Neurology in Ward 20 in 1938 [64, 66, 67].

He established a Brain Injuries Unit in Bangour General Emergency Hospital, Broxburn, Scotland, from 1939 to 1945 during World War II and was recognized for this achievement as being the recipient of the Commander of the Order of the British Empire (CBE) in 1948 [64, 65]. He was professor and Forbes chair of neurological surgery at the University of Edinburgh in 1947, co-founded a Spinal Paralysis Unit at Edenhall Ministry of Pensions Hospital, near Edinburgh, and founded and served as the first chair in the Department of Neurological Services at the Western General Hospital in 1960 [64–67].

He was elected Fellow of the Royal College of Surgeons, Edinburgh, in 1923 [64]. Dott was the founder and president (1939–1945) of the Society of the British Neurological Surgeons [64–66]. He was awarded the Freedom of the City Edinburgh in 1962 and received an honorary medical degree from the University of Edinburgh in 1969 and an honorary fellowship from the Royal College of Surgeons of Canada in 1973 [64, 67]. Dott served as vice-president of the Royal College of Surgeons in Edinburgh and President of the Edinburgh and Southeast Scotland Branch in 1969 [64, 66].

As to a description of his character as told by Phillip Harris:

> He much preferred apprenticeship training to didactic teaching, and he was a stimulating conversationalist, a great friend of young people during their medical training, and a wise counselor and adviser for those who, quite often even though senior, still sought his opinion. At all times he demanded the highest possible standards from every member of his staff. His main interest was always his patients, thus he characteristically concluded in his remarks, when he was the distinguished guest of the Congress of Neurological Surgeons in 1968 in Toronto, "When we contemplate and discuss aspects of the jungles of medical practice, education or administration, please note that all are over-topped by a striking object, the patient. This object must ever be kept in focus. We must never allow his image to become blurred. The formula 'What is best for the patient?' is the touchstone we can and should apply to all of these problems and to their solutions." An outstanding, brilliant medical man has left us, but mankind has benefited from all that he was able to do and to achieve [66, p. 71].

We were unable to identify Norman Dott's manuscript describing this sign. Hamilton Bailey referred to it as the thoracic compression test. According to Bailey:

> When it is difficult to decide whether a young child has acute appendicitis or basal lung involvement, compression of the lower thorax from side to side elicits obvious distress when the lesion is above the diaphragm, whereas in appendicitis it has no effect [68, p. 285].

We are unaware of any study that evaluated this sign's sensitivity of specificity (Table 6.1).

Table 6.1 Miscellaneous non-reflex signs in appendicitis

Name	Year	Description of the sign	Method
Hayem–Sonnenburg [10, 18]	1889	*Hayem:*	Observation
		Elevated white blood cell count is found in patients with obscure or complex intra-abdominal diseases	
	1894	*Sonnenburg:*	
		A serofibrinous exudate occurs on the surface of the peritoneum near a focus of severe infection caused by a phlegmon, perforation, or gangrene. The exudate is cloudy, contains microbes and leukocytes, and occurs more rapidly and to a greater extent in severe infections—The more severe the infection, the greater the fibrin content and soft fibrinous adhesions	
Roux [23]	1890	Early perforation and infiltration occur in the intestinal wall covered by the mesentery. The infiltrate causes thickening and rigidity of the intestinal wall making it palpable and slightly dull to percussion. The palpable resistance at the cecal wall feels similar to soft cardboard soaked in hot water	Palpation / Percussion
Mannaberg [27]	1894	Increased intensity of the second pulmonary sound	Auscultation
Filatov [31]	1904	A circumscribed hardening immovable mass, *painful upon pressure* in the right iliac region at a point precisely corresponds to the caecum	Palpation
Klemm [33]	1906	Local gaseous dilation of the cecum persists even after evacuation. In thin patients with a scaphoid abdomen, a protrusion is present in the right lower abdominal quadrant. When palpating the abdomen, a mass of air the size of a fist is felt. On intermittent light palpation, a squeaky, cooing sound is heard	Observation / Palpation
Kahn [37]	1906	A subnormal pulse in gangrenous appendicitis	Palpation
Dubard [42]	1907	Vagal neuritis, of pulmonary origin, causes a localized ulcer and other chronic inflammatory disorders of the gastrointestinal tract in the organs innervated by this nerve. The frequency of associated lesions of the gastrointestinal tract partly explains the post-operative failure of operations limited to a single organ (appendectomy, gastroenterostomy). As a corollary to the surgeon, this observation implies the obligation to explore the patient's digestive tract as completely as possible	Observation
Williams [44]	1908	A mass in the scrotum contains a portion of the omentum and appendix	Observation
Hönck [45]	1908	The temperature of the right axilla is higher than that of the left. In some cases, a one-sided temperature increase occurs. In other cases, a temperature difference occurs only at the trunk, or there is a crossing of the temperature differences so that there is a higher temperature at the trunk on the right and a lower temperature at the left lower extremities and vice versa. A similar crossing might take place at the head	Observation

Name	Year	Description	Observation/palpation
Widmer [47]	1908	The right axilla showed a significantly higher pulse and temperature than the corresponding one on the left, and this difference remained until it returned to normal. There is also a pronounced subjective feeling of heat on the right side of the trunk, from the surgical wound upward toward the neck	Observation/palpation
Przewalsky [48]	1912	Air (or gas) within the ampullae of the rectum	Observation
Volkovich [54]	1914	In chronic appendicitis, or during intervals between attacks of acute appendicitis, there is a weakening of the abdominal wall and a noticeable softness and decrease in its volume on the right compared to the left side. These differences are determined based on the following sequence. First, palpate the abdominal wall at the iliac region. Second, continue palpating the hypochondrium and lumbar regions where the broad abdominal muscles (oblique and transversalis), have not yet merged into the tendon fibers-these, are the firmest. Now, grasp the soft tissues above the iliac crest between the fingers to determine the quality of the abdominal wall at these regions. The skin and soft tissue on the right side of the abdomen are more depressible, thinner, and easily grasped between the fingers. The reduction in the muscle volume on the right side is carefully determined visually by observing horizontally with the patient in the supine position. The right iliac region appears more depressed compared to the left side. Additionally, when examining the patient posteriorly, the muscles at the right lumbar region appear less prominent and have a more pronounced depression in the hypochondrium. The muscles on the affected side of the abdomen appear more fibrous and less elastic and have a greater softness and decreased volume	Observation / Palpation (chronic appendicitis)
Morris [58]	1917	Persistent distention of the ascending colon with gas occurs in chronic appendicitis—The "cider barrel sign." Percussion of the left side of the abdomen in chronic appendicitis reveals a normal resonance note-suggesting percussion of the cider barrel in October. If we percuss the right side of the abdomen, we obtain a percussion note suggestive of a cider barrel in January	Percussion (chronic appendicitis)
Lockwood [63]	1932	The patient lies supine with the head raised on a pillow and knees flexed to relax the superficial abdominal muscles. The examiner sits to the patient's right and palpates the right iliac region near McBurney point with the three inner fingers of the left hand. If the examiner feels a trickle of gas passing over their fingers, and *if repeated after waiting about half to one minute or longer*, either a chronically inflamed appendix or adhesions are present	Palpation
Dott [68]	[n.a.] (before 1949)	When deciding whether a young child has acute appendicitis or basal lung involvement is difficult, compression of the lower thorax from side to side elicits obvious distress when the lesion is above the diaphragm. In contrast, in appendicitis, it has no effect	Palpation

6.3   Conclusion

Non-reflex mediates eponymous signs were additional bedside tools used as a method to assist in confirming the diagnosis of acute and chronic appendicitis. The signs were detected using the time-honored techniques of the physical and laboratory examination-observation, palpation, percussion, and auscultation. Although several of these signs are antiquated, they serve as a reminder of the search that some physicians sought in order to discover novel techniques for diagnosing disease.

References

1. Verso ML. Some nineteenth-century pioneers of haematology. Med Hist. 1971;15:55–67.
2. [No author]. Les cérémonies médicales: La médaille du Professeur Hayem. Paris méd. 1911;4:707–14.
3. [No author]. Nécrologie: le professeur Georges Hayem à Paris. Archives israélites de France. 1933;94:135.
4. Landmann I, Rittenberg L, Cohen S. The Universal Jewish Encyclopedia: an authoritative and popular presentation of Jews and Judaism since the earliest times, vol. 5. New York: Universal Jewish Encyclopedia Inc.; 1941.
5. Hayem G. Études sur les diverses formes d'encéphalite: anatomie et physiologie pathologiques. Paris: V. Adrien Delahaye; 1868.
6. Hayem G. Des bronchitis. Thèse d'agrégation. Paris: Adrien Delahaye; 1869.
7. Hayem G. Des hémorragies intra-rachidiennes. Thèse présentée au concours pour l'agrégation soutenue le 26 avril 1872. Paris: V. Adrien Delahaye; 1872.
8. Delmas V, François M, Loeper M, Floderer A, Capot M, Hayem G. Comité des travaux historiques et scientifiques. Institut rattaché à l'École nationale des chartes. http://cths.fr/an/savant.php?id=105621#. Accessed 9 Nov 2022.
9. Castiglioni A. A history of medicine. (trans: E.B. Krumbhaar). New York: Alfred A. Knopf; 1941.
10. Hayem G. Du sang et des ses altérations anatomiques, tome 1. Paris: G. Masson; 1889.
11. Bernstein H. George Hayem. In: The American Jewish yearbook (October 2, 1913 - September 20, 1914). Philadelphia: The Jewish Publication Society of America; 1914. p. 221–360.
12. Mühsam R. Eduard Sonnenburg. Dtsch med Wochenschr. 1915;41:774–5.
13. Gluck TV. Eduard Sonnenburg. Berl klin Wochenschr. 1915;52:675–6.
14. [No author]. Kleine Mitteilungen: Eduard Sonnenburg. Med Klin. 1915;11:658.
15. Biografie, Eduard Sonnenburg. Wissenschaftliche Sammlungen. Humboldt-Universität zu Berlin. https://www.sammlungen.hu-berlin.de/objekte/-/18701/. Accessed 9 Nov 2022.
16. [No author]. Tagesgeschichtliche Notizen. Münch med Wochenschr. 1916;62:768.
17. [No author]. Eduard Sonnenburg. Berl klin Wochenschr. 1915;52:591.
18. Sonnenburg E. Pathologie und Therapie der Perityphlitis (Appendicitis simplex und appendicitis perforativa), Bd. 38. Leipzig: Verlag von FCW Vogel; 1894.
19. César Roux (1857–1934). Les personnages marquants dans l'histoire du service de chirurgie viscérale. Le Centre hospitalier universitaire vaudois (CHUV). https://www.chuv.ch/fr/chirurgie-viscerale/chv-home/en-bref/historique/les-personnages-marquants/. Accessed 14 Sep 2021.
20. Roux (César). Description des Archives cantonales Vaudoises sous une forme électronique (DAVEL). https://davel.vd.ch/detail.aspx?ID=31503. Accessed 14 Sep 2021.

21. Von der Mühl R. Contribution à l'étude des paragangliomes de la surrénale. Lausanne: Université de Lausanne; 1928.
22. Roux C. Chirurgie gastrointestinale. Rev Chir. 1893;13:402–3.
23. Roux C. Du traitement chirurgical de la pérityphlite suppurée. Rev Med Sui Rom. 1890;10:200–49.
24. Wyklicky H. Mannaberg, Julius. In: Neue Deutsche Biographie: Herausgegeben von der historischen Kommission bei der bayerischen Akademie der Wissenschaften, Bd. 16. Berlin: Duncker & Humblot; 1990. p. 57–8.
25. Mannaberg, Julius (1860–1941), Internist. Österreichisches Biographisches Lexikon. https://biographien.ac.at/oebl/oebl_M/Mannaberg_Julius_1860_1941.xml. Accessed 14 Sep 2021.
26. Dem Bundesminister für Kunst und Kultur, Verfassung und öffentlichen Dienst wird empfohlen, das im Dossier der Kommission für Provenienzforschung „Sammlung Dr. Julius Mannaberg". 2014. http://www.provenienzforschung.gv.at/beiratsbeschluesse/Mannaberg_Julius_2014-07-03.pdf. Accessed 14 Sep 2021.
27. Mannaberg J. Ueber Accentuirung des II. Pulmonaltones bei Perityphlitis. Zentralbl inn Med. 1894;15:209–11.
28. Filatov, Nil Fedorovich - Филатов, Нил Фёдорович. Encyclopedia. https://mewikisv.com/wiki/Филатов,_Нил_Фёдорович. Accessed 28 Aug 2022.
29. Филатов, Нил Фёдорович (Filatov, Nil Fedorovich). Летопись Московского университета (Chronicle of Moscow University). http://letopis.msu.ru/peoples/488. Accessed 28 Aug 2022.
30. Филатов, Нил Федорович (Filatov, Nil Fedorovich). Children's City Clinical Hospital. https://web.archive.org/web/2012051607325; http://13dgkb.ru/0040.shtml. Accessed 28 Aug 2022.
31. Filatov NF. Appendicitis and perityphiltis. In: Semeiology and diagnosis of diseases of children, vol. 1. (trans: G.B. Hassin). Chicago: Cleveland Press; 1904. p. 201–10.
32. Moxgis D, Sviestina I, Baltinš M, Apins P. Dr. med. Pauls Klemms-vina redzējums vairāku kirurgisko slimību gadījumā ap 19. un 20. [Miju Paul Klemm M.D. and his view on different surgical conditions at late 19th and early 20th century]. Latvia: Zinātnu Vesture un Muzejniecība; 2015. p. 82–90.
33. Klemm P. Ueber die chronische, anfallsfreie Appendicitis. Mitt Grenzgeb Med Chir. 1906;16:580–608.
34. Harvey SC. Congenital variations in the peritoneal relations of the ascending colon, caecum, appendix and terminal ileum. Ann Surg. 1918;67:641–86.
35. Hofmeister F. Ueber Thyphlektasie – Chronische perityphlitis, coecum mobile. Beitr klin Chir. 1911;71:832–46.
36. Koren N. Kahn, Maurice Guttman. In: Jewish physicians: a biographical index. Jerusalem: Israel Universities Press; 1973. p. 199.
37. Kahn M. Bradycardia in appendicitis. JAMA. 1906;47:2011.
38. [No author]. École de Médecine de Dijon. Lyon Méd. 1896;83:523.
39. [No author]. Dubard (Pierre-Marie-Maurice). J Off Rép Fr. 1921;1:2468.
40. Historique du Comité de Côte d'Or. La Ligue contre le cancer. http://www.ligue-cancer21.info/historique-du-comite/. Accessed 10 Jun 2022.
41. Dubard PM. Ulcère gastro-duodénal et appendicite chronique: signe du pneumogastrique. Lyon Chir. 1918;15:356–62.
42. Huchon F. L'ulcére de l'estomac et la névrite du pneumogastrique. J Méd Chir Prat. 1907;78:903.
43. Tennyson BD. The Canadian experience of the great war: a guide to memoirs. Lanham, MD: Scarecrow Press; 2013.
44. Williams EJ. Two interesting cases: the appendix in the inguinal canal and scrotum. Montreal MJ. 1908;37:191–3.
45. Hönck E. Ueber Unterschiede der Temperatur beider Achselhöhlen bei akuter Epityphlitis. Dtsch med Wochenschr. 1908;35:1511.
46. Hahnemann S. Organon der Heilkunst. Leipzig: Verlag von Dr. Willmar Schwabe; 1921.
47. Widmer C. Halbseitentemperaturen bei Appendicitis. Münch med Wochenschr. 1908;55:620–1.

48. Przewalsky B. Die Maximaldehnung des Mastdarmes als ein sehr frühes Symptom bei Appendicitis acuta septica. Zentralbl Chir. 1912;39:845.
49. Khokholia VP. Nikolai Markiianovich Volkovich (k 125-letiiu so dnia rozhdeniia) [Nikolai Markiianovich Volkovich (on the 125th anniversary of his birth)]. Klin Khir. 1983;12:55–6.
50. Shumada IV, Ovchinnikov GI. Nikolai Markianovich Volkovich. Ortop Travmatol Protez. 1979;2:62–4.
51. Kolomichenko MI. Vydaiushchiisia deiatel' otechestvennoi khirurgii Nikolai Markianovich Volkovich; k stoletiiu so dnia rozhdeniia [Nikolai Markianovich Volkovich, outstanding figure of Russian surgery; to the centenary of his birth]. Klin Med (Mosk). 1959;37:157–9.
52. Novitskii ST. Nikolai Markianovich Volkovich; ego zhizn', deiatel'nost' i znachenie v khirurgii [Nikolai Markianovich Volkovich, his life, activities and significance in surgery]. Vestn Khir Im I I Grek. 1954;74:76–81.
53. Karavanov GG, Rol' NM. Volkovicha v razvitii khirurgii zhelchnogo puzyria i vnepechenochnykh zhelchnykh puteĭ na Ukraine [The role of N.M. Volkovich in the development of gallbladder and extrahepatic bile duct surgery in the Ukraine]. Klin Khir. 1967;1:72–7.
54. Volkovitch NM. More about the muscular sign of chronic appendicitis. Rousskiy Vratch. 1914;17:601–4.
55. [No author]. N.M. Volkovitch. JAMA. 1914;63:1146.
56. Sachdeva A, Futta AK. Advances in pediatrics. In: Mahaveer pediatric surgery. New Delhi: Jaypee Brothers Medical Publishing; 2012. p. 1432.
57. Vogel A. Die Behandlung der Appendizitis an der chirurgischen Klinik der Universität Bern. Arch klin Chir. 1921;115:1–85.
58. Morris RT. Appendicitis and the gynecologist. JAMA. 1917;69:2036–7.
59. [No author]. Charles Barrett Lockwood, FRCS. Br Med J. 1914;2:903–4.
60. Macalister A. Obituary: Charles Barrett Lockwood, 1856–1914. J Anat Physiol. 1914/1915;49:240–2.
61. Lockwood CB, 1856–1914. Plarr's lives of the fellows. London: Royal College of Surgeons of England. http://livesonline.rcseng.ac.uk/biogs/E002562b.htm. Accessed 14 Sep 2021.
62. [No author]. Royal College of Surgeons. Lancet. 1888;2:92.
63. Colt GH. Chronic appendicitis: Lockwood's sign. Br Med J. 1932;2:942.
64. [No author]. Norman McOmish Dott. Br Med J. 1973;4:737.
65. Harris P. Norman McOmish Dott, 1897–1973. J Neurosurg. 1974;40:415–7.
66. Harris P. Obituary: Norman McOmish Dott, 1897–1973. Spinal Cord. 1974;12:70–1.
67. McOmish Dott N. The Royal College of Surgeons of Edinburgh. https://archiveandlibrary.rcsed.ac.uk/surgeon/4024173-norman-mcomish-dott. Accessed 10 Aug 2022.
68. Bailey H. Common acute abdominal conditions: special points in the examination of a young child. In: Demonstrations of physical signs in clinical surgery. 11th ed. Baltimore: Williams & Wilkins; 1949. p. 285.

Chapter 7
Liver and Biliary Signs

7.1 Introduction

The name "liver" is derived from *ípar* (ήπαρ) in ancient Greek and *hēpar* in Latin. One of the earliest accounts regarding the relationship between liver disease and ascites was written by Aulus Cornelius Celsus (fl. c. 175 AD), who related Erasistratus of Alexandria's (fl. c. 260 BC) belief that ascites is caused by liver disease:

> But if the form of the affection [i.e., hydrops] is that in which much water is drawn into the belly… [suggested remedies are listed]: if the belly is not dried up by such remedies, and in spite of them the humor is in large amount, and must be given in a quicker way, by giving issue to it through the belly itself. I am quite aware that such a way of treatment was disapproved of by Erasistratus, for he deemed the disease to be one of the liver, that therefore it was the liver which had to be rendered sound, and that it was no use to let out water which, if that organ is diseased, will continually be reproduced [1, p. 14–15].

The term liver lobule was first used by Marcello Malpighi (1628–1694) in *De Viscerum Structura Exercitatio Anatomica* (Essay on the Anatomical Structure of the Viscera), published in 1669 with the name acinus later substituted for lobule by Francis Kiernan (1800–1874) in 1833 [2, 3]. One of the earliest English pathological descriptions of a "glandulous appearance of the liver" (later termed cirrhosis) was written by John Browne (1642–1702) in 1685 [4].

Matthew Baillie (1761–1823) used the term "scirrhous" liver in cases caused by alcoholism in 1799:

> The process by which they are formed is very slow, although it varies in this respect a good deal in different individuals, and it is commonly produced by a long habit of drinking spirituous liquors. When the liver has undergone this change it is commonly said to be scirrhous, but the morbid appearance is very different from what is observed in the genuine scirrhus of other gland. It should rather be considered as a disease *sui generis*. (…) The liver in this disease is not enlarged in its size, but is, on the contrary, somewhat diminished [5, p. 101].

René Laënnec (1781–1826) coined the term "cirrhosis" to describe the appearance of the liver:

© The Author(s), under exclusive license to Springer Nature
Switzerland AG 2023
S. H. Yale et al., *Gastrointestinal Eponymic Signs*,
https://doi.org/10.1007/978-3-031-33673-7_7

> This type of growth belongs to the group of those under the name of scirrhus. I believe we ought to designate it with the name of *cirrhosis*, because of its color. Its common causes of ascites, and has the peculiarity that as the cirrhosis develops, the tissue of the liver is absorbed, and it ends often, as in the subject, by disappearing entirely; and that in all the cases, a liver which has cirrhosis becomes smaller in volume instead of increasing all the more. This type of growth develops also in other organs, and finishes by softening like all morbid growths [6, p. 196].

The earliest known account of gallstones was by Alexander of Tralles (c. 525–c. 605), a respected physician in the Byzantine Empire. Gentile da Foligno (d. 1348) was the first physician to describe gallstone with his observation recorded by Marcellus Donato in his book *De Medica Historia Mirabili Libri Sex*:

> In the gall bladder many stones were seen, Gentile himself testifies, in a certain woman, whose viscera were removed, so that the body could be embalmed they found in the duct of the gall bladder at its mouth, a stone tending to green, from which the moderns with right remark that there was jaundice present [7, p. 269].

Included are excerpts from Jean François Fernel (Ioannis Fernelii) (c. 1497–1558), who provides a clear and accurate depiction of gallstone which remains pertinent even to this day:

> Obstruction, calculus, fullness and emptiness attack the gall bladder. The obstruction is either of the duct by which the bile is led away from the liver, or of that by which it is discharged from the gall bladder into the intestine. In both, the bowels are obstinate and sluggish, feces whitish, the urine is reddish and thick so that it frequently becomes dark, the bile diffused with the blood throughout the whole body disfigures the skin with jaundice. In the former moreover, the gall bladder is entirely empty: in the latter it is distended by the larger amount of bile, and is oppressed by various symptoms of great importance [8].

By the later part of the nineteenth century, a variety of signs involving the liver and biliary system were identified through observation, palpation, percussion, and auscultation as a method for diagnosing diseases. The eponymously named signs are presented in chronological order based on the earliest date reported and depicted as initially described by the authors.

7.2 Liver and Biliary Eponymous Signs

7.2.1 *Hanot Sign*

Victor Charles Hanot (1844–1896) was born in Faubourg Saint-Antoine, Paris, France. He was appointed extern in medicine in 1869 and intern in 1871, studying under the aegis of Jean-Martin Charcot (1825–1893) [9–11]. He received his medical degree based on the thesis titled "Étude sur une forme de cirrhose hypertrophique du foie: cirrhose hypertrophique avec ictère chronique" (Study on a Form of Hypertrophic Cirrhosis of the Liver: Hypertrophic Cirrhosis with Chronic Jaundice) in 1875, which was later eponymously referred to as Hanot disease or primary biliary cirrhosis [12].

Hanot was appointed chief of the medical clinic of Professor Ernest Charles Lasèque (1816–1893) in 1876, Director for the Central Office in 1880, agrégé with his thesis "Du traitement de la pneumonie aiguë" (Treatment of acute pneumonia) at the Faculty of Medicine in 1883 and Doctor of Hospitals (Saint-Antoine) in 1884 [9–11]. He became a member of the Anatomical Society of Paris in 1873, a full member in 1875, and editor-in-chief of the *Archives Générales de Médecine* (General Archives of Medicine) [9, 11].

Hanot in collaboration with Anatole Chauffard (1855–1932) described a condition of diabetes, hypertrophic cirrhosis, and skin pigmentation in 1882, and Schachmann coined the term "diabète bronze" (bronze diabetes) in 1886. The condition was ultimately eponymously named Troisier-Hanot-Chauffard syndrome or hemochromatosis [13, 14].

As to insight into his character:

A first-class clinician, he ran an active department at the hospital. He gave close practical instructions to students, who greatly appreciated his benevolent direction. (…) A spirit of great stature disappears, admirably gifted, adorned, and cultivated. (…) Profoundly honest, fundamentally sound, a sure and faithful friend [9, p. 736–737].

Hanot described in four patients:

In most cases, jaundice and hepatic pain were accompanied initially by other symptoms, including anorexia, constipation, general malaise, fatigue, and fever. The four patients I observed clearly indicated this "febrile" state during the initial period and flares throughout the disease. (…) Several times, the pain was accompanied by a high fever of 39.5° to 39.8° and a pulse of 110 or 120. This fever did not last as long as the pain, but the attack was more violent and more prolonged when it did occur. At other times the painful episodes were completely afebrile. This initial crisis lasted from one to several weeks. Then, the disease enters a quiescent period, characterized mainly by chronic jaundice and enlarged liver. Jaundice is, therefore, one of the most significant manifestations of the disease. We have seen in some cases that this was one of the initial signs. It is hardly noticeable at first but then increases imperceptibly; at other times, it is intense as soon as it appears. However, once produced, jaundice persists throughout the course. However, during the long duration, it may present variations; sometimes veritable green jaundice, sometimes much less charged. Nevertheless, even though it may be minimum, it remains noticeable and generalized. It is always much more than the subicteric hue encountered in many other conditions [15, p. 53–54].

Hanot referred to this condition as hypertrophic cirrhosis and reported on the histopathologic findings:

But the most characteristic lesions are those of the bile canaliculi; we find, in fact, especially in this form, a proliferation of the epithelial cells of these ducts, which are often infiltrated with bile pigment, and an extreme development of the network of canals, not only outside the lobules but also probably inside the lobules [15, p. 58].

Thus Hanot sign or disease is believed to be the condition now recognized as primary biliary cirrhosis (Table 7.1).

7.2.2 Rosenbach Sign

Ottomar Ernst Felix Rosenbach (1851–1907) was born in Krappitz (Krapkowice, Silesia), studied medicine at the Universities of Breslau and Berlin, and received his medical degree in 1874 [16–18]. He served as an assistant to Wilhelm Olivier Leube (1842–1922) and Hermann Nothnagel (1841–1905) in the Polyclinic of the University of Jena from 1874 to 1877 [16].

He was appointed assistant to Julius Friedrich Cohnheim (1839–1884) at the Allerheiligen-Hospital in Breslau and an associate professor at the University of Breslau in 1878. Rosenbach was chief in the Department of Medicine at Allerheiligen-Hospital from 1887 to 1893 and an extraordinary professor in 1888 [16, 17, 19, 20]. He resigned from this hospital in 1893 and the University of Breslau in 1896, returning to the University of Berlin in 1896 [16, 17, 20].

Rosenbach described the sign of liver pulsation found in tricuspid insufficiency as well as the trembling of the eyelid when the eyes are closed in Grave disease. He is considered the founder of functional diseases of the stomach. His work spanned multiple experimental, clinic, pathological, diagnostic, and therapeutic areas.

As to his character:

> Rosenbach was an exceptional personality in every respect. Endowed with a penetrating intellect, he was at the same time of rare kindness of heart and tenderness of feeling. He practiced innumerable benevolent deeds, always in such a way that no third person knew about them, and he understood all human weaknesses. His very strongly developed sense of justice made him always stand up for all the oppressed. Only in the field of science was there no compromise for him. Here he fought for what he believed to be right, without regard for others, and his own advantage. He was cheerful, full of life, and gifted with wit and humor. (…) He had a sense of all that was good and beautiful in life, art, and science. All those who were fortunate enough to be among his friends and acquaintances looked up to him with the greatest reverence and will never forget his memory [20, p. 490].

As described by Rose:

> In every respect Rosenbach was an unusual personality, a physician the like of whom has only rarely existed. His diagnoses were remarkably clear-sighted: in the prognoses he but rarely erred, and in the domain of therapy he was remarkably successful. It is a characteristic fact that a large number of colleagues consulted him for his advice. His love and capacity for work were truly astonishing. An original thinker of rare perception, he was no slavish follower of authorities, but claimed the right of working out his problems for himself, and there were few of these, indeed, to which his reasoning failed to impart a new aspect. Endowed as he was with great power of perception, gifted with rare kindness of heart and gentleness of disposition, he did many acts of benevolence, always taking care that they did not come to the knowledge of that persons. He had a full understanding for human foibles. His sense of justice was so strongly developed that he invariably came to the aid of those ill [21, p. 858].

Rosenbach acknowledged that tricuspid insufficiency was the most common cause of liver pulsation:

> The earlier view that pulsation of the liver is most commonly directly due to the elevation and lowering of its surface in tricuspid insufficiency, similar to an arterial vessel of the pulsating inferior vena cava, is true in most cases. The observation to be reported now is intended to show that there are indeed cases in which a pulsation of the liver, which differs in no way from that caused by insufficiency of the tricuspid nerves, can occur during life and that, at autopsy, a valvular defect is absent [22, p. 498].

He reported the case of an 18-year-old typesetter apprentice with aortic insufficiency (Table 7.1):

> In no heart disease other than insufficiency of the aortic valves is there a wide difference in the initial and final pressure in the arterial system that even the smallest arteries, including the capillaries, pulsate and that the whole body shows a strong systolic shock than we must consider that in such cases distinct liver pulsations are possible [22, p. 519].

Thus, Rosenbach sign refers to liver pulsation in patients with aortic insufficiency.

7.2.3 *Courvoisier Sign*

Ludwig Georg Courvoisier (1843–1918) was born in Basel, Switzerland, and received his surgical training under the aegis of August Socin (1837–1899) and Johann Jacob Bischoff (1841–1892) in Basel and obtained his medical degree from the University of Basel in 1868 [23–25]. After graduation, he studied abroad in London and Vienna and was a military surgeon during the Franco–Prussian War at the Military Hospital in Karlsruhe, Germany, from 1870 to 1871 [23, 24, 26]. Courvoisier accepted an appointment at the Deaconess Institute, Riehen, Switzerland, where he later served as a medical director [26]. He habilitated in 1880 and moved to Basel in 1883 as a private practitioner while maintaining an appointment at the Riehen Hospital. He was an associate professor in 1888 and a full professor in 1900. Courvoisier was also president of the Federal Medical Examination Committee [23–25].

As to his character:

> As a physician, Courvoisier was extraordinarily conscientious and faithful to duty, and for many families, he was the regular resident of old and new, always friendly, sympathetic, and benevolent. As a diagnostician, he was matter-of-fact and cautious, never hasty and prejudiced, often hesitant, aware of human frailty; reassuring as a surgeon and never harsh with a sick person; his technique was not calculated for external effect, but purposeful and deliberate: "nil nocere" was his highest principle [24, p. 11].

In his discussion on the consequence of obstructive gallstones, Courvoisier found that (Table 7.1):

> [e]ctasia of the gallbladder is rare if a stone obstructs the common bile duct. (…) In other kinds of obstruction, ectasia is common, with atrophy occurring in less than half of these cases. The results of this study have been surprising. It is usually stated in the handbooks and textbooks that stone obstructing the common bile duct leads to gallbladder dilatation caused by bile stasis. I found the opposite and must point out that there is no ectasia when a gallstone blocks the duct. Dilation is indicative of other types of obstruction. If this is further confirmed, it would be an essential clue in the differential diagnosis [27, p. 58].

Courvoisier proposed a pathogenesis for the findings:

> According to an earlier account, choledochal stones usually come from the gallbladder. However, on their way, the stones, as they pass, as has just been shown, irritate the cystic duct and partly the gallbladder causing chronic inflammation of the gallbladder wall, which often ultimately results in shrinkage of the duct and gallbladder. If the gallbladder is altered, even the most severe biliary stasis prevents it from expanding. In other causes of obstructions, especially those due to tumors, bile flow shows a normal compliant gallbladder [27, p. 58].

Thus, Courvoisier sign refers to a fibrotic gallbladder secondary to chronic inflammation in cases of choledocholithiasis and a distended gallbladder in causes other than that of gallstone (e.g., tumor).

7.2.4 Rovighi Sign

Alberto Rovighi (1856–1919) was born in Modena, Italy, and received his medical degree in medicine and surgery from the University of Bologna in 1879 [28, 29]. He continued his studies in Paris under Jean-Martin Charcot (1825–1893) and Luigi Luciani (1842–1919) in Florence and was an assistant of pathological anatomy in Modena under the aegis of Carlo Foà (1880–1971), the laboratory of Friedrich Daniel von Recklinghausen (1833–1910) and clinic of Adolf Kussmaul (1822–1902) in Strasbourg in 1883 [29].

Rovighi was an assistant in the medical clinic in Bologna under the direction of Augusto Murri (1841–1932) in 1884, was appointed lecturer and chair of propaedeutic medical pathology in 1887, ordinary professor of pathology and preparatory medical clinic beginning in 1888 in Modena and subsequently Sienna, Italy in 1892 [28–31]. He accepted a position at the University of Bologna as an extraordinary professor of special demonstrative medical pathology in 1894 and was selected as a full professor in 1901 [28, 29, 31].

As to his character:

> Rovighi distinguished himself among his contemporaries because he possessed a broad physiologic and anatomopathological background in his scientific investigation and sincere love for science and education. (…) Honesty and goodness were the great virtues that adorned his life and made his memory dear to his students and colleagues [29].

Rovighi described the case of a 50-year-old man (Table 7.1):

> What was most interesting about our subject was the constancy by which the voluminous mass developed in the left hypochondrium and on the intumescence of the liver and abdomen. In addition to the hydatigenic thrill, I found a deep, low sound similar to that of a vibrating metal string. This particular resonance was felt not only on the most prominent part of the large cyst of the spleen but also at other points on the mass where the thrill was less evident. It was heard at a certain distance from the cyst while striking the mass. Investigating this sound, I defined the exact area on the spleen where the large hydatid was present. I discovered another one about the size of an apple in the abdominal cavity at the umbilicus. Then listening to the liver, I heard a distinct resonant sound when the digital or pleximetric percussion fell on the site of the hydatigenic cyst within the parenchyma of the liver and a dry and metallic sound when struck at other points in the bowel. I also ascertained that when moderate pressure was exerted with the stethoscope on the cystic tumor, resonance on percussion acquired a higher pitch. If a solid body is interposed between the stethoscope and the tumor, the sonority is still perceived distinctly, while the hydatigenic thrill is no longer felt with the hand [32, p. 518]. (…) To me and others who examined my patient with multiple hydatids in the spleen and abdomen, we were sometimes unable to perceive the thrill even though it was quite evident at other times. I was often able to elicit the thrill when provoked in various ways. I found that the best way to make it noticeable is to place the palm of the left hand firmly on the mass and strike the first phalange using the right middle finger. Thus, a vibratory tremor is felt, which should not be confused with fluctuation or other tactile sensations. As we have already seen, this thrill is neither found in ovarian cysts nor superficial abscesses of the liver [32, p. 519–520].

In summary, Rovighi identified that the best method of detecting echinococcal cysts was a vibratory tremor (thrill) detected through percussion.

7.2.5   Boas Sign

Ismar Isidor Boas (1858–1938) was born in Exin, near Bromberg, province of Posen-West Prussia. He studied medicine in Berlin under the aegis of Carl Anton Ewald (1845–1915) and at the University of Halle under Theodor Weber (1836–1906). He received his medical degree from the University of Halle in 1881 and completed his state licensure examination at the University of Leipzig in 1882 [33–36].

In Berlin, Boas was an assistant to Ewald at Augusta Hospital from 1882 to 1886, where he studied the physiology and pathology of gastric secretions and gastric function and described the guaiac test as a method for detecting occult blood in the stool, among others [33–36]. He was instrumental in being the first to establish an independent practice of gastroenterology as a medical specialty and founded a polyclinic in gastric and intestinal diseases in 1886 [33–36]. He was appointed professor of medicine in Berlin in 1907 and Geheimer Sanitätsrat (Privy Medical Councilor) in 1914 [33]. During National Socialism and anti-Jewish sentiment, he and his family fled to Vienna in 1936 [34].

He founded and served as the editor of *Archiv für Verdauungs - Krankheiten mit Einschluss der Stoffwechselpathologie und der Diätik* (Archives of Digestive Diseases including Metabolic Pathology and Dietics), the first specialty gastroenterology journal from 1895 to 1933 colloquially referred to as "Boas Archiv" and published *Allgemeine Diagnostik und Therapie der Magenkrankheiten* (General Diagnosis and Treatment of Gastric Diseases) in 1890, *Spezielle Diagnostik und Therapie der Magenkrankheiten* (Special Diagnosis and Therapy of Gastric Diseases) in 1893, *Die Lehre von den Okkulten Blutungen* (The Doctrine of Occult Bleeding) in 1894, and *Gesammelte Abhandlungen aus dem Gebiete der Verdauungskrankheiten* (Collected Treatises on Digestive Diseases) in 1906 [33, 34, 36].

He was a corresponding and honorary member of the American Gastroenterological Association [33]. He and Julius Curt Pariser (1863–1931) were instrumental in establishing the first Conference for Digestive and Metabolic Disease in Bad Homburg in 1914 [33]. The Fachgesellschaft für Verdauungs- und Stoffwechselkrankheiten (Scientific Society for Digestive and Metabolic Disease) was founded in 1925 with Boas appointed the first honorary member in 1927 [33]. He was honored by the Deutsche Gesellschaft für Verdauungs- und Stoffwechselkrankheiten (German Society for Digestive and Metabolic Diseases) with a memorial plaque in the Berlin Charité in 1992, and the Boas Medal and Boas Prize are awarded annually by the German Gastroenterological Association in recognition for outstanding achievements in gastroenterology [33, 34].

As to a description of his character:

> He was a devoted, though strict, father, giving his children the best available education. He was kind, generous, charitable, and above all, had a keen sense of integrity in both his private and professional dealings. Wherever he went, he was the life and soul of the party [36, p. 52].

Boas described a palpatory method for identifying and measuring pain using an algesimeter to distinguish a gastric ulcer, gastric neurosis, and cholelithiasis:

> The pressure points on the spinal column are of diagnostic importance, to which I first drew attention. These are either multiple pressure points, randomly distributed on both sides of the spine, or extensive painful areas, which likewise show no correspondence. This behavior is most pronounced in all gastric and intestinal neuroses but is found generally in male and female neurasthenics, even without any involvement of the digestive system. Completely isolated, generally one-sided pressure areas are clearly distinguished from these pressure points, or better, pressure areas. We can distinguish: i) the pressure points in gastric ulcers and ii) those in cholelithiasis. The former occurs in typical cases of gastric ulcer, is found in about a third of all cases, and is located to the left of the spine, on the 12th thoracic vertebral body. There are occasional deviations from this, which is not surprising given the variable location of the stomach and ulcer. For example, the pain may be higher on the 10th or 11th thoracic vertebra or lower at the level of the first lumbar vertebra. Occasionally there is a corresponding soreness on the right side, but in this case, the pressure point on the left is the more sensitive. The pressure area in cholelithiasis is also in the region of the 12th thoracic vertebra, 2-3 finger widths from the vertebral bodies. From there, it often extends further to the right, sometimes to the posterior axillary line on the left side [37, p. 73–74]. (…) The examination of the pressure points is not only of diagnostic but also of therapeutic

importance, insofar as one can use this to provide objective evidence for progressive improvement or healing of the disease [37, p. 75].

Thus, Boas identified pressure areas on the spine in gastric ulcers and cholelithiasis (Table 7.1). Boas point and Boas sign have been used to describe increased cutaneous sensitivity to light touch. Boas point refers to discomfort to the left of the 12 thoracic vertebrae. In contrast, Boas sign refers to discomfort at the right infrascapular area and right upper quadrant, which departs from Boas's description [38]. Gunn and Keddie reported increased sensitivity or hyperesthesia occurring in the abovementioned areas occurring in 7% of patients undergoing cholecystectomy [39].

7.2.6 Naunyn Sign

Bernhard Naunyn (1839–1925) was born in Berlin, Germany, and studied medicine under Nathanael Lieberkühn (1821–1887), Karl Bogislaus Reichert (1811–1883), and Friedrich Theodor von Frerichs (1819–1885) and received his medical degree from the University of Berlin in 1863 [40, 41].

After qualifying, he served as an assistant in the Frerichs Medical Clinic at Charité, Berlin. This experience influenced and imparted to him a profound appreciation of experimental laboratory medicine in understanding disease and its treatment. He habilitated at this same institution in 1867 [42–44]. He was appointed extraordinary professor and director of clinical medicine at the University of Dorpat (Tartu) from 1869 to 1871, followed by the same title at the University of Bern, Switzerland, from 1871 to 1872, and Königsberg from 1873 to 1888 [40–43, 45]. He was chair of medicine at the University of Strasbourg from 1888 to 1904 [40, 41, 45].

Naunyn co-founded with Johannes von Mikulicz-Radecki (1850–1905) *Mitteilungen aus den Grenzgebieten der Medizin und Chirurgie* (Communications from the Border Areas of Medicine and Surgery) in 1869 and with Edwin Klebs (1834–1913) and Oswald Schmiedeberg (1838–1921) *Archives fur Experimentelle Pathologie und Pharmakologie* (Archives for Experimental Pathology and Pharmacology) in Leipzig in 1871 [40–46]. Naunyn's primary interest was in clinical and experimental pathology and pathological chemistry, with an emphasis on diabetes mellitus research [42, 44]. A bronze medal commemorating Bernhard Naunyn was engraved by Josef Johann Tautenhayn (1868–1962) in 1909 [46]. Naunyn was nominated for the Nobel Prize in Physiology and Medicine for his research on gallstones in 1925 [47].

As to a description of his character and impetus:

> He has been described as "a clinician body and soul." He knew that the ultimate application of medical science must be practical, at the bedside, and that science that could not be thus applied was not worthy of the name. As far as speculation solved problems or set them apart he was not averse from it, but had no use for it in itself. He was one of the most practical research worker that there has ever been [48, p. 1132].

His farewell speech at the medical clinic in Strasbourg in 1904 provides further insights into the type of person Naunyn was:

> When I look back today, gentlemen, my closest students, and assistants always stood at the top of my clinical work. The gentlemen who gathered around and worked with me were introduced to science. The memory of this part of my work and activity is, without reservation, a happy and clear one, and I thank heaven for that. My collaboration with my students and assistants was the most important part of my life's work. It is also a source of joy for me to reflect on this part of my work with complete satisfaction. We stood together, gentlemen, like a circle of friends, where the thoughts and discoveries of each individual became the property of all through joyful sharing. Stimulating and encouraging each other, we have never worried about the demarcation of our intellectual property, neither has it been neglected, and we have all remained friends to this day. As I age, it is no small pride that I may boast of having such a circle of faithful and dependable friends [49].

Naunyn described a palpatory maneuver for examining the liver in causes of acute cholecystitis caused by gallstone (Table 7.1) (Fig. 7.1):

> If the liver is swollen as the result of the attack (i.e., recently) the organ is always tender, and often very acutely so; frequently, it is tender without being swollen. In such cases it is found that pain is induced when, during a deep inspiration, pressure is made with the hand projecting as far upwards as possible beneath the right costal border. At the moment when the liver impinges upon the tips of the fingers the patient experiences a deep–seated pain which sometimes radiates over the entire hepatic region and on to the epigastrium. Rarely, liver tenderness is only manifested by tension of the muscles of the anterior abdominal wall on the right side. In such cases the difference in tension of the right and left side respectively is best observed in the rectus abdominis [50, p. 79].

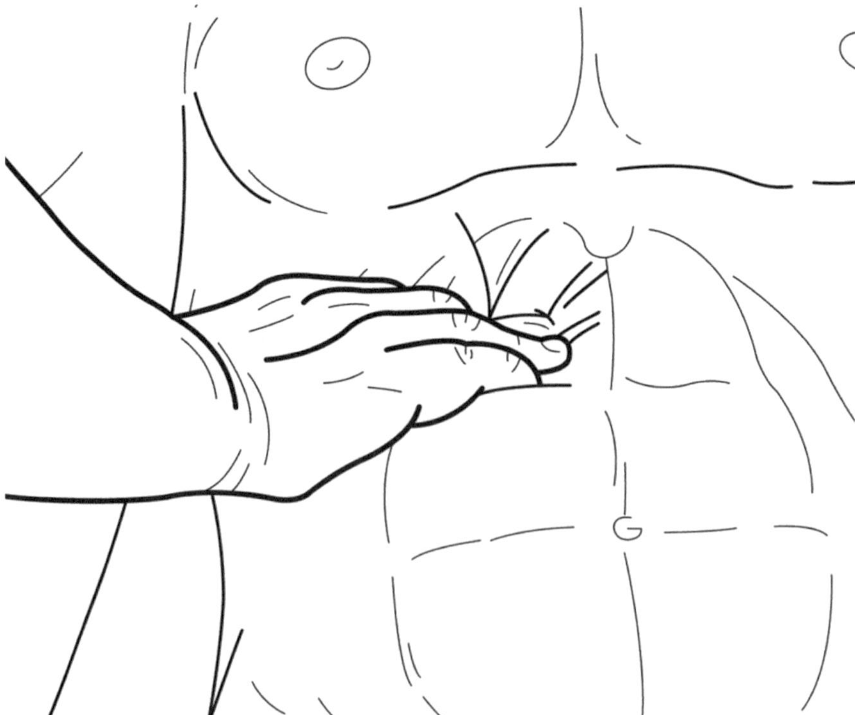

Fig. 7.1 Naunyn sign (by Ryan Yale)

Thus, Naunyn sign refers to a tender liver found on inspiratory palpation at the right costal margin.

7.2.7   *Lennhoff Sign*

Rudolf Lennhoff (1866–1933) was born in Lüdenscheid, Westfalen, Germany [51]. He served on the medical council of the Society for the Study of Social Medicine and Hygiene and as a medical statistician in Berlin [51, 52]. The purpose of this society involved the collaboration of medical practitioners and statisticians interested in political and social issues [52]. He was also a member and chairman of the Berlin-Brandenburg Medical Association and editor of the *Medizinische Reform* (Medical Reform) [52, 53].

Lennhoff described a finding found on examination of the abdomen as a method to confirm the diagnosis of an echinococcal cyst (Table 7.1):

> On inspection of the abdomen, one sees a moderate bulging of the hepatic region, projecting somewhat beyond the midline to the right. During deep inspiration, two smaller protrusions are seen on the right, by which palpation shows that they belong to the liver. The lower left edge of the liver is sharp and rough, the right edge only slightly firmer and thicker. The entire surface of the organ, including the protrusions, is smooth, and the latter feels somewhat firmer. Immediately during the initial examination, when I looked at the patient lying horizontally, I noticed the previously described furrow that formed between the rib wall and the protrusion as soon as the liver descended during deep inspiration. I then diagnosed liver echinococcus [54, p. 409].

Thus, Lennhoff sign refers to a furrow or crease found on deep inspiration below the lowest rib and echinococcal cyst.

7.2.8   *Mayo-Robson Sign*

Biographical information about Sir Arthur William Mayo-Robson (1853–1933) is found in Chap. 9—Pancreatitis. Mayo-Robson described a finding in patients with cholecystitis (Table 7.1):

> When seen there was tenderness at a point midway between the ninth costal cartilage and the umbilicus, which we have found to be almost as significant of inflammatory trouble about the gall-bladder as is tenderness at McBurney's point of appendicitis. This sign, together with slight icterus after each attack, led to the diagnosis of gall-stones, although the pain had latterly been more especially on the left side of the abdomen. The left-sided pain, as was pointed out some years ago (by the author), is always associated with adhesions between the pylorus and gall-bladder with adhesions between the pylorus and gall-bladder or bile-ducts, and from this and similar cases it almost seems as if, when this event occurs, a transference of the pain takes place from the right to the left side, as in reflected pain in other parts of the body [55, p. 153–154].

Thus, Mayo-Robson sign refers to tenderness located midway between the right ninth costal cartilage and umbilicus in patients with acute cholecystitis. He also described another sign in patients with acute pancreatitis, spontaneous pain at the left costovertebral angle (see Chap. 9).

7.2.9   Gilbert Sign

7.2.9.1   Augstin Nicolas Gilbert

Augustin Nicolas Gilbert (1858–1927) was born in Buzancy (Ardennes), France, and was appointed extern in 1878 and intern at Hôtel-Dieu under the tutelage of Hippolyte Hérard (1819–1913), Victor Charles Hanot (1837–1915), Paul Camille Hippolyte Brouardel (1837–1906), Jacques-Joseph Grancher (1843–1907), George Hayem (1841–1933), Jean Alfred Fournier (1832–1914), and Charles-Jacques (Joseph) Bouchard (1837–1915) [56]. He received his medical degree in 1886 with a gold medal distinction [56–59].

Gilbert was a physician of the Central Hospital Office in 1888 and agrégé of the Faculty of Medicine, Paris, in 1889 [56]. He was appointed to the Tenon Hospital in 1893 and Broussais Hospital in 1894 and served as head of the laboratories of Georges Hayem and Louis Théophile Joseph Landouzy (1845–1917) [56]. Gilbert was a professor of therapeutics in 1902 and a professor of clinical medicine at the Hôtel-Dieu, Paris, in 1905. He was chair of the medical clinic of the Hôtel-Dieu in 1910 [56–59].

With Paul Brouardel (1837–1906) and J. Girode, he co-edited *Traité de Médecine et de Thérapeutique (Treatise on Medicine and Therapeutics)* in 1895 and 1902 [56]. Among his awards and accolades, Gilbert was elected member of the National Academy of Medicine, Therapeutic Section in 1905 and recipient of the Commander of the Legion of Honor in 1913 [56, 58].

7.2.9.2   Pierre Émile Auguste Lereboullet

Pierre Émile Auguste Lereboullet (1874–1944) was born in Paris, France, and was an intern under the aegis of Paul Jules Tillaux (1834–1904) and Henri Barth (1853–1945) at Charité, Hôtel-Dieu with Édouard Brissaud (1852–1909), Gilbert at the Broussais Hospital in 1900, and interim-laureate of Hutinel at Hospice des enfants assistés (Assisted Children's Hospice) [59, 60]. He was appointed Doctor of Hospitals in 1907, associate professor of infant medicine in 1920, and professor of hygiene and the clinic of early childhood and director of the Childcare Institute, Paris, in 1928 [59, 60]. Lereboullet returned to Hospice des Enfants-assistés where he remained through retirement. He was elected president of the Office for Maternal and Infant Protection of the Department of Seine, National Committee for Childhood, and member of the Academy of Medicine in 1925 [59, 61].

As described by Carnot:

> Our notice of the life of Pierre Lereboullet would be incomplete and disloyal if we did not state here the great discreet, active, benevolent, and charitable piety that guided him all his life. He was largely open-minded, and one could easily remain his friend provided one strives to be like him, a "good man" [60, p. 32].

As to his character as described by Girons:

> We would omit an essential part of the pediatric work of M. Lereboullet if we did not recall, if only in a few words, what he was for his patients and pupils. He welcomed the former,

whether at his hospital or family consultations, with an affectionate gentleness that doubled the value of his advice. He knew how, even to the parents of the incurable, to lavish the encouragement which allows hope, even if the improvement is slow or nonexistent. All those he healed now realize what they have lost through his death. His pupils, students, doctors, and nurses maintain a profound recognition of his teaching. He opened up to them the various fields of pediatrics and frequently inspired their vocation. They will piously keep his memory by seeking inspiration from his example [61, p. 166].

Gilbert and Lereboullet described a phenomenon at the Biological Society in 1901, occurring in patients with cirrhosis (Table 7.1):

Examining the urine in the morning on an empty stomach or during the day after meals shows that in the physiological state, the urine is much more abundant after the meal. In cirrhosis, we observe an opposite phenomenon. The urine becomes scarce after a meal and is more abundant after fasting. This phenomenon is what M. Gilbert and Lereboullet refer to it as the inversion of the normal rhythm of aqueous elimination. This disorder in urinary secretion is an early sign of portal hypertension as it may precede ascites and is an extremely important prognostic sign. This sign is found not only in cirrhosis but also in congestions of the liver of cardiac origin and even in jaundice. Gilbert and Lereboullet explain that this symptom is caused by obstruction of the portal circulation, leading to a delay in aqueous absorption in the intestine [62, p. 400–401].

Thus, Gilbert (and Lereboullet) sign refers to the finding in hepatic cirrhosis of increased excretion of urine occurring during fasting than after a full meal (opisura).

7.2.10 Kayser–Fleischer Sign (Ring)

7.2.10.1 Bernhard Kayser

Bernhard Kayser (1869–1954) was born in Bremen, Germany, and received his medical degree from the University of Berlin in 1893 [63]. He was an intern in Tübingen and an assistant at the University Eye Clinic in Freiburg. Kayser traveled overseas and worked as a physician at the North German Lloyd Shipping Company and general practitioner in Brazil [63]. On his return to Germany, he was a general practitioner in Brandenburg and Bremen, followed by a specialty in ophthalmology in Stuttgart [63].

Kayser at the University Eye Clinic in Tübingen in 1902 described the case of a 23-year-old male with multiple sclerosis and congenital greenish discoloration of the cornea:

Even on external inspection in ordinary daylight, it is immediately noticeable in both completely non-irritated eyes that the cornea, which is clear and transparent in its central parts, shows a ring-shaped opacity in the periphery, resembling gerontoxon in form and extent. The cornea appears opaque here and has a dark green-brown color. This ring of opacity is widest above, less wide below, and very narrow outside and inside so that the area of the clear cornea is lying oval. The opacity begins immediately at the limbus and has no sharp border extending to the clear center of the cornea [64, p. 22–23].

On binocular microscopic examination:

[i]n the peripheral ring zone described above, there is a significant accumulation of fine yellow spots in the deeper layer close to the posterior wall so that the underlying iris and chamber

angle cannot be seen. The yellow spots are apparently in an area parallel to the corneal surface. (…) This accumulation of yellow spots begins in the periphery, where their arrangement is densest, and the individual spots are the largest. In general, they are smaller and less dense in the middle portion of the ring and fine in the portion nearer the corneal center so that their turbidity no longer appears patchy but diffuse, allowing more light to reach the underlying surface of the iris. While the above dense patches of turbidity give a yellow appearance at the center of the cornea, the color is different: the yellow hue gradually changes into a yellowish-green, proceeding gradually into the black of the pupil. The arrangement of the spots is entirely random. The individual spots appear under the binocular microscope as flat bodies, without sharp boundaries, that are quite irregular shaped, at least the coarser ones in the periphery. The corneal tissue does not reveal any abnormal abnormalities. There is no sign of vascular formation. The central parts of the cornea are completely normal [64, p. 23].

7.2.10.2 Bruno Fleischer

Bruno Otto Fleischer (1874–1965) was born in Stuttgart, Germany, received his medical training at the Universities of Tübingen, Geneva, and Berlin, and earned a medical degree from the University of Tübingen in 1898 [65]. He was an assistant at the University of Tübingen Eye Clinic, habilitating in ophthalmology in 1904. He was appointed chair of ophthalmology at the University of Erlangen, Germany, from 1920 to 1951 [65].

Fleischer identified, in two cases, ocular findings similar to that reported by Kayser. His first case involved a 29-year-old photographer with tremors and on ocular examination:

> The greenish discoloration of the cornea is ring-shaped in the periphery, approx. 1 mm wide and consists of small brownish-greenish dots and spots merging into one another, becoming finer towards the center of the cornea and gradually merging into the clear cornea. Fine, lighter stripes run through the discolored area irregularly. The superficial layers of the cornea are clear. The discoloration resides in the deepest layers, in an area concentric to the surface, and is quite similar in both eyes [66, p. 490].

Thus, Kayser-Fleischer sign refers to the greenish-yellow ring surrounding the cornea at the lumbus, which was later found to be caused by excessive copper deposition (Table 7.1).

7.2.11 Murphy Sign

John Benjamin Murphy (1857–1916) was born in Appleton, Wisconsin, USA, and received his medical degree from Rush Medical College in 1879. He completed an internship at Cook County Hospital, Chicago, in 1881. Murphy then traveled abroad to the Wiener Allgemeine Krankenhaus (Vienna General Hospital), continuing his medical studies under Theodor Billroth (1829–1894) in 1882 and at the University of Berlin and Heidelberg, Germany [67, 68]. Upon his return to Chicago in 1884, he served as a lecturer in surgery at Rush Medical College and an attending surgeon at Cook County Hospital and Alexian Brothers Hospital [67–70]. He was appointed professor of clinical surgery at Chicago Post-Graduate Medical School, College of

Physicians and Surgeons (later renamed the University of Illinois College of Medicine) in 1892 [70]. He was a chief surgeon and chief of staff at Mercy Hospital, Northwestern's first teaching hospital in Chicago, from 1895 to 1916 [69, 70]. Murphy later accepted a position as professor of surgery at Northwestern University Medical School from 1901 to 1905 [67, 69], returned to Rush Medical College, and was appointed co-chairman of surgery department from 1905 to 1907, and later again at Northwestern where he accepted an appointment as chairman of surgery department from 1908 to 1916 [71].

Murphy was the founder and editor of *The Clinics of John B. Murphy at Mercy Hospital, Surgical Clinics of John B. Murphy at Mercy Hospital* (later renamed *Surgical Clinics of Chicago, Surgical Clinics of North America*) and "Volume of Surgery" in the *American Year-book* [67, 68]. He also served as president of the Chicago Surgical Society in 1904, the Chicago Medical Society from 1904 to 1905, the American Medical Association from 1911 to 1912, and the Clinical Congress of Surgeons from 1914 to 1915 [67, 69]. He was the founder of the American College of Surgeons. Murphy received an honorary degree of DSc from the University of Sheffield, an LLD from the University of Illinois and Catholic University, and the Laetare Medal from the University of Notre Dame for his service to humanity and science [67, 68]. He also received the Collar and Cross of Saint Gregory the Great from the Pope in 1916 [68].

His work spanned multiple therapeutic areas, including abdominal surgery, neurology, and orthopedics. His many discoveries and contributions included end-to-end arterial anastomoses, grafting cartilage and bone, restoration of ankylosed joints, and rectal saline infusion in the treatment of peritonitis. His name is eponymously associated with the Murphy button, Murphy punch, Murphy–Lane bone skid, and Murphy drip [67–69].

As to his character as described in a memoriam by Dr. John B. Deaver:

> He was a man of unusual personal charm, striking originality, and exceptional skill [68, p. 994]. (…) [h]e was sure of himself and unafraid; abiding by his statements, radical and unusual though they may have appeared, because they were based on accurate, painstaking research, experimentation and observation [68, p. 995]. (…) He was a powerful, vigorous public speaker, full of enthusiasm and earnestness, which, coupled with an attractive personality and delightful humor, at once gained for him the attention of his hearers, young and old alike [68, p. 996].

Murphy described a maneuver for identifying patients with acute cholecystitis secondary to gallstone and infection of the gallbladder (Fig. 7.2):

> Hypersensitiveness of the gall-bladder is present in all varieties of *infection* and *calculous* obstruction, but not in the neoplastic, torsion, flexion, cicatricial or valvular obstructions. The hypersensitiveness is elicited by deep palpation just below the right ninth costal cartilage, or in a line from that point to the middle of Poupart's ligament, as this is the common track of gallbladder enlargement. Deep percussion along the same line, with patient in forced inspiration gives pronounced pain. The most characteristic and constant sign of gallbladder hypersensitiveness is the inability of the patient to take a full, deep inspiration, when the physician's fingers are hooked up deep beneath the right costal arch below the hepatic margin. The diaphragm forces the liver down until the sensitive gall-bladder reaches the examining fingers, when the inspiration suddenly ceases as though it had been shut off. I have never found, this sign absent in a calculous or infectious case of gall-bladder, or duct disease [72, p. 827–828].

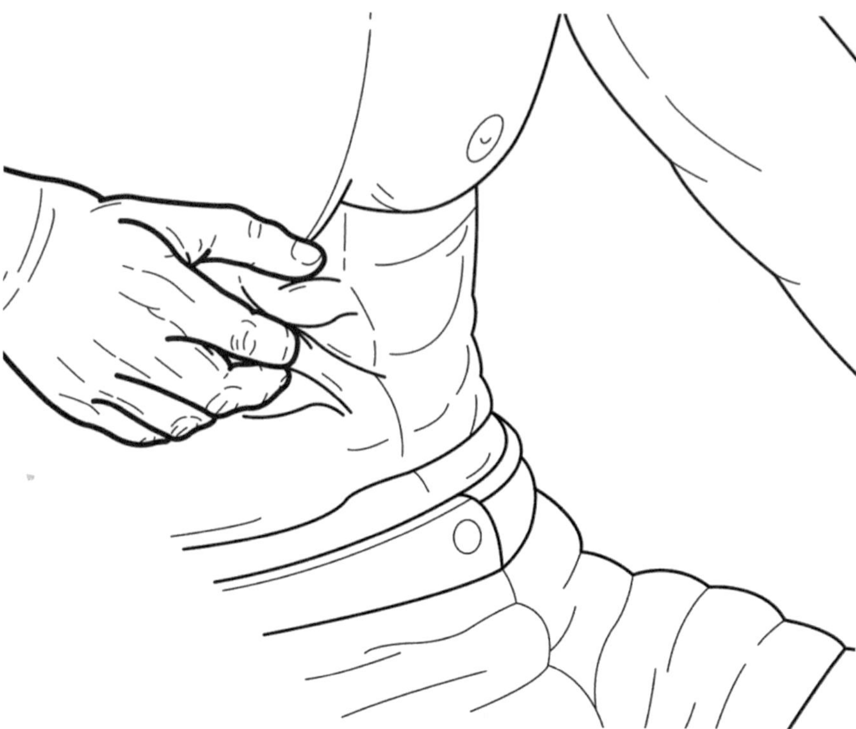

Fig. 7.2 Murphy sign I (by Ryan Yale)

Murphy discussed another technique for examining the gallbladder during a symposium on the gallbladder, gall ducts, and liver at the Chicago Medical Society on April 20, 1910. During this maneuver, the middle finger of the left hand is flexed perpendicularly at the tip of the ninth costal cartilage, and "[t]he finger struck with the right hand when the patient is in deep inspiration. This causes great pain if the gallbladder is distended or inflamed" [73, p. 278] (Fig. 7.3). Thus, Murphy sign refers to the palpable technique in which the patient is unable to take a deep inspiratory breath secondary to pain when the examiner hooks their fingers below the right costal margin and deeply beneath the hepatic margin in patients with acute cholecystitis (Table 7.1).

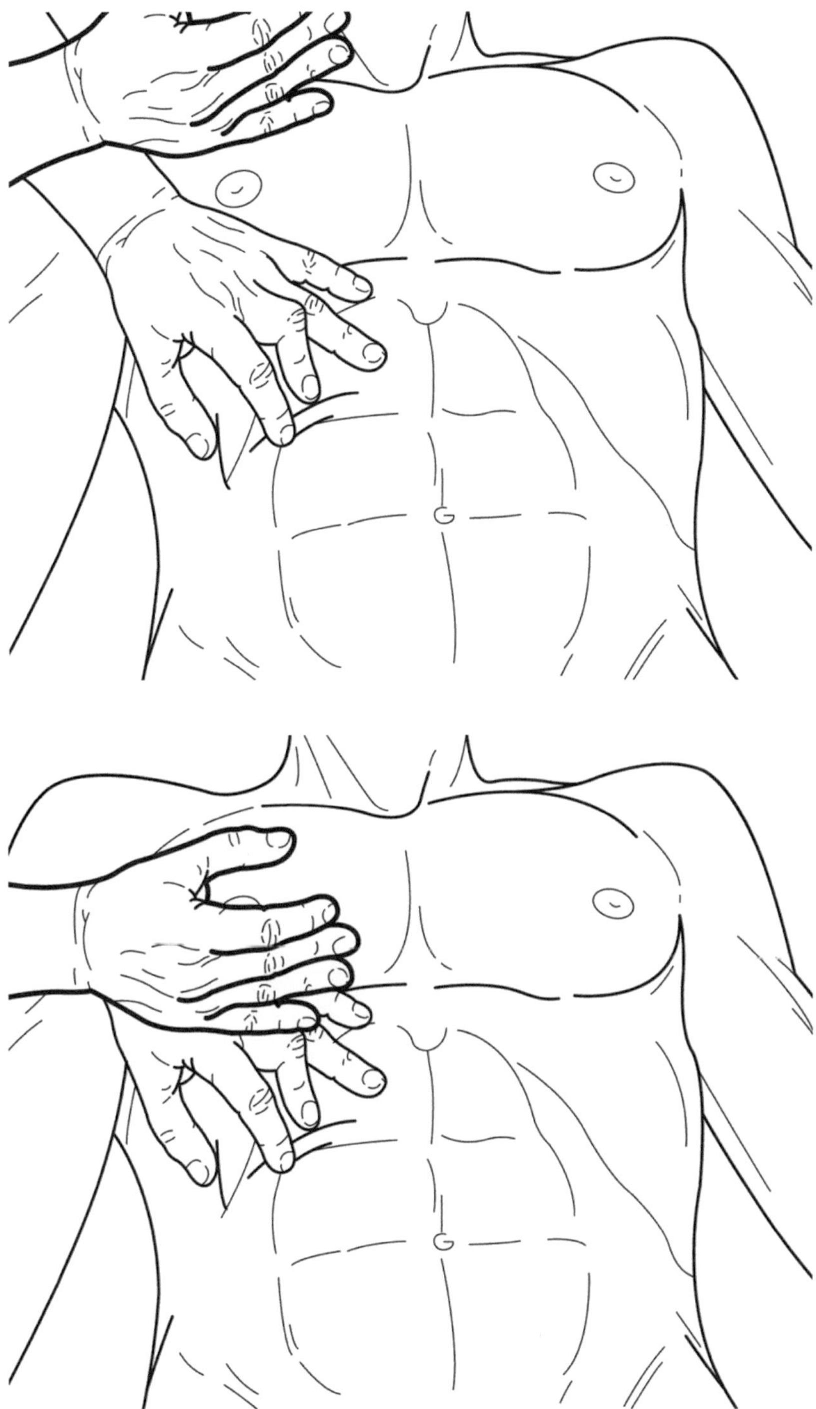

Fig. 7.3 Murphy sign II (by Ryan Yale)

7.2.12   *Abrahams Sign*

Robert Abrahams (1861–1935) was born in Russia and immigrated to the USA in 1880. He received his medical degree from the College of Physicians and Surgeons, Columbia University (currently Columbia University Vagelos College of Physicians and Surgeons), and after graduation, was a private practitioner [74]. He was a member of the Board of the New York Manhattan State Hospital, Ward's Island, beginning in 1913, and served as president of the Board of Managers [75]. He was also an adjunct professor of medicine at Postgraduate School and Hospital and attending physician at the Home of the Daughters of Jacob, New York [74].

Abrahams described a pathognomonic sign to assist in the bedside diagnosis of cholelithiasis (Table 7.1) (Fig. 7.4):

> The sign consists in a painful point midway between the umbilicus and the costal cartilage of the ninth rib in the right hypochondriac. The method of eliciting it is as follows: Place the patient in the recumbent position with the arms and legs extended. Ascertain a point midway between the umbilicus and ninth costal cartilage, then with a sudden thrust press the index and middle fingers of the right hand into that point. The effect on the patient is like an electric shock, there is either a grimace on the face denoting suffering or a quick involuntary jump of the abdomen as if it were struck with a pointed instrument. (…) In an acute attack with a diffuse area of hyper asthenia, the midway point mentioned is the point of maximum pain. In chronic cases the painful point is present at all times while the whole area around it may enjoy freedom from sensitiveness [76, p. 74].

Abrahams believed this painful point corresponds to the location on the fundus of the inflamed gallbladder. Although he did not expressly state, this location corresponds to the region where the inflamed distended fundus of the gallbladder contacts the parietal peritoneum causing a somatosensory reflex. Thus, Abraham sign refers to pain occurring when palpable pressure is applied midway between the ninth right costal cartilage and the umbilicus.

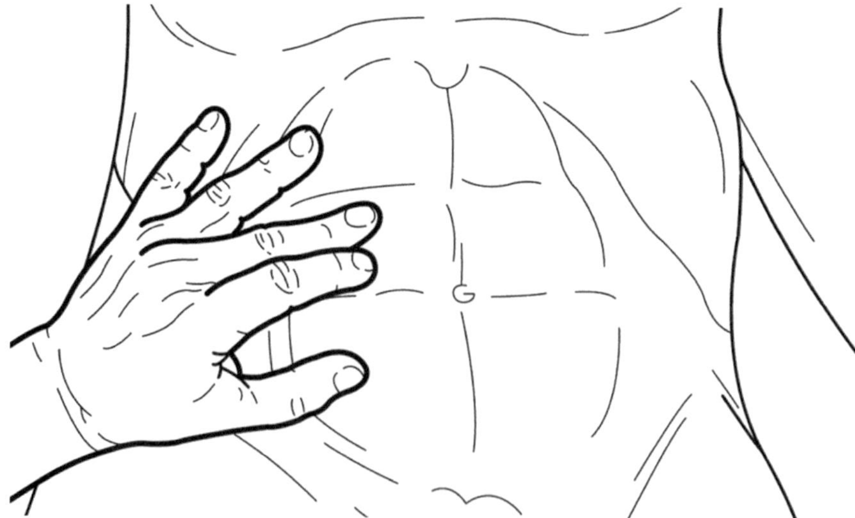

Fig. 7.4 Abraham sign (by Ryan Yale)

7.2.13   *Finsterer Sign*

Hans Finsterer (1877–1955) was born in Weng, Austria, and received his medical degree from the University of Vienna in 1902 [77–79]. He was a surgeon at the University of Vienna Surgical Clinic under the aegis of Julius von Hochenegg (1859–1940) in 1906 and assistant to Viktor Ritter von Hacker (1852–1933) from 1907 to 1909 in Graz, Austria [78, 79].

He returned to the University of Vienna Hochenegg Surgical Clinic, where he was appointed assistant in 1910 and received venia legendi (authorization to teach) in 1913. During World War I, he was a surgeon in the Russian Front's Deutsch-Ordensspital (German Order Hospital) and served in the Garrison Hospital from 1915 to 1918 [77, 79]. He was appointed associate professor in 1919 and headed the Kaiser-Franz-Joseph-Ambulatorium Outpatient Clinic, followed by Krankenhaus der Barmherzigen Brüder (Brothers of Charity Hospital) Surgical Department, returning to the Kaiser-Franz-Joseph-Ambulatorium Outpatient Clinic from 1924 to 1935 [77, 79].

Finsterer was awarded the titles of extraordinary professor in 1919, ordinary professor in 1940, and full professor of surgery in 1948 at the University of Vienna [79]. He was chief physician in the surgical department of the Vienna General Hospital in 1935 and head of the surgical department at the University of Vienna from 1935 until 1951. His name is eponymously associated with a sign and two surgical procedures: Finsterer–Drüner operation and Hoffmeister–Finsterer operation [77, 79].

Finsterer described the case of a 27-year-old man who sustained a self-inflicted gunshot wound and tissue injury involving the left lobe of the liver. He found that:

> [t]he patient presents with a symptom that I believed had never previously been mentioned or appreciated in abdominal injuries-bradycardia in acute anemia. I observed that the pulse in our patient had dropped to 52, and significant bleeding was found at laparotomy. (…) Review of the literature shows that my observation is not unique in that a striking slowing of the pulse has been found in twelve other cases [80, p. 1751].

Finsterer believed that bradycardia in patients with injury to the liver has prognostic importance in that a high pulse rate and pallor are more likely to be found in cases of severe hemorrhage compared to patients with a lower pulse (Table 7.1).

7.2.14   *Milkó Sign*

Vilmos Milkó (1878–1956) was born in Óbecse, Serbia, and received his medical degree from the University of Budapest in 1900 [81]. He was a physician in the Pathology Institute and Surgical Clinic in 1901 and surgery department at Szent Rókus Hospital in Budapest in 1903 [81].

He was appointed chief surgeon at the Park Sanatorium, Orsz, Budapest, in 1908, Németvölgy út State Pulmonary Hospital and Hospital for Disabled People from

1920 to 1928, Madarász út Children's Hospital in 1929, and Maglódi út Hospital from 1933 to 1943 [81]. He maintained an appointment since 1928 as a surgical expert for the Social Insurance Institute and Social Insurance Center of the Trade Unions. His last appointment was as a Capital City Council's Disability Assessment Committee member [81].

Milkó was co-editor of *Orvosi Hetilap* (Medical Weekly) and editor-in-chief of *Magyar Sebészet* (Hungarian Surgery). Among his appointments, he was president of the Surgical Group of the Medical Trade Union. The focus of his research was on general, military, and pediatric surgery [81].

Finsterer, in his paper "Zur Diagnose der Leberverletzungen," spoke of a communication by Milkó that he could only access in a report. Milkó found that:

> In the early diagnosis of abdominal injuries, reflex tension in the abdominal wall is the most important symptom. The behavior of the pulse, even in the most severe abdominal injuries and in general peritonitis, may remain normal longer than expected. In several cases of severe intestinal injury, Milkó found marked bradycardia lasting 8 to 10 hours [82, p. 378].

Thus, Milkó sign refers to bradycardia occurring in abdominal injuries (Table 7.1).

7.2.15 Grocco Sign

Pietro Grocco (1856–1916) was born in Albanese, Piemonte, Province of Pavia, Italy. He studied medicine at the Faculty of Medicine and Surgery at the University of Pavia, receiving his medical degree in 1879 [83]. He was assistant to Francesco Orsi (1828–1899), followed by a teaching appointment in clinical propedeutics at the Faculty of Medicine in Pavia [83]. He continued his training with Jean-Martin Charcot (1825–1893) at the Salpêtrière, Paris, and with Hermann Nothnagel (1841–1905) and Moritz Rosenthal (1833–1889), Vienna, in 1882 [83–86].

Grocco was appointed chair of special medical pathology at the University of Perugia in 1884, chair of the medical clinic at the University of Pisa from 1887 to 1889, and finally director of clinical medicine at the Istituto di Studi Superiori (Institute of Higher Studies), Florence, Italy, in 1892 [83, 85, 86]. He founded the Instituto Antirrabico and Montecatini thermal baths used to treat rheumatism [83, 84, 86]. He was appointed Senator of the Kingdom in 1905. Among his many accolades, he was Knight of the Order of the Crown of Italy [84]. He also described another sign that eponymously bears his name, the paravertebral or "Grocco triangle," a triangular-shaped area of dullness occurring in patients with pleural effusion.

As to his character and teacher:

> Anyone fortunate to know Grocco as a clinical teacher could learn a good amount about him by scrolling through his book of clinical lessons. A book without vain documentation or useless information that contained historical comparisons and elegance of style, and not philosophical digressions. A simple, practical, honest book written by a great doctor for his students to make them physicians in his form based on comparable experience. The style of this book is the mirror of his spirit: in those pages, you see him, you hear him speak; short,

jerky, nervous, clear, intelligent, very eloquent, all the more so as stripped of any artifice [83, p. 11]. (…) The best reward for his long labor as Master was his gift to Tuscany and Italy, educating a whole generation of physicians who were aware of their duties and rigidly trained based on his honest, objective, simple and practical method [83, p. 13].

Grocco emphasized that percussion should extend from the last dorsal vertebral and left paravertebral zone to determine whether there is an enlargement of the left lobe of the liver. He reported a systematic method of percussion of the liver (Table 7.1):

In order to detect this finding, percussion must be applied with sufficient force. Practice is required before it can be easily and confidently detected. Percussion is performed in a methodical manner moving from the top to bottom, first along the right paravertebral line a, then along the spine b and to the left of it, corresponding to lines c, d, e, etc., so that each time where the thoracic sound ends and liver dullness begins is marked. In this way, one finally arrives at line f, which delimits the almost horizontal section of liver dullness to the left of the spinal column. Once line f is reached, it is advisable to percuss from left to right, along the horizontal line i-g, in the direction of arrow 1, in order to pinpoint point g, the outer limit of the left portion of the hepatic dullness [87, p. 668].

Thus, Grocco sign refers to a percussion dullness technique to detect enlargement of the left lobe of the liver. Percussion begins to the right of the last dorsal vertebral and right paravertebral zones, extends from the top to bottom, moves from right to left and finally left to right.

7.2.16 *Lesieur Sign*

Charles Lesieur (1876–1919) was born in Cousance, Jura, France, in 1876, received his medical training in Lyon, and served as an extern in 1894, intern in 1897, and in the Laboratory of Experimental and Comparative Medicine of Saturnin Arloing (1846–1911) in 1897 [88]. He served in the Hygiene Laboratory of Jules Courmont (1865–1917) from 1900 to 1909. During this period, he was chief of the anti-rabies services at the Bacteriological Institute of Lyons and a physician at the anti-tuberculosis dispensaries [88].

Lesieur was agrégé beginning in 1907 and was chair of the medical clinic from 1908 to 1910, the position previously held by Raphaël Lépine (1840–1919) [88]. He was director of the office of hygiene in Lyon in 1909 and succeeded Gabriel Roux as chair of pathology and general therapeutics in 1912 [88]. During World War I, he organized the Municipal Hospital and Joffe School for the Disabled in Lyon [88]. He was also stationed in Verda, Bar-le-Duc, and Bouges, France, the latter where he was director of the health service of the eighth region [88]. Lesieur was awarded the Vernois Prize from the Academy of Medicine in 1904, was the recipient of the cross of the Legion of Honor, and was appointed chair of hygiene, the position occupied by his former mentor Jules Courmont in 1918 [88].

Lesieur's work involved multiple therapeutic areas, including infectious diseases. (e.g., diphtheria, typhoid fever, tuberculosis, pneumococcus, rabies), poisonings (e.g., alcoholism), neurology, and gastrointestinal [88]. At the time of the publication of his sign, coauthored with J. Marchand who was former substitute intern at Lyon Hospitals [89].

Lesieur and Marchand described a pulmonary percussion finding in patients with typhoid fever caused by liver hypertrophy (Table 7.1):

> In two previous communications, one at the Congress of the French Association for the Advancement of Science in Dijon (August 1911) and the other at the National Society of Medicine of Lyon (meeting December 11, 1911), one of us was attracted the attention to a "very clear and frequent" sign of typhoid fever, of which he gave the description and showed the value while trying to explain its pathogenic mechanisms. During ordinary classic fever, he wrote, if one superficially percusses the right base of the thorax, one notices almost always a noticeable dullness, which we do not find at the left base, which is generally not explained by pleuro-pulmonary lesion and whose observation appears to have a real value in diagnosis, prognosis, and treatment [89, p. 625]. Hypertrophy of the liver seemed capable of explaining the existence of a zone of sub-dullness at the right base of the thorax in typhoid patients [89, p. 626].

Thus, Lesieur sign refers to decreased auscultatory breath sounds at the right base in typhoid fever caused by hepatic hypertrophy.

7.2.17 Frank Sign

Alfred Erich Frank (1884–1957) was born in Berlin, Germany, and studied medicine in Breslau (Wroclaw, Poland). He passed his state examination in 1907, completed his internship at the Wiesbaden Municipal Hospital, and received his doctorate from the University of Strasbourg in 1908 [90]. He was involved in diabetes and metabolic research under the aegis of Wilhelm Weintraud (1866–1920) at the medical clinic at the Wiesbaden Municipal Hospital from 1908 to 1911 [90].

Frank was an assistant in Oskar Minkowski's (1858–1931) Clinic for Internal Diseases at the University of Breslau beginning in 1911, habilitated in 1913, and an extraordinary professor in internal medicine in 1919 [90]. He was a senior physician at the University of Breslau in 1918 and, in 1926, was chief physician in the medical department of the Municipal Wenzel-Hancke Hospital, Breslau. Among his many accomplishments, he was the first to recognize the association between the posterior pituitary gland and diabetes insipidus [90].

He fled during National Socialism to Turkey in 1934 and was granted a position at the University of Istanbul, where he was director of the second chair of the internal department of the Faculty of Medicine at Gureba Hospital [90]. He founded *Istanbuler Zeitschrift für klinische Medizin* (Istanbul Journal for Clinical Medicine) in 1951 [90].

Frank coined the term pseudohemophilia to describe the clinical features that distinguish true hemophilia from other causes that resemble this condition (Table 7.1):

> There is no doubt that acute and chronic liver disease, if sufficiently advanced, results in a significant prolongation of blood coagulation. However, it must be emphasized that it is not found in all cases of severe hepatic insufficiency [91, p. 457]. (…) The cause of hypocoagulability is the disappearance of the fibrinogen, through lack of formation and increased

destruction [91, p. 457]. (…) I now imagine that even in severe hepatic insufficiency, the delay in coagulation is merely an indicator of a process that prevents platelet thrombus formation. (…) The mechanism of hemorrhage in hepatic pseudohemophilia is, therefore, similar to that in thrombocytopenia: it is based on the absence or the excessively loose structure of the platelet thrombus. It is, therefore, a question of thrombocytopenia in the truest sense of the word; but since the name thrombocytopenia has already been assigned, I would prefer to refer to the absence of thrombus formation when there is a numerically sufficient number of platelets as athrombia [91, p. 458].

Frank recognized the finding of hypocoagulability in patients with chronic liver disease is caused by hypofibrinogenemia and platelets that may be normal in number but fail to cause blood clotting—a condition he referred to as athrombia, currently known as thrombasthenia.

7.2.18   Ortner Sign

Ritter Norbert Ortner von Rodenstätt (1865–1935) was born in Linz, Austria, and received his medical degree from the University of Vienna in 1888 [92]. He was a physician at the Crown Prince Rudolf Children's Hospital and, subsequently, the Rudolf Foundation Hospital until 1893 [90]. He was appointed assistant to Edmund von Neusser (1852–1912) at the second medical clinic in 1893. Ortner was primaries at the Kaiser-Franz-Josef Hospital in 1900 and a full professor of internal medicine at the University of Innsbruck in 1907 [92]. He returned to the University of Vienna in 1911 as a professor of special medicine and pathology, and therapy at the third medical clinic and the second medical clinic (a position previously held by Neusser) [92].

Ortner described two signs. One involves hoarseness due to vocal cord paralysis caused by compression of the recurrent laryngeal nerve in patients with an enlarged left atrium. He also described the physical examination findings in patients with biliary colic (Table 7.1):

Objectively, we find tenderness in the region of the incisura, at least on deep inspiration, pressure against the liver during inspiration, and on bimanual palpation of the liver with one hand on the incisura and the other pressing against it from the lumbar region. There is hyperesthesia of the skin over the gallbladder region and posteriorly between the lower border of the right lung and posterior costal arch. The lowest part of the thorax and right hypochondrium is tender on rapid, sharp percussion of these regions with the ulnar part of the hand. (…) Not uncommonly, the patient complains of increased pains which last several hours after palpation of the gallbladder [93, p. 164–165].

Thus, Ortner sign refers to the (1) palpable technique for detecting cutaneous hyperesthesia over the gallbladder region and posteriorly between the lower right lung and posterior costal arch and (2) percussion tenderness using the ulnar aspect of the hand located over the lower thorax and right hypochondrium in patients with acute cholecystitis.

7.2.19   *Riesman Sign*

David Riesman (1867–1940) was born in Thuringia, Germany, received his medical training at the University of Michigan and the University of Pennsylvania, and earned his medical degree from the latter in 1892 [94]. He completed an internship at the Philadelphia General Hospital and was appointed demonstrator in pathology until 1901. He held subsequent positions as instructor in clinical medicine in 1901, assistant professor of clinical medicine in 1905, and professor of clinical medicine from 1912 to 1933 at the University of Pennsylvania [94]. He also held teaching posts from 1901 to 1918 as a professor of clinical medicine in the Polyclinic Hospital and at the College for Graduates in Medicine. He was appointed the first professor of medical history in the Graduate School of Medicine at the University of Pennsylvania [94].

As to a description of his character and teaching:

> He was kindly and wise, forceful and stimulating, tolerant, versatile, cultivated and amazingly industrious. (…) His life and teaching will always stand as an inspiration to all of us who had the rare privilege of knowing David Riesman personally, and to those countless members of the profession who knew him only through his works [94, p. 303].

Riesman described ulnar percussion as a method for diagnosing cholecystitis where conventional examination methods for eliciting tenderness remain obscure (Table 7.1) (Fig. 7.5):

> The method of employing it simple: The patient is asked to take as deep a breath as possible and to hold it. The suddenly one strikes a quick but not hard blow over the upper part of the right rectus muscle, with the ulnar side of the hand. If there is any disease of the gallbladder, the blow will cause a sharp pain. If one is in doubt as to whether this pain is superficial and due to the blow on the integument, all that is necessary is to perform the test on the left side [95, p. 1963].

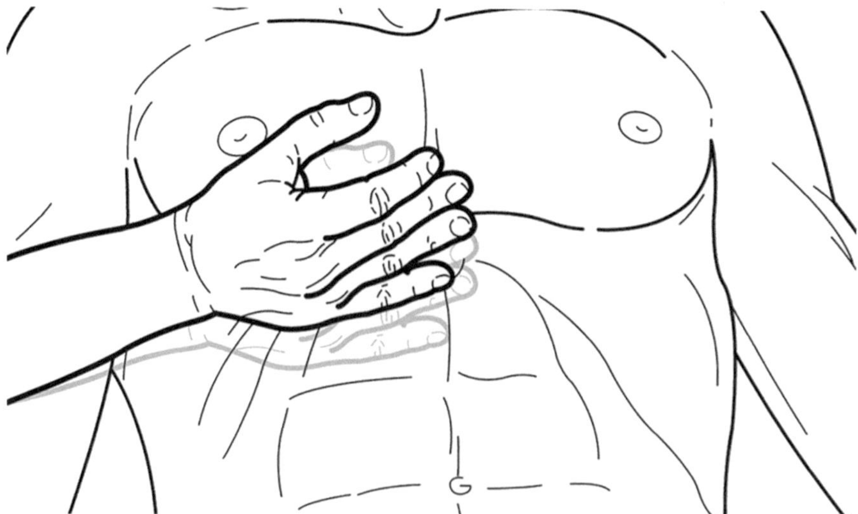

Fig. 7.5 Riesman sign (by Ryan Yale)

Thus, Riesman sign refers to the pain located along the upper portion of the right rectus muscle while the patient holds their breath after deep inspiration and strikes this region using the ulnar aspect of the hand.

7.2.20 Carmalt-Jones Sign

Dudley William Carmalt-Jones (1874–1957) was born in London, England, and received his Bachelor of Medicine degree from St. Mary's Hospital, London, in 1903 [96, 97]. He continued as house surgeon and house physician at St. Mary's Hospital and subsequently was appointed senior house physician at the National Hospital for the Paralyzed at Maida Vale [94]. He returned to St. Mary's and worked as an assistant in Sir Almroth Wright's (1861–1947) Laboratory of Therapeutic Inoculation [97]. Carmalt-Jones was an assistant physician at the Seamen's Hospital, Greenwich, in 1907 and Westminster Hospital, London, and honorary director of the department of bacterio-therapeutics from 1910 to 1913, where he later was full physician and dean of the Westminster Hospital Medical School in 1912 [96, 97]. He received his Doctorate of Medicine degree from Oxford in 1911 [94]. During World War I, he served in the Royal Army Medical Corps, where he was stationed in France from 1914 to 1918, and as a temporary colonel and a consulting physician of the expeditionary forces to Egypt from 1918 to 1919 [96, 97].

Carmalt-Jones was the Mary Glendinning professor and chair of systemic medicine at the University of Otago School of Medicine, New Zealand, in 1920, whose primary responsibility was teaching medical students at Dunedin Hospital [96–98]. He was a member of the Royal College of Physicians, London, in 1907 and a fellow in 1914 [96]. Carmalt-Jones was editor of the *Proceedings of the University of Otago Medical School* [96, 98]. He served as president of the New Zealand Branch of the British Medical Association in 1935 [96]. He was appointed foundation fellow, vice-president, and member of the first council of the Royal Australian College of Physicians [96].

As articulated by his former student regarding Carmalt-Jones character:

> Carmalt-Jones was beloved by all, who recognized him the scholar and gentleman in addition to the physician. Maybe he was a little "old school," but he strove to keep us abreast of developments. He was fine company, and lost no chance of introducing us to Plato and the Greeks through Sir Richard Livingstone's little books. His own history of the Otago School is a valued bequest. Those who were fortunate to meet him latterly in his retirement near London found him the same kindly interested "C.J." of thirty years ago in Dunedin [99, p. 661].

Carmalt-Jones identified in patients with cholecystitis a sharp pain involving the rib cartilage in the right hypochondrium (Table 7.1):

> I found a tender spot upon the eight right costal cartilage, on its lower edge (not its anterior surface), which could have been found by approaching the patient from behind and hooking one's right-hand fingers round the costal margin. (…) The sign is sought for with the hand flat on the upper abdomen; the third finger-tip is brought into firm contact with the costal

margin, inch by inch along its whole length from without inwards, beginning on the left side, saying nothing and watching the patient's face. (…) On the right, in a case of cholecystitis, a single tender spot, indicated by the patient's expression, is found, generally on the eight rib edge, sometimes a little higher or lower, and just covered by the finger-tip. Occasionally, but by no means always, the skin of the whole eight dorsal segment on the same side is hyperalgesia to pin-prick [100, p. 615].

He postulated that the etiology was due to:

I would suggest that spasm of the sphincter of Oddi, which is believed to be controlled by the sympathetic, induces this tender spot on the body wall, and sometimes hyperalgesia of a whole segment in the areas of corresponding somatic innervation [100, p. 616].

Thus, Carmalt-Jones sign refers to a tender spot located on the eighth right costal cartilage below the costal margin elicited by hooking the fingers of the right hand around the costal margin.

7.2.21   Kenawy Sign

There is limited historical information available on Mohammed Radwan Kenawy. He served in the medical unit as a medical tutor at the Qasr al-Aini Hospital, University of Cairo, Egypt, in 1939 and in the Faculty of Medicine at Fuad I. University, Cairo, in 1947 [101, 102].

Kenawy described in 1939 an auscultatory finding, the continuous venous hum, in patients with cirrhosis (Table 7.1):

The venous hum is usually heard over a localized area over just below the xiphoid process of the sternum. It is continuous and is accentuated by deep inspiration. (…) i) Over the site of the hum and in a strictly localized area a continuous thrill could be felt, especially on applying very lightly the tip of one finger; ii) careful inspect of the site of the thrill showed an elevation of the skin, which is probably due to an underlying vein; iii) when light pressure was applied over the elevation, the thrill disappeared; and iv) when the stethoscope was applied to the xiphoid process and the hum listened to, the application of light pressure over the site of the thrill caused the hum to disappear. When the pressure was released, the hum returned [102, p. 821–822].

Thus, Kenawy sign refers to a continuous venous hum in patients with hepatic cirrhosis.

7.2.22   Čičovački Sign

We were unable to identify any historical information on Danilo Čičovački. At the time of his publication, he held an appointment under Professor Nikolaus V. Jagić (1875–1956) at the Second Medical University Clinic in Vienna.

Čičovački further expanded upon the cutaneous condition found in patients with cirrhosis (Table 7.1):

Star-shaped skin telangiectasias in cirrhosis of the liver, first described by Eppinger, were reported in 23 out of 41 cases. They are predominantly located on the skin of the upper half of the body and increase in number and size as the disease progresses. Their presence has been found exclusively in liver cirrhosis, although not in every case, and their diagnostic importance is emphasized accordingly. As far as the development of vasodilatation is concerned, a common significant constitutional cause is assumed for both liver cirrhosis and telangiectasia. Liver disease significantly influences their shape, size, and appearance [103, p. 483].

Thus, Čičovački sign refers to the star-shaped cutaneous telangiectasis in patients with hepatic cirrhosis.

7.2.23 Gruenwald Sign

Peter Gruenwald (Grünwald) (1912–1979) was born in Schoenwald, Bohemia (Czech Republic), and received his medical degree from the University of Vienna in 1936 [104, 105]. He was appointed demonstrator and instructor of histology and embryology at the University of Vienna from 1936 to 1938 [102]. During World War II, he immigrated to the USA, where he was a research fellow at the Cook County Hospital in Chicago [104, 105]. He was an instructor of anatomy at the Chicago Medical School from 1939 to 1942; assistant professor of histology and embryology at Middlesex University at Waltham, Massachusetts from 1942 to 1944; New York State fellow in pathology Mount Sinai Hospital from 1944 to 1945; assistant professor of pathology at Long Island College of Medicine from 1945 to 1951; and assistant professor Department of Obstetrics and Gynecology (pathology) State University of New York College of Medicine from 1951 to 1954 [104, 105]. He was appointed pathologist and director of laboratories Margaret Hague Maternity Hospital, New Jersey, in 1955 and in the Department of Obstetrics and Gynecology at Johns Hopkins School of Medicine, Baltimore, Maryland, in 1958. He was named assistant professor in 1961 and associate professor in 1964 in the Department of Pathology at Johns Hopkins University [104, 105].

His academic interests included placental development, developmental and comparative anatomy, placental and fetal pathology, fetal malnutrition, and respiratory distress syndrome [105]. He served as an associate professor of pathology at the University of Pennsylvania and Veterans Administration Hospital in 1969. His final appointment was at Hahnemann Medical College and Hospital in Philadelphia, where he accepted the associate professor of pathologist position in 1970 [104].

He was a member of the American Association of Anatomists, American Society of Human Genetics, and a fellow of the New York Academy of Science, Teratology Society, and American Association for the Advancement of Science [104].

Gruenwald reported eight cases of hepatic rupture with associated hemoperitoneum occurring during vaginal delivery. He proposed a mechanism for this phenomenon (Table 7.1):

Pressure on the thorax is an important factor in the production of these lesions. By such pressure, the organs of the upper abdomen are squeezed out of the hollow of the diaphragm, and undue tension on the ligaments of the liver and spleen then produce part of the lesions. Others are the result of direct pressure of the costal margin on the anterior surface of the liver. A minority of the lesions of the liver in the present group of cases are not obviously related to these mechanisms and are probably due to direct trauma [106, p. 201].

This mechanism was proposed to account for the locations of the lacerations of the spleen at the phrenicolienale, liver at the coronary and hepatoduodenal ligaments, and umbilical vein in infants.

7.2.24   Tanyol Sign

7.2.24.1   Hasib Tanyol

Hasib (Hasip) Tanyol (1916–1999) was born in Eskisehir, Turkey, and received his medical degree from the University of Istanbul Faculty of Science [107, 108]. He completed his internship at the Universities of Vienna and Freiburg [107]. He was a research fellow at Jefferson Medical College and an assistant professor of anatomy at Hahnemann Medical College in 1951 [107]. He was a private practitioner in Lafayette Hill and subsequently Fort Washington in the mid-1960s and was appointed to the medical staff at Germantown Hospital, Philadelphia, and Montgomery Hospital, Norristown, Pennsylvania [107].

His primary areas of interest were hypertension and vascular aspects of liver cirrhosis. He was a founding member of the American Society of Hypertension. He received the Honors Achievement Award from the Angiology Research Foundation [107, 108].

7.2.24.2   Hyman Menduke

Hyman Menduke (1921–1999) received his Ph.D. in economic statistics at the University of Pennsylvania in 1952 [109]. He was appointed assistant professor of biostatistics at Thomas Jefferson University in 1953 and professor of preventive medicine (biostatistics) in 1963 [109]. Menduke served as professor of pharmacology (biostatistics) in the Faculty of Medicine at Thomas Jefferson University in 1978 [109].

Among his other appointments, Menduke was an adjunct professor of statistical evaluation of clinical data at Philadelphia College of Pharmacy and Science. He also served as past president of the Philadelphia Chapter of the American Statistical Association [109]. The Hyman Menduke Research Prize is awarded annually to the graduating senior for excellence in research [110].

Tanyol and Menduke measured the distance between the lower edge of the xiphoid and umbilicus and umbilicus and upper edge of the pubic symphysis in patients with cirrhosis without ascites or obesity and age and race match controls without liver disease and found that (Fig. 7.6):

In noncirrhotic individuals the distance from the umbilicus to the xiphoid process is almost equal to the distance from the umbilicus to the symphysis. In cirrhotic patients, however, the upper distance is much greater than the lower [111, p. 422–423].

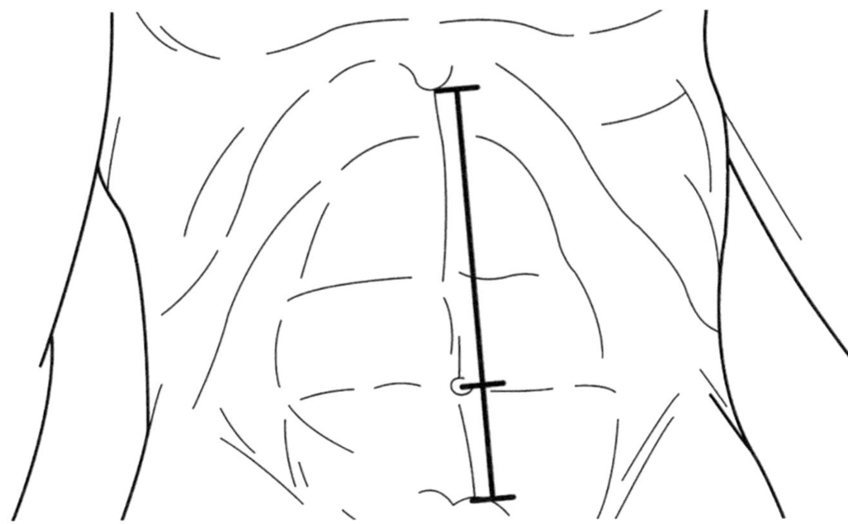

Fig. 7.6 Tanyol sign (by Ryan Yale)

They coined the term "umbilical ptosis" to signify the lengthening of the distance between the xiphoid process and the umbilicus in patients with portal cirrhosis (Table 7.1).

7.2.25 *Coronel Sign*

Armando Pareja Coronel (1896–1965) was born in Guayaquil, Ecuador, and received his medical degree from the Faculty of Medicine of the University of Guayaquil in 1920 [112, 113]. He was head of the women's tuberculosis service at Guayaquil Hospital in 1924 and appointed professor of internal medicine at the University of Guayaquil in 1929 [112]. Coronel was chief physician of the women's service at Santa Elena Hospital in 1931 [112]. He was elected president of the Municipality of Guayaquil in 1908, appointed governor of Guays in 1922, and the province of Guayaquil in 1926 [112, 114]. Coronel was president of the Surgical Medical Society of Guayas, the Ecuadorian Anti-tuberculous League in 1940, a member of the council in 1946, and the Sports Federation of Guays and the National Federation of Ecuador [112, 113]. He received the Medal of Civic Merit from the Municipality of Guayaquil in 1956 [112].

The phrenic nerve pressure point of sensitivity described by Coronel is: [a] painful spot in front of the scalenus muscle corresponding to the area of the phrenic nerve [115, p. 119]. Coronel believed that the phrenic nerve pressure point was diagnostic of acute malaria and that the pain was due to hepatosplenic syndrome (Table 7.1).

Table 7.1 Liver and biliary signs

Name	Year	Description of sign	Significance
Hanot [15]	1876	Jaundice and hepatic pain are accompanied initially by anorexia, constipation, general malaise, fatigue, and fever. Fever was present initially, during flares, and throughout the disease course. Several times, the pain was accompanied by a high fever of 39.5–39.8° and a pulse of 110 or 120. This fever did not last as long as the pain, but the episode was more intense and prolonged. At other times the painful episodes were completely afebrile. This initial crisis lasts from one to several weeks. Then, the disease enters a quiescent period, characterized by chronic jaundice and enlarged liver. Jaundice is one of the major manifestations of the disease and, in some cases, the initial symptom. Jaundice, once present, persists throughout the disease course. However, there is a variable intensity of jaundice during its long duration. Even though it may be minimum, it is generalized and apparent and always more intense than the subicteric hue encountered in other conditions	Primary biliary cirrhosis
Rosenbach [22]	1878	Pulsatile liver in aortic insufficiency	Aortic insufficiency
Courvoisier [27]	1890	A stone obstructing the common bile duct leads to contraction of the cystic duct and gallbladder, while a normal complaint gallbladder is found in other causes of obstruction (e.g., tumor)	Gallstones
Rovighi [32]	1894	A distinct resonant sound is heard at a site on a hydrogenic cyst of the liver using digital or pleximetric percussion. When moderate pressure is applied with the stethoscope on the cystic mass, resonance on percussion acquires a higher pitch. The sonority remains distinct if a solid body is interposed between the stethoscope and the mass, while the hydrogenic thrill is no longer palpable. In cases where the thrill is not apparent, it can be elicited by placing the palm of the left hand firmly on the mass and striking it with the right hand's middle finger on the left hand's first phalanges. Thus a kind of vibratory tremor is felt, which cannot in any way be confused with fluctuation or other tactile sensations	Echinococcal cyst
Boas [37]	1894	1. Pressure points are present to the left of the 12th thoracic vertebral body in gastric ulcers. The painful area can be higher on the 10th or 11th thoracic vertebra or lower at the level of the first lumbar vertebra. Occasionally there is a corresponding soreness on the right side, but in this case, the pressure point on the left is the more sensitive	Gastric ulcer
		2. The pressure area in cholelithiasis is also found 2–3 finger widths from the 12th thoracic vertebra, often extending to the right, and sometimes to the posterior axillary line	Cholelithiasis
Naunyn [50]	1896	Pain occurs during deep inspiration when pressure is applied with the hand direct superiorly beneath the right costal border. When the liver impinges upon the tips of the fingers, the patient experiences deep-seated pain, which sometimes radiates over the entire hepatic region and epigastrium. The liver tenderness is associated with tension involving the right rectus abdominis muscle	Acute gallstone cholecystitis

Lennhoff [54]	1898	On inspection of the abdomen, a moderate bulging of the hepatic region is seen, projecting beyond the midline to the right. During deep inspiration, two smaller protrusions are seen on the right. They are found within the liver during palpation. The lower left edge of the liver is sharp and rough, with the right edge slightly harder and thicker. The entire surface of the organ, including the protrusions, is smooth, with the latter feeling firmer. With the patient supine, the furrow formed between the rib wall and the protrusion is perceived as soon as the liver descends during deep inspiration	Echinococcal cyst
Mayo-Robson [55]	1900	Tenderness at a point midway between the ninth costal cartilage and the umbilicus. A transference of pain takes place from the right to the left side. The left-sided pain is associated with adhesions between the pylorus and gallbladder or bile ducts	Cholecystitis with adhesions
Gilbert [62]	1901	In patients with cirrhosis, the urine becomes scarce after a meal and more abundant after fasting. This disorder in urinary excretion is an early sign of portal hypertension and may precede the development of ascites	Cirrhosis
Kayser [64]	1902	The cornea, clear and transparent in its central parts, shows a ring-shaped opacity in the periphery, resembling gerontoxon. The cornea appears opaque with a dark green-brown ring color widest above, less wide below, and very narrow laterally and medially so that the area of the clear cornea is oval. The opacity begins immediately at the limbus and has no sharp border at the clear center of the cornea. On binocular microscopic examination in the peripheral ring zone described above, there is a significant accumulation of fine yellow spots in the deeper layer close to the posterior wall so that the underlying iris and chamber angle cannot be seen. The yellow spots are apparently in an area parallel to the corneal surface. This accumulation of yellow spots begins in the periphery, where their arrangement is densest, and the individual spots are the largest. In general, they are smaller and less dense in the middle portion of the ring and fine in the portion nearer the corneal center so that their turbidity no longer appears patchy but diffuse, allowing more light to reach the underlying surface of the iris. While the above dense patches of turbidity give a yellow appearance, the color at the center of the cornea is different. The yellow hue changes into a yellowish-green, proceeding gradually into the black of the pupil. The arrangement of the spots is completely random. The individual spots appear under the binocular microscope as flat bodies without sharp boundaries that are quite irregular, at least the coarser ones in the periphery. The corneal tissue does not reveal any abnormal abnormalities. There is no sign of vascular formation. The central part of the cornea is completely normal	Ocular finding in Wilson disease

(continued)

Table 7.1 (continued)

Name	Year	Description of sign	Significance
Fleischer [66]	1903	Greenish discoloration of the cornea is ring-shaped in the periphery, approximately 1 mm wide, and consists of small brownish-greenish dots and spots merging into one another, which become finer toward the center of the cornea and very gradually merge into the clear cornea. Fine, lighter stripes run through the discolored area irregularly. The superficial layers of the cornea are translucent; the discoloration resides in the deepest layers, in an area concentric to the surface, and is quite similar in both eyes	Ocular finding in Wilson disease
Murphy [72]	1903	Hypersensitiveness of the gallbladder is elicited by deep palpation just below the right ninth costal cartilage or in a line from that point to the middle of the inguinal ligament. Deep percussion along the same line, with the patient in forced inspiration, gives pronounced pain	Acute cholecystitis
		Maneuver 1	
		The most characteristic and constant sign of gallbladder hypersensitiveness is the inability of the patient to take a full, deep inspiration when the physician's fingers are hooked up deep beneath the right costal arch below the hepatic margin. The diaphragm forces the liver down until the sensitive gallbladder reaches the examining fingers, which causes inspiration to cease suddenly	
		Maneuver 2	
		The right hand is elevated with the middle finger of the left hand flexed perpendicularly at the tip of the ninth costal cartilage. The finger is struck with the right hand when the patient is in deep inspiration, causing severe pain if the gallbladder is distended or inflamed	
Abrahams [76]	1910	A painful point is located midway between the umbilicus and the costal cartilage of the ninth rib in the right hypochondriac. Place the patient in a recumbent position with the arms and legs extended—a point is located midway between the umbilicus and the ninth costal cartilage. Press the index and middle fingers using the right hand into that point, applying a sudden thrust. This causes either a grimace on the face or a quick involuntary jump of the abdomen. In an acute attack with a diffuse area of hyperesthesia, the midway point is the point of maximum pain	Cholelithiasis
Finsterer [80]	1910	Bradycardia	Liver injury
Milkó [82]	1911	In severe abdominal injuries or general peritonitis, the pulse may be normal. In severe intestinal injury, marked bradycardia lasts 8–10 h	Intestinal injury

Grocco [87]	1911	Percussion should extend from the last dorsal vertebral and left paravertebral zone to determine whether there is an enlargement of the left lobe of the liver. Percuss with sufficient force in a systematic manner moving from the top to bottom, first along the right paravertebral line a, then along the spine b, and to the left of it, corresponding to lines c, d, e, etc., so that each time where the thoracic sound ends and liver dullness begins is marked. In this way, one finally arrives at line f, which delimits the almost horizontal section of liver dullness to the left of the spinal column. Once line f is reached, it is advisable to percuss from left to right, along the horizontal line i–g, in the direction of arrow 1, to pinpoint point g, the outer limit of the left portion of the hepatic dullness	Hepatomegaly
Lesieur [89]	1913	Dullness on superficial percussion at the right base of the thorax is caused by liver hypertrophy	Typhoid fever
Frank [91]	1915	Acute and chronic advanced liver disease results in impaired blood coagulation. The cause is hypofibrinogenemia, due to either the lack of its formation or increased destruction. Even in severe hepatic insufficiency, the delay in coagulation is merely an indicator of a process that prevents platelet thrombus formation. Sometimes, a coagulation abnormality is not detectable, and there is no platelet aggregate. The mechanism of hemorrhage in hepatic pseudohemophilia is similar to that in thrombocytopenia—the absence or the excessively loose structure of the platelet thrombus	Liver disease
Ortner [93]	1922	*Maneuver 1* Tenderness is present in the region of the hepatic incisura during deep inspiration, with pressure against the liver during inspiration and on bimanual palpation of the liver while applying one hand on the incisura and the other pressing against it from the lumbar region *Maneuver 2* There is hyperesthesia of the skin over the gallbladder region and posteriorly between the lower border of the right lung and posterior costal arch. The lowest part of the thorax and right hypochondrium is tender on rapid, sharp percussion using the ulnar aspect of the hand in these regions. The patient complains of increased pains which last several hours after palpation of the gallbladder	Biliary colic
Riesman [95]	1922	Ask the patient to take a deep breath and hold it. Using the ulnar side of the hand, apply a quick but not hard blow over the upper part of the right rectus muscle. If there is disease involving the gallbladder, the blow causes sharp pain. If in doubt as to whether this pain is superficial and caused by the blow, perform the same maneuver on the left side	Cholecystitis

(continued)

Table 7.1 (continued)

Name	Year	Description of sign	Significance
Carmalt-Jones [100]	1932	While approaching the patient posteriorly, hook the fingers of the right hand around the costal margin; a tender spot is present on the inferior edge of the eighth right costal cartilage. The hand is flat on the upper abdomen. The third fingertip is brought into firm contact with the costal margin, inching along its whole length, beginning laterally on the left side and moving medially while observing the patient's facial expression. In cholecystitis, a single tender spot over the fingertip on the right eighth rib edge, sometimes slightly superiorly or inferiorly, is confirmed by the patient's expression of the pain. Occasionally, the skin of the eighth dorsal segment on the same side is hyperalgesia to pinprick	Cholecystitis
Kenawy [102]	1939	The venous hum is usually heard over a localized area over just below the xiphoid process of the sternum. It is continuous and accentuated by deep inspiration. Over the site of the hum and in a strictly localized area, a continuous thrill could be felt, especially on applying the tip of one finger very lightly. Inspection of the thrill site showed an elevation of the skin, probably due to an underlying vein. Applying light pressure over the elevation causes the thrill to disappear. The venous hum also disappears when light pressure of the stethoscope is applied over the site of the thrill at the xiphoid process. The venous hum returned when the pressure was released	Hepatic cirrhosis
Čičovački [103]	1940	Star-shaped skin telangiectasias are located predominately over the skin of the upper half of the body and increase in number and size as the disease progresses	Liver cirrhosis
Gruenwald [106]	1948	Hepatic rupture and hemoperitoneum occur in newborns during vaginal delivery	Hepatic rupture
Tanyol [111]	1956	In patients with cirrhosis without ascites or obesity, the distance from the umbilicus to the xiphoid process is greater than that from the umbilicus to the pubic symphysis. In noncirrhotic, the distance from the umbilicus to the xiphoid process is nearly equal to the distance from the umbilicus to the symphysis in cirrhotic patients	Hepatic cirrhosis
Coronel [115]	[n.a.]	A painful spot in front of the scalenus muscle corresponds to the phrenic nerve	Hepatosplenic syndrome and acute malaria

7.3 Conclusion

Murphy sign is the most highly recognized sign involving the liver and biliary tract. Even today, clinicians still use it as a bedside maneuver despite its wide sensitivity and specificity in diagnosis. For the remainder of the signs, their sensitivity and specificity have yet to be studied, and their utility in clinical practice remains to be discovered. They are important to recognize and further study to better understand their role, if any, in clinical practice.

References

1. Celsus AC. On medicine, vol. 3. (trans: W.G. Spencer). Cambridge: Harvard University Press; 1971.
2. Malpighii M. De Viscerum Structura Exercitatio Anatomica. Amstelodami: Petrum le Grand; 1669.
3. Kiernan F. The anatomy and physiology of the liver. Philos Trans R Soc Lond. 1833;123:711–70.
4. Browne J. A remarkable account of a liver, appearing glandulous to the eye. Philos Trans R Soc Lond. 1685;15:1266–8.
5. Baillie M. Plate II. In: The morbid anatomy of some of the most important parts of the human body. London: W. Bulmer Co.; 1799. p. 101.
6. Laënnec RTH. Traité de l'auscultation médiate et des maladies des poumons et du cœur, tome 2. Paris: J.S. Chaudé; 1826.
7. Donato M. De Medica Historia Mirabili Libri Sex. Mantua: Fr. Osanna; 1586.
8. Ambiani FI. Universa Medicina. Francofurti: Andreas Wechel; 1581.
9. D'Heilly M. Discours prononcé sur la tombe de M. Victor Hanot. Bull et Mém Soc Méd Hôp Paris. 1896;13:735–7.
10. Dureau A. Nécrologie: Hanot. Chron méd. 1896;3:702.
11. Delmas V, François M, Hanot VC. Comité des travaux historiques et scientifiques. 2011. https://cths.fr/an/savant.php?id=105618. Accessed 5 Jan 2022.
12. Hanot V. Thèse pour le doctorat en médecine: Étude sur une forme de cirrhose hypertrophique du foie. Paris: Imprimeur de la Faculté de Médecine; 1875.
13. Hanot VC, Chauffard A. Cirrhose hypertrophique pigmentaire dans le diabète sucré. Rev méd. 1882;2:385–403.
14. Hanot V, Schachmann M. Sur la cirrhose pigmentaire dans le diabète sucré. Arch Physiol Norm Pathol. 1886;7:50–87.
15. Hanot V. Étude sur une forme de cirrhose hypertrophique du foie: cirrhose hypertrophique avec ictère chronique. Paris: J.-B. Baillière et fils; 1876.
16. Pagel JL. Biographisches Lexikon, hervorragender Ärzte des neunzehnten Jahrhunderts. Berlin: Urban & Schwarzenberg; 1901.
17. Singere I, Haneman FT. The Jewish Encyclopedia. https://www.jewishencyclopedia.com/articles/12837–rosenbach–ottomar–ernst–felix. Accessed 30 Jan 2022.
18. Voswinckel P, Rosenbach O. Deutsche Biographie. https://www.deutsche–biographie.de/gnd11759475X.html#ndbcontent. Accessed 30 Jan 2022.
19. Eschle FCR, Rosenbach O. Münch med Wochenschr. 1907;54:734–5.
20. Guttmann W, Rosenbach O. Berl klin Wochenschr. 1907;44:490–1.
21. Rose A. Ottomar Rosenbach: character traits of his life, collected from tributes paid to his memory. Med Brief. 1907;35:857–60.

22. Rosenbach O. Ueber arterielle Leberpulsation. Dtsch med Wochenschr. 1878;4:498–500; 509–11; 519–23.

23. Veillon E. Professor Dr. med. L.G. Courvoisier. Schweiz med Wochenschr. 1918;43:1314–9.

24. Veillon E. Prof. Dr. med. L.G. Courvoisier. In: Basler Stadtbuch. Basel: Helbing & Lichtenhahn; 1920. p. 1–14.

25. Buess H. Courvoisier, Ludwig Georg (Louis). In: Neue Deutsche Biographie, Bd. 25. Berlin: Duncker & Humblot; 1957. p. 384.

26. [No author]. Ludwig Courvoisier (1843–1918): Courvoisier's sign. JAMA. 1968;204:627.

27. Courvoisier LG. Folgen der Choledochus–Obstructionen. In: Casuistisch-statistische Beiträge zur Pathologie und Chirurgie der Gallenwege. Leipzig: Verlag von F.C.W. Vogel; 1890. p. 55–69.

28. Cantelli O. Prof. Alberto Rovighi. Riforma Med. 1919;35:844.

29. Viola G, Alberto Rovighi. Historical archives of the University of Bologna. https://archivios-torico.unibo.it/System/27/618/rovighi_alberto.pdf. Accessed 12 Feb 2022.

30. Alberto Rovighi, professor of special medical pathology at the university. 1894. https://www.bibliotecasalaborsa.it/bolognaonline/cronologia–di–bologna/1894/alberto_rovighi_profes-sore_di_patologia_speciale_medica_alluniversit. Accessed 12 Feb 2022.

31. Piccinini G. Alberto Rovighi. Il Policlin. 1919;26:1079–80.

32. Rovighi A. Del fremito e della risonanza idatigena. Il Policlin. 1894;1:512–23.

33. In memory of Prof. Dr. med. Ismar Boas, 1858–1938. Commemoration of the German Society of Gastroenterology. https://www.dgvs–gegen–das–vergessen.de/en/biografie/ismar–boas/. Accessed 23 Aug 2022.

34. Ismar Isidor Boas, 1859–1938. 100 Jahre Deutsche Gesellschaft für Verdauungs-und Stoffwechselkrankheiten. August Dreesbach Verlag. https://www.dgvs.de/epaper/100–jahre–dgvs/files/assets/common/downloads/publication.pdf. Accessed 22 Aug 2022

35. Boas I. Deutsche Biographie. https://www.deutsche–biographie.de/pnd118660322.html#indexcontent. Accessed 23 Aug 2022.

36. Avery H. Tribute to Ismar Boas (1858–1938). Gastroenterologia. 1958;90:49–53.

37. Boas I. Die Palpation des Magens. In: Diagnostik und Therapie der Magenkrankheiten nach dem Heutigen Stande der Wissenschaft. Leipzig: Verlag von Georg; 1894. p. 69–90.

38. Iyer HV. Boas' sign revisited. Ir J Med Sci. 2011;180:301.

39. Gunn A, Keddie N. Some clinical observations on patients with gallstones. Lancet. 1972;2:239–41.

40. [No author]. Bernhard Naunyn (1839–1925). Nature. 1939;144:410.

41. Naunyn B. Historisches Lexikon der Schweiz. https://hls–dhs–dss.ch/de/arti-cles/042576/2007–08–02/. Accessed 22 Aug 2022.

42. Medvei VC. Naunyn, Bernhard, 1839–1925. In: The history of clinical endocrinology: a comprehensive account of endocrinology from earliest times to the present day. New York: The Parthenon Publishing; 1993. p. 458.

43. [No author]. Death of Bernhard Naunyn. JAMA. 1925;85:602.

44. [No author]. Bernhard Naunyn. Dtsch med Wochenschr. 1925;51:1493–5.

45. Woodyatt RT. Bernhard Naunyn. Diabetes. 1952;1:240–1.

46. Tautenhayn J. Bernhard Naunyn Bronze Medal commemorating his 70th birthday (Sept. 2, 1909). Tulane University Digital Library. https://digitallibrary.tulane.edu/islandora/object/tulane%3A50482. Accessed 26 Aug 2022.

47. Naunyn B. Nomination archive. Nobel Prize. https://www.nobelprize.org/nomination/archive/show.php?id=13246. Accessed 26 Aug 2022.

48. [No author]. Bernhard Naunyn. Lancet. 1925;209:1131–2.

49. Naunyn B. Projekt Gutenberg. https://www.projekt–gutenberg.org/ebstein/arztrede/chap014.html. Accessed 24 Aug 2022.

50. Naunyn B. A treatise on cholelithiasis. (trans: A.E. Garrod). London: New Sydenham Society; 1896.

51. Walk J. Lennhoff, Rudolf. In: Kurzbiographien zur Geschichte der Juden, 1918–1945. Jerusalem: Leo-Baeck-Institute; 1988. p. 221.

52. [No author]. Medical sociology. Echoes News Gen. 1905;86:310.

53. [No author]. Prof. Dr. Rudolf Lennhoff. Med Klin. 1934;30:40.

54. Lennhoff R. Ueber Echinococcen und syphilitische Geschwülste. Dtsch med Wochenschr. 1898;24:407–11.

55. Mayo-Robson AW. Gallstone or cholelithiasis. In: Diseases of the gallbladder and bile ducts including gallstones. 2nd ed. London: Baillière, Tindall and Cox; 1900. p. 150–65.

56. Gleu E, Floderer NA, Capot M. Gilbert, Nicolas Augustin. Comité de travaux historiques et scientifiques. https://cths.fr/an/savant.php?id=3679. Accessed 12 Apr 2022.

57. Haubrich WS. Biographical sketch: Gilbert of Gilbert's syndrome. Gastroenterology. 1998;115:821.

58. Chabrol EA. Gilbert (1858–1927). Bull Acad Nat Méd. 1956;140:632–42.

59. Perrot E, Carnot P, Floderer A. Lereboullet, Pierre Emile Auguste. Comité des travaux historiques et scientifiques. https://cths.fr/an/savant.php?id=4093. Accessed 12 Apr 2022.

60. Carnot P. Pierre Lereboullet (1874–1944). Bull Acad Méd. 1945;129:25–32.

61. Girons FS. L'oeuvre pédiatrique du Professeur Pierre Lereboullet. Paris méd. 1944;34:165–6.

62. Gilbert A, Lereboullet P. Inversion du rythme normal de l'évacuation des urines (des urines retardées) dans les cirrhoses. L'Art méd. 1901;92:400–1.

63. Firkin BG, Whitworth JA. Kayser–Fleischer ring. In: Dictionary of medical eponyms. Boca Raton: Parthenon Publishing; 1987. p. 269.

64. Kayser B. Über einen Fall von angeborener grünlicher Verfärbung der Kornea. Klin Mbl Augenheilkd. 1902;40:22–5.

65. Fleischer B. Gastroenterología. https://articulos.sld.cu/gastroenterologia/archives/4196. Accessed 12 Jul 2022.

66. Fleischer B. Zwei weitere Fälle von grünlicher Verfärbung der Kornea. Klin Mbl Augenheilkd. 1903;41:489–91.

67. [No author]. Report of Committee of Necrology: John B. Murphy. Trans Meet Am Surg Assoc. 1918;36:xlii–v.

68. Andrews EW. In memoriam [John B. Murphy]. In: The clinics of John B. Murphy, MD, vol. 5. Philadelphia: W.B. Saunders; 1916. p. 989–1001.

69. [No author]. John B. Murphy, MD. Br Med J. 1916;2:343.

70. Pace EA, Pallen CB, Shahan TJ, Wynne SJ, et al. Murphy, John Benjamin. In: The Catholic Encyclopedia, vol. 17 (Supp. 1). New York: The Encyclopedia Press; 1922. p. 520–1.

71. Hannan C. Murphy, John Benjamin. In: Wisconsin biographical dictionary. Hamburg, MI: State History Publications; 2008. p. 285–7.

72. Murphy JB. The diagnosis of gall-stones. Med News. 1903;82:825–33.

73. Murphy JB. Gallstone disease and its relation to intestinal obstruction. Ill Med J. 1910;18:272–80.

74. [No author]. Hold rites today for Abrahams. Jewish Daily Bull. 1935;12:3.

75. [No author]. Annual report of the Board of Directors, vol. 31. New York: Manhattan State Hospital; 1936. p. 7.

76. Abrahams R. Two signs of diagnostic value: on in cholelithiasis, the other in incipient tuberculosis. N Y Med J. 1910;91:74.

77. Leu M. Prof. Dr. med. univ. Hans Finsterer. In: Medizinethik im Spiegel der Zeitschrift, Arzt und Christ – Zur Frühgeschichte der Institutionalisierung der Medizinethik in Deutschland, Österreich und der Schweiz. Göttingen: Georg-August-Universität zu Göttingen; 2016. p. 41.

78. Walterskirchen M. Professor Hans Finsterer. Bol Soc Cir Uruguay. 1955;26:707–14.

79. Jantsch M. Finsterer, Hans. Deutsche Biographie. https://www.deutsche–biographie.de/sfz16143.html. Accessed 15 May 2022.

80. Finsterer H. Ein geheilter Fall von Leberschuss. Wien klin Wochenschr. 1910;49:1749–51.

81. Milkó V. Hungarian Biographical Lexicon. https://www.arcanum.com/hu/online–kiad-vanyok/Lexikonok–magyar–eletrajzi–lexikon–7428D/m–76AF9/milko–vilmos–76E44/. Accessed 5 Sep 2022.

82. Finsterer H. Zur Diagnose der Leberverletzungen. Arch klin Chir. 1911;95:376–80.

83. Levi E. In morte di Pietro Grocco, commemorazione letta alla Società "Leonardo da Vinci" in Firenze il di 21 febbraio 1916. Firenze: G. Ramella; 1916.

84. [No author]. Obituary: Pietro Grocco. Lancet. 1916;190:546–7.

85. [No author]. Notes. Nature. 1916;97:42–3.

86. Grocco P. Treccani. https://www.treccani.it/enciclopedia/pietro–grocco_(Dizionario–Biografico). Accessed 24 Aug 2022.

87. Grocco P. Über vertebrale und linksseitige paravertebrale Leberdämpfung. Wien klin Wochenschr. 1911;19:667–9.

88. Rochaix A. Charles Lesieur (1876–1919). Ann Hyg. 1919;31:129–38.

89. Lesieur C, Marchand J. La submatité de la base droite (submatité retro-hépatique) signe de fièvre typhoid. Presse Méd. 1913:625–6.

90. Prof. Dr. med. Erich Frank, 1884–1957. Deutsche Gesellschaft für Gastroenterologie, Verdauungs- und Stoffwechselkrankheiten. https://www.dgvs–gegen–das–vergessen.de/bio-grafie/erich–frank/. Accessed 3 Feb 2022.

91. Frank E. Die essentielle Thrombopenie. Berl klin Wochenschr. 1915;52:454–8.

92. Collective. Ortner von Rodenstätt. In: Österreichisches biographisches Lexikon, 1815–1950, Bd. 7. Wien: Verlag der Österreichischen Akademie der Wissenschaften; 1978. p. 256.

93. Ortner N. Colicky pains in the region of the gallbladder and right hypochondrium. In: Abdominal pain. (trans: W.A. Brams, P.A. Luger). New York: Rebman Company; 1922. p. 163–91.

94. Cooper DA. Transactions of the seventeenth annual meeting of the American Association of the History of Medicine. Bull Hist Med. 1941;10:299–304.

95. Riesman D. Some points in physical diagnosis. JAMA. 1922;78:1962–3.

96. [No author]. D.W. Carmalt Jones DM, FRCP. Br Med J. 1957;1:649–50.

97. Trial RR. Dudley William Carmalt-Jones. Royal College of Physicians. https://history.rcplon-don.ac.uk/inspiring–physicians/dudley–william–carmalt–jones. Accessed 16 Mar 2022.

98. Early research at the Otago Medical School. Otago Medical School Research Society. https://www.otago.ac.nz/omsrs/about/history/index.html. Accessed 16 Mar 2022.

99. [No author]. Dudley William Carmalt Jones. Med J Australia. 1957;44:661.

100. Carmalt-Jones DW. Tender rib-cartilage as a sign of cholecystitis. Lancet. 1932;219:615–6.

101. Anrep GV, Kenawy MR, Barsoum GS, Misrahy G. Therapeutic uses of khellin: method of standardisation. Lancet. 1947;249:557–8.

102. Kenawy MR. Venous hum in bilharzial cirrhosis of the liver. Lancet. 1939;233:821–2.

103. Čičovački D. Ueber sternförmige Hautteleangiektasien bei der Lebercirrhose und ihre diag-nostische Bedeutung. Wien klin Wochenschr. 1940;53:478–83.

104. Amenta PS. Peter Gruenwald (1912–1979). Anat Rec. 1980;198:306.

105. [No author]. Dr. Peter Gruenwald. Bull Margaret Hague Mat Hosp. 1955;8–9:82.

106. Gruenwald P. Rupture of liver and spleen in newborn infant. J Pediatr. 1948;33:195–201.

107. January 1992 - Part III. Postgraduate Alumni (pp. 793–896). Thomas Jefferson University Jefferson Digital Commons. https://core.ac.uk/download/pdf/46965476.pdf. Accessed 18 Aug 2022.

108. Tanyol H. Find a grave. https://www.findagrave.com/memorial/54781305/hasib–tanyol. Accessed 28 Aug 2022.

109. January 1989 - Part II: Basic sciences - Chapter 8. Department of Pharmacology (pp. 222–232). Thomas Jefferson University Jefferson Digital Commons. https://jdc.jefferson.edu/cgi/view-content.cgi?article=1008&context=wagner2. Accessed 18 Aug 2022.

110. The Hyman Menduke Research Prize. Awards to graduating students. https://jdc.jefferson.edu/cgi/viewcontent.cgi?article=1015&context=skmcclassday. Accessed 18 Aug 2022.

111. Menduke H, Tanyol H. Umbilical ptosis: frequent physical sign in portal cirrhosis. Am J Dig Dis. 1956;1:417–23.
112. Pareja Coronel A. Rodolfo Perez Pimentel. https://rodolfoperezpimentel.com/pareja–coronel–armando–2/. Accessed 20 May 2022.
113. Evocación a Abel Gilbert y Armando Pareja. 2015. https://www.eluniverso.com/vida–estilo/2015/05/25/nota/4909761/evocacion–abel–gilbert–armando–pareja/. Accessed 20 May 2022.
114. [No author]. Medical news: Dr. Armando Pareja Coronel. JAMA. 1926;86:209.
115. Robertson WME, Robertson HF. Diagnostic signs, reflexes, and syndromes. 3rd ed. Philadelphia: F.A. David Company; 1947.

Chapter 8
Spleen Signs

8.1   Introduction

The word spleen—σπλήν (splín) in Ancient Greek and splen in Middle English—dates back to Hippocrates in the fourth century BC [1]. Marcello Malpighi (1628–1694), in 1659, was the first to describe the white pulp, later eponymously named Malpighian corpuscles in his book *De Viscerum Structura Exercitatio Anatomica* (An Anatomical Study on Structure of the Viscera) [2]. Rudolf Albert Kölliker (1817–1905), in *A Manual of Human Microscopic Anatomy*, proposed the concept of the normal phagocytic destruction of nascent red blood cells in the spleen [3]:

> For these considerations, I was forced (as early as 1854) to abandon the view, that the changes of the blood discs in the splenic pulp belonged to the series of physiological appearances; I conceived that such changes, to be normal, must occur in the interior of vessels, and in this opinion I find myself supported by the great majority of physiologists. I am still of opinion that a solution of blood-cells actually does go on within the spleen, and in this organ much more than in the liver. But I have conclusively given up the grounds on which I originally regard the occurrence of decomposed blood-cells in the pulp as establishing such a view [3, p. 367].

Eponymous signs related to the spleen were first reported in the late nineteenth century by Georges Maurice Debove, who described splenomegaly and its associated clinical features. It was in the mid-twentieth century that Robert K. Nixon and Donald O. Castell reported percussion methods to determine splenic dimensions and enlargement. Other signs described during the physical examination by Pitts, Ballance, Saegesser, and Hedri were involved in devising methods for detecting splenic injury. This chapter contains brief biographical information of physicians who reported splenic signs and the sign as initially described.

S. H. Yale et al., *Gastrointestinal Eponymic Signs*,
https://doi.org/10.1007/978-3-031-33673-7_8

8.2 Splenic Eponyms

8.2.1 *Debove Sign*

Georges Maurice Debove (1845–1920) was born in Paris, France, was a hospital intern in 1869, and received his medical degree from the Faculty of Medicine, Paris, in 1873 [4–6]. He was head of the Germain Sée Clinic, a hospital doctor in 1877, and agrégé of the Faculty of Medicine in 1878 [4–6]. Debove was professor of the second chair of medical pathology in the Faculty of Medicine from 1890 to 1900; appointed the second chair at Charité; taught medicine at the Beaujon Hospital, Paris, from 1901 to 1908; and was dean of the Faculty of Medicine, Paris, in 1906 [5–7].

He was president of the French National League against Alcoholism and was a staunch critic of alcohol and its adverse effect on human health [7]. Debove was elected member of the French National Academy of Medicine, member of the section of therapeutics in 1893, later permanent secretary from 1913 to 1920, and titular of the Anatomical Society of Paris in 1873 [4, 6]. He was honorary president of the National Council of Hygiene and presided over the Medical Society of Hospitals in 1897 [4]. In collaboration with Charcot, they wrote *Bibliothèque Médicale Charcot-Debove* in 1892 and with Achard, *Manuel de Médecine* in eight volumes and *Manuel de Thérapeutique* in three volumes [7].

Debove described the entity, primary splenomegaly, a condition previously recognized by Gaucher in 1882 (Table 8.1):

> Primary splenomegaly, which I believe should be separated from other splenic hypertrophies, is characterized by hypertrophy or an increase in spleen volume and progressive anemia without an increase in the number of leukocytes or alteration of the lymph nodes. The onset is sometimes insidious, and hypertrophy of the spleen is present during the initial examination. At other times the disease is announced by local phenomena, including weight loss, uneasiness, and pain in the left side, sometimes even by painful crises analogous to visceral colic, which is probably the expression of an attack of localized peritonitis. Finally, the disease begins at other times with general phenomena: weakness, pallor, apathy, asthenia, and weight loss. After a variable time, the spleen becomes greatly enlarged, to the point of sometimes occupying the entire left half of the abdomen. Its shape is preserved, but its consistency is increased, assuming a woody hardness on palpation. The liver protrudes one to two fingerbreadths from the false ribs. However, there is neither ascites, jaundice, or dilation of veins on the abdominal wall. The spleen, thus hypertrophied, may cause heaviness, tightness, and soreness in the region. Sometimes the pain resembles intercostal neuralgia and is so severe as to recommend a splenectomy. There is no relationship between the size of the spleen and the degree of anemia. The examination of the blood reveals marked hypoglobulism with decreased hemoglobin. There are variable digestive disorders. Hematemesis is often observed, most likely due to congestion of the portal vein. This hematemesis recurs, in some cases, several times and, if frequent enough, can be life-threatening [8, p. 506].

Thus, Debove described the condition splenomegaly. Although he classified this as primary splenomegaly, hepatomegaly with splenomegaly is consistent with portal hypertension (secondary splenomegaly).

8.2.2 *Pitts Sign*

Bernard Pitts (1848–1914) was born in Sowerby, Yorkshire, England, studied medicine under the tutelage of Joseph Lister (1827–1912) in Edinburgh; and at Scotland and Cambridge in 1873, and was a clinical clerk and dresser at St. Thomas's Hospital in 1873 [9]. He earned his Bachelor of Medicine and Master of Art degrees from Cambridge in 1875 and served as a resident clinical assistant at Bethlehem Hospital that same year [10].

Pitts was a house surgeon at St. Thomas's Hospital in 1876 and under the Red Cross Society as a surgeon during the Serbo-Turkish War (1876–1877) that same year [9]. Upon his return to St. Thomas's Hospital after the war, he was appointed resident *accoucheur*, demonstrator of anatomy in 1877, resident assistant surgeon in 1878, resident assistant surgeon in 1878, and extra assistant surgeon in 1882 [9]. At the Hospital for Sick Children, Great Ormond Street, he was an assistant surgeon in 1882, a surgeon in 1892, and consulting surgeon in 1912 [9, 10].

He was a lecturer on practical surgery at St. Thomas's Hospital and examiner in surgery for Cambridge, the Durham Society of Apothecaries, and the Royal College of Surgeons from 1899 to 1909. Within the Royal College, he was a Hunterian professor of surgery in 1983 [9]. Pitts was also a member of the Council of the Nurses' Cooperation, serving as an advocate for the welfare of nurses [10].

As to a description of his character:

> He was one of those all too rare men who hate anything in the way of pretense or sharp practice, and did not hesitate to speak his mind freely and without fear when occasion seemed to demand plain speaking. (…) Those who knew him will retain an affectionate remembrance of his strong character and his unselfish devotion to the interest of others [10, p. 123].

Pitts and Sir Charles Alfred Ballance (1856–1936) reported on three cases of splenic rupture where:

> The diagnosis in these cases was arrived at from the locality of the injury, from the evidence of internal hemorrhage, from the great increase in the fixed dullness in the splenic region, and from the fact, though both flanks were dull on percussion, the right flank alone became entirely resonant on change of position [11, p. 95–96].

Thus, Pitts sign refers to the presence of percussion dullness in the splenic region in patients with splenic rupture (Table 8.1). Pitts name is assigned separately to this sign, presumably because he was the primary author of the publication.

8.2.3 *Ballance Sign*

Sir Charles Alfred Ballance (1856–1936) was born in London, UK, studied medicine at St. Thomas's Hospital, and received his Bachelor of Medicine degree from London University in 1881 with first-class honor and gold medal. He was elected fellow of the Royal College of Surgeons (FRCS) in 1882 [12].

He was appointed assistant aural surgeon at St. Thomas's Hospital in 1888, followed by an assistant surgeon at the West London Hospital [13]. Ballance was appointed on staff to the National Hospital for Paralysed and Epileptic Queen Square, London, from 1891 to 1908 and returned to St. Thomas's Hospital as a chief surgeon in 1900 and consulting surgeon in 1919 [12–16]. He was chief surgeon to the Metropolitan Police from 1912 to 1926 [12, 13, 16]. During World War I, he was consulting surgeon with the rank of colonel stationed in Malta [12, 13, 15].

Ballance was president of the Medical Society of London in 1906 and the Society of British Neurological Surgeons in 1927 [13–15]. In the Royal College of Surgeons, he was an examiner in anatomy from 1887 to 1891, a member of the Court of Examiners from 1900 to 1919, and elected vice-president in 1920 [14, 15].

Among his many accolades, he was the recipient of the Knight Commander of the Order of St. Michael and St. George (KCMG) in 1918 and Knight of Grace and Order of St. John of Jerusalem for his consulting work during the War [12, 15]. He was also the recipient of honorary degrees from the Universities of Glasgow and Malta and elected as an honorary fellow of the New York Academy of Medicine [12, 13, 16, 17].

As to a description of his character:

> His sincerity and enthusiasm gained him many admirers and friends among his colleagues at home and abroad. (…) He had a genial personality and a fine presence, and even at an advanced age his enthusiasms for and sincerity in his work were undiminished. He had an impelling drive to search for truth, and this and his accomplishments ensure him of a niche in the Hall of Fame [13, p. 148–149].

Ballance described the features of splenic rupture based on the following (Table 8.1):

> i) The locality of the injury, ii) the evidence of internal hemorrhage, and iii) the large fixed dullness in the left flank. The fixed dullness in the left loin and splenic region is not present in intra-abdominal hemorrhage from other organs, and is caused by this region being occupied by large quantities of clot. The dullness, therefore, cannot change with position, and is pathognomonic of this injury [18, p. 357].

Thus, Ballance sign refers to fixed dullness in the left loin and splenic region in patients with splenic rupture. This is the same sign reported by Pitts and Ballance two years earlier.

8.2.4 Pagniello Sign

There is limited historical information on Rafael Pagniello. At the time of the publication of his sign in 1920, he was a state railway physician in Melfi, Italy [19]. Pagniello identified a characteristic finding in patients with malaria (Table 8.1):

> If with the tip of the index or middle finger of the right hand, moderate pressure is applied at the ninth left intercostal space between the midline and posterior axillary line. The patient reports a painful sensation located at this point. The pain is associated with a reflex muscular contraction of the trunk or face or verbal communication that the patient is experiencing pain. (…) Pain may rarely occur when pressure is applied at the eighth, ninth, or tenth

intercostal space. (…) It is best to cautiously apply this maneuver in patients who are sensitive to pain. In this case, the entire palm is applied to the splenic region, starting with the fingertips at the twelfth rib and gradually moving proximally to the location where the patient reports that pain is greatest. If continuous pressure is applied to this region, the pain eventually resolves [19, p. 830].

Thus, Pagniello sign refers to palpatory tenderness at the ninth intercostal space between the clavicular and posterior axillary lines in patients with malaria.

8.2.5 Castronuovo Sign

Giovanni Castronuovo (1873–1944) was born in Sant'Arcangelo, Italy, began his medical studies in 1889, and received his medical degree from the University of Naples [20]. He was an assistant to De Renzi at the First Medical Clinic and Institute of Hygiene and Pathological Anatomy. He was a lecturer in special medical demonstrative pathology in 1903. He qualified by ministerial decree, free lecturing in the Royal University of Naples medical clinic and was an assistant at the first clinic and Ospedale degli Incurabili (Hospital of the Incurables) [20, 21]. He served as head of the free external polyclinic at the first clinic and was chief physician at Ospedali Riuniti (United Hospitals) [20]. At the time of the publication of his sign in 1927, he was head of hospitals and director of the L. Armanni Anatomo-Pathological Institute in charge of the clinic and atology of exotic and tropical diseases at the Royal University of Naples [22]. Castronuovo was a member of the Royal Medical-Surgical Academy of Naples and president of the Order of Doctors in the Province of Naples [20].

Castronuovo described the case of a 21-year-old male with a smooth, non-fixed enlarged spleen measuring >14 cm at the seventh left rib at the posterior axilla over Traube area. The most striking features were (Table 8.1):

> [t]he plastic modeling, as if it were made of wax or clay so an imprint of the pressing fingers sink into it and persists without being painful. I believe that this characteristic finding of plastic modeling or malleability of the splenic tissue is caused by anatomical changes that are important to recognize for differential and pathogenetic diagnostic reasons [22, p. 554].

Castronuovo postulated that this phenomenon was caused by splenic hyperemia and accentuated by gastrointestinal bleeding resulting in specific fibrous changes to the spleen. These alterations included hyperplastic changes involving the splenic follicles and pulp that increased cortical thickening, consistency, and increased plasticity of the spleen.

8.2.6 Sailer Sign

Joseph Sailer (1867–1928) was born in Philadelphia, Pennsylvania, and received his medical degree from the University of Pennsylvania in 1891 [23]. He interned at Presbyterian and Philadelphia General Hospitals and pursued additional training in neurology and pathology in Zurich, Paris, and Vienna [23]. Sailer served as a demonstrator of morbid anatomy in the Department of Pathology at the University of Pennsylvania [23]. He transitioned to pursue a career in clinical medicine, where he was appointed instructor, followed by an associate, assistant, and professor at the Philadelphia General Hospital in 1912 [23, 24]. He was appointed professor of clinical medicine at the University of Pennsylvania Medical School and chair of the Department of Gastroenterology at the Philadelphia Polyclinic [23, 24].

Sailer was involved in forming the Philadelphia Heart Association and Pennsylvania State Heart Association and was co-founder of the American Heart Association in 1924, the latter of which he was a member of the executive committee [24, 25]. He was also a member of the American Gastro-Enterological Association beginning in 1907 and was elected president of this organization in 1920 and chief promoter of the Philadelphia Children's Heart Hospital [23, 26].

As to a description of his character Joseph Riesman, a friend and colleague, writes:

> As a teacher Sailer commanded the respect of the students in an unusual degree. His thorough knowledge of medical literature and his vast experience made his lectures important events in the life of the students of the University of Pennsylvania. (…) In Joseph Sailer the American Gastro-Enterological Association has lost more than a mere member, it has lost an influence for progress and an inspiration to higher ideals. His name will live in our annals and in the annals of American medicine [23, p. 578].

Sailer reported the case of a 27-year-old man with aortic insufficiency as well as his review of three other cases and stated (Table 8.1):

> If one can draw conclusions from four cases described in detail, the conditions necessary to cause the pulsation of the spleen are a severe type of aortic insufficiency and an infectious process. (…) Pulsation, of the spleen, owing to its rarity, can be of no great importance, and even if it were more common, would probably prove to be nor more than an additional sign of aortic insufficiency, for it is doubtful whether or not it can occur in any other condition [27, p. 452].

It is to be noted that Carl Adolph Christian Jacob Gerhardt (1833–1902) previously described splenic pulsation in patients with rheumatic fever and aortic insufficiency in his 1882 publication titled "Pulsierender Milztumor" [28, 29]:

> [a] surprising phenomenon was the marked pulsation in which the hard mass swelled with each heart systole, expanding on all sides, and shrinking again during systole. One heard a dull double tone above the mass only at the upper edge of the heard sound. (…) The pulsation of the swollen spleen was so clear in this case that it could be demonstrated to numerous observers. As one could grasp the spleen tip with the fingers it was easy to prove that it was not a displacement of the spleen by the movement of the apex, but a true systolic swelling of the organ [29, p. 449].

Thus, Sailer and Gerhardt signs refer to the presence of splenic pulsation in patients with aortic insufficiency.

8.2.7 Saegesser Sign

Max Saegesser (1902–1975) was born in Langenthal, Switzerland, studied medicine in Geneva, Zurich, Bern, Munich, Paris, and Basel, and received his medical degree from the latter in 1927 [30, 31]. He habilitated in surgery in Bern from 1935 to 1937 and was chief physician at the Frutigen District Hospital in 1937, followed by an appointment at the Viktoriaspital, Bern [30, 31]. He was an associate professor in 1947 and a full professor at the University of Bern in 1973 [30].

He published the book *Spezielle chirurgische Therapie für Studierende und Ärzte* (Special Surgical Therapy for Students and Doctors) beginning in 1946 through 11 editions with translations in Spanish and Italian [32]. Saegesser described a finding in patients with splenic rupture and those with subcapsular hematoma (Table 8.1):

> It has been shown that all of our patients with splenic injuries have pronounced left-sided phrenic nerve pressure pain. We owe this fact to the observation that a person with a splenic injury reported severe shoulder pain interpreted as phrenic nerve pain. Subsequently, attention to every splenic injury and phrenic nerve tenderness was routinely found. The examination is performed by applying pressure with the thumb of the right hand posteriorly on the left side of the neck between the sternocleidomastoid and anterior scalene muscles and directed towards the larynx and spine. As a control, the phrenic nerve pressure pain on the right side is tested with the same hand movement. The presence of shoulder pain and clearly detectable pressure pain on the left side provides compelling evidence for splenic injury [33, p. 2179–2180].

Saegesser proposed a pathogenesis for this finding:

> The anatomical basis of this hyperesthesia of the phrenic nerve in injuries to the spleen is that the phrenic nerve leads to sensory branches, which run from the splenic capsule via sympathetic branches and celiac ganglion to the phrenic plexus and phrenic ganglion, from where the phrenic-abdominal rami also run in the phrenic nerve sensory fibers to the area of origin (IV. cervical nerve with anastomoses from 3, 4, 5 and 6). It is, therefore, a viscero-sensitive pain reflex [33, p. 2180].

Thus, Saegesser sign refers to shoulder pain occurring after pressing using the thumb of the right hand posteriorly on the left neck between the sternocleidomastoid and anterior scalene muscles in patients with splenic rupture and subcapsular hematoma.

8.2.8   *Nixon Sign*

Robert Kenneth Nixon Jr. (1921–1997) was born in Santa Barbara, California, USA, and received his medical degree from Northwestern University Medical School in 1946 [34]. He completed an internship and residency at Cook County Hospital in Chicago, Illinois, followed by a hematology fellowship at the Hektoen Institute in Chicago, Illinois, from 1951 to 1952 [34]. He joined Henry Ford Hospital in 1954 and rose to the rank of head of the second medical division in 1966 and acting chairman of the Department of Medicine from 1984 to 1985 [35].

He was a physician volunteer in the Cabrini Clinic in the inner City of Detroit, Michigan, beginning in 1955 and chief of medicine on the SS Hope from 1962 to 1972 [34]. He was appointed chairman of the Henry Ford Hospital medical board in 1973 and clinical professor of medicine at the University of North Carolina School of Medicine in 1986 [34].

As to a description of his character by R.J. Priest, "Henry Ford Hospital has been fortunate to have distinguished service from a doctor of such clinical and research acumen and social responsibility. Dr. Nixon's career has touched us with pride and gratefulness" [34, p. 292].

Nixon in 1954 described a method for determining spleen size (Table 8.1, Fig. 8.1):

> The patient is placed in the right lateral recumbent position with the left arm extended forward and upward sufficiently to clear the left lower part of the thorax. In this position the spleen lies above the stomach and colon, permitting determination of its upper and lower borders of dullness. After palpation for the lower border on inspiration, percussion is initiated at the lower level of pulmonary resonance in approximately the posterior axillary line and carried downward obliquely on a general perpendicular line toward the lower midanterior costal margin. Normally the upper border of dullness is measured 6 to 8 cm above the costal margin. Dullness increased over 8 cm is indicative of splenic enlargement in the adult [35, p. 166].

Thus, Nixon sign refers to the percussion technique for delineating spleen size. Nixon believed this technique was helpful in patients with a muscular and rigid abdominal wall with minimal splenic enlargement and those unable to cooperate by taking a deep breath during palpation.

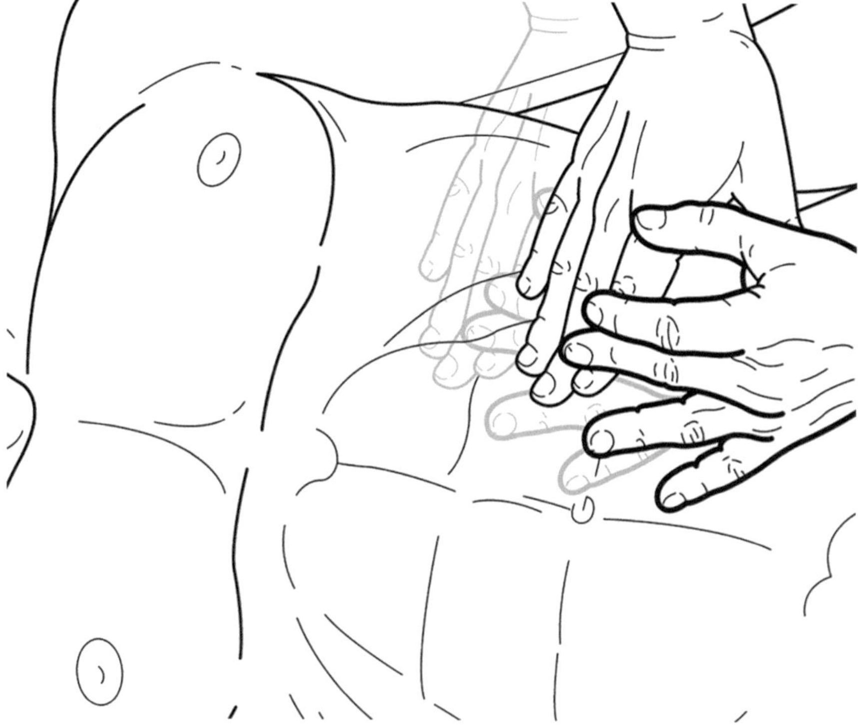

Fig. 8.1 Nixon sign (by Ryan Yale)

8.2.9 Castell Sign

Donald Overton Castell (1935–2021) was born in Washington, D.C., USA, and received his medical degree from George Washington School of Medicine in 1960 [36]. He was a medical intern from 1960 to 1961 and a resident from 1962 to 1965 at the National Naval Medical Center, Bethesda, Maryland [36–38].

He was appointed staff internist and consultant in gastroenterology from 1965 to 1967 at the Great Lakes Naval Hospital, Chicago, Illinois. He pursued a gastroenterology fellowship at Shattuck Hospital Tufts, followed by additional training at Boston University, Boston, Massachusetts, from 1968 to 1969 [37]. Castell was chief and later director of the Philadelphia Naval Hospital's clinical investigation service, chief of the gastroenterology division, and director of gastroenterology research and faculty at Jefferson Medical College, Philadelphia, Pennsylvania [37, 39].

He was captain and chairman of medicine at the National Naval Medical Center; professor and vice chairman of medicine at the Uniform Services University (USU) of the Health Sciences, Bethesda, Maryland; and professor of medicine at George Washington University from 1975 until 1979 when he retired from the navy but continued his position at USU [37–39]. Castell was chief of gastroenterology at Bowman Gray School of Medicine at Wake Forest, North Carolina in 1982; Rohrer Professor of Medicine and chief of the division of gastroenterology and hepatology at Thomas Jefferson Hospital and Graduate Hospital in Philadelphia in 1989; Kimbel professor and chairman of the Department of Medicine at the Graduate Hospital of the University of Pennsylvania; and director of the esophageal disorders program at the Medical University of South Carolina at South Carolina in 2001 [36, 37, 39, 40].

He was president of the American Gastroenterological Association (AGA) in 1999 [36, 38, 40]. From the AGA, he received the AGA Distinguished Teacher Award, Kirsner Award for Clinical Research in 1992, Baker Presidential Leadership Award in 1995, and Julius Friedenwald Medal [36]. He was recognized for his excellence in teaching with the Outstanding Civilian Educator Award from USU and Basic Science Teaching Excellence Award from Bowman Gray [36, 37, 39, 40].

A description of Castell's character as articulated by Barbara Frank at his inauguration as the 92nd president of the AGA:

> Now we will have the benefit of his talents as a leader, not just his organizational and administrative skills but his "people skills," the warmth, sincere concern, rigorous honesty, and enthusiasm that characterize his interactions with others and the insight and sound judgment that he brings to difficult issues [37, p. 1091].

Castell described a percussion method for determining the size of the spleen. Percussion is performed using the middle finger of the left hand (Table 8.1, Fig. 8.2):

> With the patient in the supine position percussion in the lowest intercostal space (eighth or ninth) in the left anterior axillary line usually produces a resonance note if the spleen is normal in size. Furthermore, the resonance persists with full inspiration. As the spleen enlarges the lower pole of this organ is displaced inferiority and medially. This may produce a chain in the percussion note in the lowest left interspace in the anterior axillary line from resonance to dullness with full inspiration. The percussion note is considered positive, therefore, when such a change is noted between full expiration and full inspiration [41, p. 1265].

Thus, Castell sign or the splenic percussion sign refers to a change in the percussion note of the spleen between deep inspiration and expiration in the lowest left intercostal space on the anterior axillary line when the patient is in the supine position. Ten males with a positive percussion sign and ten controls underwent a spleen scan. Castell found a positive concordance between a positive percussion sign and slight to moderate degrees of splenic enlargement, as confirmed through a spleen scan.

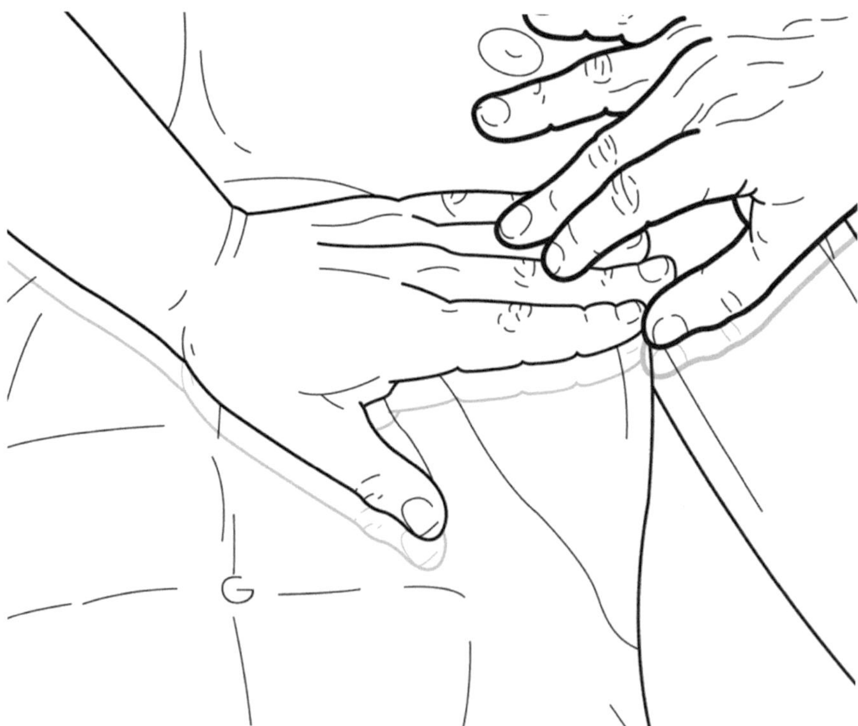

Fig. 8.2 Castell sign (by Ryan Yale)

8.2.10 Hedri Sign

Endre Hedri (1893–1962) was born in Gradiška, Bosnia and Herzegovina, and received his medical degree from Semmelweis University in Budapest, Hungary [42, 43]. His first appointment after obtaining his medical certificate was as an assistant in the Department of Surgery under the aegis of Manó Herczel (1862–1918) at the Szent Rókus Hospital from 1914 to 1918, interrupted during World War I, where he was a physician at the Gyáli út Garrison Hospital [42, 43].

Hedri was an assistant surgeon in Vienna, Leipzig, the surgical clinics of Kamiló Vidákovits in Szeged, Hungary, from 1918 to 1923, and József Ferenc Pulmonary Clinic in Budapest from 1924 to 1927 [42–44]. He was a clinical assistant professor at Országos Társadalombiztosítási Intézet (OTI) at the Ursoki Utcai Kórház Hospital from 1927 to 1933 and chief physician of Baleseti Sebészeti Osztályának from 1933 to 1945 [44].

Hedri was a chief trauma surgeon at OTI Baleseti Sebészeti Kóháza Hospital from 1945 to 1947 and a public professor of Trauma Surgery at Pázmány Péter University and Budapest Medical University, the latter of which he was appointed professor in 1952 [44]. He was a director of the third surgical clinic at Koltói Anna Baleseti Kórházban from 1947 to 1949 and director of the first surgical clinic at Budapest Medical University from 1949 to 1962 [42, 44]. Hedri was a corresponding member of the German Surgical Society, recipient of an honorary doctorate from the University of Leipzig, and president of the Sándor Korányi Society [44, 45].

As a tribute to Hedri's life by Babics:

> We thank him for his tireless zeal, the exemplary care he gave to his patients, the enthusiasm with which he devoted himself to promoting scientific life, and the boundless diligence with which he always worked to solve the most complex surgical problems [45, p. 1].

His character as described by Zsebök:

> One of his most characteristic qualities is his concern for patients. He was a humanist, a good man, for whom surgery was only a means to be his fellow man; help him with the most concrete tools of medicine and the methods of surgical intervention. This ability to help drove him to take on many, often almost impossible, surgical tasks. Even in the most challenging moments of life, he remained a human being whose main law was to help others [44, p. 2306].

Keleman, in his book *Physical Diagnosis of Acute Abdominal Diseases and Injuries*, described Hedri's sign of thoracic compression:

> [p]ressure of the sternum elicits pain in the left costal arch in splenic rupture; whereas pain in the right costal arch indicates liver injury. This is a particularly valuable sign in differentiating non-penetrating injuries causing abdominal hemorrhage if fracture of the lower ribs can be excluded [46, p. 94].

Thus, Hedri sign is the method for determining splenic rupture or hepatic injury.

8.3 Summary of Bedside Methods to Determine Spleen Size

Direct (single-finger) and mediate (two-finger) techniques have been used to percuss the spleen to determine its size. The authors typically position the patient in the supine position. Hoover (1901) recommended using a direct technique in which "the patient should lie on his back so as to bring the spleen in intimate contact with the ribs. The lower border of the lung in the posterior axillary line is first determine and then percuss gently in the intercostal space toward the median line at right angles to the costal border" [47]. A study compared splenic percussion (Nixon and Castell) with palpation using scintigraphy as the gold standard to confirm splenic enlargement ($\geq$12 cm in length and/or >7 cm in width). The sensitivity and specificity were for Nixon (59%, 94%), Castell (82%, 83%) and palpation (71%, 90%) [48, 49]. Combining both palpation and percussion techniques identified, up to 88% of spleens were enlarged by scintigraphy [48]. In a comprehensive review of prior studies on the splenic percussion sign, a sensitivity of 25–85%, specificity of 32–94%, positive likelihood ratio of 1.7, and negative likelihood ratio of 0.7 were identified for Castell sign, and a sensitivity of 25–66%, specificity of 68–95%, positive likelihood ratio of 2.0, and negative likelihood ration of 0.7 for Nixon sign. In contrast, the sensitivity, specificity, and likelihood ratio for detecting an enlarged spleen by palpation were 18–78%, 89–99%, 8.5, and 0.5, respectively [49]. A false negative percussion sign may occur in patients with marked splenomegaly or fluid in the stomach or stool in the adjacent colon. Palpation is more likely to detect splenic enlargement than percussion techniques.

There is poor intraobserver agreement using percussion alone to measure spleen size. Applying a strategy that incorporates pre-test clinical suspicion of splenomegaly improves the performance of the test and provides a rationale for obtaining an ultrasound to confirm splenic enlargement [50, 51]. Using this strategy, if the pretest probability is <10%, neither percussion nor palpation is sufficiently sensitive to rule out splenomegaly, and the specificity is not sufficiently high to rule in splenomegaly. If the clinical suspicion is >10%, then percussion and palpation can rule in splenomegaly. If either percussion or palpation, but not both, detects an enlarged spleen, an ultrasound is recommended to confirm spleen size. Because of the lower sensitivity of percussion or palpation, an ultrasound is required to rule out splenomegaly [50, 51].

Table 8.1 Splenic eponyms

Name	Year	Description of eponym	Significance
Debove [8]	1892	Splenomegaly, hypertrophy, or an increase in spleen volume	Portal hypertension
Pitts [11]	1896	Fixed dullness in the splenic region	Splenic rupture
Ballance [18]	1898	Fixed dullness in the left flank	Splenic rupture

(continued)

Table 8.1 (continued)

Name	Year	Description of eponym	Significance
Pagniello [19]	1920	Moderate pressure is applied at the ninth left intercostal space between the midline and posterior axillary line using the index or middle finger of the right hand. The patient reports a painful sensation located at this point associated with a reflex muscular contraction of the trunk or face, or the patient tells you that they are experiencing pain. Pain may also rarely occur when pressure is applied at the eighth, ninth, or tenth intercostal space. In patients sensitive to pain, it is best to cautiously apply this maneuver, using the entire palm to the splenic region, starting with the fingertips at the twelfth rib and gradually moving proximally to the location where the patient reports that pain is greatest. If continuous pressure is applied to this region, the pain eventually resolves	Malaria
Castronuovo [22]	1927	The spleen is soft, so a non-painful imprint occurs when palpating this organ	Splenic hyperemia
Sailer [27]	1928	Splenic pulsation	Aortic insufficiency
Saegesser [33]	1938	Pressure is applied with the thumb of the right hand posteriorly on the left side of the neck between the sternocleidomastoid and anterior scalene muscles and directed toward the larynx and spine. The phrenic nerve pressure point on the right side is evaluated using the same hand movement. A positive sign is the presence of left shoulder pain	Splenic rupture
Nixon [35]	1954	The patient is placed in the right lateral recumbent position with the left arm extended forward and upward sufficiently to clear the left lower part of the thorax. After palpation to identify the lower border on inspiration, percussion is initiated at the lower level of pulmonary resonance in approximately the posterior axillary line and moved downward obliquely on a general perpendicular line toward the lower mid-anterior costal margin. Normally the upper border of dullness measures 6–8 cm above the costal margin. Dullness extending over 8 cm is indicative of splenic enlargement in the adult	Splenomegaly
Castell [41]	1967	With the patient supine, percuss in the lowest intercostal space (eighth or ninth) in the left anterior axillary line. A resonance note is present and persists throughout inspiration if the spleen is normal in size. As the spleen enlarges, the lower pole of this organ is displaced inferiorly and medially causing further dullness on percussion in the lowest left interspace during full inspiration. The test is positive if percussion dullness is present over a larger area on full inspiration compared to full expiration	Splenomegaly
Hedri [46]	[n.a.]	Pressure over the sternum causes pain at the left costal arch	Splenic rupture

8.4 Conclusion

Signs of the spleen were identified prior to the advent of advanced imaging techniques, including ultrasonography which can now detect splenic enlargement, rupture, and portal hypertension at the bedside. They remain of historical interest as they provide insight into the discovery of novel methods used for diagnosing disease. The physical examination is moderately sensitive but nonspecific in detecting splenomegaly. Thus, its absence does not exclude the presence of disease. The examination should still be taught as splenic enlargement, or other maneuvers used to detect conditions involving the spleen assist in diagnosis when used concomitantly with other clinical aspects of disease.

References

1. Skinner HA. The origin of medical terms. Baltimore, MD: Williams & Wilkins; 1949.
2. Malpighii M. De liene praefatio. In: De viscerum structura exercitatio anatomica. Amsterdam: Apud Petrum Le Grand; 1669. p. 96–145.
3. Kölliker A. Vessels of the spleen. In: A manual of human microscopic anatomy. London: John W. Parker and Son; 1860. p. 358–72.
4. [No author]. Décès de M. Debove, secrétaire perpétuel. Bull Acad Méd. 1920;84:238–42.
5. Delmas V, Achard C, Janes J. Debove George Maurice. Comité Trav Hist Sci. http://cths.fr/an/savant.php?id=105493. Accessed 25 Nov 2022.
6. [No author]. Professor G.M. Debove. Br Med J. 1920;2:955.
7. Cherrington EH. Georges Maurice Debove. In: Standard encyclopedia of the alcohol problem, vol. 2. Westerville, OH: American Issue Publishing Company; 1924. p. 775.
8. Debove GM. De la splénomégalie primitive. France Méd. 1892;30:506–7.
9. Pitts B. Plarr's lives of the fellows. London: Royal College of Surgeons of England; 2012. https://livesonline.rcseng.ac.uk/client/en_GB/lives/search/detailnonmodal/ent:$002f$002fSD_ASSET$002f0$002fSD_ASSET:375144/one?qu=%22rcs%3A+E002961%22&rt=false%7C%7C%7CIDENTIFIER%7C%7C%7CResource+Identifier. Accessed 3 Nov 2022.
10. [No author]. Bernard Pitts, MC, FRCS, consulting surgeon to St. Thomas's Hospital and to the Hospital for Sick Children, Great Ormond Street. Br Med J. 1914;2:1122–3.
11. Pitts B, Ballance CA. Three cases of splenectomy for rupture. Clin Soc. 1896;29:77–104.
12. [No author]. Sir Charles Ballance, KCMG, CB MS, FRCS. Br Med J. 1936;1:339.
13. Elsberg CA. Obituary: Charles Alfred Ballance, 1856–1936. Bull N Y Acad M. 1936;12:146–9.
14. Ballance CA. Plarr's lives of the fellows. London: Royal College of Surgeons of England; 2013. https://livesonline.rcseng.ac.uk/client/en_GB/lives/search/detailnonmodal/ent:$002f$002fSD_ASSET$002f0$002fSD_ASSET:375978/one?qu=%22rcs%3A+E003795%22&rt=false%7C%7C%7CIDENTIFIER%7C%7C%7CResource+Identifier. Accessed 20 Nov 2022.
15. Manché A. Sir Charles Ballance: a pioneer surgeon in Malta. Malta Med J. 2014;26:56–9.
16. Turner A. Ballance, Sir Charles Alfred (1856–1936). London: Royal College of Surgeons of England; 2008. https://aim25.com/cats/9/9914.htm. Accessed 20 Nov 2022.
17. [No author]. Sir Charles Ballance, KCMG, CB, MVO. Nature. 1936;137:350.
18. Ballance CA. On splenectomy for rupture without external wound. Practitioner. 1898;60:347–58.
19. Pagniello R. Medio fácil y rápida para el diagnóstico de la infección malárica. Sem Méd. 1920;27:830–1.

20. Tomasulo B. Giovanni Castronuovo. La Basilicata nel Mondo. 1924;1:212–3.
21. [No author]. Giovanni Castronuovo. Rome: Bollettino Ufficiale del Ministero della Istruzione Pubblica; 1907. p. 2504.
22. Castronuovo G. Milza plastica o malleabile nell'anemia fibroadenica, tipo Griesinger-Banti. Riforma Med. 1927;43:554.
23. Riesman J. Joseph Sailer. Am J Surg. 1929;7:576–8.
24. [No author]. Joseph Sailer. Am Heart J. 1929;6:367–8.
25. [No author]. AHA elections. Bull Am Heart Assoc. 1928;3:5.
26. [No author]. Former officers: President Joseph Sailer. Annu Meet Am Gastroenterol Assoc. 1926;28:8.
27. Sailer J. Pulsating spleen in aortic insufficiency. Am Heart J. 1928;3:447–53.
28. Yale SH, Tekiner H, Mazza JJ, Yale ES, Yale RC. Aortic regurgitation murmurs. In: Cardiovascular eponymic signs: diagnostic skills applied during the physical examination. Cham: Springer; 2021. p. 105–42.
29. Gerhardt C. Pulsierender Milztumor. Ztschr klin Med. 1882;4:449–50.
30. Saegesser M. (16 Feb 1902–17 Oct 1975). Google arts & culture. https://artsandculture.google.com/entity/g1215vkg6?hl=es. Accessed 12 Nov 2022
31. Weisser C. Max Saegesser. In: Chirurgenlexikon: 2000 Persönlichkeiten aus der Geschichte der Chirurgie. Berlin: Springer; 2019. p. 281.
32. Vierhaus R. Max Saegesser. In: Deutsche biographische Enzyklopädie. Munich: K.G. Saur; 2005. p. 669.
33. Saegesser M. Der linksseitige Phrenikusdruckpunkt als diagnostisches Merkmal bei Milzverletzungen. Zentralbl Chir. 1938;65:2179–80.
34. Priest RJ, Robert K. Nixon. Henry Ford Hosp Med J. 1996;34:291–2.
35. Nixon RK Jr. The detection of splenomegaly by percussion. NEJM. 1954;250:166–7.
36. Richter JE, Katz PO, Katzka DA. In memoriam: Donald O. Castell, MD. Gastroenterology. 2021;160:1905–7.
37. Frank BB. Our new president: Donald O. Castell, MD. Gastroenterology. 1998;114:1091–4.
38. DeVault K, Katz P, Richter J. Donald O. Castell (1935–2021): a life dedicated to investigation, mentoring, and education. Am J Gastroenterol. 2021;116:444.
39. Castell DO, emeritus Professor of Medicine, 1935–2021. MUSC remembers Donald O. Castell, MD. Medical University of South Carolina. 2021. https://medicine.musc.edu/departments/dom/news-and-awards/2021/january-2021/remembering-don-castell. Accessed 2 Nov 2022.
40. Rattan S, Cao W, Katz PO, Goyal RK. In memory of our following colleagues, and friends. J Neurogastroenterol Motil. 2022;34:e14393.
41. Castell DO. The spleen percussion sign: a useful diagnostic technique. Ann Intern Med. 1967;67:1265–7.
42. Endre H. Arcanum. https://www.arcanum.com/en/online-kiadvanyok/Lexikonok-magyar-eletrajzi-lexikon-7428D/h-75B54/hedriendre-75CDE/. Accessed 23 Nov 2022.
43. Endre H. Nemzeti Örökség Intézete. https://intezet.nori.gov.hu/nemzeti-sirkert/budapest/farkasreti-temeto/hedri-endre-1919-igschossberger-endre/. Accessed 23 Nov 2022.
44. Zsebök Z. Hedri Endre Dr. (1893–1962). Orv Hetil. 1962;103:2305–6.
45. Babics A. Prof. Endre Hedri (1893–1962). Acta Chir Acad Sci Hung. 1963;4:1.
46. Keleman E. Physical diagnosis of acute abdominal diseases and injuries. Budapest: Akadémiai Kiadó; 1964.
47. Hoover CF. The diagnosis of typhoid fever. Cleve Clin J Med. 1901;6:5–8.
48. Sullivan S, Williams R. Reliability of clinical techniques for detecting splenic enlargement. Br Med J. 1976;2:1043–4.
49. McGee SR. Evidence-based physical diagnosis. 3rd ed. Philadelphia, PA: Elsevier; 2012. p. 428–40.
50. Grover SA, Barkun AN, Sackett DL. Does this patient have splenomegaly? JAMA. 1993;270:2218–21.
51. Barkun AN, Grover SA. Splenomegaly. In: Simel DL, Rennie D, editors. The rational clinical examination: evidence based clinical diagnosis. New York, NY: McGraw Hill; 2009. p. 610–3.

Chapter 9
Pancreas Signs

9.1 Introduction

While a clinical description of acute pancreatitis was first presented in the seventeenth century by Nicolaes Tulp (1593–1674), the word pancreatitis is believed to have first appeared in the literature by Robley Dunglison (1798–1869) in 1842, but clearly, the disease had been further described as early as 1804 by Antoine Portal (1742–1832) [1, 2]. Felix Victor Birch-Hirschfeld (1842–1899) described chronic pancreatitis in 1895, while Reginald Heber Fitz's description of acute suppurative gangrenous hemorrhagic pancreatitis with fat necrosis presented at the New York Pathological Society in 1889 remains notable even today [3, 4]. Fitz's paper brought attention to the significance of this gland, including its frequency, pathology, and treatment. His name is eponymously ascribed in honor of his description of the clinical features of acute pancreatitis and thus, in the strictest sense, represents symptoms and not a sign [4].

There are few signs of acute and chronic pancreatitis, presumably due to the limited access of this organ to palpation and percussion. With the advent of radiographic imaging, other patterns and associated findings in acute pancreatitis were recognized, including isolated dilation of the transverse colon by Josef Goblet in 1913 and the "inverted figure 3" sign by Nils Frostberg in 1938. Furthermore, their role in clinical practice is unknown since they have never been studied. We present these signs as a tribute to their keen observation and meticulous examination techniques to better define the diseases of acute and chronic pancreatitis.

9.2 Eponymic Signs

9.2.1 Fitz Sign

Reginald Heber Fitz (1843–1913) was born in Chelsea, Massachusetts, USA. He was a house officer at Boston City Hospital in 1867 and received his medical degree from Harvard Medical School in 1868 [5–7]. He continued his studies abroad primarily with Rudolph Virchow (1821–1902) in Berlin; Carl von Rokitansky (1804–1878), Johann Ritter von Oppolzer (1808–1871), and Joseph Škoda (1805–1881) in Vienna; Victor André Cornil (1837–1908) in Paris; and Charles Murchison (1830–1879) in London [5–10].

Fitz served in Boston as an instructor in pathological anatomy at the Harvard Medical School from 1870 to 1873, was a physician to the Boston Dispensary, a microscopist at Massachusetts General Hospital in 1871, and assistant professor of pathology from 1873 to 1878 and chair of pathological anatomy at Harvard Medical School in 1878 (renamed Shattuck Professor of Pathological Anatomy in 1879) [5, 6, 9, 10]. He was appointed visiting physician to the Massachusetts General Hospital in 1887 and Hersey Professor of the Theory and Practice of Physic at Harvard Medical School in 1892 [5, 9, 10].

Among his numerous accolades, Fitz was elected fellow of the American Academy of Arts and Sciences, associate fellow of the College of Physicians in 1892, honorary member of the Medical and Chirurgical Faculty of Maryland in 1893, and honorary fellow of the New York Academy of Medicine. He received an honorary degree of L.L.D. from Harvard College in 1905 [5]. He was president of the Association of American Physicians in 1894 and was elected corresponding member of the Gesellschaft für innere Medizin und Kinderheilkunde (Society of Internal Medicine and Pediatrics), Vienna, and president of Congress of American Physicians and Surgeons in 1907 [5, 8].

As to his character as described by Stone:

> The work that Dr. Fitz has done during his active period of life has been largely critical and judicial, though always with a constructive tendency. He has formed his opinions for himself, and then bravely stood by them, even at times when they were in opposition to those of a majority of his friends or to the potent influence of the president of the university [11, p. 12].

Fitz, in his Middleton-Goldsmith Lecture on patients with acute suppurative pancreatitis, delivered before the New York Pathological Society in 1889, described the symptoms found in this disease:

> The cases of acute, suppurative pancreatitis usually began suddenly, with severe generally intense, gastric, epigastric or abdominal pain, vomiting, and sometimes great prostration. The vomiting might be incessant and distressing, or it might give temporary relief to the pain. The ejected fluid was sometimes stringy and brown. The bowels were usually constipated, although diarrhea might occur within the first twenty-four hours. This latter symptom was not infrequent at a later date of the disease. Fever usually slight, was the next conspicuous symptom, being manifested about the third day. At the same time the upper abdomen, especially the epigastrium, was likely to become distended, tympanitic, and sensitive. Hiccough, sometimes quite obstinate, was not infrequent at this state, and occasionally chills were to be met with. The abdomen, in general, then became moderately swollen, tense, and tympanitic [4, p. 56].

Thus, Fitz enumerated the symptoms of acute pancreatitis, which include the sudden onset of severe vomiting, epigastric abdominal pain, and abdominal swelling (Table 9.1).

9.2.2 *Körte Sign*

Werner Friedrich Emil Körte (Koerte) (1853–1937) was born in Berlin, Germany, studied medicine in Berlin, Bonn, and Strasburg, and received his medical degree in 1857 [12, 13]. He was an assistant at the University Surgical Clinic from 1874 to 1876 and Max Wilms (1867–1918) at the Bethanien Hospital, Berlin, from 1877 to 1879 [13, 14]. Körte was director of the surgical division of Städtisches Krankenhaus am Urban zu Berlin (Berlin Urban Hospital) from 1889 to 1924 [12–14]. During World War I, he was a consultant to the Third Reserve Corps. At Berlin University, he was a Geheimer Sanitätsrat (honorary title of Privy Medical Advisor) and titular professor [13].

Körte was a recipient of the Iron Cross (first class) for his valor during World War I, president of Deutsche Gesellschaft für Chirurgie (German Society of Surgery), and president and honorary chairman of Berliner Gesellschaft für Chirurgie (Berlin Society for Surgery) [12–14].

As to a description of his character by Brentano:

> He was a brilliant orator who surprised his audience, lecturing with clarity and conciseness and socially with wit and spirit. (…) He possessed a warm, gentle, virtuous heart not always hidden under a rough shell. This heart corresponded to an unsurpassable love of truth, which he found expression in his scientific work and everyday life, making it so valuable [15, p. 1923].

Körte described his experience with palpation of the pancreas in cases of acute pancreatitis:

> A symptom that confirms the diagnosis beyond the realm of suspicion and is of major interest for surgical treatment is feeling a tumor in the epigastrium at the site of the pancreas. Due to its protected position, the organ is not easily accessible for palpation. However, it is possible to feel the gland and its granular structure in the epigastrium in front of the spine if the abdominal wall is relaxed and not obese and the stomach and intestines are empty [16, p. 153]. Only when epigastric distension has subsided or eliminated by gastric lavage and when the tension in the abdominal muscles is overcome after reducing the pain or using anesthesia can the swollen organ be felt. After the stomach and intestines have been emptied, possibly under anesthetic, can a tumor be observed in the epigastrium, corresponding to the location of the pancreas. In that case, it must be borne in mind that there remain various possibilities for error. (…) After the stomach is reduced, it can be established that the mass is felt behind the stomach, but it cannot be ruled out that it originates from the posterior wall of the stomach. Complete certainty that the tumor is felt in the pancreas cannot be achieved in all cases, nor can it be determined with certainty after the pus has erupted whether the resistance felt lies in the pancreas or is located either retroperitoneally or intraperitoneally in the omental bursa. As a rule, the swelling can only be felt when the acute stage of the disease is over and the pain and distention of the epigastrium have subsided. If one feels resistance in the epigastrium behind the stomach or between the stomach and colon in patients who present the clinical picture outlined above, then one can consider the diagnosis of pancreatitis [16, p. 154].

Thus, Körte sign refers to the palpable epigastric mass in patients with acute pancreatitis (Table 9.1).

9.2.3 Halsted Sign

William Stewart Halsted (1852–1922) was born in New York City, USA, received his medical degree from Columbia University College of Physicians and Surgeons (currently Columbia University Vagelos College of Physicians and Surgeons), New York, in 1877, and was an intern at the fourth surgical division at Bellevue Hospital [17–20]. He traveled abroad for two years to Vienna, Leipzig, and Würzburg in 1878 to further his medical training [18–20]. He served as a demonstrator of anatomy at the College of Physicians and Surgeons and established the outpatient department at Roosevelt Hospital in 1880 [18, 21]. Halsted was appointed first at the Charity Hospital as attending surgeon and director of the outpatient departments from 1881 to 1887, surgeon-in-chief to Emigrant Hospital Ward's Island, and visiting physician to Bellevue and Presbyterian Hospitals from 1885 to 1887 [19, 21]. He worked at William Henry Welch's (1850–1934) Laboratory at Johns Hopkins University, followed by appointments as associate professor of Surgery, head of the outpatient department, acting surgeon to the hospital in 1889, surgeon-in-chief in 1890, and professor of surgery in 1892 at Johns Hopkins Hospital [18, 19].

As described his character by MacCallum:

> In attempting to estimate the significance of Dr. Halsted's work it seems that his greatest service was not so much his surgical discoveries and inventions, many and important as these were, as his attitude in operating upon the human body which must forever be the proper attitude of the surgeon. It was simply the recognition of the normal or physiological condition of the tissues which one should attempt to restore, realizing their natural defense and the reasons for their vulnerability. (…) He was not inflated with self-esteem, he did not advertise and he was not a politician, the things which lead to present but not to permanent fame. But he made lasting contributions to the world's knowledge and his name will endure [19, p. 162].

As reported in an obituary in the *California State Journal of Medicine*:

> This philosopher-surgeon was ever intent on extending the bounds of medical knowledge, and devoted himself whole-heartedly to qualifying and enriching the minds of his many pupils. We are grateful for this legacy, which he so bountifully distributed during his lifetime, "teaching what he had learned, and learning in order that he might teach." We glory in his tireless energy, his quiet, simple and unostentatious manner, and in the splendid accomplishment of his many tasks. He was truly a great man, a daring and brilliant pioneer of surgery, and his single-hearted and self-sacrificing devotion to the cause of scientific research had its reward in achievements of the most vital and far-reaching nature [22, p. 420].

Halsted made significant contributions to surgery, with those most highly coveted involving the surgical management of breast cancer, use of rubber gloves, inguinal herniorrhaphy, thyroid and parathyroid glands, and subclavian artery aneurysms. He is the recipient of several honorary degrees, including the L.L.D. from Yale (1904) and Edinburgh (1905) as well as a D.Sc. from Columbia (1904) University [17, 21]. Additionally, he was an honorary fellow of the Royal College of Surgeons of England and Edinburgh [17, 21].

Halsted, in his description of a case of acute hemorrhagic pancreatitis involving an 18-year-old male, described on physical examination that:

> He was sensitive to pressure over the epigastrium, but not exquisitely, the point of greatest tenderness being a little above and, I thought, to the right of the umbilicus. (…) I have thought that it might be well to represent graphically the only sign which this obscure case presented, the white print of the fingertips in a slightly cyanosed field just over the site of greatest pain [23, p. 180].

Thus, Halsted sign refers to the blanching of the skin when the fingertip is applied to the cyanotic abdomen in patients with hemorrhagic pancreatitis (Table 9.1).

9.2.4 Mayo-Robson Sign

Sir Arthur William Mayo-Robson (1853–1933) was born at Filey, Yorkshire, England, studied at Leeds School of Medicine and received his membership of the Royal College of Surgeons in 1874 and licentiate of the Royal College of Physicians in 1875 [24]. He was appointed demonstrator in anatomy and lecturer from 1876 to 1886 at Leeds School of Medicine. He was a fellow of the Royal College of Surgeons in 1879 [24–26]. Mayo-Robson was appointed assistant surgeon in 1882 and surgeon in 1884 to the General Infirmary, Leeds, followed by professor and chair of surgery at Yorkshire College (Victoria University) from 1890 to 1899 [25, 26]. During World War I, he was consulting surgeon to the Mediterranean Expeditionary Force with the rank of temporary lieutenant colonel Royal Army Medical Corps stationed in Egypt and Gallipoli in 1915 [24, 26]. He served as a consultant to the medical counsel of the Southern Command Ward Office in 1917, as inspector of the Military Orthopedic Hospital in London in 1918, followed by consulting surgeon to the King Edward VII Hospital, Windsor and Dreadnought Hospital, Greenwich [24, 26].

Mayo-Robson served as president of the British Gynecological Society and Leeds and West Riding Medico-Chirurgical Society, vice-president of the Royal College of Surgeons, and member of the British Medical Association [24, 25]. He was knighted in 1908, Knight Commander of the Order of the British Empire in 1919, and Companion of the Royal Victorian Order in 1911 [24, 25].

As to a tribute to his character as articulated by Moynihan:

> He possessed industry the like of which I have seen matched in only one other among those with whom I have worked. He had a radiant, quenchless enthusiasm. His capacity for seizing upon relevant features in a new problem, of capturing the essential principle, and neglecting specious non-essentials seemed like wizardry. All these qualities and many more were at once in his service [27, p. 948].

Mayo-Robson described in patients with pancreatitis:

> The more acute inflammations are characterized by excessive tenderness on pressure, the presence of a tender spot just above and to the right of the umbilicus, rigidity of the recti, and pain of an agonizing character [28, p. 314].

Thus, Mayo-Robson sign refers to pain in acute pancreatitis above and to the right of the umbilicus (Table 9.1).

9.2.5 Löwi Sign

Otto Löwi (Loewi) (1873–1961) was born in Frankfurt am Main, Germany, and received his medical degree from the University of Strasburg in 1896 [29–32]. He worked with Hans Horst Meyer's (1853–1939) Laboratories at the Pharmacologic Institute at the University of Marburg, continuing his work with Meyer in Vienna from 1898 to 1908 [30]. During this period, he was appointed and rose to the rank of assistant and associate professor [30]. He served as a lecturer in pharmacology in Marburg in 1900, was appointed extraordinary professor in Vienna in 1904, and was chair of pharmacology at the University of Graz, Austria, in 1909 [30, 32]. He is best recognized for his work on the autonomic nervous system and the role of the vagus, acetylcholine release, and sympathetic nerves in the heart [32]. He and Sir Henry Hallett Dale (1875–1968) were awarded the Nobel Prize in Physiology and Medicine in 1936 [29–31, 33]. He was imprisoned by the Nazis in 1938, fled Austria, and served as a visiting professor at the Free University of Brussels and the Nuffield Institute in Oxford [29, 31, 33]. While in England, he received an appointment as a research professor in pharmacology from New York University College of Medicine in 1940 [29, 30].

As to a description of his character:

> A man with an irrepressible zest for life, thoughtful optimism, and sense of humor. These surely are some of the outstanding traits which comes to mind to the many friends who knew Otto Loewi. (…) A chance meeting with Otto Loewi could be a memorable occasion. One drew readily a spark of enthusiasm from his ever-searching mind. His eyes would shine, his remarkable kaleidoscopic face would light up as he took hold of ideas and developed them [29, p. 451].

Löwi received numerous awards, honorary degrees, and memberships throughout his career, recognizing his outstanding accomplishments and contributions to physiology and medicine. His image was honored through a stamp issued in Austria in 1973 in recognition of the centenary of his birth [33, 34].

Löwi presented a finding at the Vienna Medical Society in 1907 in patients with pancreatic insufficiency:

> By injecting a solution of adrenaline into the conductive sac of animals whose pancreas had been removed, he observed a marked pupillary mydriasis, which he never found in the control animals. [I]n healthy individuals, installing a few adrenaline drops never produced any phenomenon. However, in patients with diabetes, it produces marked pupillary mydriasis [35, p. 934].

Löwi believed that mydriasis occurred due to the absence of nerves that inhibits pupillary dilation. Thus, a positive Löwi sign is the presence of marked pupillary mydriasis after the installation of three to four drops of adrenaline into the conjunctival sac in patients with diabetes mellitus caused by pancreatic insufficiency (Table 9.1).

9.2.6   Goblet Sign

We could only identify limited historical information on Josef Goblet (1878–1944). At the time of his publication titled "Beiträge zur akuten Pankreasnekrose" (Contributions to acute pancreatic necrosis), he was a surgical ordinary at the Gewerkschaftlichen Krankenhause (Union Hospitals) in Orlau, Czech Republic [36].

Goblet described a finding in pancreatic necrosis:

> In my experience, I observed in my first published case isolated distension of the transverse colon, I have already discussed its possible significance as an early symptom of acute pancreatic necrosis prompting von Faykiss to designate the name Goblet's symptom. (...) Based on my observations and the perceptions of other authors, I have to emphasize again that isolated distension of the transverse colon represents an early symptom of acute pancreatic necrosis, which in the absence of other symptoms, is characteristic of pancreatic necrosis [36, p. 1387].

Thus, Goblet sign refers to the gaseous distension (meteorism) of the transverse colon in acute pancreatic necrosis (Table 9.1).

9.2.7   Frostberg (Inverted 3) Sign

Nils Johan Frostberg (1905–1972) was born in Lund, Sweden, and received his medical license in 1934 [37]. He was chief physician of the Provincial (District) Hospital in Hässleholm, Sweden, in 1949 and senior physician in the Department of Radiology at Kristianstad, Sweden, in 1957 [37].

Nils Frostberg summarized the radiographic findings in three cases of pancreatic carcinoma and other inflammatory conditions involving the head of the pancreas:

> The author is recording three cases of a similar and peculiar deformity of the descending part of the duodenum, assuming the shape of an inverted figure "3". On the strength of the radiographic examination, growths in the head of the pancreas were considered the most probable explanation. However, autopsy findings have shown that pancreatitis and edema may also give rise to such deformities [38, p. 172].

Thus, Frostberg sign refers to the radiographic appearance seen on barium examination of the small bowel whereby there are two adjacent rounded or bud-shaped depressions involving the concave portion of the descending portion (second part) of the duodenum (Table 9.1). This radiographic finding represents an infiltrative process that distorts or effaces the mucosal pattern on the medial wall of the duodenum originating from the head of the pancreas due to tumor, edema, inflammation, or duodenal carcinoma [39].

9.2.8 Mallet-Guy Sign

Pierre Albert Mallet-Guy (1897–1995) was born in Beaune, France, and received his medical degree from the University of Lyon in 1925. At the University of Lyon, he served as head of the surgical clinic in 1927, associate professor in 1939, and professor of surgical pathology in 1946 [40]. He was appointed professor of the surgical clinic A and director of the surgical research unit of the National Institute of Health and Medical Research at the Edouard Herriot Hospital in Lyon in 1958 [40]. He served as mission officer by the General Directorate of Cultural Affairs to numerous countries, including the USA, in 1948 and later annotated an honorary foreign member for his distinguished service [40].

Among his many accolades, Mallet-Guy was recognized for his valor by being decorated with the War Cross, officer of the Legion of Honor, and commander of the Order of the Yugoslav Star, Doctor honoris causa at the University of Giessen and member of the French Association of Surgery Board of Directors [40]. He was also a member of the Academies of Medicine and Surgery, the American College of Surgeons, and the Belgian Society of Surgery, to name a few. He was editor-in-chief of *Lyon Chirurgical* [40].

Mallet-Guy described, in 1943, a maneuver used to detect a painful point in chronic pancreatitis (Fig. 9.1):

> The fasting patient is placed in the right lateral decubitus position, with the legs semi-flexed on the abdomen. The tips of the fingers are placed 3 to 4 cm along the costal margin at the 9th cartilage and are easily inserted under the costal arch by depressing the anterior abdominal wall in the lateral direction toward the vertebra. This position allows the pancreas to be more easily explored. The examiner identifies a palpatory point causing sharp pain that confirms the diagnosis [41, p. 175].

He further clarified precisely the location and direction of the fingers:

> Place the extended fingers beneath the costal margin and directed them superiorly. When the fingertips are deep under the diaphragm, raise the heel of the hand and palpate the pancreas under the fingers. This maneuver displaces the stomach inferiorly and medially [41, p. 175].

Mallet-Guy reported his experience with this sign:

> This is a sign of pancreatitis. My personal experience with 34 patients suffering from chronic pancreatitis (in 23 the disease was confined to the left side of the pancreas) allows me to use this sign in cases where the diagnosis was unclear [41, p. 174–175].

He called for the need to evaluate this finding further in order to confirm its ability to distinguish chronic pancreatitis from other conditions in this abdominal region:

> I would like to see a systematic investigation of this symptom. It is always present when the disease is located on the left side of the pancreas. It is often possible to distinguish this condition from renal disease, post-operative peptic ulcer disease, and splenic vein thrombosis [41, p. 175].

Thus, Mallet-Guy sign is the technique for identifying the painful point in chronic pancreatitis (Table 9.1).

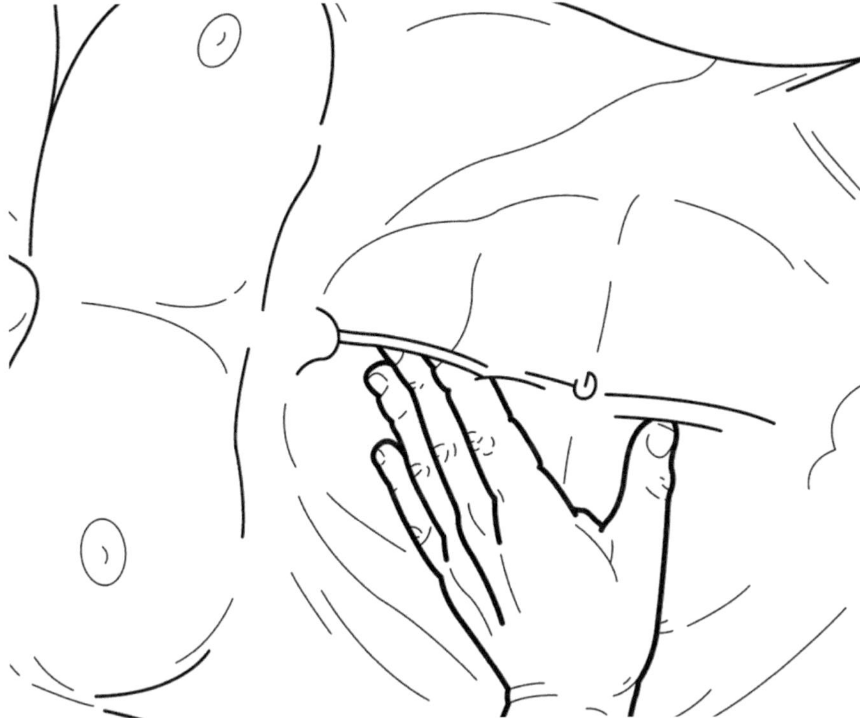

Fig. 9.1 Mallet-Guy sign (by Ryan Yale)

9.2.9   Imrie Sign

Clem William Imrie (1943–) graduated from the University of Glasgow Medical School with a Bachelor of Medicine and Bachelor of Surgery degree in 1967 [42]. He completed his surgical residency in the West of Scotland, at St. George's Hospital with Sir Rodney Smith (1914–1998), and fellowship training in Europe and the USA [43]. Imrie was a surgeon at the Glasgow Royal Infirmary from 1969 to 2007, rising to consultant surgeon in 1977 and professor of surgery Lister Department of Surgery at the University of Glasgow, UK, from 1996 to 2007 [44]. He was elected a fellow of the Royal College of Physicians and Surgeons in 2002. He is currently professor emeritus, Department of Surgery at the Glasgow Royal Infirmary, National Health Service Greater Glasgow and Clyde [42].

He served as president of the International Society of Pancreatology from 1994 to 1996, the European Pancreatic Club from 1989 to 1990, the Pancreatic Society of Great Britain and Ireland from 1990 to 1991, and the International Pancreatic Association from 1994 to 1996 [42, 43]. He is the recipient of the George E. Palade

Prize from the International Association of Pancreatology [44]. His name is eponymously ascribed to a score devised to determine the severity and predict mortality in acute pancreatitis (Glasgow–Imrie Criteria for Severity of Acute Pancreatitis) [44].

Imrie described a finding occurring in patients with acute pancreatitis (Table 9.1):

> Facial flushing in the absence of pyrexia is a frequently observed clinical sign in the initial 48 hours after the onset of acute pancreatitis. (…) The flushing was readily observed in the initial 12 hours after admission in most patients, but a minority developed the striking appearance between 12 and 36 hours after admission. It is unusual for the flushing to be present for approximately a day [45, p. 593].

He postulated that the cause of the flushing was due to the release of vasoactive peptides into the blood, secondary to the inflammation of the pancreas.

9.2.10   Baid Sign

Jai Chand Baid (1947–) received his surgical training in Rajasthani, India, in 1970. He was an associate professor at Jawaharlal Nehru (JLN) Hospital in Rajasthani in 1991 [46]. He also was a general surgeon at the Gheesibai Memorial Mittal Hospital and Research Centre, St. Francis Hospital, Ajmer, Rajasthan, and professor and head of the Department of Surgery at JLN Medical College Ajmer, Rajasthan [47].

Baid served as president of the Association of Surgeons of India (ASI) Rajasthan Chapter and member of the Governing Council of ASI. He was the former vice-president of the Association of Colon and Rectal Surgeons of India (ACSRI) and a member of the International Society of Coloproctology. He is an honorary fellow of the ACSRI [47].

Baid described a bedside method for detecting a pancreatic pseudocyst. He noted that in patients with a Ryle tube (nasogastric tube) (Table 9.1):

> I have noted a physical sign that can help immediately in the clinical diagnosis. A Ryle tube is palpated over the lump in the epigastrium in thin patients suffering from pancreatic cyst because it provides the counter force to the palpating hand, and as the cyst enlarges and becomes tense it pushes the stomach forward. This results in the obliteration of the gastric lumen and the space between the stomach and the parietes [48, p. 1167].

Baid noted that the tube is more likely to be palpated if the cyst is located behind the stomach and in patients with a thin abdominal wall. In patients with a thick abdominal wall, the test is more likely to be negative because the abdominal wall fat impedes the ability to palpate the tube. No studies have evaluated the sensitivity or specificity of this sign.

Table 9.1 Pancreas signs

Name	Year	Description of sign	Significance
Fitz [4]	1889	Sudden, generally severe, and intense gastric or epigastric abdominal pain, vomiting, and sometimes great prostration. Initially, the upper abdomen, especially the epigastrium, is distended, tympanitic, and sensitive. Later, the entire abdomen is moderately swollen, tense, and tympanitic	Acute pancreatitis
Körte (Koerte) [16]	1898	A palpable mass is felt in the epigastrium at the site of the pancreas when the abdominal wall is slack and thin; the stomach and intestines are empty; abdominal distention has improved or is eliminated by gastric lavage; or when the tension in the abdominal muscles has improved or the pain reduced through anesthesia. Pancreatic swelling is also felt when the acute stage of the disease has resolved, and the pain and distention of the epigastrium have subsided	Acute pancreatitis
Halsted [23]	1901	The white print of the fingertips is seen in a slightly cyanosed field just over the site of greatest pain, located slightly above and to the right of the umbilicus	Acute hemorrhagic pancreatitis
Mayo-Robson [28]	1907	Acute inflammation is characterized by a tender spot above and to the right of the umbilicus	Acute pancreatitis
Löwi (Loewi) [35]	1907	In patients with diabetes mellitus installing adrenaline drops in the eyes causes marked pupillary mydriasis	Pancreatic insufficiency
Goblet [36]	1913	Isolated distension of the transverse colon	Necrotizing pancreatitis
Frostberg [38]	1938	Deformity of the descending part of the duodenum, which radiographically assumes the shape of an inverted figure "3"	Inflammatory and benign or malignant process involving the head of the pancreas
Mallet-Guy [41]	1943	The fasting patient is placed in the right lateral decubitus position, with the legs semi-flexed on the abdomen. The tips of the fingers are placed 3–4 cm along the costal margin at the ninth cartilage. The fingers are inserted under the costal arch by depressing the anterior abdominal wall in the lateral direction toward the vertebra. The examiner identifies a palpatory point causing sharp pain, confirming the disease	Chronic pancreatitis
Imrie [45]	1974	Facial flushing without fever	Acute pancreatitis
Baid [48]	1976	A Ryle tube is palpable over the lump in the epigastrium in patients with a thin abdominal wall if the cyst is located behind the stomach	Pancreatic pseudocyst

9.3 Conclusion

Körte, Mayo-Robson, and Mallet-Guy reported three palpatory signs of acute pancreatitis. Körte described a palpatory mass, while Mayo-Robson and Mallet-Guy a tender abdominal point. Advanced computer tomographic imaging and laboratory tests have altered how physicians diagnose this disease. These historical signs shed light and provide a better perspective of how physician diagnosed disease at a time without sophisticated diagnostic tools.

References

1. Portal A. Cours d'anatomie médicale, tome 3. Paris: Baudouin; 1803.
2. Dunglison R. The practice of medicine, or a treatise on special pathology and therapeutics, vol. 2. Philadelphia, PA: Lea & Blanchard; 1842.
3. Birch-Hirschfeld FV. Lehrbuch der pathologischen Anatomie. Leipzig: FCW Vogel; 1895.
4. Fitz RH. Acute pancreatitis: a consideration of pancreatic hemorrhage, hemorrhagic, suppurative, and gangrenous pancreatitis and of disseminated fat-necrosis. Boston, MA: Cupples and Hurd; 1889.
5. [No author]. Reginald Heber Fitz. Bost Med Surg J. 1913;169:625–6.
6. Kelly HA. American medical biographies: Fitz, Reginald Heber (1843–1913). Bost Med Surg J. 1919;180:75–7.
7. Morrison H. Reginald Heber Fitz's contribution to the development of medical education and practice in America. Bull Hist Med. 1951;25:60–5.
8. Morrison H. Reginald Heber Fitz. Bull Hist Med. 1941;10:250–9.
9. [No author]. Deaths. JAMA. 1913;61:1471–2.
10. [No author]. Reginald Heber Fitz. JAMA. 1963;185:210–1.
11. Stone AK. Reginald Heber Fitz. In: Medical papers dedicated to Reginald Heber Fitz. Boston, MA: Boston Medical and Surgical Journal Publications; 1908. p. 7–12.
12. Winkelmann O. Körte, Werner. In: Neue Deutsche Biographie, Bd. 12. Munich: Duncker & Humblot; 1980. p. 395–6.
13. Körte W (1853–1937). Plarr's lives of the fellows. London: Royal College of Surgeons of England; 2013. https://livesonline.rcseng.ac.uk/client/en_GB/lives/search/detailnonmodal/ent:$002f$002fSD_ASSET$002f0$002fSD_ASSET:376508/one?qu=%22rcs%3A+E004325%22&rt=false%7C%7C%7CIDENTIFIER%7C%7C%7CResource+Identifier. Accessed 24 Oct 2022.
14. Körte W. Ein großer Chirurg seiner Zeit. Neuruppin: Berliner Chirurgische Gesellschaft; 2003. https://bchirg.de/2003/08/werner-korte-ein-groser-chirurg-seiner-zeit/. Accessed 16 Oct 2022.
15. Brentano A. Zum Gedächtnis Werner Körtes. Dtsch med Wochenschr. 1937;63:1923.
16. Körte W. Die eitrige Pankreasentzündung, Pankreasabscesse und peripankreatische Eiterung. In: Die chirurgischen Krankheiten und die Verletzungen des Pankreas. Stuttgart: Verlag von Ferdinand Enke; 1898. p. 147–55.
17. [No author]. Obituary: W.S. Halsted MD. Har; FRCS. Eng. and Edin. Br Med J. 1922;2:663.
18. Rankin JS. William Stewart Halsted: a lecture by Dr. Peter D. Olch. Ann Surg. 2006;243:418–25.
19. MacCallum WG. Biographical memoir of William Stewart Halsted, 1852–1922. In: National Academy Biographical Memoirs, vol. 17. Washington, DC: National Academy of Sciences; 1933. p. 151–70.
20. Halsted WS (1852–1922). Plarr's lives of the fellows. London: Royal College of Surgeons of England; 2012. https://livesonline.rcseng.ac.uk/client/en_GB/lives/search/detailnonmodal/

ent:$002f$002fSD_ASSET$002f0$002fSD_ASSET:374280/one?qu=%22rcs%3A+E002097%22&rt=false%7C%7C%7CIDENTIFIER%7C%7C%7CResource+Identifier. Accessed 15 Oct 2022.

21. [No author]. William Stewart Halsted, 1852–1922. Science. 1922;56:461–4.

22. [No author]. Obituary: William Stewart Halsted. Cal State J Med. 1922;20:420.

23. Halsted WS. Retrojection of bile into the pancreas: a cause of acute hemorrhagic pancreatitis. Johns Hopkins Hosp Bull. 1901;12:179–82.

24. [No author]. Sir Arthur Mayo-Robson, KBE, CB. Br Med J. 1933;2:761–2.

25. [No author]. Sir Arthur Mayo-Robson, KBE, CB, CVO, FRCS. Ann R Coll Surg Engl. 1952;11:330–2.

26. Mayo-Robson AW (1853–1933). Plarr's lives of the fellow. London: Royal College of Surgeons of England; 2013. https://livesonline.rcseng.ac.uk/client/en_GB/lives/search/detailnonmodal/ent:$002f$002fSD_ASSET$002f0$002fSD_ASSET:376857/one?qu=%22rcs%3A+E004674%22&rt=false%7C%7C%7CIDENTIFIER%7C%7C%7CResource+Identifier. Accessed 2 Feb 2022.

27. [No author]. Obituary: Arthur William Mayo-Robson, KBE, CB, FRCS. Lancet. 1933;222:948–9.

28. Mayo-Robson AW, Cammidge PJ. The pancreas, its surgery and pathology. Philadelphia, PA: Saunders; 1907.

29. Kuffler SW. Otto Loewi, 1873–1961. J Neurophysiol. 1962;25:451–3.

30. Dale HH. Otto Loewi, 1873–1961. Biogr Mem Fellows R Soc. 1962;8:67–89.

31. Engel M. Loewi, Otto. In: Neue Deutsche Biographie, Bd. 15. Munich: Duncker & Humblot; 1987. p. 108–9.

32. Loewi O. Treccani. 1938. https://www.treccani.it/enciclopedia/otto-loewi/. Accessed 15 Oct 2022.

33. Loewi O. Biographical. The Nobel Prize. https://www.nobelprize.org/prizes/medicine/1936/loewi/biographical/. Accessed 16 Oct 2022.

34. Haas LF. Otto Loewi (1873–1961). J Neurol Neurosurg Psychiatry Res. 2003;74:843.

35. Quadrio RG. Intorno ad un nuovo segno dell'insufficienza pancreatica. Il Policlin. 1908;15:933–5.

36. Goblet J. Beiträge zur akuten Pankreasnekrose. Wien klin Wochenschr. 1913;26:1381–9.

37. Frostberg NJ. Vem är det: Svensk biografisk handbok. 1963. http://runeberg.org/vemar-det/1963/0350.html. Accessed 17 Oct 2022.

38. Frostberg N. A characteristic duodenal deformity in cases of different kinds of peri-vaterial enlargement of the pancreas. Acta Radiol. 1938;19:164–73.

39. Goodman P, Anaya LN, Gourley WK. "Reverse-figure 3" sign in duodenal adenocarcinoma arising in a villous adenoma: radiographic demonstration. Clin Imaging. 1991;15:283–5.

40. Mallet-Guy P. Académie royale de Médecine de Belgique. http://old.armb.be/index.php?id=3567. Accessed 18 Oct 2022.

41. Mallet-Guy P. Le point douloureux sous-costal gauche des pancréatites chroniques. Presse Méd. 1943;13:170–5.

42. Imrie CW. Surgeon. Medical educator. Prabook. https://prabook.com/web/clement_william.imrie/550124. Accessed 10 Oct 2022.

43. [No author]. Editorial Board of the British Journal of Surgery. Br J Surg. 1983;80:409.

44. Glasgow. Imrie criteria for severity of acute pancreatitis. MDCalc. https://www.mdcalc.com/calc/3287/glasgow–imrie–criteria–severity–acute–pancreatitis. Accessed 10 Oct 2022.

45. Imrie CW. Facial flushing in acute pancreatitis. Br Med J. 1974;4:593.

46. Collective. Baid, Jai Chand, MB, BS, MS. In: American College of Surgeons Yearbook. Chicago, IL: American College of Surgeons; 1995. p. 237.

47. Kochar SK. Common surgical emergencies. 2nd ed. New Delhi: Jaypee Brothers Medical Publishers; 2009.

48. Baid JC. Clinical diagnosis of pancreatic tumor. Arch Surg. 1976;111:1167.

Chapter 10
Intra-Abdominal and Diaphragm Signs

10.1   Introduction

Intra-abdominal signs within the abdomen may involve the peritoneum and primarily, or secondarily, the diaphragm. The word "diaphragm" originated from ancient Greek and was used by Galen of Pergamon (129–c. 216 AD) in reference to that structure that partitions the thorax from the abdomen [1]. This chapter includes signs found extra-abdominally that should raise suspicion for an intra-abdominal process (e.g., Oehlecker and Kehr signs) and intra-abdominal processes, including intestinal perforation and hemorrhage, adhesions, ascites, peritonitis, and subphrenic abscess. The signs are listed chronologically, beginning from the earliest date of the discovery. They serve as the method for diagnosis before the advent of computer tomography and ultrasonographic imaging of the abdomen. These signs have not been well studied; thus, their utility in clinical practice remains unknown. They are historically significant as a hands-on approach to diagnosis as they provide the learner with a better understanding and appreciation of the underlying pathophysiologic process.

10.2   Eponymic Signs

10.2.1   Hippocratic Facies (Sign)

Hippocrates (c. 460 BC–c. 370 BC), a Greek physician, was born on the Aegean Island of Cos. Little historical information is available about his life as it is challenging to distinguish which writings were attributed to him since physicians at that time did not sign their works. He is recognized as the "father of medicine," using the constructs of philosophy as the basis for medical diagnosis, separating philosophy from medicine, and cultivating both the art and science of medicine [2, 3].

S. H. Yale et al., *Gastrointestinal Eponymic Signs*,
https://doi.org/10.1007/978-3-031-33673-7_10

Hippocrates described the physical appearance of the patient with acute peritonitis during the agonal state in the *Book of Prognostics* (Table 10.1):

> [f]or if they shun the light, or weep involuntarily, or squint, or if the one be less than the other, or if the white of them be red, livid, or has black veins in it; if there be a gum upon the eyes, if they are restless, protruding, or are become very hollow; and if the countenance be squalid and dark, or the color of the whole face be changed—all these are to be reckoned bad and fatal symptoms. (…) [b]ut if the eyelid be contracted, livid, or pale, or also the lip, or nose, along with some of the other symptoms, one may know for certain that death is close at hand [4, p. 237].

The observations by Hippocrates were used to describe acute and progressive disease, and a "Hippocratic facies" is still used today to describe the morbid appearance of patients in an advanced disease state such as that caused by untreated peritonitis.

10.2.2 *Stokes Sign*

William Stokes (1804–1878) was born in Dublin, Ireland, and received his medical degree from the University of Edinburgh, Scotland, in 1825 [5]. His first appointment was as a physician at the Dublin General Dispensary, followed by Meath Hospital in 1826. He served as president of the King and Queen's College of Physicians of Ireland in 1849 [5, 6].

Stokes was a co-founder of the Pathological Society of Dublin in 1838 and president of the British Medical Association and Royal Irish Academy in 1847 [7]. Among his many honors and accolades, he received an honorary medical degree from the University of Dublin in 1839, a D.C.L. from Oxford, and an L.L.D. from Cambridge and Edinburgh [6]. He was nominated by the crown as a representative of Ireland on the General Medical Council, a position he served from 1858 to 1877, honorary member of the National Institute of Philadelphia, and recipient of the insignia of the Prussian Order of Merit from the Emperor of Germany [6, 8].

He is best recognized for his works titled *A Treatise on the Diagnosis and Treatment of Diseases of the Chest* (1837), *The Diseases of the Heart and Aorta* (1854), and *Lectures on Fever* (1876) [6, 8].

As to a description of his character:

> As a hospital physician and clinical teacher, he was pre-eminent, setting an example to all—colleagues, practitioners, and students alike—of painstaking accuracy and faithfulness. He was remarkable for grace of manner, courtesy, earnestness, and felicity of language. He was a man of taste and literary attainments; and as one who seems to have known and admired him testifies, "his social qualities were of the most genial and agreeable nature; his benevolence was unbounded, and his kindliness of heart and disposition endeared him to all with whom he came in contact." [9, p. 765].

Stokes, in his discussion of enteritis, described the following finding:

> In cases of this kind where the diagnosis depends as much on negative as on positive cir-
> cumstances, it is of importance to have a direct sign by which we may be able to ascertain,
> with some degree of certainty, the existence of a suspected enteric inflammation, and I think
> I have discovered one, which I believe has not been as yet noticed; this is increased pulsa-
> tion of the abdominal vessels [10, p. 181]. From these circumstances I was led to conclude,
> that, in cases of acute inflammation of the digestive tube, there would be increased pulsation
> of the abdominal aorta; and on following up the investigation by examining several persons
> who had distinct and well-marked intestinal inflammation, I found that my conclusions
> were well grounded [10, p. 182]. I drew your attention at my last lecture to the increased
> pulsation of the abdominal aorta and its immediate branches and stated that I look upon this
> as a direct sign of abdominal inflammation. (…) What I wish to draw your attention to, is
> this: where we have this symptom in addition to other signs of inflammation of the digestive
> tube, it is of considerable value as a diagnostic [10, p. 183].

Thus, Stokes sign refers to the marked pulsation of the abdominal aorta and its immediate larger arterial branches in patients with enteritis (Table 10.1).

10.2.3   Duchenne Sign

Guillaume-Benjamin-Amand Duchenne (1806–1875) was born in Boulogne, France, and qualified in medicine from the University of Paris in 1831 [11, 12]. He initially returned to Boulogne as a general practitioner in 1831 and subsequently Paris to pursue further clinical opportunities in 1842 [11–13]. Interestingly, Duchenne never sought out an academic appointment or committees. Duchenne's interests were in electrophysiology and neuromuscular disorders [14, 15]. He described progressive muscular atrophy (Duchenne–Aran disease), glosso-labio-laryngeal paralysis and coined the term pseudo-hypertrophic muscular paralysis and locomotor ataxia [13, 14]. He published *De l'électrisation localisée et de son application à la pathologie et à la thérapeutique* (Localized electrification and its application to pathology and therapy) in 1855 and *Physiologie des mouvements, démontrée à l'aide de l'expérimentation électrique et de l'observation clinique et applicable à l'étude des paralysies et des déformations* (Physiology of movements, demonstrated using electrical experimentation and clinical observation and application to the study of paralysis and deformities) in 1867 [15, 16].

As to his character as described by Collins:

> But the fruit of his labors he submitted with confidence to the medical profession at home
> and abroad, who, not distracted by the sight of the travail or prejudiced by the aggressive-
> ness of the creator, sat in clam judgement upon it and bestowed praise whenever it was
> merited and gave credit whenever it was due. Indeed, there is much in Duchenne that
> reminds of Plato. The self-belief, the equanimity, the desire to abide by the collective judg-
> ment of his fellow men, the willingness to argue his contention with every corner, and his
> abiding faith in his own observations and deductions, all suggest the immortal Æginian [11,
> p. 51]. (…) [h]e combined the moral qualities of perseverance, endurance, and self-reliance,
> which are the possession of some many obscure heroes of the seas for whom the accom-
> plishment of dity is adequate reward. (…) He was independent, ardent, tenacious. These
> were his dominant racial qualities, and they were the foundation of his whole career. He was

not easily discouraged and pursued his research and experiments with a patience and perseverance unbounded [11, p. 54].

Duchenne described a finding observed in the abdomen in cases of diaphragmatic paralysis:

> These are noticeable during respiration and are as follows: At the moment of inspiration the epigastric and hypochondriac regions are depressed although the chest dilates; during expiration, these movements are reversed. When the diaphragm is merely weak these signs are seen only during forced respiration, but during tranquil breathing the bulging of the belly and the expansion of the chest, and vice versa, occur together, as in health. When the diaphragm is palsied on one side only, these signs are seen only on the palsied side. Respiration is quicker than usual, but is without serious difficulty during repose [17, p. 330].

Thus, Duchenne sign refers to the depression of the epigastrium and hypochondrial regions during inspiration in the case of diaphragmatic paralysis (Table 10.1).

10.2.4   Pfuhl–Jaffé Sign

10.2.4.1   Eduard Pfuhl

Johann Eduard Pfuhl (1852–1917) was born in Berszienen (Kirchspiel Grünheide) Insterburg district, Russia, and received his medical degree from Kaiser Wilhelm Academy in 1876 [18]. He was an assistant physician at Mercy Hospital, Königsberg, from 1878 to 1881; professor at the Kaiser Wilhelm Academy from 1886 to 1891, the Institute for Infectious Disease in Berlin from 1891 to 1894, and Strasbourg from 1894 to 1898 [18]. He returned to Kaiser Wilhelm Academy in 1898 where he later served as professor of the Hygienic Chemical Laboratory until 1908 [18].

Pfuhl reported the case of a right-sided pyopneumothorax and a method for distinguishing a subphrenic abscess from pyopneumothorax:

> The following observation concerns a case of purulent exudate, which occurred due to a perforating duodenal ulcer and formed between the convexity of the liver and the lower surface of the right half of the diaphragm. Like liver abscesses and echinococcus tumors, it had risen into the right thoracic space, pushing the diaphragm upwards, the heart upward to the left, and the liver downwards, enlarging the right thoracic space. Eventually, the lungs were perforated, and air leaked into the pus-filled cavity. These conditions caused complex symptoms to develop, consistent with a right-sided pyopneumothorax [19, p. 57]. (…) In the case of a thoracentesis, the behavior of the respiratory movements visible on the manometer should provide a point of reference. Within the pleural space, the pressure falls during inspiration and rises during expiration; accordingly, we see the mercury in the manometer rise on expiration and fall on inspiration. Conversely, findings below the diaphragm behave differently: during inspiration, where the diaphragm descends, the pressure (and thus the mercury) must rise. In our case, unfortunately, not enough attention was paid to this moment because we had no suspicion of an error. Slight respiratory excursion commonly causes only a 2 mm deflection on manometry. It is typically greater, although not consistently, between 3 to 6 mm in patients with pleuritic exudates and at least 10 mm in severe dyspneic movements [19, p. 60].

10.2.4.2   Karl Jaffé

There is limited historical information on Karl Jaffé (1854–1917). Born in Hamburg, Germany, he studied medicine in Hamburg and Strasbourg and practiced gynecology in Hamburg. In 1881 he was an assistant physician at the Hamburg General Hospital [20].

In a lecture delivered to the Hamburg Medical Society on December 14, 1880, Jaffé described two cases of subphrenic abscess extending to the thorax causing a pleural empyema and reported on a physical examination method to distinguish these two entities:

> Next to the history, the physical examination comes into consideration, and it is here that the clinician can prove his reputation as a diagnostician. Suppose we have found an inflammatory exudate in the lower part of the thorax, and the test puncture has revealed a pus-like consistency. The question arises: Is the abscess cavity above or below the diaphragm? (…) Pfuhl drew attention to another physical symptom that can support the diagnosis. During the respiratory movements of the thorax, the pressure conditions in the thoracic cavity must be exactly the opposite of those in the abdominal cavity. In the latter, inspiration produces an increase, and expiration a diminution of pressure. In the thorax, the reverse relationship occurs. If a manometer attached to the puncture cannula is inserted into the abscess, the pressure fluctuations occurring during respiration movements will allow a direct conclusion as to whether the cannula is above or below the diaphragm [21, p. 215].

Thus, Pfuhl–Jaffé sign refers to the increase in manometric pressure during inspiration and the decrease in subdiaphragmatic manometric pressure during expiration in a subphrenic abscess (Table 10.1).

10.2.5   Federici Sign

Cesare Federici (1838–1892) was born at Serravalle di Chienti (Province of Macerata), Italy, and studied medicine at the Universities of Camerino, Bologna, and Florence, Italy [22–24]. He was appointed lecturer on materia medica and clinics at the University of Camerino in 1861, full professor in 1863, and chair of special pathology at the propaedeutic medical clinic in 1886 [22–24]. He was a professor and director of the medical clinic at the University of Palermo in 1870 [22, 23]. Here, he was promoted to professor extraordinary in 1872 and professor ordinary of physic in 1873 [22, 24]. He was elected chair and professor of clinical medicine at the Institute of Higher Studies and Specialization, Florence, in 1883. He was also appointed as director-in-chief of the government's baths at Montecatini [22, 24].

Among his many appointments, he served on the boards of the Superior Council of Public Education; the administrative council of the Hospital of Santa Maria Nuova, and the Provincial Health Council, Florence; and was a member of the town council of which he provided services involving issues related to hygiene, education, and health to Tuscany, Italy [22–24].

A description of his character as articulated by Grocco:

> Precise, clear, and complete in describing and assessing symptoms and distinguishing the experimental from the clinical sciences. He was stringent in diagnostic inductions and could confirm a disease based on vast exceptional knowledge and personal experience. Federici was also likable and impressive, arousing genuine enthusiasm in his pupils. With a candid soul, fierce patriotism, exuberance in family affections, and loyal friendships, Federici left an everlasting impression of himself wherever he went. The proof of this is the strong echo of pain that reverberated from Florence and in every part of Italy at the announcement of his death [24, p. 121].

Federici wrote in his paper titled "Istoria di una rara oppilazione dell'intestino" (History of a rare oppilation of the intestine), regarding the finding he reported in his paper "La propagazione dei suoni del cuore in ordine alla diagnosi fisica dello stomaco" (The propagation of heart sounds in order to the physical diagnosis of the stomaco):

> In my other writing, I distinctly spoke of a precious sign to define the size of the stomach. That is the transmission of heart sounds within an area that is precisely the size of the ventricle. I found that air entering the peritoneal cavity formed a wide space bounded and enclosed by the diaphragm. The air in this space could be heard as perfectly as stomach air. Here is a sign of the clearest evidence for intestinal perforations [25, p. 92–93].

He believed this was caused by air within the peritoneal cavity. However, the pathophysiologic mechanism involves a fluid exudate within the peritoneum. Thus, Federici sign refers to auscultation of normal cardiac sound in the abdomen in intestinal perforation (Table 10.1).

10.2.6 *Thomayer (Toma) Sign*

Josef Thomayer (1853–1927) was born in Trhanov, Domažlice District (today Czech Republic), and received his medical degree from the Charles-Ferdinand University in Prague at Karlova, in 1876 [26–28]. He completed an internship at Garrison Hospital in Prague and was a demonstrator at the Institute for Pathology and Anatomy at the General Hospital. Thomayer was an assistant at Jan Nepomuk Eiselt's (1805–1868) internal medicine clinic, habilitated and appointed head of the first Czech University Polyclinic in 1885, extraordinary professor in 1886, and full professor in 1897 [26–29]. He was head of the second internal clinic of the Faculty of Medicine, Charles-Ferdinand University, Prague, from 1902 to 1921 [26–28].

He wrote literary works under the pseudonym "R.E. Jamot." Thomayer Hospital is named in his honor in the Prague district of Krč. He co-founded *Sborník Vyděčíky* (Collected Papers), first published in 1885 [27, 29].

As to his character as described by Jedlička:

> Thomayer made the polyclinic famous both in terms of medicine and teaching. The polyclinic was highly sought after by patients, as Thomayer devoted much of his energy to it and was there even on Sunday mornings. Medical students also diligently visited the polyclinic. There, the extraordinary didactic talent of Thomayer shone. He lectured in a sonorous voice amid deep silence and with listeners' greatest attention. He was an excellent speaker and

instilled a clear picture of the disease in the brains of his students by drawing attention to the main characteristic signs of the disease, by which it can be more easily recognized [29, p. 554].

Thomayer identified a method for differentiating inflammatory conditions of the peritoneum (e.g., carcinomatosis, tuberculosis) from non-inflammatory conditions (e.g., simple ovarian cysts):

> If we now consider the five cases of carcinoma and three cases of tuberculosis of the peritoneum, which is always filled with more or less copious amounts of fluid, we see a peculiar finding on percussion of the abdominal cavity. Instead of the crescent-shaped muffled area which we find in ordinary ascites without inflammatory complications on the part of the peritoneum over the fluid-filled space, we see in our cases that the dimensions and localization of both the tympanitic and the muffled districts are quite different. In all cases, the tympanitic intestinal sound was predominantly found over the abdomen's right half. In contrast, the dull liquid sound was predominantly found over the abdomen's left half. (…) As has already been remarked and partly explained, the anatomist has not always emphasized this relationship. However, it is certain that in other cases of tuberculosis and carcinomas of the peritoneum, the small intestine loops often stick together due to inflammatory changes in the intestinal serosa and are pushed together like a ball. However, the same changes in the rest of the peritoneum must mean that the intestinal loops, glued together like a ball, are shifted to the right half of the abdomen. It is well-known what changes occur in the mesentery and omentum in both forms of the disease [30, p. 404].

As to the proposed pathogenesis of this clinical and autopsy findings:

> Based on these conditions, it is self-evident why, especially in the case of scirrhous forms of cancer, the lump of the small intestine is shifted more to the right side. In this form of the disease, however, the mesentery often shrinks to an extraordinary degree; consequently, the bundle of small intestine must follow the shrinking mesentery, and as this originates on the right side, the small intestine must then be found more in the right than in the left half, provided that particular circumstances do not prevent it from such displacement. The outpouring of the liquid exudate into the abdominal cavity and the shrinking of the mesentery sometimes happens simultaneously since the liquid exudate, the free ascites fluid, depends on the anatomical changes in the peritoneum. Because of this, it happens that as long as the ascites fluid is not extraordinarily copious and does not owe its formation to the compression of blood vessels, the effusion surrounds the loops of the small intestine and, as they are displaced to the right, accumulates primarily on the left. Based on these conditions, it is clear that under such circumstances, the result of percussion is different from that in ordinary free ascites. Although the preceding arguments concern only carcinoma of the peritoneum, the same applies, mutatis mutandis, to tuberculosis. In tuberculous peritonitis, shrinking processes occur both in the omentum and mesentery, resulting in the loops of the small intestine experiencing a fate similar to that of carcinoma. For this reason, the schemes showing the percussion ratios are very similar and analogous in both diseases [30, p. 405–406].

Thus, Thomayer (Toma) sign refers to the findings of tympanitic sounds on percussion located over the right side and dullness to percussion on the left side of the abdomen in patients with tuberculosis peritonitis and peritoneal carcinoma (Table 10.1). Contraction of the mesentery causes the intestines to be drawn to the right causing a tympanic percussion sound. At the same time, ascitic fluid collects on the left side of the abdomen, causes a dull percussion sound.

10.2.7   Clark Sign

Alonzo Clark (1807–1887) was born in Chester, Massachusetts, USA, and received his medical degree from the College of Physicians and Surgeons (currently Columbia University Vagelos College of Physicians and Surgeons), New York City, in 1835. He was an intern at the New York Hospital until 1837 and studied abroad in London and Paris in 1837 [31–34].

Clark was appointed professor of pathology and materia medica at the University of Vermont Medical School, Burlington [31, 34]. He served as chair of physiology and pathology at the College of Physicians and Surgeons from 1848 to 1885, as visiting physician at Bellevue Hospital, New York City, in 1847 (later consulting physician), and as professor and chair of pathology and practical medicine at the College of Physicians and Surgeons from 1855 to 1885 [31–33]. He was appointed the dean and president of the College of Physicians and Surgeons from 1875 to 1885. He also served as consulting physician at St. Luke's and Roosevelt Hospitals in New York City [34].

He was a member of the pathological society and was elected president of the New York Academy of Medicine and State Medical Association in 1853 [31, 34]. The Alonzo Clark Scholarship Fund was established as a memorial endowment at the College of Physicians and Surgeons [35].

His character as described by Delafield:

> In looking back over Dr. Clark's life, it seems to me that, perhaps, one of its most useful results was the influence it exerted on the medical profession. Here was a man whom everyone knew, who had attained to the highest honors in the profession, and the largest success in practice, and yet no one could accuse him of a mean or an unworthy act-no man was his enemy. He shunned publicity and notoriety in every form; medical politics were unknown to him; he appeared but rarely in the medical societies or the journals; and yet everything came to him. He never tried to do anything but to learn all he could about the science and art of medicine, and to communicate this knowledge to others; and behold, honors, practice, wealth, were added to him. How many a struggling and discouraged physician had looked at Dr. Clark and taken heart once more to walk in the narrow and straight way of integrity [33, p. 124].

As described by Elliot:

> His commanding and graceful presence, his pleasant manners, his mastery of the English language, his distinct and elegant enunciation, the knowledge of his subject, apparently inexhaustible, and his scholarly methods, command instant and persistent attention [36, p. 501].

In Clark's discussion of intestinal perforation in typhoid fever, he reported:

> Suddenly severe pain sets in, oftenest in the lower part of the abdomen, and spreads rapidly; the pulse is quickly accelerated and becomes small. And it has been lately stated that in this and other intestinal perforations the gases of the bowels, escaping into the peritoneal cavity will give resonance to percussion over the lower part of the liver [37, p. 1136].

Thus, Clark sign represents resonance on percussion over the lower hepatic region in cases of intestinal perforation and intraperitoneal air (Table 10.1).

10.2.8 Fürbringer Sign

Paul Walther Fürbringer (Fuerbringer) (1849–1930) was born in Delitzsch, Prussian Province of Saxony, near Leipzig, and studied medicine in Jena and Berlin, Germany [38]. He was an assistant in the Pathological Institute under the aegis of W. Müller in Jena from 1872 to 1874 and assistant to Nikolaus Friedreich (1825–1882) at the clinics of the University of Heidelberg, Germany [38].

Fürbringer habilitated in pharmacology and medicinal chemistry in 1876 and was appointed extraordinary professor and chief of the district polyclinic in Jena in 1879 [38]. He was a professor of dermatology at the University of Jena in 1883 and director of the Municipal Hospital at Friedrichshain, Berlin, from 1886 to 1903 [38–40]. Fürbringer was appointed to the Geheimrat (Privy Medical Councilor) in Berlin in 1890 and was a member of the Royal Medical College of the province of Brandenburg from 1890 to 1921 [38, 39].

During a discussion on subphrenic abscesses, Fürbringer commented that:

> The presence of a serous exudate in an upper and a purulent in a lower intercostal space on puncture is a valuable finding for diagnosing a subphrenic pyothorax but is not pathognomonic. Redner observed the same in two cases on autopsy, which later revealed multilocular pleurisy. Critical in diagnosis is the aspiration of pus after the puncture needle has passed the diaphragm or when the needle moves during respiration [41, p. 288].

Thus, Fürbringer sign refers to the movement of the subdiaphragmatic portion of the needle upward during inspiration and downward during expiration (Table 10.1).

10.2.9 Bolognini Sign

Pirro Bolognini (1860–1918) was born in Bologna, Italy, and received his medical degree from the University of Bologna in 1855 [42, 43]. He was appointed assistant at the Major Hospital of Bologna and physician at the Condotta di Borgo, Panigale, where he taught in the pediatric clinic in 1902 [42]. During World War I, he was a medical lieutenant of the Italian Red Cross stationed at Rovigo and Bologna and director of the Military Hospitals [43]. He was appointed colonel in Bari and inspector of the province of the department of the Red Cross [42, 44].

Bolognini served as director of the Civic Hospital, Rovigo, in 1913 [44]. He was president of the Polesana section of the National Association of Hospital Doctors and honorary president of the Order of Midwives. He was also the founder of the Italian Society of Pediatrics [44].

As described by his colleague:

> He was a man of great ingenuity, a good soul, endowed with profound culture. He leaves some valuable works in general medicine and pediatrics. He was generally loved and esteemed [42, p. 209].

Bolognini described in 1895 a finding occurring in patients during the prodromal phase and disappearing with the onset of the cutaneous eruption in measles. He emphasized that during the maneuver, the physician should attempt to calm the patient to avoid abdominal muscle contraction:

> The patient is placed in a supine position with the thighs flexed to relax the abdominal muscles. Place the hands on the abdomen using the three middle fingers, alternate between the hands light touch followed by increasing pressure. A tactile thrill is felt, giving the impression that rubbing is occurring under the fingers, slightly produced by two rough surfaces sliding over each other. The sensation is not uniform throughout the abdomen and is only detectable in specific abdominal regions. Sometimes the rubbing is restricted to a specific point on the abdomen. The rubbing may be present for only a brief period. It is difficult to reproduce the phenomenon where it was previously found. In order to prolong the detection of this finding, especially for those performing this maneuver for the first time, it is recommended that only slight pressure be initially applied because by applying increasing pressure, the sensation will disappear [45, p. 111].

Bolognini reported that the finding was present in 198 of 200 children examined with measles.

He postulated that the finding was caused by an exanthema on the serosa of the visceral and parietal peritoneum. Thus, Bolognini sign refers to the presence of a tactile thrill over the middle finger in patients with peritoneal inflammation caused by measles (Table 10.1).

10.2.10   Cushing Sign

Harvey Williams Cushing (1869–1939) was born in Cleveland, Ohio, USA, and received his medical and master's degrees from Harvard Medical School in 1895 with cum laude [46, 47]. He was a surgical house staff at Massachusetts General Hospital from 1895 to 1896 and subsequently at Johns Hopkins Hospital under the aegis of William S. Halsted (1852–1922) from 1896 to 1900 [46–49]. He studied abroad at the physiology laboratories of Emil Theodor Kocher (1841–1917) and Hugo Kronecker (1839–1914) in Berne, Switzerland, and Charles Scott Sherrington (1857–1952) in Liverpool, England. Upon his return to Johns Hopkins, he established the Hunterian Laboratory in honor of John Hunter (1728–1793) from 1900 to 1912 [46–48]. He was appointed associate professor of neurosurgery in 1903, ascending to the rank title of Moseley professor of surgery at Harvard Medical School and surgeon-in-chief at Peter Bent Brigham Hospital in 1912 [46–48, 50].

He served during World War I, initially with the French Army at the American Ambulance Hospital, Paris, at the United States Base Hospital No. 5 from 1917 to 1919, neurosurgery consultant to the Royal Army Medical Corps, Camiers and Boulogne, and subsequently, the medical headquarters of the American Expeditionary Force [46–48].

After mandatory retirement, he accepted a position as Sterling professor of neurology at Yale University from 1933 to 1937 and subsequently as director of studies in the history of medicine [46–48, 50].

He founded the Society of Neurological Surgeons [48]. Among his many awards and accomplishments, he received the United States Distinguished Service Medal, from Great Britain; the Order of Companion of Bath; and France, officer of the Legion of Honor, for his service during the war [47, 48]. He received numerous honorary degrees, including the Doctor of Science and Law. Notably, he was elected an honorary fellow of the Royal College of Physicians, London, and the Royal College of Surgeons, England, in 1917 [46, 47]. He received the Cameron Prize from the University of Edinburgh in 1924 and Lister Medalist from the Royal College of Surgeons, England, in 1930. He was elected president of the American College of Surgeons in 1922, the American Neurological Association in 1923, and the American Surgical Association in 1927 [46, 47].

As to his character as described by MacCallum:

> In Harvey Cushing everyone recognized a person of brilliant intellect and of great personal charm. His influence upon all who came in contact with him was deep and inspiring and especially to his students and associates this had a lasting effect upon their lives. His extreme and rigid dominance over his assistants during his operations was only part of his care for the welfare of his patients and throughout the course of their illness under his supervision his devotion to their every comfort and attention to their slightest needs for the sake of their successful recovery was part of his profound interest in their good [47, p. 53].

As described in an editorial:

> Essentially an aristocrat and a perfectionist, he always evinced the highest sense of obligation to his profession, and if his critical attitude, which tolerated nothing but the best, was difficult for some colleagues from time to time it was magnificently good for the world at large. Imbued with great vitality and enormous energy, he became the foremost surgeon of his day, a master-teacher, a profound and prolific investigator, and the most accomplished medical writer in our country [49, p. 623].

Among his many accomplishments and contributions to medicine and surgery, his name is undoubtedly best known in association with pituitary dysfunction or Cushing disease.

Cushing described a finding occurring during the early stage of typhoid fever:

> A sudden acute onset of increased abdominal pain is an all-important symptoms which unfortunately may be absent or owing to a patient's stupor be overlooked. Any complaint of pain, however, of less abrupt onset, associated with tenderness, must arouse the greatest suspicion on the part of the attendant. I cannot but believe that the condition which has been spoken of above as a pre-perforative stage of ulceration often exists. A little localized inflammation of the serosa, with or without the passage of microorganisms and leading to a slight adhesive peritonitis, usually of omentum, can give rise to these symptoms and produce an associated slight leucocytosis. This is precisely analogous to what occurs in the pre-perforative stage of appendicitis, which, however, is of less urgent nature because in the case of appendix which is fixed and does not move about freely in the general cavity, as do the coils of ileum, the adhesions are less likely to be dislocated and a general peritonitis, which would result from this separation, is avoided [51, p. 266].

Thus, Cushing sign refers to sudden non-fixed pain in the abdomen during the pre-perforation stage of small bowel perforation (Table 10.1).

10.2.11 Strauss Sign

Hermann Strauss (1868–1944) was born in Heilbronn am Neckar, Germany, studied medicine at the Universities of Würzburg and Berlin, and received his doctorate in Berlin in 1890 [52–54]. In 1893 he worked at the Medical University Hospital, and from 1895 to 1906, he served as a senior physician at the Berlin University III. Medical Clinic of Charité, Berlin [52]. At Kaiserin-Augusta Hospital in Berlin, Strauss trained and conducted digestive physiology research with Carl Anton Ewald (1845–1915) at the Medical University Clinic in Giessen under the auspices of Franz Riegel (1843–1904) from 1893 to 1895 [53, 54]. He was appointed assistant and senior physician at the III. Medical Clinic and polyclinic at Charité, Berlin, under Hermann Senator (1834–1911) from 1895 to 1905 [53, 54]. Strauss habilitated with the medical faculty at the Friedrich Wilhelm University of Berlin in internal medicine in 1897 and was appointed a professor extraordinarius at the University of Berlin from 1902 to 1934. He was relieved of all office duties, prohibited from teaching, and had his medical license revoked under National Socialism in 1938 [53–55]. In 1906, he established a private polyclinic and, in 1910, served as chief physician of internal medicine at the Jewish Hospital in Berlin. Beginning in 1910, he served as director of the Department of Internal Medicine at the Jewish Hospital in Berlin and was appointed to the Privy Medical Council [53]. The Gestapo deported him to the Theresienstadt ghetto, Terezin, in 1942 [53, 56]. Here he was a member of the Council of Elders and head of the science committee in the concentration camp's health care service [53].

Among his many outstanding accomplishments, he developed an intravenous venous cannula (Strauss cannula) in 1898, introduced a low-salt diet to treat renal insufficiency, and designed the Strauss proctosigmoidoscope for examination of the rectum and sigmoid in 1903 [52, 53]. He was appointed head physician in the Department of Internal Medicine at the Jewish Hospital in Berlin from 1910 to 1942 [53]. Among his other accolades, he served as congress president of the Hufeland Society for Digestive and Metabolic Disease and was decorated with the Iron Cross for his service to his country during World War I [56]. He was co-editor of *Archiv für Verdauungs-Krankheiten* (Digestive Diseases Archives) in 1910 [53].

In his discussion of an operative case of carcinoma of the stomach, Strauss remarked:

> Carcinoma metastases were found in the liver, retroperitoneal tissue, and Douglas pouch; the latter was the site where we repeatedly found metastases. Consideration should be made to investigate this site because it is commonly found and readily accessible for digital exploration [57, p. 584–585].

In 1899 he again spoke of a diagnostic method for detecting metastatic gastric carcinoma in cases where pathognomonic symptoms are absent:

> I have already pointed out earlier that it is possible to detect cancerous nodules in the Cavum Douglasii as an early or sole metastasis in isolated cases. In the meantime, I have again observed two cases of this kind, of which one was of particular interest because only

by the detection of metastases in Douglas' space could the differential diagnosis be made between gastric ulcer and carcinoma ventriculi (ex ulcere natum) [58, p. 874].

Thus, palpating a mass in the pouch of Douglas during a rectal exam suggests metastatic gastric carcinoma (Table 10.1). We are unaware of any studies evaluating this sign's sensitivity or specificity.

10.2.12   Landau Sign

Leopold Landau (1848–1920) was born in Warsaw, Poland, and studied medicine at the Universities of Breslau, Würzburg, and Berlin and received his medical degree from the University of Berlin in 1870 [59, 60]. He was an assistant surgeon during the Franco-Prussian War from 1870 to 1871. He habilitated and was an assistant to Otto Spiegelberg (1830–1881) at the clinic for gynecology and obstetrics at the University of Breslau in 1872 and became an associate professor in 1874 [59–62]. He was a faculty member at the University of Berlin in 1876, titular professor in 1893, appointed as the Privy Medical Councilor in 1895, and an assistant professor in 1902 [59–62].

Landau was elected member in 1894, deputy chairman in 1919, and an honorary member of the Berlin Medical Society in 1918 [60, 62]. He served as an alderman of Berlin's City Council in 1901 and founded the Berlin Academy for the Science of Judaism [59, 60, 62].

As to his character:

> A very popular academic teacher, he has trained many students over the years who have taken his teachings around the world. Despite his great practical and scientific activity, he always found time to participate in the social endeavors of doctors. A rich, industrious life came to an end with the death of Leopold Landau. But what he created will remain in our science for all time [61, p. 128].

Landau described a novel sign for the early detection of ascites in females (Table 10.1, Fig. 10.1):

> The sign consists of the inability to grasp the uterus in the usual or pathognomonic way, even with a small amount of free fluid. With the patient in a horizontal position, the fingers of the two palpating hands do not meet on the sides of the uterus. The slightly depressed uterus feels to the palpating fingers as if it were lying on a cushion of air or water. If the patient is examined with the pelvis elevated and the abdominal wall relaxed as much as possible by adduction of the thighs and flexion of the knees bimanual examination provides a different result. Now the fingers meet on the side of the uterus so it can be grasped. The findings on bimanual palpation have entirely changed since the fluid directly flows toward the diagram when the pelvis is elevated [63, p. 1202].

Thus, Landau sign refers to the method for identifying ascitic fluid in the abdomen in women.

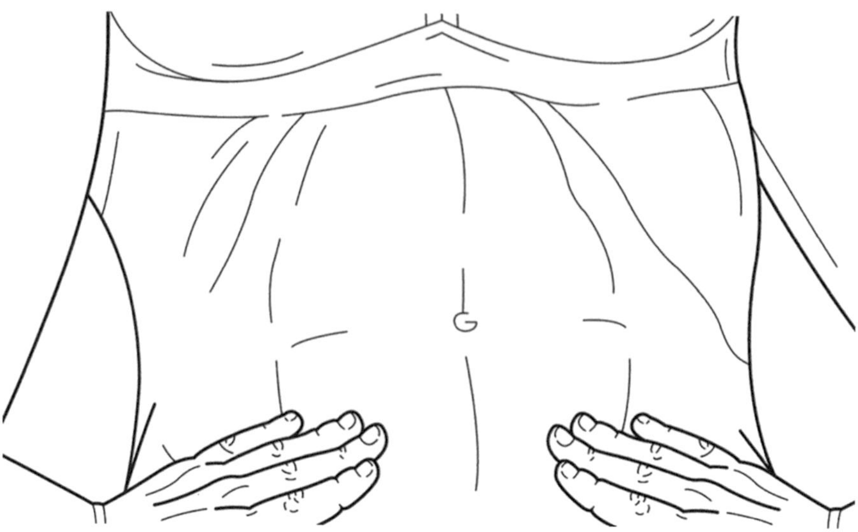

Fig. 10.1 Landau sign (by Ryan Yale)

10.2.13 Lennander Sign

Karl Gustaf (Gustav) Lennander (1857–1908) was born in Kristianstad, Sweden, and received medical training at the University of Uppsala and Karolinska Institute and Serafimerlasarettet (Seraphim Hospital), Stockholm [64, 65]. He served as an associate professor in surgery and obstetrics at the University of Upsala, Sweden, in 1888, was appointed professor of surgery at the University of Uppsala in 1891, and subsequently chief surgeon of the Uppsala Hospital [64, 65].

Lennander was an honorary fellow of the Royal College of Surgeons in 1900 and recipient of the Doctor of Law from the University of Edinburgh [64–66]. Among his many awards and honors, he was a member of the Swedish Academy of Science, Science and Academy Society of Gothenburg in 1902, and the Royal Academy of Sciences in 1905.

As to his character:

> At Uppsala and in his operating theatre, one came to know the man fully. Of medium height and figure, his head first caught the eye and called forth admiration of its massive powerfulness. Brusque in manner and careful of words, he lacked the polish of the Swede and reminded one somewhat of the Norwegian type of Scot. The testimony of his patients showed that he never lacked kindliness and consideration. (…) He was a good teacher, and his clinic was always well attended [64, p. 1086].

Lennander observed in patients with peritonitis (Table 10.1):

> A large number of diffuse as well as circumscribed infections of the peritoneum during their course occur without elevation of temperature. Usually, however, there is a temperature elevation. In order to detect it with certainty, the temperature must be measured in the rectum. In fact, the axillary temperature is often abnormally low. The difference between the temperature in the rectum and the axilla, which under normal conditions is about 0.6 °C,

can be much greater in peritonitis. As a rule, the larger it is, the worse the patient's general condition when the temperature is taken. A large difference in temperature between the rectum and axilla is, in most cases, is due to collapse with feeble blood flow in the skin, not infrequently in conjunction with profuse sweating ("cold sweat"). It is not uncommon for the difference to be 2-3 times or more degrees when death is imminent. Simultaneous measurement in the axilla and the rectum can therefore be of great importance from a prognostic point of view. (…) Even an insignificant rise in temperature can be of great diagnostic importance. If you suspect organ perforation and diffuse peritonitis without having a clear picture, you must measure it every hour. In such cases, an increase in the temperature of the rectum by a few tenths of a degree and increasing sensitivity to pressure on palpation from the rectum establish the diagnosis of diffuse peritonitis [67, p. 35–36].

As stated by Propping:

It is known that Madelung was the first to point out that one could diagnose peritonitis by comparing the temperature of the axilla with that of the rectum. The difference in suppurative peritonitis is always greater than normal and can even go up to 1.5°. Considering the extreme importance of a symptom with such reliability, the often-difficult diagnosis of peritonitis can be established with certainty. However, no agreement has yet been reached, and there has been no confirmation of this temperature change. While Lennander in 1893 regarded the abnormal temperature difference as pathognomonic for purulent peritonitis with exudation in the lower part of the abdomen, he also found in 1901 that the difference between the rectal and axillary temperatures was not frequently significantly greater than usual [68, p. 506].

Thus, Madelung and Lennander sign srefer to the difference between the axillary and rectal temperatures in peritonitis.

10.2.14 Bryant Sign

John Henry Bryant (1876–1906) was born in Ilminster, Somerset, England, and received his bachelor of medicine and bachelor of science degrees from Guy Hospital in 1890 with the distinction of earning first-class honors, a gold medal in medicine, first-class honors in forensic medicine, and a medical degree in 1891 [69–71]. He was appointed house physician and resident obstetric assistant, elected medical register from 1892 to 1898, and subsequently assistant physician to Guy Hospital [69–71]. Bryant was appointed demonstrator of morbid anatomy in 1899 and lecturer on materia medica and therapeutics in 1903. He was the co-editor of *Guy's Hospital Reports* [69–71]. He received fellowship in the Royal College of Physicians in 1901 [69].

As to his character:

As a physician the same conscientious care and thoroughness characterized his work in all departments. In the investigation of cases his systematic method enabled him often to come to definite conclusions where haphazard work would have signally failed. His knowledge of the world too, was not the least of his assets as a consultant enabling him at all times to take a human interest in his patients quite apart from their professional aspect. It was no doubt this trait in his characters which endeared him to patients, for although, a man of few words, he had a large fund of sympathy, which showed itself in many small unostentatious ways. (…) Always strenuously opposing deceit in any form, he said freely what he thought, perhaps sometimes to his own detriment, and he always pursued the course which he considered right. It would be hard to find a man of more upright character, who ran straight at all times, and thus endeared himself to everyone who really knew him [69, p. 1319].

Bryant described a series of patients with abdominal aortic aneurysms. He reported:

> In one case blood was effused into the right spermatic cord, and the corresponding half of the scrotum was much ecchymosed [72, p. 75]. When blood is extravasated into the anterior abdominal wall ecchymosis may appear, and in one case which I have already mentioned, in which blood was effused into the spermatic cord, the scrotum on the same side became much ecchymosed [72, p. 79].

Thus, Bryant sign refers to scrotal ecchymosis caused by intra-abdominal hemorrhage (Table 10.1).

10.2.15 Morel Sign

There is limited historical information on Louis Morel (1876–?). He was an intern at the Hospitals of Paris in 1904, appointed agrégé in 1926, and was a professor at the Faculty of Medicine, Toulouse, France [73–75].

Morel described an observation found in a patient with intraperitoneal rupture of the bladder:

> We noticed a second peculiarity: instantaneousness engorgement of the bladder, which should be sought in the following way: The wounded lying down is probed; the catheter brings back a certain amount of urine and empties the bladder. The injured person is then asked to stand and remain upright for a few minutes. He is then put back down and probed a second time. The bladder fills again through the intraperitoneal effusion with a quantity equal to the first evacuation withdrawn. This observed finding occurs because the urine, which leaves the bladder freely through the ruptured bladder, reenters it with the same capacity and manner as to fill the urinary reservoir with urine collected in the small pelvis by standing. The urine collects in the iliac fossae and between the intestinal loops [74, p. 809–810].

Thus, Morel sign refers to intraperitoneal fluid filling the bladder in the standing position after the bladder is emptied in bladder rupture (Table 10.1).

10.2.16 Kehr Sign

Johannes Otto Kehr or Hanes Kehr (1862–1916) was born in Waltershausen, Thuringia, Germany, and received his medical training in Freiburg, Halle, Berlin, and Jena, and his medical degree from the latter in 1885 [76, 77]. He was appointed assistant to Ernst Meusel (1843–1914) in Gotha and continued his surgical training with Eduard Albert (1841–1900) and Theodor Billroth (1829–1894), earning the

Specialist for Surgery and Orthopedics degrees in 1888. He was a surgeon in a private clinic in Halberstadt, a professor in 1895, and a privy councilor in 1905. He later moved and worked at the private clinic of Ernst Unger (1875–1938) in Berlin in 1910 [76, 77]. In 1913, he published his two-volume book *Die Praxis der Gallenwege Chirurgie in Wort und Bild* (The Practice of Bile Duct Surgery in Words and Pictures) [78]. His most significant contributions were in the surgical management of gallbladder and biliary diseases.

Kehr sign has traditionally been described as pain in the left shoulder associated with splenic rupture. Klimpel, in a review of the literature, found a lack of compelling evidence that this sign should be attributed to Johannes Otto Kehr (1862–1916) [79]. We found on the contrary, upon further review of the literature, that Kehr stated in his discussion on splenic rupture in *Handbuch der praktischen Chirurgie* (Manual of Practical Surgery):

> There is no pathognomonic symptom for injuries to the spleen. In contusions, pain and enlargement of the spleen are typical symptoms. When rupture occurs, all other signs and symptoms of internal bleeding are less critical. In subcutaneous injury, the affected person usually experiences pain, initially on the left side, quickly spreading to the entire abdomen. The signs of collapse (pronounced pallor, small pulse, feeling cold and faint) appear. In rare cases, the injured person does not experience anything from splenic rupture, and collapse may not be present. Left shoulder pain is not common. Other manifestations involve the lungs, heart, and larynx (hoarse voice up to complete lack of voice). The latter indicates an alteration of the vagus involving the splenic plexus through the semilunar ganglion [80, p. 689].

Levy referenced Kehr's publication on splenic injuries and left shoulder pain symptoms and presented the case of a 29-year-old man with internal hemorrhage secondary to splenic injury and severe left shoulder pain, emphasizing its diagnostic significance [81].

Interestingly, Kehr, in his book *Introduction to the Differential Diagnosis of the Separate Forms of Gallstone Disease*, described a patient with recurrent cholecystitis or cholangitis (accompanying inflammatory jaundice), adhesive peritonitis, and adhesions between the gallbladder and omentum or colon, and "with this several attacks of colic and inflammation in the left-shoulder-joint" [82]. He also reported, "The pain of gallstone colic is more to the right and localized in the gallbladder region, whence it frequently radiates to the back, and the right should blade and breast" [82].

A study by Lowenfels (1966) showed that nine out of ten patients with splenic rupture had a positive Kehr sign at presentation [83]. Studies reported this sign in patients with splenic abscess, spontaneous phrenic artery rupture, infectious mononucleosis, and following colonoscopy [84–90]. Irritation of the diaphragm by the abdominal contents, including free blood, results in the transmission of pain sensation through the phrenic nerve to the C3-C4 nerve roots. The supraclavicular nerve supplying the left shoulder shares the origin with the phrenic nerve innervating the diaphragm; thus, pain is referred to as the left shoulder [83, 84]. There are no studies that defined the sensitivity and specificity of this sign.

Thus, Kehr sign refers to pain in the left shoulder in splenic rupture (Table 10.1).

10.2.17 Barnard Sign

Harold Leslie Barnard (1868–1908) was born in Highbury, London, England, and received his bachelor of medicine degree from the University of London with first-class honors; fellowship from the Royal College of Surgeons of England in 1895; and master of science degree in 1896 [91–94]. He was appointed sequentially as senior dresser to outpatients, receiving room officer; house physician, and house surgeon at the London Hospital to Drs. Samuel Fenwick (1821–1902) and Edwin Hurry Fenwick (1856–1944), respectively; surgical registrar in 1897; assistant demonstrator of anatomy; demonstrator of physiology to Leonard Hill (1866–1952) in 1897; and surgical tutor in 1899 [91–93].

He held a full-time staff appointment and was an assistant at the surgical office at the Metropolitan Hospital until 1900, followed by serving as a surgical tutor at the London Hospital from 1900 to 1904. His last position was demonstrator of surgical pathology and surgeon in charge of outpatients at the London Medical School and Hospital in 1907 [91–93].

His character as described by Hill:

> Mr. Barnard was a man of enormous mental energy, which continually carried him beyond his bodily strength. His enthusiasm for his profession, his untiring zeal, have I fear led to the great loss we have sustained by his early death. He was a man possessed with the simple faith of living a life devoted to his work and the search after truth, and his great spirit has overdriven a body too frail for the tasks he set it [91, p. 539].

With Leonard Hill they described the armlet method of determination of blood pressure by the sphygmomanometer, the technique simultaneously described by Riva Rocci [94].

Barnard defined the clinical features of a subphrenic abscess:

> The abdominal swelling formed by a subphrenic abscess does not descend on respiration, because it is adherent. The part of the swelling formed by peritoneal adhesions is rigid, tender, and dull on percussion. The part formed by pus in contact with the abdominal wall is scarcely tender, bulges and fluctuates, and is dull on percussion [95, p. 432].

In his description of the temperature:

> Pyrexia was always present. As a rule, it was low (100 to 101), sustained and rocked night and morning. In several cases, however, it frequently reached normal, and was never above 100 F. These cases were well localized or had ruptured into the stomach or intestines. On the other hand, in the diffuse and a cause stages temperatures as high as 104 to 105 F, were often recorded [95, p. 431].

Thus, Barnard sign refers to the absence of pain and hectic temperature in some patients with subphrenic abscesses (Table 10.1).

10.2.18 Blumer Sign

George Blumer (1872–1962) was born in Darlington, County Durham, England, and received his medical degree from Cooper Medical College (Leland Stanford University), San Francisco, in 1891 [96–99]. He completed an internship at San

Francisco City and County Hospitals and became a surgical officer and house officer while conducting postgraduate work in bacteriology and pathology at Johns Hopkins Hospital until 1893. He was appointed assistant to the surgical staff under William Stewart Halsted (1852–1922) and then Sir William Osler (1849–1919) from 1893 to 1895, followed by an assistantship in the Department of Pathology under William Henry Welch (1850–1934) from 1895 to 1896 [96–99]. He was director of the Bender Hygienic Laboratory in Albany, New York, from 1896 to 1903 [96, 100].

He served on the faculty initially as an adjunct professor, followed by a professor of pathology and bacteriology at Albany Medical College until 1903 [99]. While in Albany, he also maintained positions as a pathologist at St. Peter's and Childs' Hospitals, Cohoes Hospitals in Cohoes, New York; Troy and Samaritan Hospital in Troy, New York; and director of the Bureau of Pathology and Bacteriology for the New York State Board of Health [98].

He was an associate professor of pathology at Cooper Medical College San Francisco from 1904 to 1905 and an assistant in the medical schools at the University of California from 1905 to 1906 [98, 99]. Blumer was appointed the John Slade Ely professor of theory and practice medicine from 1906 to 1910 and subsequently dean of the Yale Medical School beginning in 1910 and named the David P. Saith professor of clinical medicine at Yale University Medical School in 1920. He was the director of the New Haven Hospital and Dispensary [96–99].

In a paper read before the Troy and Vicinity Medical Association on April 6, 1909, Blumer reported:

> The sign which I wish to bring to your attention is one which I have been observing for the past two or three years. It is not, as I shall presently show you, a new sign, but for some reason it seems never to have gotten into the textbooks, and scarcely at all into the periodical literature. I prefer to call it the rectal shelf because that best describes its feel [101, p. 362–363]. (…) It is evident from these observations that under certain conditions malignant neoplasms within the abdomen metastasize to Douglas pouch and that in certain inflammatory conditions of an infectious nature the infective agent may set up marked localized changes in the same region. (…) The effect of this malignant or inflammatory infiltration of Douglas' cul-de-sac is the formation of the palpable rectal tumor which I have described as the rectal shelf [101, p. 363].

Blumer described the method for examination of the rectal shelf:

> If one passes the finger into the rectum in these cases the lower portion of the bowel is usually normal, it is not until the prostate gland has been passed that any abnormality is detected. Just above the prostate in some cases, in others at the limit of palpability, 2 to 4 cm above, if the finger is passed along the anterior rectal wall it impinges upon a shelf of almost cartilaginous feel which projects into the rectal cavity. In some cases, further palpation shows that the whole rectum is involved in an annular zone of infiltration more marked anteriorly and tapering off toward the posterior wall, a signet ring stricture, as Schnitzler calls it. In such cases the infiltration is no longer confined to Douglas' pouch but has involved the submucosa of the rectum in which the new formation may spread quite widely. The infiltrated area is more or less fixed, it is shelf-like or peg-like, at the most prominent portion, and there is no ulceration of the mucous membrane over it. The lack of ulceration of the overlying mucosa, together with the peculiar shape, is what distinguished the rectal shelf from a primary rectal neoplasm [101, p. 364–365].

Thus, Blumer sign refers to the palpable, fixed, rectal shelf signifying a malignant or infiltrative process occurring at the pouch of Douglas (Table 10.1).

10.2.19　Brown Sign

Alfred Jerome Brown (1878–1960) was born in New York, USA, and studied medicine at the College of Physicians and Surgeons of Columbia University (currently Columbia University Vagelos College of Physicians and Surgeons) in 1903 [102–105]. He completed an internship at Presbyterian Hospital, New York City, from 1903 to 1905 and was an assistant in surgery at Columbia University College of Physicians and Surgeons. This was followed by appointments as surgical director of the first surgical division at Columbia University Division of Bellevue Hospital, New York, and assistant at Presbyterian Hospital and Vanderbilt Clinic Dispensaries [103, 104]. Brown was a visiting surgeon at New York and New Jersey Orthopedic Hospitals, assistant surgeon lieutenant junior grade first battalion in 1906, and assistant in anatomy in 1909 [104–107].

During World War I, Brown was an instructor in the War Department Surgeon General's Office and major in the United States Army as chief of the surgical service at Debarkation Hospital in Staten Island, New York, and the Base Hospital at Brest, France, chief of surgical services and consulting surgeon from 1917 to 1919 [102, 104].

Brown was appointed assistant professor to the College of Medicine at the University of Nebraska in 1919 and was a professor of surgery from 1934 to 1943 [102, 105]. He was also a division, district, or local surgeon to four railroads and a physician to the Federal Security Board of the United States and Civil Service Commission [104].

Brown was president of the Western Surgical Association, Omaha-Douglas County Medical Society, and Omaha Midwest Clinical Society. He was a member of many other surgical and medical societies and organizations [104, 105].

His character as described by R.R. Best:

> Dr. Brown was the author of many articles in the field of general surgery and frequently these publications as well as basic statements on the embryology or anatomy pertaining to the subject. Students, internes, residents, and younger surgeons had a tremendous admiration for and remembrance of this quality, so readily noted in lectures, conferences and during ward rounds. His memory was phenomenal and once he saw, read, or heard, he never forgot. In spite of this mass of information pertaining to history, anatomy and embryology, he was not one to take the floor at a meeting and relate his knowledge, and he seldom openly criticized or corrected a misstatement by others [104, p. 348].

Brown identified and described two signs occurring in patients with intestinal perforation secondary to typhoid fever:

> The first sign, for want of a better description, I have designated as the "dipping crackel" sound. At the first examination, which took place a few minutes after the perforation on placing the bell of the stethoscope over the right iliac fossa and dipping suddenly with it as in dipping palpation, a very fine crackle was heard which sounded much like a fine crepitant rale, or as if two sticky surfaces were being drawn apart. It seems to be due to the fact that in dipping suddenly the parietal and visceral layers of the peritoneum come in contact for an instant and apparently, the inflamed surfaces stick together for a moment and then pull

apart. I have never found this sign present over an area of more than two inches in diameter and never later than four hours after the initial symptoms, presumably because the accumulated gas prevents the surfaces from coming in contact [108, p. 695].

The second sign involved the following:

> The patient was examined immediately, and a small area of tenderness found low down in the right iliac fossa. He was turned on his left side and in half an hour the areas of tenderness had moved toward that side about two inches [108, p. 695]. (…) The explanation of the sign is simple. At the time of perforation there is a greater or lesser amount of the contents of the intestine extruded into the peritoneal cavity, and this extravasation tends to flow in the direction of least resistance, that is, downward, and its extension is marked by the indication of local peritonitis, pain, tenderness, and rigidity. By turning the patient over on the unaffected side that side is made the lowermost, and if there be a perforation with extravasation the sign of the extension of the local peritonitis will pass to that side which is lowermost [108, p. 696].

Thus, Brown sign refers to the auscultatory "dipping-crackle" sound in acute peritonitis and tenderness found in the lower right iliac fossa, extending approximately 2 in. to the left when the patient is turned toward the left side (Table 10.1).

10.2.20 Chilaiditi Sign

Demetrius Chilaiditi (1883–1975) was born in Vienna, Austria, and received his medical degree from the University of Vienna in 1908 [109, 110]. He worked as an internist and radiologist at the III. Medical University Clinic and Central Roentgen Institute in Vienna. He moved to Istanbul, Turkey, where he established a Radiologic Institute and co-founded the Turkish Radiological Society [109, 110].

Chilaiditi reported three cases, as confirmed fluoroscopically and on X-ray, where there was partial temporary displacement of the liver from the dome of the diaphragm as a result of the interposition of the transverse colon between the liver and dome of the diaphragm:

> The type and severity of displacement vary depending on the quantity and degree of distension of the interposed loop of the bowel and secondarily on the behavior of the hepatic ligaments. During the displacement, there were no symptoms or dysfunction of the relevant organs, and the patient could not detect the transition. The change in the shape of the liver during displacement and the assumption of a normal shape during reduction can be explained by the softness, the plasticity, and the changing blood content in vivo, which can also be seen in the X-ray images but is particularly evident during fluoroscopy. The percussion findings usually, but only sometimes, coincide with the X-ray findings. The palpation finding is sometimes uncertain, especially when bowel loops are in front of the edge of the displaced liver. (…) The term hepatoptosis or wandering liver for this type of displacement needs to be specified insofar as it is a ptosis in the narrower sense, in contrast to the much larger number of cases of hepatoptosis in which the liver does not give up its direct contact with the diaphragm or can speak of an interposition ptosis (insofar as certain organs interpose between the liver and the diaphragmatic dome). One could also refer to this condition as a "wandering liver." If used, the term should not be interpreted as having the same meaning as hepatoptosis (which is what most authors are currently doing). The wandering liver

would, therefore, only constitute a relatively rare form of hepatoptosis. The liver displacement is partial in all three cases since, even with severe displacement, the median parts of the liver remain in direct contact with the diaphragm to varying degrees, despite possible damage to all the ligaments. This partial ptosis does not become total because of the more resistant attachment of the median parts of the liver, the physically explicable behavior of the intestine pushing off, and the nature of the liver tissue, which protects the median fixation apparatus. Even if the ligamentous attachments are damaged, the ptosis can remain partial [111, p. 205–206].

Thus, Chilaiditi sign refers to the interposition of the transverse colon between the liver and diaphragm (Table 10.1).

10.2.21 Oehlecker Sign

Franz Oehlecker (Öhlecker) (1874–1957) was born in Hamburg, Germany, studied medicine in Leipzig, Tübingen, Kiel, Berlin, and Strasburg, and received his medical degree in 1901 [112, 113]. He was an assistant physician at the Pathological Institute from 1902 to 1903, Friedrichshain City Hospital from 1903 to 1905, and a scientific assistant at Imperial Health Office in Berlin-Dahlem, conducting research on tuberculosis from 1905 to 1907 [112]. He trained in surgery under the tutelage of Wilhelm Körte (1853–1937) in Berlin and Hermann Kümmell (1852–1937) at the University Hospital of Eppendorf, Hamburg. He was a senior physician in the I. surgical department of Hamburg-Barmbek General Hospital from 1914 to 1947 [112, 114]. Oehlecker was an associate professor in 1923 and a professor in 1931 at the University of Hamburg [114].

He is best recognized for devising a direct method to determine blood compatibility for blood transfusion (Oehlecker test) [112]. He was a member of the German Society of Surgery in 1957 [115]. An award medal has been named for Franz Oehlecker by the German Society for Transfusion Medicine and Immunohaematology [116]. He was elected an honorary member of the German Society for Blood Transfusions at the fifth Conference in Bochum in 1955 [114]. Oehlecker is also the recipient of the Federal Cross of Merit and an honorary doctorate from the Faculty of Natural Sciences at the University of Hamburg [114].

Oehlecker's name should not be used in medical discourse to describe his sign or test because he signed the Confession of German professors declaring loyalty to Adolf Hitler in 1933. He was a member of the National Socialist German Workers' Party and was involved in forced male sterilization [117].

Oehlecker reported his experience of left or right shoulder pain in various acute intra-abdominal diseases:

Shoulder pain is triggered not only by inflammatory processes but also by mechanical stimuli involving phrenic nerve endings. Irritation of the phrenic nerve endings causes shoulder pain not only on the convexity of the liver but also on the diaphragm and the area supplied by the phrenic-abdominal rami. If the disease is in the abdominal cavity, and we observe right or left shoulder pain, we can conclude that the disease process, which can be quite different, occurs near the diaphragm. In many cases, the shoulder symptom is overlooked.

The patient, like the doctor, often attaches no importance to the pain in the shoulder; sometimes, it is regarded and treated as rheumatism when it represents a distant symptom of the phrenic nerve. The shoulder symptom is common in acute diseases of the abdomen and is frequently overlooked because of the presence of severe symptoms and pain in the abdominal cavity [118, p. 853–854].

Thus, Oehlecker sign refers to left or right shoulder pain caused by subdiaphragmatic inflammation (Table 10.1).

10.2.22 Claybrook Sign

Edwin Booth Claybrook (1871–1931) was born in Westmoreland County, Virginia, USA, and received his medical degree from the University College of Medicine, Richmond, Virginia. He co-founded the Allegheny General Hospital in Cumberland, Maryland, where he practiced surgery [119, 120]. He was also a surgeon for the Baltimore-Ohio (B&O) and Western Maryland railroads [120]. He was a member of the Cumberland Board of Health, a fellow of the American College of Physicians, and several societies, including the Southern Medical Society and Allegany-Garrett Medical Society [120].

Claybrook described an auscultatory sign in patients who sustained intestinal perforation. The sign:

[c]onsisted in the transmission of the heart and respiratory sound, so that they could be heard all over the abdomen almost as well as over the chest. The ear was all that was needed to elect the symptom, and if it was of any special value, it was doubly valuable on that account, for often the very life of these patients depends upon the attitude of the doctor who first sees them [121, p. 105–106].

Claybrook postulated that the sign was caused by sound transmitted by bowel content, blood, and urine in the abdominal cavity and irritating the parietal peritoneum. The sign was absent in case of abdominal wall injury, extraperitoneal bladder rupture, and a small hepatic rupture confined to the liver. It was present regardless of whether the abdomen was rigid or soft. Claybrook erroneously believed that fluid is less effective for sound transmission than air or gas, and that its presence was an indication for proceeding to an immediate laparotomy.

Thus, Claybrook sign refers to the transmission of heart and respiratory sounds through the abdominal wall in cases of intestinal perforation (Table 10.1).

10.2.23 Drachter Sign

There is limited historical information on Richard Drachter (1883–1936). Drachter was an associate professor, followed by a senior surgeon in 1922 at the University Children's Hospital, Munich, where he served from 1914 to 1936 [122, 123]. With Josef Rudolf Gossmann, he published the book *Chirurgie des Kindesalters* (Pediatric

Surgery) in 1930. The Richard Drachter Prize for pediatric surgery is the highest prize established by the German Society for Pediatric Surgery [124, 125].

Drachter described a maneuver for examining a child with suspected peritonitis (Fig. 10.2):

> With the patient lying on his back, the examiner slightly raises one leg (the right one) by gasping the front foot with the left hand with the knee extended. The sole of the right foot is tapped lightly with the right fist. When examining for peritonitis, we intend to use this technique to cause the visceral peritoneum to move, albeit minimally, against the parietal peritoneum and thereby induce pain in the presence of inflammatory conditions in the abdomen. An advantage of this examination method over others is that when it is performed, one can separate oneself from the diseased part of the body, which only the patient can touch. (…) If the patient suffers abdominal pain from the impact, or if previously existing pain suddenly increases, the patient will express this in some way; This often happens—which is very characteristic—by the child grasping the body with one or both hands. If there is no abdominal pain, or if the pain is not due to an inflammatory condition of the peritoneum, a similar pain sensation or increased pain from the impact does not occur [122, p. 599].

Thus, Drachter sign refers to abdominal pain produced by tapping on the plantar aspect of a child's foot (Table 10.1).

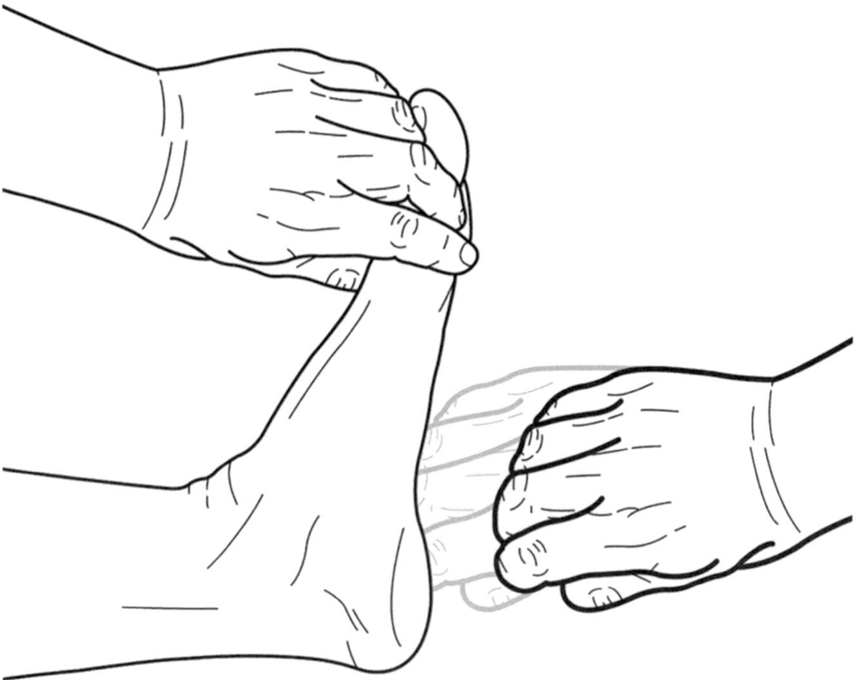

Fig. 10.2 Drachter sign (by Ryan Yale)

10.2.24 Douglas Sign (Douglas Cry)

Douglas sign or cry was named by Henri Alphonse Albertin (1860–1939) after the Douglas cul-de-sac or pouch, the anatomical structure initially described by James Douglas (1675–1742). We were able to identify limited historical information on Henri Albertin. He received his medical degree in 1887 based on the thesis titled "Des injection intra-utérines au point de vue obstétrical sous la méthode antiseptique" (Intrauterine Injections from an Obstetric Point of View under the Antiseptic Method) [126]. Albertin served as an intern at the Lyon Hospital, a surgeon at the Charité Hospital, Lyon, and later as a prosecutor at the Faculty of Medicine, Lyon [127]. He received the Legion of Honor in 1912 [128].

Albertin described a finding that he identified during laparotomy and digital rectal examination in women:

> Since that time, the notion of a cause and effect between touching Douglas pouch and the characteristic inspiratory reflex accompanied by the "oh" has become common in Lyon. There is no surgeon or assistant who has not observed this finding if he remembers to perform this aspect on examination [129, p. 479].

Albertin reported on how to perform and reproduce what he referred to as an inspiratory reflex at the pharyngo-laryngeal region:

> To produce it, it is necessary to touch the cul-de-sac of Douglas, which causes traction on the uterus similar to that occurring during a hysterectomy. Palpation causes straining of the uterosacral ligaments, an inspiratory reflex, and the cry. The reflex can be reproduced rhythmically by touching the uterus at regular intervals [129, p. 480].

In a comment to this paper, Tixier noted this reflex in men causes prostate-rectal dilation. Thus, Douglas cry sign as described by Albertin refers to the painful expression caused by palpation of the Douglas pouch in cases of peritonitis (Table 10.1).

10.2.25 Danforth Sign

William Clark Danforth (1878–1949) was born in Chicago, Illinois, USA, and received his medical degree cum laude from Northwestern University in 1903, followed by an internship at Cook County Hospital that same year [130, 131]. He worked at the General Hospital, Vienna, from 1906 to 1907. Danforth was a private practitioner in Evanston, Illinois, and was appointed chief of obstetrics and gynecology at Evanston Hospital in 1908 [131].

He was president of the Chicago Gynecological Society in 1921, the Evanston Branch of the Chicago Medical Society, the Chicago Gynecological Society, the Institute of Medicine of Chicago, the American Gynecological Society, and a charter member of the Central Association of Obstetricians and Gynecologist to name a few [131, 132].

As to his character as articulated by Grier:

> He was by nature direct, analytical, and adamant in matters of principle. Yet, all who knew him well will recall his keen sense of humor, his hearty laugh, and his seemingly limitless repertoire of anecdotes. (…) He was a most generous contributor to many charitable causes and was ever ready to give freely of his time to civic programs and to the care of the indigent sick [131, p. 139–140].

Danforth reported two cases of patients who presented with bilateral shoulder pain, found during surgery to have an intra-abdominal hemorrhage secondary to a ruptured tubal pregnancy (Table 10.1). He described the pathophysiology of this process:

> In rupture of the pregnant tube, particularly if considerable intrabdominal hemorrhage occurs, blood may enter the subphrenic space and cause traction upon the falciform ligament in the same manner as it is produced by gas. This is especially apt to be so if the bleeding is large in amount and if the rupture of the tube is followed by faintness. The patient then is likely to lie flat for a time and often the foot of the bed is elevated. This allows the fluid blood to run upward along the colon on both sides, particularly the right side, and to find its way into the subphrenic space [133, p. 883–884].

Thus, the shoulder pain represents a referred pain from the third, fourth, and fifth cervical cord segments of the phrenic nerve.

10.2.26   D'Amato Sign

There is limited historical information on Hugo Julio D'Amato. He served as Secretary General of the Ministry of the Interior National Department of Hygiene, president of the editorial commission of the *Boletín Sanitario* (Health Bulletin), and vice-president and official delegate of the Argentina Republic at the first Latin American Congress of Hospitals [134–136].

D'Amato reported on 13 patients with infrahepatic adhesions and a positive Novaro-Bermúdez sign. This paper titled "Consideration on a sign of adherence of the infrahepatic area" was presented by Raul Novaro and Bermúdez Zolezzi at the 21st session of the Society of Internal Medicine and was based on nine cases observed at the Institute of Professor Agote. As reported by D'Amato:

> It is opportune to transcribe her the words with which the authors of the sign have so brilliantly described. "The procedure is simple. The first investigation is performed with the patient in the supine position. Palpate the duodenum and gallbladder area, applying direct pressures toward the spine. Once the point of greatest pain is found, and with the fingers remaining in this position, place the patient in the left lateral decubitus position with legs flexed. In the case of adhesions, gentle pressure causes intense unbearable pain. Pain is absent even when firm pressure is applied with the patient placed in the right lateral decubitus position. The sign is so prominent that there is no uncertainty about the pain provoked. When referring to the explanation of the phenomenon, the authors said, "in the left lateral decubitus, there is a tendency to separate the duodenum and the gallbladder from the lower surface of the liver. The evidence for this finding is that frequently the patient cannot adopt such a position due to immediate pain. With manual pressure, the organs separate immediately, causing intense pain due to the pulling. Contrary, in the opposite position (right lateral decubitus), the named organs are in close contact and cannot be separated regardless of how much pressure is applied." [137, p. 18].

Thus, D'Amato sign refers to palpatory pain in the infrahepatic region in the supine and left lateral decubitus position in patients with intrabdominal adhesions (Table 10.1).

10.2.27 Chapman Sign

Limited historical information is available on Charles Leopold Granville Chapman (1871–1951). He was a medalist and prizemen for the Arthur Durham Third- and Fourth-Year Prize for Dissection in 1896 and 1897 at Guy Hospital, London, England [138, 139]. Chapman was a member of the Royal College of Surgeons of England. At the time of the publication of his sign, he was a surgeon at the District Hospital, Grimsby, England [140].

Chapman reported a method for identifying an acute abdomen which he called the "Rising test." The maneuver is performed as follows:

> [t]he patient putting both hands down by the side of the thighs and then raising himself in bed by means of the abdominal muscles. This produces pain immediately, and the patient fails to raise himself or complains of pain in doing so. This test will prove positive when there is little or no tenderness in the abdomen. In my hands it has frequently proved he presence of acute abdomen and is often the decisive factor in doing an immediate operation. The test is a sign of an acute abdominal condition, not necessarily appendicitis, and applies equally well in any acute abdomen [140, p. 786].

Thus, Chapman sign refers to the inability of the patient to raise themself in the supine position without using their hands in cases of acute peritonitis (Table 10.1).

10.2.28 Blaxland Sign

Athelstan Jasper Blaxland (1880–1963) was born in London, England, and received his bachelor of medicine and bachelor of science degrees from Westminster School and University College Hospital in 1904 [141]. He was appointed house physician under the aegis of Sidney Martin (1860–1924) at the University College Hospital; to Sir Archibald Garrod (1857–1936) at the Hospital for Sick Children, Great Ormond Street; and house surgeon to Gilbert Benjamin Mower White (1866–1952) at the Great Northern Central Hospital, London. He served initially as a house surgeon rising to the rank of assistant surgeon at Norfolk and Norwich Hospital, England, in 1909 [141, 142]. He became captain of the Second London Casualty Clearing Station and surgeon in the Royal Army Medical Corps (RAMC) stationed in France during World War I [141, 143]. On his return, he became a full surgeon in 1925 at Norfolk and Norwich Hospital [141, 142].

Blaxland was elected fellow of the Royal College of Surgeons (RCS), England, and earned his master of science degree in 1908 [141, 144]. He was honorary secretary to the Norfolk Branch of the British Medical Association from 1922 to 1928 and its president from 1930 to 1931, chairman of the Norwich Division from 1923 to 1924, vice-president of the Medical Defense Union, and chairman of the nursing committee of the Norfolk and Norwich Hospitals [141, 142].

As to a description of his character:

> Jasper was a whimsical, lovable character who retained his impish sense of fun to the end. (…) His provocative interventions in committee frequently aroused impatience-quickly to be dissolved by an ingenuous aside [141, p. 123].

Blaxland described a method for distinguishing an ovarian cyst from ascites:

> To elicit the sign, the fingers of the two hands are pressed—one hand on either side of the lower abdomen—firmly and steadily backwards towards the lumbar spine. In the case of an ovarian cyst the pulsation of the abdominal aorta can be felt. Presumably the tension in the cyst, caused by the pressure of the fingers, permits the transmission of the pulsation. This sign can be accentuated—and also be made evident to onlookers—by inserting one end of a flat ruler (or a long pencil) under the fingers of one of the hands pressing on the abdomen. The free end of the ruler will then show the pulsation magnified. I have never been able to obtain this sign in a case of pure ascites [145, p. 839].

Thus, Blaxland sign refers to pulsation of an ovarian cyst in the absence of ascites (Table 10.1).

10.2.29   Butler–Carlson Sign

10.2.29.1   Edmund Butler

Edmund Butler (1886–1952) was born in Davenport, Iowa, USA, and received his medical degree from Cooper Medical College in 1911 [146]. He served as assistant to Stanley Stillman (1861–1934) from 1911 to 1914. During World War I, he was a lieutenant in the navy. He was appointed chief surgeon at San Francisco Emergency Hospital in 1919 [146]. Butler was an associate professor at Stanford University and a member of the American Medical Association, American College of Surgeons, and San Francisco County Medical Society. He was a secretary of general surgery at the 1922 meeting of the California State Surgical Society and president of the San Francisco Surgical Society in 1943 [146–148].

10.2.29.2   Everett Carlson

Everett Carlson (1896–1983) received his medical degree from Stanford University in 1924 and served as a house officer in surgery at the San Francisco County Hospital and resident physician administrator of the Stanford University staff in 1926 [149, 150]. He was a fellow of the American College of Surgeons and vice-president of the San Francisco Surgical Society in 1956 [151].

Butler and Carlson reported the case of a 24-year-old male with acute abdominal and bilateral testicular pain occurring after sustaining a traumatic upper abdominal contusion. On laparotomy, they found a rupture involving the posterior wall of the third portion of the duodenum. They concluded that:

> Early excruciating pain in the testicles following a severe trauma to the upper abdomen indicates a retroperitoneal rupture of the duodenum with a spreading out of bile beneath the

peritoneum so as to irritate the testicular nerves, the sympathetic chain accompanying the spermatic artery [152, p. 118].

Thus, Butler–Carlson sign refers to intense testicular pain in retroperitoneal duodenal rupture (Table 10.1).

10.2.30 Leotta Sign

Nicola Leotta (1878–1967) was born in Acireale, Sicily, Italy, and received his medical degree from the University of Rome in 1901 [153, 154]. He was elected assistant surgeon to the United Hospitals, Rome, in 1901 and at the University of Rome Clinic, rising to the rank of assistant of the surgical clinic in 1907. He was a lecturer in special surgical pathology in 1908 and a teaching surgeon from 1909 to 1928 [154].

Leotta was an assistant physician first class to the Italian Red Cross in 1906 and later the recipient of the bronze medal for his service assisting victims of earthquakes in Reggio Calabria in 1908 and Marsica in 1915 [154, 155]. During World War I, he served as a medical captain organizing the surgical service of the Second Army in 1916 and was promoted to lieutenant colonel in 1918 and later colonel [154, 155]. He was appointed to Castrense University of San Giorgio di Nogaro in 1918, returning to the University of Rome after the war. He was appointed extraordinary professor of special surgical pathology at the Institute of Clinical Surgery, University of Palermo [154].

He assisted in the recruitment of the faculty of medicine; served as director of the surgical clinic in 1925; full professor of the surgical clinic and operative medicine in 1926; and rector from 1927 to 1929 at the University of Bari [154, 155]. Leotta was appointed director of the University of Palermo Surgical Institute in 1929, dean from 1932 to 1934, and rector magnifico from 1939 to 1943 [154].

He was president of the Medical Academy of Palermo and Apulian Academy of Sciences, secretary of the Italian Society of Surgery, and member of the Higher Council for Public Education [154, 155]. Among his many awards and honors, he was a recipient of the title of honorary professor of surgery from the University of Argentina, Great Officer of the Crown of Italy, Knight of the Order of Saints Maurice and Lazarus, Greater Officer of Merit of the Republic, and a Gold Medal for his contributions to the school, culture, and art [154].

Leotta reported at the 38th Surgical Congress at Bari, Italy, a physical sign for identifying the presence of adhesions arising from inflammatory conditions involving the gallbladder, duodenum, stomach, and transverse colon. The sign cause pain, elicited by applying indirect traction by longitudinally stretching the abdominal wall in the right upper abdominal quadrant. He referred to this as a "stretching maneuver" which involves:

1) To establish the existence of adhesions in the upper crossroads, i.e., between the colon at the bottom and the liver and gallbladder at the tip; the maneuver of stretching at the bottom

is applied, i.e., the fingers are placed in the right upper abdominal quadrant and pressed downward. The traction pushing the colon downward will be painful if adhesion adheres to the gallbladder or the liver. The pain increases if the patient forcibly exhales while the hand is maintained in the lower traction position because the diaphragm rises, stretching the liver and gallbladder upwards.

2) To establish the existence of adhesion between the ascending colon and parietal peritoneum, the maneuver involving stretching inside the right half of the abdomen is used. Traction and pressure are applied with the hand in a transverse direction, starting from the lateral abdomen, moving towards the midline, and from the midline outwards. This maneuver stretches the adhesions, if they exist, in the ascending colon and the nearby parietal peritoneum, causing more or less severe pain [156, p. 119].

Thus, Leotta sign refers to the palpatory method for detecting adhesions between the colon at the bottom, the liver and gallbladder tip, and ascending colon and parietal peritoneum (Table 10.1).

10.2.31   Lian–Odinet Sign

10.2.31.1   Camille Lian

Camille Lian (1882–1969) was born in Treigny (Yonne), France, studied medicine in Paris, was an intern, and conducted research at Laennec Hospital and François Franck's Physiology Laboratory, graduating in 1909 based on a thesis on mitral incompetence [157]. He was a battalion medical officer during World War I in 1914. Lian served as a doctor of Hôpitaux de Paris (Paris Hospitals) in 1919, associate professor of the Faculty of Medicine, Paris, in history of medicine in 1923, and clinical professor of medicine in 1942 [157, 158]. During World War II, he served as a medical officer in the army as head physician and cardiologist at Stanislas Hospital, Nantes, France, in 1940 [159]. He was appointed physician to Tenon Hospital, France, in 1926 and chair of La Pitié, France, until 1952 [157].

Among his many accolades and accomplishments, he was president of the French Society of Cardiology from 1948 to 1950, founding president of the International Cardiological Week of La Pitié, and a member of the National Academy of Medicine of France, Spain, and Italy [158].

He was selected commander of the Legion of Honor, grand officer of the Order of Research and invention and international Order of Public Welfare and Public Health, Polonia Restituta; Knight of the Order of St. Sava, and Commander of Order of the Flag [158, 159]. He received the Medal of Honor and War Cross for his work during an epidemic during the war years [159]. He received the Golden Stethoscope Award from the International Cardiology Foundation in 1965. He invented with Minot a phonocardiograph which was instrumental in recording cardiac murmurs and abnormal heart sounds [157].

As to his character as described by Bedford:

> He was a prodigious worker, a prolific writer, and an active participant in scientific meetings and congresses. As a teacher, he spoke clearly, and emphatically, and his lecture at the Pitié on triple rhythm still ranks in my memory as a masterly exposition [157, p. 789].

On a plaque affixed to the residence where he lived from 1926 to 1969 is inscribed:

> In this house lived from 1926 until his death Professor Camille Lian (1882–1969), member of the National Academy of Medicine who was the first author of the clinical description of myocardial infarction [160].

10.2.31.2 Jacques Odinet

There is limited historical information on Marie Jacques Odinet (1903–1998). He was born in Paris, France, was an intern at the Hospitals of Paris, and defended his thesis titled "Recherches anatomiques et physiologiques sur le thymus, leurs applications cliniques et thérapeutiques" (Anatomical and Physiological Research on the Thymus, Their Clinical and Therapeutic Applications) in 1934. He was a hospital doctor at Tenon Hospital, Paris [161].

Lian and Odinet reported a technique whereby percussion in patients with ascites and hydatid cysts of the liver causes a distant auscultatory double sound (Table 10.1). Normally, percussion with a curved finger or hammer causes a single, brief, high-pitch auscultatory noise which varies depending on the compliance and distention of the abdominal wall:

> However, in ascites, the acoustic sound is different. Instead of one unique noise, two distinct juxtaposed sounds are heard. The first corresponds to the one heard in normal persons, while the second one is more intense and longer, reflecting the presence of peritoneal effusion [162, p. 1337]. (…) However, with minimal ascites, the double noise is not heard when the patient is in the recumbent position. In this case, the double noise should be searched for in the standing position. This last position is useful in that it provides decisive results. Indeed, this sign significantly increases the intensity of the sound in the standing position because this position increases the contact between the surface of the ascites and abdominal wall [162, p. 1338].

Two symmetrical points at the iliac or flanks are chosen to determine the distance between the percussion and auscultatory sounds and confirm the diagnosis of ascites.

10.2.32 Pitfield Sign

Robert Lucas Pitfield (1870–1942) was born in Germantown, Pennsylvania, USA, received his medical degree from the University of Pennsylvania in 1892, and was a resident at the Germantown Hospital from 1892 to 1893 [163, 164]. He was a special assistant to Joseph MacFarland, a researcher at the Henry K. Mulford Company, a private pharmaceutical company, and appointed demonstrator of bacteria at the Medico-Chirurgical College (merged with the University of Pennsylvania) from 1902 to 1904 [163, 164]. He was appointed pathologist at the Widener Memorial Hospital for Crippled Children in 1906 [165]. At the time of the third edition of his book titled *A Compend on Bacteriology: Including Pathogenic Protozoa* in 1917, he was a pathologist at the Germantown Hospital, Philadelphia, and visiting physician at St. Timothy's Hospital beginning in 1908, and Chestnut Hill Hospital, Philadelphia [163, 166].

Pitfield described a method for detecting ascites:

> It might well be called the diaphragm sign since this organ of respiration plays the most important part in its mechanism. It consists first in collecting the fluid into as limited a space as possible on the diaphragm by having the patient sit up in bed. The patient should now lean forward a little. The back of thorax over the suspected areas is percussed with the fingertips of one hand, the other hand palpates the quadratus lumborum muscle on the same side. This will cause the collected fluid to vibrate, and the vibrations are felt by the palpating hand on the muscle [167, p. 984].

This finding is based on the anatomical juxtaposition of the diaphragm and quadratus lumborum muscle and its attachment to the twelfth ribs. Pitfield postulated that percussion of the chest in the presence of ascitic fluid causes the chest to vibrate, which is transmitted to the diaphragm and quadratus lumborum muscle and felt by the palpating hand. Based on these principles, Pitfield explained that this sign is absent with deep inhalation and breath hold, pulmonary consolidation or neoplasm in the lower lobe of the lung, and pulmonary adhesions attached to the diaphragm. A false negative sign may be due to acute pneumonia [167, p. 983–984].

Pitfield also reported another method for detecting fluid in the abdomen. In this method, the patient is requested to:

> [s]it upright in bed rather than to lie flat on his back. The fluid is thus gathered into one place, and presses upon the entire circumference of the abdominal wall; the intestines are floated up out of the way and cannot absorb the percussion impulses; and lastly, no third hand is needed to compress the abdomen and the floating bowels as when the patient lies supine. The height of the fluid may be noted from time to time by this method by marking the lowest place where the percussion impulse is felt [167, p. 984].

Thus, Pitfield sign refers to the ability to detect the height of the fluid in the abdomen in the supine position (Table 10.1).

10.2.33 Rob Sign

Charles Granville Rob (1913–2001) was born in Weybridge, England, and received his medical degree from Cambridge University in 1937 [168]. While at Cambridge, he joined the air squadron training as a pilot, obtaining a reserve commission in the Royal Air Force [169, 170]. He was an intern in surgery at St. Thomas Hospital,

London, and a junior surgical resident at Royal Victoria Hospital, Montreal, during World War II. Rob was appointed a fellow of the Royal College of Surgeons (FRCS) in 1939, followed by a mastership of surgery in Cambridge [168–170]. He served as resident assistant surgeon upon the acquisition of Hydestile Hospital by St. Thomas Hospital [169].

Rob enlisted in the Royal Army Medical Corps and was a combat surgeon during the war in 1942. He was the recipient of the Military Cross for bravery and service and rose to the rank of lieutenant colonel [170]. He returned to St. Thomas Hospital in 1946 and was appointed professor of surgery at Mary's Hospital, London, in 1950 [168, 169].

He received an appointment at the University of Rochester Medical School in 1960, rising to the rank of professor and chair of the Department of Surgery until 1978 [168, 170]. Subsequent appointments include professor of surgery at East Carolina University Medical School, Greenville, North Carolina, from 1978 to 1983 and finally as distinguished professor of surgery as a surgical professor and senior adviser in the Department of Surgery at the Uniformed Services University of the Health Sciences, Bethesda, Maryland in 1995 [168, 170].

He is best recognized for his pioneering work in vascular surgical repair of blood vessels and performing a carotid endarterectomy [168, 170]. Rob was president of the International Society for Cardiovascular Surgery and the North American Chapter of the International Cardiovascular Society, as well as vice-president of the American Surgical Association [168, 170]. He co-edited with Sir Edwin Rodney Smith (1914–1988) the eight-volume set of *Operative Surgery* in 1956 [170].

Rob reported an auscultatory finding found in 250 patients with an acute abdominal emergency and 150 patients with an abdominal wound:

> In this series intestinal peristalsis was abolished by the presence, in the peritoneal cavity, of intestinal contents, pus, bile, hemorrhagic exudate from strangulated intestine, and exudate from an acutely inflamed pancreas. It was not abolished by the presence of blood or urine in the peritoneal cavity [171, p. 721].

Thus, Rob sign refers to the absence of intestinal peristalsis when intestinal contents, pus, bile, hemorrhagic, and exudate occur intraperitoneally.

10.2.34 Robertson Sign

William Egbert Robertson (1869–1956) was born in Camden, New Jersey, USA, and received his medical degree from the University of Pennsylvania in 1892 [172, 173]. After a brief internship at Episcopal Hospital in Philadelphia and Cooper Hospital in Camden, New Jersey, he furthered his studies abroad, pursuing postgraduate training in pathology in Heidelberg and Vienna. He returned to Philadelphia, was appointed medicine instructor, and worked under the auspices of Milton Howard Fussell (1855–1921) at the University of Pennsylvania outpatient clinic [172, 173].

He served as an instructor of bacteriology and microscopic pathology, with later appointments as an instructor in physical diagnosis and medicine and assistant professor of clinical medicine at the Medico-Chirurgical College and Hospital in Philadelphia [172, 174]. He was a pathologist at Episcopal Hospital from 1897 to 1904, maintaining an appointment as a visiting physician until 1931 [172, 173].

Robertson was appointed professor and chair of the Department of Medicine at Temple University and visiting physician at Samaritan Hospital, Philadelphia, from 1916 to 1933 [172]. He was a physician and chief of staff at Philadelphia General Hospital; visiting physician at Garrison Hospital; chief of St. Luke's and Children's Hospital Medical Center; and a consultant at Rush; Kensington Hospital for Women; and Northeastern Hospital [172, 173].

He was a fellow of the College of Physicians of Pennsylvania in 1903 and took an active role in the college's library committee, serving as its chairman and member of the council overseeing the work of the section of general medicine and medical history [173]. Robertson was appointed a fellow of the American College of Physicians in 1920, was its president, and served on the board of directors and censors of the Philadelphia County Medical Society in 1937 [173].

As a description of his character by Kern:

> His charm of personality, his grace of manner, his steadfastness of purpose, the deliberate thoroughness with which he did things, his meticulous attention to detail. He was soft-spoken and courteous, patient and forbearing, but let no one think that his mildness of manner betokened any weakness of resolution or vacillation in action [172, p. 57].

In co-authorship with his son Harold Frederick Robertson in their book *Diagnostic Signs, Reflexes and Syndrome*, they described a bedside maneuver for determining a smaller quantity of ascitic fluid:

> When a patient is recumbent, and no fluid exists in the abdominal cavity, one hand of the examiner being placed under the flank of each side will elicit no tension or fullness, and often a slight concavity, dependent upon the mount of adipose possessed by the patient. When fluid is present, however, the flank of each side presents a sensation of fullness, more or less tension, and a quick upward thrust of the fingers by momentarily displacing fluid will result in a form of ballottement. In small effusions, when the patient is recumbent, the vertebral column separates the fluid which therefore tends to collect in the form of a pool in the posterior portions of the abdomen, hence the possibility of this sign [175, p. 286–287].

Thus, Robertson sign refers to ballottement at the flanks when ascites is present (Table 10.1).

10.2.35   Way Sign

Stanley Albert Way (1913–1988) was born in Portsmouth, England, and qualified from Middlesex Hospital in 1936 [176, 177]. He served as registrar at Princess Mary Maternity Hospital and consultant in the Department of Gynecology at the

Royal Victoria Infirmary, Newcastle-upon-Tyne, in 1939 [176]. He also served as a consultant for the Newcastle Regional Cancer Organization. After a brief appointment at Shotley Bridge General Hospital, he was appointed consultant to the Queen Elizabeth Hospital, Gateshead, in 1947. He founded the oncology unit designed to manage and conduct research on gynecological cancers [176, 177]. Way is perhaps best recognized for his work on the study of the lymphatic drainage of the vulva, which led to pioneering work on radical vulvectomy and lymph node dissection in women with vulvar carcinoma.

Way was a Hunterian Professor of the Royal College of Surgeons from 1947 to 1948, Victor Bonney Prizeman and lecturer from 1964 to 1966, and with the Royal College of Obstetricians and Gynecologists the Blair Bell Lectureship from 1947 to 1948 [176, 177]. He was elected fellow of the Royal College of Obstetricians and Gynecologists in 1953 and appointed an honorary fellow of the American Association of Gynecologists and Obstetricians and the International Association of Cytology and a fellow of the Royal College of Surgeons (FRCS) in 1974 [176, 177].

Way in a consecutive series of 113 cases of tubal pregnancy reported on a frequently overlooked symptom of shoulder tip pain (Table 10.1):

> To my mind this is one of the most important symptoms in ectopic gestation and for some reason or other it has been completely neglected in gynecological textbooks. Its mechanism is well understood, namely-irritation of the under surface of the diaphragm and the reference of pain through the phrenic nerve and its connections with the third, fourth and fifth cervical segments, these same segments supplying the skin over the tip of the acromion. (…) [e]xcluding 15 of my cases in which there was no information it was found to be present in 60% of ruptured ectopic gestations and in 41% of the whole series [178, p. 551–552].

Way found a lack of correlation between the side of the ruptured ectopic pregnancy and the involved shoulder. Of the 24 patients with shoulder pain, the pain was referred to the right shoulder in 13 and the left shoulder in four. In seven cases, the pain was present in both shoulders.

10.2.36 Dew Sign

Harold Robert Dew (1891–1962) was born in Reservoir, Victoria, Australia, and received his medical degree from the University of Melbourne in 1914 [179–181]. He served during World War I as a temporary lieutenant in the Royal Army Medical Corps (RAMC) in England in 1915 and with the field ambulance in France and Egypt [180, 182]. He commanded the cholera laboratory at the Egyptian Stationary Hospital in Kantara in 1918 and received the accommodation of the Epidemics Medal of Honor for his work from the French government in 1917 [181–183].

Dew was elected Fellow of the Royal College of Surgeons (FRCS), England, in 1920 [180, 182]. He served as assistant director of the Walter and Eliza Hall Institute of Medical Research and had joint appointments with the surgical staff as a clinical assistant in 1922, becoming an honorary surgeon in 1923 at the Royal Melbourne Hospital [179].

He was a founding fellow of the Royal Australasian College of Surgeons in 1928, a professor of surgery and Bosch Chair at the University of Sydney, and a surgeon at the Royal Prince Alfred Hospital from 1930 to 1956 [179–181, 183]. Dew served as dean of the faculty of medicine at the University of Sydney from 1936 to 1938 and from 1940 to 1952 and president of the Royal Australasian College of Surgeons from 1954 to 1955 [179, 181, 183]. He was a foundation member of the National Health and Medical Research Council and was chair of the research advisor committee from 1946 to 1956 [180, 184].

His many honors included the Jacksonian Prize from the Royal College of Surgeons in 1924, the David Syme Research Prize from Melbourne University in 1927, and Hunterian Professorship in 1930 and at the Royal College of Surgeons in 1953 [180, 183]. He is the recipient of an honorary doctorate degree from Cambridge University and an honorary fellow at Edinburgh Royal College of Surgeons. Dew was knighted in 1955 [182]. The Ormond College of Sir Harold Dew Medical Scholarship is sponsored by the University of Melbourne, and the Sir Harold Dew Prize at the University of Sydney was established in 1957 [185, 186].

As to a description of his character:

> His sound clinical and operative work was based on an enviable familiarity with the fundamental preclinical aspects of surgery, and naturally this approach made him an excellent expositor both to undergraduate and to colleagues. His complete sincerity and unselfish devotion to surgery made him a wise adviser in both professional and educational manners [185, p. 1478].

Dew described a method for differentiating hydatid cysts in the right lung base and those in a subdiaphragmatic location (Table 10.1):

> Hydatid cysts of the right lung must be distinguished from cysts of the superior quadrants. Radiography shows elevation, fixation, or distortion of the diaphragm, with or without patches of calcification in the one, and a thoracic opacity in the other, and a thoracic opacity in the other, although a co-existent pleural effusion may mask the real state of affairs. A useful method is to compare the area of air entry and resonance at the right base in the sitting and in the hands and knee positions [187, p. 783].

In the case of a hydatid cyst located beneath the right cupola (subdiaphragmatically), a resonance area moves caudally when the patient assumes the hand and knee position [188].

Table 10.1 Intra-abdominal and diaphragm signs

Name	Year	Description of sign	Significance
Hippocratic facies [4]	Fourth century BC	The eyes are sensitive to light, involuntarily tear, squint, or one eyelid is more closed than the other. The conjunctiva is red and livid, has black veins, and is crusty. The eyes are restless, protruding, or become very hollow. The countenance is squalid and dark, or the color of the whole face is changed. All these are considered harmful and fatal symptoms. However, if the eyelids are contracted, the lip and nose livid or pale, along with the other symptoms, one knows that death is imminent	Peritonitis-agonal state
Stokes [10]	1842	Increased pulsation of the abdominal aorta	Enteritis
Duchenne [17]	1873	At the beginning of inspiration, the epigastric and hypochondriac regions are depressed, and the chest dilates. During expiration, these movements are reversed. When the diaphragm is weak, this signs is seen only during forced respiration. During quiet breathing, abdominal protrusion and chest expansion, and vice versa, occur in unison as during normal health. When the diaphragm is paralyzed on one side, this signs is seen only on the paralyzed side. Respiration is more rapid but is normal during rest	Diaphragmatic paralysis
Pfuhl-Jaffé [19, 21]	1877, 1881	During respiration, the pressure conditions in the thoracic cavity are exactly the opposite of those in the abdominal cavity. If a manometer attached to a cannula is inserted into the abscess, pressure fluctuations occur during respiration. In the abdomen, inspiration produces an increase and expiration a diminution of pressure. In the thorax, the reverse relationship occurs	Subphrenic abscess
Federici [25]	1883	Transmission of heart sounds at a space bounded and enclosed by the diaphragm	Peritonitis
Thomayer [30]	1884	In ascites, without peritonitis, a crescent-shaped muffled area is found during percussion. In peritoneal tuberculosis and malignancy, the dimensions and localization of both the tympanitic and the muffled areas are distinct. In all cases, the tympanitic intestinal sound was predominantly found over the right side, and the dull liquid sound was over the left side of the abdomen	Tuberculous and malignant ascites
Clark [37]	1885	Sudden, severe pain is most commonly found in the lower abdomen and spreads rapidly. The pulse is accelerated and becomes small. The bowel gas escapes into the peritoneal cavity and is resonant to percussion over the lower part of the liver	Intestinal perforation
Fürbringer [41]	1889	On needle puncture, a serous exudate is found in an upper and a purulent exudate in a lower intercostal space. Pus is aspirated after the needle has passed the diaphragm or when the needle moves during respiration	Subphrenic abscess

(continued)

Table 10.1 (continued)

Name	Year	Description of sign	Significance
Bolognini [45]	1895	The physician should quiet the patient to avoid abdominal muscle contraction. The patient is supine with the thighs flexed to relax the abdominal muscles. Place the hands on the abdomen wall and, using the three middle fingers, alternate between the fingers of the hands, applying light touch followed by increasing pressure. A tactile thrill is felt, giving the impression that rubbing is occurring under the fingers, slightly produced by two rough surfaces sliding over each other. The sensation is not uniform throughout the abdomen and is only detectable in specific regions. Sometimes the rubbing is restricted to a specific point on the abdomen. The rubbing may be present for only a brief period. It is not easy to reproduce the phenomenon where it was previously found. For those performing this maneuver for the first time, it is recommended that only slight pressure be applied initially. By applying increasing pressure, the sensation will disappear	Peritonitis
Cushing [51]	1898	Sudden acute onset of increased abdominal pain. Any complaint of pain of less abrupt onset associated with tenderness should raise suspicion for a localized inflammation of the abdominal serosa with adhesive peritonitis	Peritonitis
Strauss [58]	1899	Carcinoma metastases occurring at Douglas pouch	Peritoneal carcinomatosis
Landau [63]	1900	With the patient in a horizontal position, the fingers of the two palpating hands fail to meet on the sides of the uterus. The slightly depressed uterus feels to the palpating fingers as if it were lying on a cushion of air or water. If the patient is examined with the pelvis elevated and the abdominal wall relaxed as much as possible by adduction of the thighs and flexion of the knees bimanual examination provides a different result. Now the fingers meet on the side of the uterus so it can be grasped	Ascites
Lennander [67]	1902	The difference between the temperature in the rectum and the axilla, which normally is about 0.6 °C, is greater in peritonitis	Peritonitis
Bryant [72]	1903	Blood effused into the right spermatic cord while the corresponding half of the scrotum is ecchymosed	Abdominal aortic aneurysm rupture
Morel [74]	1906	The patient is supine, and the bladder is catheterized and emptied. The injured person is told to stand up immediately and remain upright for 2 min. The patient is now placed in the supine position, and the bladder is again catheterized. The bladder fills again with intraperitoneal fluid based on a quantity equal to the first evacuation	Perforated bladder

Kehr [80]	1907	Left shoulder pain in splenic injury	Subdiaphragmatic inflammation
Barnard [95]	1907	The abdominal swelling formed by a subphrenic abscess does not descend on respiration, because it is adherent. The part of the swelling formed by peritoneal adhesions is rigid, tender, and dull on percussion. The part formed by pus in contact with the abdominal wall is scarcely tender; it bulges, fluctuates, and is dull on percussion	Subphrenic abscess
Blumer [101]	1909	On digital rectal examination, 2–4 cm above the prostate gland, the finger is passed along the anterior rectal wall and impinges on a cartilaginous shelf that projects into the rectal cavity. In some cases, further palpation shows that the whole rectum is involved in an annular zone of infiltration more marked anteriorly and tapering off toward the posterior wall (a signet ring stricture). In such cases, the infiltration is no longer confined to Douglas' pouch but involves the submucosa of the rectum. The infiltrated area is fixed, shelf-like, or peg-like at its most prominent portion, without ulceration of the overlying mucous membrane. The lack of ulceration of the overlying mucosa and the peculiar shape distinguishes the rectal shelf from a primary rectal neoplasm	Peritoneal carcinomatosis or peritonitis
Brown [108]	1909	Two signs of intestinal perforation secondary to typhoid fever: 1. The "dipping–crackle" sound. The first exam takes place a few minutes after the perforation. On placing the bell of the stethoscope over the right iliac fossa and depressing suddenly, a very fine crackle is heard, which sounded similar to a fine crepitant rale (as if two sticky surfaces were drawn apart) 2. The patient is examined immediately, and a small area of tenderness is found low in the right iliac fossa. The patient is then placed in the left decubitus position. Within 30 min, the area of tenderness moves about 2 in. toward that side	Peritonitis
Chilaiditi [111]	1910	The large bowel is located between the diaphragm and the liver. The type and severity of displacement vary depending on the quantity and degree of distension of the interposed loop of large bowel and laxity or elongation of the falciform ligaments of the liver or suspensory ligament of the transverse colon	Interposition of the bowel between the liver and diaphragm
Oehlecker[a] [118]	1913	Right and left shoulder pain is due to inflammatory processes and mechanical stimuli involving the phrenic nerve endings of the diaphragm	Subdiaphragmatic inflammation
Claybrook [121]	1914	Transmission of heart and respiratory sounds over the abdomen and chest	Peritonitis

(continued)

Table 10.1 (continued)

Name	Year	Description of sign	Significance
Drachter [122]	1914	Slightly raise one leg (the right one) with the patient lying on his back with the knee extended and grasp the foot with the left hand. The sole of the right foot is hit lightly with the right fist	Peritonitis
Douglas (cry) [129]	1922	Palpating Douglas pouch causes traction on the uterus and causes the patient to express pain	Peritonitis
Danforth [133]	1926	The patient lies flat, and the foot of the bed is elevated, causing blood to run upward along the colon, particularly the right side, and to the subphrenic space causing traction on the falciform ligament	Subdiaphragmatic inflammation in ectopic pregnancy
D'Amato [137]	1926	The patient is in the supine position. Palpate the duodenum and gallbladder area toward the spine by applying direct pressure. Once the point of greatest pain is found, and with the fingers remaining in this position, the patient is placed in the left decubitus position with the legs flexed. Gentle pressure causes intense unbearable pain. When the patient is placed in the right decubitus position, there is no pain when firm pressure is applied	Adhesions
Chapman [140]	1927	The patient places his hand down at the side of the thighs and then raises himself in the bed utilizing his abdominal muscles. Pain occurs immediately, causing the patient to be unable to raise themselves	Peritonitis
Blaxland [145]	1930	The fingers of the two hands are pressed, one on either side of the lower abdomen, firmly and steadily backward toward the lumbar spine. In patients with an ovarian cyst, the pulsation of the abdominal aorta is felt. Presumably, the tension in the cyst, caused by the pressure of the fingers, permits the transmission of the pulsation. This sign can be accentuated and made evident to onlookers by inserting one end of a flat ruler (or a long pencil) under the fingers of one of the hands pressing on the abdomen. The free end of the ruler will then show the pulsation magnified	Ascites
Butler–Carlson [152]	1931	Early excruciating pain in the testicles following severe trauma to the upper abdomen indicates a retroperitoneal rupture of the duodenum with bile throughout the peritoneum irritating the testicular nerves, sympathetic chain, and spermatic artery	Peritonitis

Leotta [156]	1934	1. The maneuver involves stretching the abdomen to confirm the presence of adhesions between the colon, liver, and gallbladder. The fingers are placed in the right upper abdominal quadrant and pressed downward. This traction pushes the colon downward and is painful if adhesions adhere to the gallbladder or the liver. The pain increases if the patient forcibly exhales while the hand is maintained in the lower traction position because the diaphragm rises, stretching the liver and gallbladder upwards	Adhesions
		2. The maneuver of stretching inside the right half of the abdomen is applied to establish the existence of adhesion between the ascending colon and parietal peritoneum. Traction and pressure with the hand are applied in a transverse direction, starting from the lateral abdomen and moving toward the midline and from the midline outwards. This maneuver causes pain by stretching the adhesions, if they exist, in the ascending colon and the nearby parietal peritoneum	
Lian–Odinet [162]	1934	Depending on the compliance and distention of the abdominal wall, percussion with a curved finger or hammer normally causes a single, brief, high-pitch noise to be auscultated. In ascites, two distinct juxtaposed sounds are heard, with the first corresponding to the one heard in normal persons, while the second one is more intense and longer, reflecting the presence of peritoneal effusion. However, in patients with minimal ascites, the double noise is heard in the standing, not supine position, because this position enhances the contact between the surface of the ascites and the abdominal wall	Ascites
Pitfield [167]	1936	*Method 1*	Ascites
		The "diaphragm sign" consists in collecting fluid into as limited a space as possible on the diaphragm by having the patient sit in bed and leaning slightly forward. The posterior thorax over the suspected areas is percussed using the fingertips of one hand, while the other hand palpates the quadratus lumborum muscle on the same side. This causes the collected fluid to vibrate which is felt by the palpating hand on the muscle	
		Method 2	
		The patient sits upright in bed. The height of the fluid is identified by marking the lowest place where the percussion impulse is felt	
Rob [171]	1947	Absent intestinal peristalsis is caused by intestinal contents, pus, bile, hemorrhagic exudate from a strangulated intestine, and exudate from an acutely inflamed pancreas, but not by blood or urine in the peritoneal cavity	Abdominal trauma

(continued)

Table 10.1 (continued)

Name	Year	Description of sign	Significance
Robertson [175]	1947	With ascites, the flanks present a sensation of fullness and tension. With the patient recumbent, a quick upward thrust of the fingers at the flanks results in a form of ballottement	Ascites
Way [178]	1949	Irritation of the undersurface of the diaphragm causes pain over the tip of the acromion	Subdiaphragmatic
Dew [187]	1961	If the hydatid cyst is located beneath the right cupola (subdiaphragmatically), an area of resonance moves caudally when the patient assumes the hand and knee position compared to the sitting position	Subdiaphragmatic cyst

[a] Denotes an individual who supported anti-Semitism, racial acts, or committed crimes against humanity

10.3   Conclusion

A variety of signs were identified using the physical examination skills of observation, palpation, and percussion as a mechanism to identify conditions occurring intra-abdominally. Some of these indirectly involved the diaphragms leading to sub-diaphragmatic inflammation, causing pain referred to the shoulder (Oehlecker, Way). Eponymic signs of ascites described the various means to detect this condition and, in some cases, distinguish it from ovarian cysts (Blaxland). Douglas sign or "cry" represents an interesting divergence from eponyms as it was described by Henri Alphonse Albertin but in reference to the anatomical structure named by James Douglas (1675–1742). These signs have not been studied; thus, their utility in clinical practice remains unknown. They provide the learner with an appreciation of the bedside examination as a method to diagnose disease.

References

 1. Skinner HA. Diaphragm. In: The origin of medical terms. Baltimore, MD: Williams & Wilkins; 1949. p. 118.
 2. Beckett WA. A universal biography: including scriptural, classical and mythological memoirs, together with accounts of many eminent living characters, vol. 2. London: Isaac, Tuckey, and Co.; 1836. p. 636.
 3. Skinner HA. Hippocrates. In: The origin of medical terms. Baltimore, MD: Williams & Wilkins; 1949. p. 177.
 4. Adams F. The genuine works of Hippocrates, vol. 1. London: Sydenham Society; 1849.
 5. Stokes SW. William Stokes: his life and work. London: T. Fisher Unwin; 1898.
 6. [No author]. Obituary: William Stokes. Lancet. 1878;1:108–9.
 7. [No author]. Obituary: William Stokes. N Y Med J. 1878;27:330–1.
 8. [No author]. Obituary: William Stokes. Med Times Gaz. 1878;1:51–2.
 9. [No author]. Medical news: William Stokes MD, FRS. Edin Med J. 1878;22–23:764–5.
10. Stokes W, Bell J. Lectures on the theory and practice of physic, vol. 1. 2nd ed. Philadelphia, PA: Barrington & Haswell; 1842.
11. Collins J. Duchenne of Boulogne: a biography and appreciation. Med Rec N Y. 1908;73:50–4.
12. Breighton P, Breighton G. Duchenne, Guillaume (1806–1875). In: The man behind the syndrome. Berlin: Springer; 1986. p. 44–5.
13. Keith A. Duchenne of Boulogne as orthopedist. In: Menders of the maimed. London: H. Frowde; Hoddler & Stoughton; 1919. p. 91–105.
14. Brissaud E. L'Oeuvre scientifique de Duchenne de Boulogne. Rev Sci. 1899;4:449–60.
15. Collective. Duchenne, Guillaume Benjamin Amand. In: The Encyclopaedia Britannica: a dictionary of the arts, sciences, literature and general information, vol. 8. Cambridge: Cambridge University Press; 1910. p. 629.
16. Mottet A. Duchenne (de Boulogne) et son œuvre. Rev Int Électrothérapie. 1896;6:257–70.
17. Duchenne GBA. Paralysis and contraction of the diaphragm. In: Poore GV, editor. Selections from the clinical works of Dr. Duchenne (de Boulogne). London: The New Sydenham Society; 1873. p. 325–33.
18. Pfuhl E. Wiki. https://second.wiki/wiki/eduard_pfuhl. Accessed 5 Oct 2022.
19. Pfuhl E. Ein oberhalb der Leber gelegenes peritonitisches Exsudat in die rechte Lunge perforirt mit den Zeichen eines rechtsseitigen Pneumothorax. Berl klin Wochenschr. 1877;14:57–60.

20. Schomerus G. Jaffé Karl (1854–1917). In: Ein Ideal und sein Nutzen: Ärztliche Ethik in England und Deutschland, 1902–1933. Frankfurt: Peter Lang; 2001. p. 184.

21. Jaffé K. Ueber subphrenische Abscesse nebst Bemerkungen über die Operation des Empyems. Dtsch med Wochenschr. 1881;7:213–7.

22. [No author]. Obituary: Professor Cesare Federici. Lancet. 1892;1:1278.

23. [No author]. Morte di Socieo corr. Bull Sci Med. 1892;63:496–8.

24. Grocco P. Cesare Federici. In: Annuario per l'anno accademico. Firenze: R. Istituto di Studi superiori pratici di perfezionamento in Firenze; 1893. p. 120–1.

25. Federici C. Istoria di una rara oppilazione dell'intestino. In: Revista Clinica. Bologna: Francesco Vallardi; 1883. p. 84–93.

26. Thomayer J (23.3.1853–18.10.1927). Akademický bulletin. Oficiální časopis Akademie věd ČR. 2008. http://abicko.avcr.cz/archiv/2003/3/obsah/josef-thomayer-23.-3.-1853%2D%2D18.-10.-1927-.html. Accessed 25 Oct 2022.

27. Thomayer J. Ps. R.E. Jamot (1853–1927), Mediziner und Schriftsteller. Österreichisches Biographisches Lexikon. 2014. https://www.biographien.ac.at/oebl/oebl_T/Thomayer_Josef_1853_1927.xml. Accessed 25 Oct 2022.

28. Mašek F. Prof. MU Dr. Josef Thomayer. Zdrav Prac. 1975;25:170–1.

29. Jedlička J. Profesor MU Dr. Josef Thomayer, klasik české lékařské vědy, národní kulturní buditel, mecenáš a člověk. Cas Lék čes. 1972;111:551–6.

30. Thomayer J. Beitrag zur Diagnose der tuberkulösen und karzinomatösen Erkrankungen des Bauchfells. Zeitschr klin Med. 1884;6:378–408.

31. [No author]. Obituary: Alonzo Clark, MD, LLD. Bost Med Sci J. 1887;117:296.

32. [No author]. Biography: Alonzo Clark, AM, MD, LLD. Gaillard Med J. 1887;45:379.

33. [No author]. Alonzo Clark, MD: a memorial read before the Academy of Medicine on January 5, 1888. Med Rec. 1888;33:122–4.

34. Echols M, Arbittier D. Alonzo Clark, MD. Medical Antiques. https://www.medicalantiques.com/civilwar/Medical_Authors_Faculty/Clark_Alonzo.htm. Accessed 10 Sep 2022.

35. Special funds: Alonzo Clark scholarship fund. Catalogue, 1900–1901. Columbia University in the City of New York. 1901. https://www.google.com/books/edition/Catalogue/0RsZAAAAYAAJ?hl=en&gbpv=1&dq=Alonzo+Clark+1887&pg=PA54&printsec=frontcover. Accessed 20 Oct 2022.

36. Elliot E. Memoir of Dr. Alonzo Clark, MD, LLD. N Y Acad Med. 1887;4:499–510.

37. Pepper W, Starr L. A system of practical medicine: General diseases (continued) and diseases of the digestive system, vol. 2. Philadelphia, PA: Lea Brothers & Co.; 1885.

38. Stürzbecher M. Fürbringer, Paul. In: Neue Deutsche Biographie, Bd. 5. Berlin: Duncker und Humboldt; 1961. p. 690–1.

39. Fürbringer P. Biographisches Lexikon hervorragender Ärzte. http://www.zeno.org/Pagel-1901/A/F%C3%BCrbringer,+Paul. Accessed 22 Oct 2022.

40. [No author]. Veränderungen im Personalbestand der Akademie. Leopoldina. 1882;18:202.

41. Fürbringer P. Ueber Pyothorax subphrenicus. Berl klin Wochenschr. 1889;26:287–8.

42. [No author]. Prof. Dott. Pirro Bolognini. In: Annuario della R. Università degli studi di Padova per l'anno accademico. Padova: Università di Padova; 1921. p. 209–10.

43. [No author]. Necrologio: Pirro Bolognini. L'università italiana rivista dell'istruzione superiore. Bologna: Zamorani e Albertazzi; 1918. p. 48.

44. [No author]. Nuova sezione Polesana della ANMO. Rivista Ospedaliera Giornale. 1913;4:153.

45. Bolognini P. Di un segno precoce del morbillo. Pediatria. 1895;3–4:110–6.

46. Cannon WB. Obituary notices: Harvey (Williams) Cushing, 1869–1939. Biogr Mem Fellows R Soc. 1941;3:277–90.

47. MacCallum WG. Biographical memoir of Harvey Cushing, 1869–1939. Nat Acad Sci. 1940;22:49–70.

48. Trail RR. Harvey Williams Cushing. London: Royal College of Physicians. https://history.rcplondon.ac.uk/inspiringphysicians/harvey-williams-cushing. Accessed 30 Oct 2022.

49. [No author]. Editorials: Harvey Cushing. NEJM. 1939;221:623–5.

50. Cushing H. 1869–1939. Social Networks and Archival Context. https://snaccooperative.org/view/55679341. Accessed 29 Oct 2022.
51. Cushing HW. Laparotomy for intestinal perforation in typhoid fever: a report of four cases, with a discussion of the diagnostic signs of perforation. Bull Johns Hopkins Hosp. 1898;9:257–69.
52. Strauss H. Charité Memorial Site. Berlin: Charité – Universitätsmedizin Berlin. https://gedenkort.charite.de/en/people/hermann_strauss/. Accessed 22 Oct 2022.
53. In memory of Prof. Dr. med. Hermann Strauss, 1868–1944. Deutsche Gesellschaft für Gastroenterologie, Verdauungs- und Stoffwechselkrankheiten. https://www.dgvs-gegen-das-vergessen.de/en/biografie/hermann-strauss/. Accessed 26 Oct 2022.
54. Wormer EJ. Strauss, Hermann. In: Neue Deutsche Biographie, Bd. 5. Berlin: Duncker & Humblot; 2013. p. 511–2.
55. [No author]. Prof. Hermann Strauss, noted physician commits suicide in Berlin. JTA Daily News Bull. 1942;9:1.
56. Prof. Dr. Hermann Strauss. Institut Terezinské iniciativy. https://www.holocaust.cz/en/database-of-victims/victim/46922-hermann-strauss/. Accessed 26 Oct 2022.
57. Strauss H. Zur genaueren Kenntniss und Würdigung einer im milchsäurehaltigen Magensaft Massenhaft vorkommenden Bakterienart. Ztschr klin Med. 1895;28:578–85.
58. Strauss H. Ueber Eiter im Magen: nebst Bemerkungen über die Bedeutung des Befundes von Eiter und Blut im Magen sowie gewisser wenig beachteter Krebs – Metastasen für die Diagnose des Magencarcinoms. Berl klin Wochenschr. 1899;36:870–4.
59. Haneman FT. Landau, Leopold. In: The Jewish Encyclopedia: a descriptive record of the history, religion, literature and customs of the Jewish people from the earliest times to the present day, vol. 7. New York, NY: Funk and Wagnalls; 1925. p. 609.
60. Pagel J. Landau, Leopold. In: Biographisches Lexikon: Hervorragender Ärzte des neunzehnten Jahrhunderts. Berlin: Urban & Schwarzenberg; 1901. p. 942–4.
61. Abel K. Leopold Landau. Mschr Geburtsh Gynak. 1921;54:127–30.
62. [No author]. Death of Leopold Landau. JAMA. 1921;76:463–4.
63. Landau L. Ueber den frühen Nachweis von freier Bauchwassersucht. Zentralbl Gynakol. 1900;24:1202.
64. [No author]. Karl Gustaf Lennander, MD, professor of surgery and obstetrics, Uppsala. Br J Med. 1908;1:1085–6.
65. Lennander KG (1857–1908). Plarr's lives of the fellows. London: Royal College of Surgeons of England; 2012. https://livesonline.rcseng.ac.uk/client/en_GB/lives/search/detailnonmodal/ent:$002f$002fSD_ASSET$002f0$002fSD_ASSET:374696/one?qu=%22rcs%3A+E002513%22&rt=false%7C%7C%7CIDENTIFIER%7C%7C%7CResource+Identifier. Accessed 20 Oct 2022
66. Lennander KG (1857–1908). Svenska kyrkan. Uppsala Kyrkogårdar. https://kulturpersoner.uppsalakyrkogardar.se/en/karl-gustaflennander/. Accessed 20 Oct 2022
67. Lennander KG. Acute (eitrige) Peritonitis. Dtsch Ztschr Chir. 1902;63:1–74.
68. Propping K. Ueber die klinische Bedeutung der Differenz zwischen Rektal- und Axillartemperatur, speziell bei Peritonitis. Münch med Wochenschr. 1908;55:506–9.
69. [No author]. John Henry Bryant. Br Med J. 1906;1:1319–20.
70. [No author]. John Henry Bryant, MD, Lond, FRCP. Lancet. 1906;1:1575.
71. Brown GH. John Henry Bryant. London: Royal College of Physicians. https://history.rcplondon.ac.uk/inspiring-physicians/johnhenry-bryant. Accessed 5 Oct 2022
72. Bryant JH. Two clinical lectures on aneurysm of the abdominal aorta: lecture 1. Clin J. 1903;23:71–80.
73. Lorenz OH. Morel (le docteur Louis). Catalogue Général de la Librairie Française, 1906–1909. Paris: D. Jordell; 1911. p. 251.
74. Morel L. Contribution à l'étude des ruptures traumatiques de la vessie. Ann Mal Org Génito-urin. 1906;24:801–10.

75. Morel L (1876-19..). BnF Data. Bibliothèque nationale de France. https://data.bnf.fr/fr/13008682/louis_morel/. Accessed 10 Oct 2022.

76. Firkin BG, Whitworth JA. Kehr sign. In: Dictionary of medical eponyms. London: Parthenon Publishing; 1987. p. 270.

77. Schmidt R. Professor Hans Kehr, 1862–1916. https://gehlberg-chronik.de/index.php/startoffcan. Accessed 4 Oct 2022.

78. Kehr H. Die Praxis der Gallenwege: Chirurgie in Wort und Bild. Munich: J.F. Lehmann; 1913.

79. Klimpel V. Does Kehr's sign derive from Hans Kehr? A critical commentary on its documentation? Chirurg. 2004;75:80–3.

80. Kehr H. Die Chirurgie der Milz. In: Bergmann EV, Burns PV, editors. Handbuch der praktischen Chirurgie, Bd. 3. Stuttgart: Verlag von Ferdinand Enke; 1907. p. 685–701.

81. Levy L. Zur Diagnose der Milzverletzungen. Zentralbl Chir. 1910;37:1577–9.

82. Kehr H. Introduction to the differential diagnosis of the separate forms of gallstone disease: based upon his own experience gained from 433 laparotomies for gallstones. Philadelphia, PA: P. Blakiston's Son & Co.; 1901.

83. Lowenfels AB. Kehr's sign: a neglected aid in rupture of the spleen. NEJM. 1966;274:1019.

84. Sutton CD, Marshall LJ, White SA, Berry DP, Dennison AR. Kehr's sign - a rare cause: spontaneous phrenic artery rupture. ANZ J Surg. 2002;72:913–4.

85. Söyüncü S, Bektas A, Cete Y. Traditional Kehr's sign: left shoulder pain related to splenic abscess. Ulus Travma Acil Cerrahi Derg. 2012;18:87–8.

86. Skipworth JRA, Raptis DA, Rawal JS, Damink SO, Shankar A, Malago M, Imber C. Splenic injury following colonoscopy: an underdiagnosed, but soon to increase, phenomenon? Ann R Coll Surg Engl. 2009;91:W6–11.

87. Shah PR. Splenic rupture following colonoscopy: rare in the UK? Surgeon. 2005;3:293–5.

88. Sachdev S, Thangarajah H, Keddington J. Splenic rupture after uncomplicated colonoscopy. Am J Emerg Med. 2012;30:515.e1–2.

89. Steele DC, Mohamed AM, Kaza A, McCarthy D. Splenic rupture following colonscopy. Dig Dis Sci. 2017;62:72–5.

90. Bonsignore A, Grillone G, Soliera M. Occult rupture of the spleen in a patient with infectious mononucleosis. G Chir. 2010;31:86–90.

91. [No author]. Obituary: Harold Leslie Barnard. Br Med J. 1908;2:538–9.

92. [No author]. Harold Leslie Barnard, MB, MS Lond, FRCS Eng, LRCP Lond. Lancet. 1908;2:984.

93. Barnard HL (1868–1908). Plarr's lives of the fellows. London: Royal College of Surgeons of England; 2009. https://livesonline.rcseng.ac.uk/biogs/E000762b.htm. Accessed 7 Oct 2022.

94. O'Connor WJ. Harold Leslie Barnard (1868–1908). In: British Physiologists, 1885–1914: a biographical dictionary. Manchester: Manchester University Press; 1991. p. 280.

95. Barnard HL. An address on surgical aspects of subphrenic abscess: delivered before the Surgical Section of the Royal Society of Medicine, January 14th, 1907. Br Med J. 1908;1:371–5, 430–6.

96. [No author]. George Blumer, MD, 1872–1962. Dis Colon Rectum. 1980;23:445–60.

97. Hill EG. George Blumer, MD. In: A modern history of new haven and eastern new haven county, vol. 2. New York, NY: S.J. Clarke Publishing; 1918. p. 334–7.

98. [No author]. Professor George Blumer. Yale Med J. 1906;13:32–3.

99. White FA. George Blumer. In: Physical signs in medicine and surgery: an atlas of rare. Lost and forgotten physical signs. Ocala, FL: Museum Press; 2009. p. 676.

100. Gorham GE. History of the bender hygienic laboratory. Studies from the Bender Hygienic Laboratory. 1904;1:1–5.

101. Blumer G. The rectal shelf: a neglected rectal sign of value in the diagnosis and prognosis of obscure malignant and inflammatory disease within the abdomen. Albany M Ann. 1909;30:361–6.

102. Schleicher J. From the archives: Bookplates. Leon S. McGoogan Health Sciences Library. University of Nebraska Medical Center. https://blog.unmc.edu/library/2018/02/19/3574/. Accessed 22 Oct 2022.

103. Brown AJ. Alfred Jerome Brown bookplate collection, ca. 1890–ca. 1960. Archivegrid. 1878. https://researchworks.oclc.org/archivegrid/data/53342607. Accessed 22 Oct 2022.

104. Best RR. In memoriam: Alfred Jerome Brown, 1878–1960. Trans West Surg Assoc. 1960;48:347–9.

105. Alfred JB. Columbia University Irving Medical Center Augustus C. Long Health Sciences Library. Archives and Special Collections. https://www.library-archives.cumc.columbia.edu/obit/alfred-jerome-brown. Accessed 22 Oct 2022.

106. [No author]. Casualties. In: Annual report of the adjutant-general of the state of New York for the year 1906, vol. 2. New York, NY: James B. Lyon; 1907.

107. [No author]. Catalogue and general announcement, 1909–1910. New York, NY: Columbia University; 1910.

108. Brown AJ. The diagnosis of intestinal perforation in typhoid fever. JAMA. 1909;52:695–7.

109. Weißer C. Chilaiditi, Demetrius. In: Chirurgenlexikon: 2000 Persönlichkeiten aus der Geschichte der Chirurgie. Berlin: Springer; 2019. p. 55.

110. Maizlin ZV, Cooperberg PL, Clement JJ, Vos PM, Coblentz CL. People behind exclusive eponyms of radiologic signs (Part I). Can Assoc Radiol J. 2009;60:201–12.

111. Chilaiditi D. Zur Frage der Hepatoptose und Ptose im Allgemeinen im Anschluss an drei Falle von temporarer, partieller Leberverlagerung. Fortschr Geb Rontgenstr Nukl Erganzungsband. 1910;11:173–208.

112. Vierhaus R. Oehlecker, Franz. In: Deutsche Biographische Enzyklopädie, Bd. 7. Munich: K.G. Sauer; 2007. p. 541.

113. Heim W, Schulten H, Dahr P. Nekrologe: Franz Oehlecker. Dtsch med Wochenschr. 1958;83:514.

114. Oehlecker F. Universität Hamburg. https://www.hpk.uni-hamburg.de/resolve/id/cph_person_00000056. Accessed 20 Oct 2022.

115. Oehlecker F. Prof. Dr. med., Hamburg, 16.11.1957. Deutsche Gesellschaft für Chirurgie. https://www.dgch.de/index.php?id=85. Accessed 20 Oct 2022.

116. Franz-Oehlecker-Medaille. Deutsche Gesellschaft für Transfusionsmedizin und Immunhämatologie e.V. https://www.dgti.de/gesellschaft/dgti/gesellschaft/preise/franz-oehlecker-medaille. Accessed 20 Oct 2022.

117. Schmoock M. Anwohner fühlen sich bei Straßenumbenennung übergangen. Hamburger Abendblatt. 2015. https://www.abendblatt.de/hamburg/hamburg-nord/article206808261/Anwohner-fuehlen-sich-bei-Strassenumbenennung-uebergangen.html. Accessed 20 Oct 2022.

118. Oehlecker F. Zur Klinik und Chirurgie des Nervus phrenicus. Zentralbl Chir. 1913;40:852–9.

119. Dr. Edwin Booth Claybrook. The Tabb Family in the United States. Descendants of Humphrey Tabb. https://tabbfamilyhistory.com/p60.htm. Accessed 2 Oct 2022.

120. [No author]. Death of Dr. Edwin Brown Claybrook, B & O surgeon at Cumberland for thirty-on years. B O Mag. 1930;18:31.

121. Claybrook EB. A new diagnostic sign in injuries of the abdominal viscera. Surg Gynecol Obstet. 1914;18:105–6.

122. Drachter R. Zur Diagnose der Peritonitis im Säuglings- und Kindesalter. Münch med Wochenschr. 1914;61:599–600.

123. Hecker WC, Prévot J, Spitz L, Stauffer UG, Wurnig P. Historical aspects of pediatric surgery. Berlin: Springer; 1986.

124. Adams B. Richard-Drachter-Preis für Kinderchirurgie geht nach Leipzig. Universität Leipzig. 2008. https://www.uni-leipzig.de/newsdetail/artikel/richard-drachter-preis-fuer-kinderchirurgie-geht-nach-leipzig-2008-09-19. Accessed 3 Oct 2022.

125. Carachi R, Young DG, Buyukunal C. A history of surgical paediatrics. Singapore: World Scientific Publishing; 2009.

126. Albertin HA. Des injections intra-utérines au point de vue obstétrical sous la méthode anti-septique. Thèse présentée à la Faculté de Médecine et de Pharmacie de Lyon pour obtenir le grade de docteur en médecine. Lyon: J. Gallet; 1887.

127. Albertin HA. Bibliothèques d'Université Paris Cité. https://www.biusante.parisdescartes.fr/histoire/biographies/?refbiogr=130. Accessed 5 Oct 2022.

128. Albertin HA. Archives nationales. République Française. https://www.leonore.archives-nationales.culture.gouv.fr/ui/notice/2334. Accessed 5 Oct 2022.

129. Albertin HA. Le "cri du Douglas" chez la femme. Lyon Chirurg. 1922;19:479–82.

130. Collective. Bulletin of Northwestern University Annual Catalogue, 1903–1904. Evanston, IL: Northwestern University; 1904.

131. Grier RM. A tribute to William Clark Danforth. Q Bull Northwest Univ Med Sch. 1950;24:138–40.

132. Past Presidents: W.C. Danforth, MD, 1921. The Chicago Gynecological Society. https://chicagogyn.org/PAST-PRESIDENTS. Accessed 20 Oct 2022.

133. Danforth WC. Referred pain in the shoulder in ruptured tubal pregnancy. Am J Obst. 1926;12:883–5.

134. [No author]. Comision de redaccion. Boletín Sanitario. 1942;6:ii.

135. Collective. Memoria del Ministerio de Relaciones Exteriores y Culto. Buenos Aires: Ministerio de Relaciones Exteriores y Culto; 1942.

136. D'Amato HJ. Primer Congreso Latino Americano de Hospitales. Boletín Sanitario. 1940;4:362.

137. D'Amato HJ. El signo de las adherencias infrahepáticas. Sem Med. 1926;33:17–35.

138. [No author]. The Arthur Durham Prize for Dissection: medalists and prizemen [Charles Leopold Granville Chapman, Grimsby, Certificate]. Guy's Hosp Rep. 1896;52:215.

139. [No author]. The Arthur Durham Prize for Dissection: medalists and prizemen [Charles Leopold Granville Chapman, Grimsby]. Guys Hosp Rep. 1898;53:297.

140. Chapman CLG. The "rising test" for acute abdomen. Br Med J. 1927;2:786.

141. [No author]. Obituary: A.J. Blaxland, MS, FRCS. Br Med J. 1964;1:123.

142. Blaxland AJ (1880–1963). Plarr's lives of the fellows. London: Royal College of Surgeon of England; 2014. https://livesonline.rcseng.ac.uk/client/en_GB/lives/search/detailnonmodal/ent:$002f$002fSD_ASSET$002f0$002fSD_ASSET:377089/one?qu=%22rcs%3A+E004906%22&rt=false%7C%7C%7CIDENTIFIER%7C%7C%7CResource+Identifier. Accessed 22 Oct 2022.

143. [No author]. Territorial force [Athelstan Jasper Blaxland]. J Roy Army Med Corps. 1915;24:82.

144. [No author]. Universities and colleges [Athelstan Jasper Blaxland]. Br Med J. 1908;2:1846.

145. Blaxland AJ. Ovarian cyst or ascites. Br Med J. 1930;1:839.

146. Edmund W. Butler, MD. San Francisco County Biographies. https://freepages.rootsweb.com/~npmelton/genealogy/sfbbutl.htm. Accessed 10 Oct 2022.

147. [No author]. General session and section officers for the 1922 meeting of the state society. Cal State J Med. 1921;19:419.

148. Past Presidents. San Francisco Surgical Society. http://sanfranciscosurgical.org/past-presidents-and-officers. Accessed 10 Oct 2022.

149. [No author]. News. Stanford Illustrated Review. 1924;26:104.

150. Schecter W, Lim R, Sheldon G, Christensen N, Blaisdell W. The history of the surgical service at San Francisco General Hospital. Wilmington, NC: Broadfoot; 2008.

151. Vice-Presidents: Everett Carlson. San Francisco Surgical Society. 1956. http://sanfrancisco-surgical.org/past-presidents-and-officers. Accessed 10 Oct 2022.

152. Butler E, Carlson E. Pain in the testicles: a symptom of retroperitoneal traumatic rupture of the duodenum. Am J Surg. 1931;11:118.

153. Nicola L. Archivio Storico – Università degli Studi di Cagliari. https://archiviostorico.unica.it/persone/leotta-nicola. Accessed 8 Oct 2022.

154. Nicola L. Treccani. https://www.treccani.it/enciclopedia/nicola-leotta_%28Dizionario-Bio-grafico%29/. Accessed 8 Oct 2022.
155. Nicola L. Bio. Centro Interuniversitario di Ricerca Seminario di Storia della Scienza. https://www.seminariodistoriadellascienza.uniba.it/index.php/il-centro/item/566-nicola-leotta-bio. Accessed 8 Oct 2022.
156. Rabboni F. Sul segno semeiologico di Leotta per le aderenze periviscerali. Il Policlin. 1934;41:118–23.
157. Bedford E. Camille Lian, 1882–1969. Br Heart J. 1969;31:789–90.
158. Lian C. Académie royale de Médecine de Belgique. http://old.armb.be/index.php?id=3420. Accessed 20 Sep 2022.
159. Alain S. La petite maison du grand cardiologue. L'Yonne Républicaine 2014. https://www.lyonne.fr/treigny/sante/2014/03/20/la-petite-maison-du-grand-cardiologue_1925697.html. Accessed 20 Sep 2022.
160. Lian C (1882–1969). BnF Data. Bibliothèque nationale de France. https://data.bnf.fr/fr/10912043/camille_lian/. Accessed 20 Sep 2022.
161. Odinet MJ. Recherches anatomiques et physiologiques sur le thymus: leurs applications cliniques et thérapeutiques. Thèse pour le doctorat en médecine. Faculté de Médecine de Paris. Paris: Librairie Louis Arnette; 1934.
162. Lian C, Odinet J. Le double bruit ascitique et le signe de la matité horizontale dans la station debout: leur importance dans le diagnostic des petites ascites. Presse Méd. 1934;42:1337–8.
163. Marquis AN. Pitfield, Robert Lucas. In: Who's who in America: a biographical dictionary of notable living men and women of the United States, vol. 6. Chicago, IL: A.N. Marquis & Company; 1910–1911. p. 1524.
164. Poupar JA. Robert Lucas Pitfield. In: A history of microbiology in Philadelphia: 1880 to 2010. Philadelphia, PA: Xlibris Co; 2010. p. 52–3.
165. [No author]. Scientific notes and news. Science. 1906;23:518.
166. Pitfield RL. A compend on bacteriology, including pathogenic protozoa. Philadelphia, PA: P. Blakiston's Son; 1947.
167. Pitfield RL. New methods for detecting fluid in the serous cavities. Lancet. 1936;228:983–4.
168. Saxon W. Dr. Charles Granville Rob, 88, surgeon who aided Churchill. The New York Times. 2001. https://www.nytimes.com/2001/07/29/us/dr-charles-granville-rob-88-surgeon-who-aided-churchill.html. Accessed 27 Sep 2022.
169. Cherry N. Lieutenant-Colonel Charles G. Rob. Airborne Assault – ParaData. https://www.paradata.org.uk/people/charles-g-rob. Accessed 27 Sep 2022.
170. Estrada L. Surgeon Charles Rob, 88, dies. Washington Post. 2001. https://www.washingtonpost.com/archive/local/2001/07/29/surgeon-charles-rob-88-dies/d5027a7f-64f1-4975-84c9-8404196f9fac/. Accessed 27 Sep 2022.
171. Rob CG. Auscultation in acute abdominal disease. Lancet. 1947;250:720–1.
172. Kern RA. Memoir of William Egbert Robertson, 1869–1956. Trans Stud Coll Physicians Phila. 1958;26:56–8.
173. McMillan TM. Submission of titles for ACP 1957 session: Dr. William Egbert Robertson. ACP College News Notes. 1956;45:lxviii–lxix.
174. [No author]. Robertson, William Egbert. JAMA. 1956;161:637.
175. Robertson WME, Robertson HF. Diagnostic signs, reflexes and syndrome. 3rd ed. Philadelphia, PA: F.A. Davis Company; 1947.
176. [No author]. Obituary: S.A. Way. Br Med J. 1988;297:550.
177. Way SA (1913–1988). Plarr's lives of the fellows. London: Royal College of Surgeons of England; 2015. https://livesonline.rcseng.ac.uk/client/en_GB/lives/search/detailnonmodal/ent:$002f$002fSD_ASSET$002f0$002fSD_ASSET:379891/one?qu=%22rcs%3A+E007708%22&rt=false%7C%7C%7CIDENTIFIER%7C%7C%7CResource+Identifier. Accessed 28 Sep 2022
178. Way S. A clinical survey of 113 consecutive cases of tubal pregnancy. J Int Coll Surg. 1949;12:550–5.

179. [No author]. Obituary: Sir Harold Dew MBBS, FRCS, FRACS. Br Med J. 1962;2:1478.
180. Carmody J. Dew, Sir Harold Robert (1891–1962). In: Australian dictionary of biography, vol. 13. Melbourne, VIC: Melbourne University Press; 1993. p. 210–1.
181. Dew HR. The University of Sydney School of Medicine Online Museum. https://www.sydney.edu.au/medicine/museum/mwmuseum/index.php/Dew,_Harold_Robert. Accessed 28 Sep 2022.
182. Dew HR, Kt Medaille d'Honneur. Scotch College - World War I Honours and Awards. https://www.scotch.vic.edu.au/ww1/honour/dewHR.htm. Accessed 28 Sep 2022.
183. Dew HR (1891–1962). Plarr's lives of the fellows. London: Royal College of Surgeons of England; 2014. https://livesonline.rcseng.ac.uk/client/en_GB/lives/search/detailnonmodal/ent:$002f$002fSD_ASSET$002f0$002fSD_ASSET:377184/one?qu=%22rcs%3A+E005001%22&ic=true&rt=false%7C%7C%7CIDENTIFIER%7C%7C%7CResource+Identifier. Accessed 28 Sep 2022.
184. Dew HR (1891–1962). Encyclopedia of Australian Science and Innovation. https://www.eoas.info/biogs/P000363b.htm. Accessed 28 Sep 2022.
185. Scholarship Care. Ormond College Sir Harold Dew Medical Scholarship. https://www.scholarshipcare.com/ormond-college-sir-harold-dew-medical-scholarship/. Accessed 28 Sep 2022.
186. Calendar. The Sir Harold Dew Prize. 1964. p. 504. https://www.google.com/books/edition/Calendar/wKSgAAAAMAAJ?hl=en&gbpv=1&bsq=Harold%20Dew%20. Accessed 28 Sep 2022.
187. Dew H. Hydatid disease of the abdomen. In: Maingot R, editor. Abdominal operations. 4th ed. New York, NY: Appleton-Century-Crofts; 1961. p. 782–3.
188. Bailey H. Demonstration of physical signs in clinical surgery. Bristol: John Wright and Sons; 1944.

Chapter 11
Abdominal Wall Signs

11.1 Introduction

Imaging has been the mainstay in evaluating the etiology of abdominal pain. Chronic abdominal wall pain is frequently incorrectly misattributed to visceral pain leading to delayed diagnosis, unnecessary diagnostic testing, and high cost of medical care. Signs of the abdominal wall are those that primarily or secondarily involve the abdominal wall. They include the physical examination techniques of observation and palpations. These signs provide clinical cues to an underlying disease process occurring within the abdomen and the organ system. They are reported chronologically based on the date of their initial description.

11.2 Eponymous Signs

11.2.1 Auenbrugger Sign

Leopold Auenbrugger (1722–1809) was born in Graz, Styria, Austria, and studied medicine at the University of Vienna under the aegis of Baron Gerard van Swieten (1700–1772) [1–5]. He was a resident medical assistant and later physician at the Spanish Military Hospital from 1751 to 1762 and Holy Trinity Hospital in 1753, renamed the "United Hospital" in 1760 [1–5]. Auenbrugger was an associate physician in 1755 and an attending physician in 1761 [4].

Auenbrugger published his historical book *Inventum Novum Ex Percussione Thoracis Humani Ut Signo Abstrusos Interni Pectoris Morbos Detegendi* (A New Discovery that Enables the Physician from the Percussion of the Human Thorax, to Detect the Diseases Hidden within the Chest) in 1761 [4]. The method of chest percussion in clinical diagnosis was not initially well received or adopted by physicians.

© The Author(s), under exclusive license to Springer Nature
Switzerland AG 2023
S. H. Yale et al., *Gastrointestinal Eponymic Signs*,
https://doi.org/10.1007/978-3-031-33673-7_11

It was Baron Jean-Nicolas Corvisart des Marets (1755–1821) who is credited for translating Auenbrugger's writing from Latin to French under the title *Nouvelle méthode pour reconnaitre les maladies internes de la poitrine par la percussion de cette cavité* (New Method for Recognizing Internal Diseases of the Chest by Percussion of this Cavity). It was because of Corvisart that this method of physical examination gained notoriety as an important tool in clinical medicine and physical diagnosis [3].

Auenbrugger spent the remainder of his career as a private practitioner and developed a reputation for treating diseases of the chest [1, 4]. He was a member of the court at Vienna and was conferred the title "Elder von Auenbrugger" by Josef II for recognition of his public service and skills as a physician [4].

To gain some insights into his character, Clar wrote:

> He was a tireless and undeterred as a doctor and full of goodness and philanthropy to his last days; the bells went form the front door into his living room, and a small hand lantern was always ready, with which he often used to light his way to the remotest suburbs on his way to the sick at night. He was the most sought-after doctor of chest diseases [6, p. 29].

In the preface of *Inventum Novum*, the reader can further gain a glimpse of his profound humility, sincerity, and careful investigation devoted to chest percussion:

> What I have written I have proven again and again by the testimony of my own senses, and amid laborious and tedious exertions; —still guarding, on all occasions, against the seductive influence of self-love. (…) I think it is necessary candidly to confess, that there still remain many defects to be remedied—and which I expect will be remedied by careful observation and experiences [7, p. 379]. In submitting this to the public, I doubt not that I shall be considered, by all those who can justly appreciate medical science, as having thereby rendered a grateful service to our art inasmuch as it must be allowed to throw no small degree of light upon the obscure diseases of the chest, of which a more perfect knowledge has hitherto been much wanted [7, p. 380].

Under the twelfth observation of dropsy of the chest in *Inventum Novum* Auenbrugger described the finding of "Swelling of the abdomen, more especially in the epigastrium and particularly in that point on which the incumbent water gravitates" (Table 11.1) [7, p. 399]. Thus, Auenbrugger sign refers to abdominal swelling secondary to a pericardial effusion.

11.2.2   Rosenbach Sign

For historical information regarding Ottomar Rosenbach (1851–1907), see Chap. 7, Liver and Biliary System Signs. We included for the interested reader additional information describing his profound, extraordinary character:

As expressed by W. Guttmann:

> He possessed a personality that was striking and extraordinary in every respect. He was not only an excellent doctor, scholar, and researcher of lonely greatness but also a great noble, a free and proud spirit, and a man of rare integrity and purity of character. All who were fortunate enough to be among his friends and acquaintances looked up to him and held him

in the greatest reverence. Moreover, even from afar, only a few could escape the magic of his personality. His penetrating mind and knowledge made him recognize all weaknesses, whether abstract things or people he had encountered. He was of such extraordinary goodness, benevolence, and tenderness of sentiment that he, far from becoming a misanthrope to all who approached him with a request, provided advice, comfort, and support. His powerful sense of justice always made him stand up for those who were weaker or poorly treated. He could forgive everything, just not the oppression of others. (…) Unrelenting in severity towards himself, he was full of consideration for others and always had understanding and forgiveness for human weaknesses. Only in the field of knowledge were there no compromises for him. Here he defended what he recognized as true and correct with the most extraordinary energy and, if necessary, with cutting edge, without regard to the personal sensitivity of others and their advantage. Science was sacred to him. The courage with which he, often alone, opposed the prevailing dogmas and trends on essential questions (e.g., tuberculin, diphtheria serum, bacteriology, syphilis) when he considered them wrong and disastrous was truly admirable [8, p. 5–6].

Rosenbach described the absence of the superficial abdominal reflex in patients with cerebral hemiplegia (Table 11.1):

> It is well known that stroking the abdomen produces a reflex retraction. Based on the contraction of the abdominal muscles, these indentations can be induced on one side since the skin stimuli do not cross the midline. The depression occurs most clearly when the nail is quickly run over the abdominal surface, regardless of the direction of the stroke. Contact with cold objects can also often produce the sign, but the stroke with the fingernails works best. If the procedures described are applied to those with cerebral hemiplegia, no abdominal reflex, as I would like to call the phenomenon, occurs on the paralyzed side. In contrast, the same occurs promptly and unchanged on the healthy side. As mentioned above, the failure of the abdominal reflex is always present in patients with acute hemiplegia. If the hemiplegia is subacute, the contraction occurs weakly. Even in chronic cases, a difference on both sides of the body is observed, in these cases. As far as I can tell, it always remains weaker on the diseased side [9, p. 846].

Thus, Rosenbach sign refers to the absence of the abdominal skin reflex in cerebral hemiplegia.

11.2.3 Simon Sign

There is limited historical information on Jules Simon (1831–1899). He served as a physician at the Hôpital des Enfants Malades (Hospital of the Sick Children) in Paris throughout his career [10]. As to his character as described by Pierre Merklen:

> To speak of his laborious life, his high professional capacity, and the value and success of his teaching, is to repeat things known to all. Those who have seen him at work and have had the pleasure of living in his intimacy can add that his grand notoriety was based on his work and personal qualities [10, p. 769]. Jules Simon had given himself entirely to medical practice, sacrificing pleasure and rest to it and finding joy only in the exercise of his profession. Endowed with a spirit of penetrating observation and open to all progress, with great common sense, animated by a lively and convincing faith in the effectiveness of hygiene and therapy, he inspired boundless confidence in his patients and their families. He pleased them with his attention full of solicitude, refined good nature, and often playful and picturesque conversation [10, p. 770].

Simon described a finding occurring during the early phase of meningitis in children (Table 11.1):

> I especially wish to insist on the disharmony, the dissociation of the movements of the diaphragm of the rib cage appearing from the first days of meningitis. This finding reveals this disease even in complex and misleading cases. (…) If you do not entirely bare the chest and abdomen in the epigastric region, you will be unable to observe the sign I am showing. If you are fortunate to examine a child with meningitis early in the disease course, hyperesthesia of the skin, brought into contact with the air, causes brief involuntary reflex movements of the chest and abdomen. Proceed slowly by first observing the region of choice covered with the child's shirt. Gradually try to lift it, and put it back without jerks, and you will find yourself in the presence of a curious finding [11, p. 250].

Simon sign is ascribed to two phenomena occurring in early meningitis. First, the dyssynchrony between the diaphragm and thorax movements, and second, involuntary reflex contraction of the chest and abdomen. Although not explicitly stated by Simon, it is because of this dissociation of movement that the umbilicus remains fixed or retracted during inspiration [12].

11.2.4   Guinard Sign

Marie Aimé Désiré Guinard (1856–1911) was born in Saint-Étienne, France, and studied medicine in Paris under the aegis of Aristide Auguste Stanislas Verneuil (1823–1895) at La Pitié Hospital and Paul Jules Tillaux (1834–1904) at Beaujon Hospital [13, 14]. He was head of the surgical clinic at La Pitié and Tillaux of the Paris Faculty of Medicine in 1885 and 1886, respectively, and appointed hospital surgeon and assistant to Peyrot in 1892 [13]. Guinard was director of the surgical department at the Ivery, Bicêtre in 1900, Dubois Municipal House of Health, Paris in 1901, Tenon in 1903, Saint-Louis Hospital in 1904, and the Hôtel-Dieu, Paris in 1906 [13, 14].

He was president of the Union of Doctors, Seine, vice-president of the Anatomical Society in 1896; secretary general of the French Society of Surgery and editorial secretary of *Bulletin général de thérapeutique* (General Bulletin of Therapeutics); and secretary and first-class medical officer of the Territorial Army [13]. He was anointed knight of the Legion of Honor in 1907 and received a prize for his research on surgical diseases of the abdomen from the French Academy of Medicine in 1911 [13, 14].

In a presentation of a paper titled "De la laparotomie dans les contusions de l'abdomen" (Laparotomy for abdominal contusions), presented at the French Surgical Congress in October 1896, Guinard reported two symptoms diagnostic for intestinal perforation:

> [t]wo symptoms, which are essential from the point of view of the diagnosis of perforation. It is first the prehepatic tympanic tone and, secondly, a contracture of the abdominal muscles that prevents deep manual exploration. Unfortunately, apart from these two signs, it is often impossible to confirm the diagnosis [15, p. 874].

Thus, Guinard, Demons, and Hartmann reported rigidity of the abdominal wall in intestinal perforation (involuntary guarding) caused by intra-abdominal injury. Guinard also identified the prehepatic tympanitic percussion sound found in intestinal perforation.

11.2.5   Demons Sign

Jean Octave Albert Demons (1842–1920) was born in Saint-Ciers-de-Canesse, France, and received his medical degree from Bordeaux University in 1868 [16, 17]. He spent his entire medical career at the Faculty of Medicine, Bordeaux, being appointed surgeon to the hospitals of Bordeaux in 1869 and was responsible for directing the surgical department of the Children's Hospital, followed by Saint-André Hospital [17]. Demons was appointed assistant professor in 1871, associate professor in 1879, chair of the surgical clinic, and professor and chair of the surgical clinic from 1886 to 1911 [16–18]. He was a surgeon during the Franco-Prussian War in 1870 and served on the Girondine Ambulance Francis de Luze [18].

Demons founded the Tastet Girard Hospital and contributed to the foundation of the Protestant Nursing Home in Bordeaux [16, 19]. He was editor of the *Archives Provinciales de Chirurgie* (Provincial Archives of Surgery); was a national correspondent for the division of surgical pathology of the French Academy of Medicine from 1892 to 1920; and founded, chaired, and presided over a session of the French Congress of Surgeons in 1891 [16–20]. He received the Knight's Cross in 1873 and was an officer in the Legion of Honor in 1894 [17, 18].

In his presentation on abdominal wall trauma and the involvement of visceral organs, he reported at the French Surgical Congress in October 1897 that:

> A more frequently encountered and decisive symptom is abdominal wall rigidity. The marked rigidity of the wall is sometimes accompanied by moderate distension or, in some cases, by flattening or even excavation of the abdomen. This physical finding suggests visceral involvement and properly accompanies ruptures of the hollow viscera [21, p. 976; 22, p. 385].

Thus, Guinard, Demons, and Hartmann reported that rigidity of the abdominal wall (involuntary guarding) is a sign of intra-abdominal injury and intestinal perforation (Table 11.1).

11.2.6   Hartmann Sign

Henri Albert Charles Antoine Hartmann (1860–1952) was born in Paris, France, studied medicine at the Sorbonne, Paris, was an interne at Hôtel-Dieu from 1881 to 1882, demonstrator of anatomy in 1884, and prosecutor of anatomy at the Faculty of Medicine, Paris, in 1886 [23].

He received his medical degree in 1887 and the Argenteuil Prize for his thesis titled "Des cystitis douleureuses" (Painful cystitis) from the Faculty of Medicine, Paris [23–25]. Hartmann was chief of the urology clinic at the Lariboisière Hospital in 1892, appointed agrégé of surgery in 1895, taught at the surgical clinics at Pitié Salpêtrière Hospital, was deputy director of operative surgery at Lariboisière Hospital in 1898, professor and chair of clinical surgery at Bichat Hospital in 1909, and professor of surgery at Hôtel-Dieu. He was head of the first surgical clinical chair at Hôtel-Dieu from 1914 to 1930 [23–28].

Hartmann was editor of the Journal *Gynécologie et Obstétrique* (Gynecology and Obstetrics) and co-founder of Ligue nationale contre le cancer (French National Cancer League) [23, 28]. He was vice-president of the Anatomical Society in 1892 and the French Association of Surgery in 1922 [25]. He was a founding member of the French Association of Urology and the Society of Obstetrics, Gynecology, and Pediatrics [25]. Hartmann was elected member of the Academy of Medicine in 1918, served as its president in 1936, and was the Grand Officer of the Legion of Honor in 1946 [23–26]. Among his many appointments, he was president of the French Society of Surgery and was president of the French Surgery Congress in 1919, to name a few [23]. Hartmann was elected to the French Academy of Sciences in 1945 and received an honorary degree of a fellowship from the Royal College of Physicians, England, in 1913 [23]. His name is best recognized eponymously for his description of the procedure involving oversewing the rectal or distal colonic stump after resectioning the colonic segment (Hartmann procedure and pouch) [25].

As to a description of his character by Moulonguet:

> His curiosity for exact and precise facts and humility before them were most striking. We have often spoken of his complex character, but we still need to sufficiently note the contrast between his aggressiveness towards men and his docility towards things and events. Through examples, it is easy to show how his practice and teaching have always obediently followed the lesson of facts without bias and pride [26, p. 169]. (…) No less remarkable were his qualities as an observer. It has often been recalled how he interviewed a patient, interrupting the explanations and comments to hear the story of the raw fact, the statement of the pure symptom [26, p. 170]. (…) Docility in the face of facts, admirable gift of observation, solid erudition, meticulous awareness during the operation, these qualities can be given as examples. They justify what his pupil, Lecène, said of him: "It was with Hartmann that I understood what surgery should be, elevated to the height of true science and carried out with respect for others." [26, p. 170].

In a report by Hartmann, he stated (Table 11.1):

> In October 1898, I told you that in the presence of a contusion of the abdomen, I considered, in the absence of any other symptom, the existence of contracture of the wall, not limited to the contused point, as a clear indication for an immediate celiotomy. In the absence of contracture, whatever the reason, I abstain from any intervention [29, p. 234–235].

Thus, Guinard, Demons, and Hartmann reported that abdominal wall rigidity (involuntary guarding) is a sign of intestinal perforation from an intra-abdominal injury.

11.2.7 Sergent Sign

Émile-Eugène-Joseph Sergent (1867–1943) was born in Paris, France, and served as an extern of the Hôpitaux de Paris (Hospitals of Paris) from 1890 to 1891, intern in 1892, and a hospital physician in 1903 [30, 31]. He became head doctor at the Charité Hospital in 1911 and rose to the rank of professor and chair of propaedeutics in 1921 [30]. During World War I, Sergent was a medical lieutenant colonel head of the tuberculosis service, Le Vésinet, France, and during World War II, he served as chief at Boucicaut Hospital. He was chair at Broussais Hospital in 1933 and an honorary doctor in 1937 [30].

Among his accolades, he was honorary doctor of the Faculties of Quebec and Montreal, an honorary professor of the faculties of Bucharest and Montevideo, and an honorary member of the Academy of Medicine, Buenos Aires [30]. He was awarded Grand Officer of the Legion of Honor for his outstanding service in 1943. For his work on adrenal insufficiency, he received the Saintour Prize for his research on syphilis and tuberculosis. Among his other awards, he was Grand Officer of the Crown of Romania and Yugoslavia, to name a few [30].

He was elected member of the National Academy of Medicine, the section of medical pathology in 1919, and served as its president in 1941; president of the Medical Society of Paris Hospital and the Society of the Study of Tuberculosis in 1924; and member of the Supervisory Board for Public Assistance [30, 32].

Sergent described what he believed to be a pathognomonic finding in patients with acute adrenal insufficiency (Table 11.1):

> This pathognomonic sign, which I previously discussed, would remove any doubt about the diagnosis. I encountered this diagnostic finding in a previous case to which I have already alluded in connection with acute adrenal insufficiency. I have described this symptom as the adrenal white line phenomenon. When a line is traced with the fingernail on the patient's skin, this line grows pale and outlined, by its whiteness, the path followed by the finger [33, p. 383].

Sergent postulated that the "white line" was caused by reflex capillary spasm. This sign has been inconsistently described in the literature as taking place on the chest or abdomen [34, 35]. However, Sergent did not specify in his publication the region of the body where the skin is scratched.

11.2.8 Beevor Sign

Charles Edward Beevor (1854–1908) was born in London, England, and received his medical degree from the University College Hospital London in 1881 [36, 37]. He was elected master of the Royal College of Physicians in 1882 and fellow in 1888 [36, 38, 39]. He served as a house physician at the University College Hospital and resident medical officer at the National Hospital for the Paralyzed and Epileptic at Queens Square, Bloomsbury, London [36]. This was followed by an appointment as an assistant physician at National Hospital for the Paralyzed and Epileptic in 1883 and 1885 as an assistant physician at the Great Northern Central Hospital [38]. He rose to the rank of physician at both hospitals [36–38].

Beevor contributed most extensively to the field of neurology, with his most classic works including *Diseases of the Nervous System: A Handbook for Students and Practitioners* in 1898, *Muscular Movements and Their Representation in the Central Nervous System* published in 1904, *The Diagnosis and Localisation of Cerebral Tumours* published in 1907, and *The Distribution of the Different Arteries Supplying the Human Brain* published in 1908 [40, 41]. The last work was significant because it provided precise blood supply localization to various brain regions. His areas of interest, expertise, and crowing achievements were the diagnosing and localization of cerebral tumors and arterial supply to the brain [42, 43].

He was elected president of the Neurological Section of the Royal Society of Medicine from 1907 to 1908, officer and trustee of the Medical Society of London, and honorary secretary to the Association for the Advancement of Medicine by Research [36].

A description of his character as articulated by Sir Victor Horsely, who first worked with him as a clinical clerk, "His extraordinary good nature, his never-failing graceful courtesy, and his untiring efforts to help us made an ineffaceable impression and inaugurated an unbroken friendship of exactly thirty years." [36, p. 1785].

Another friend and colleague wrote:

> Beevor's character was singularly winning and attractive. Sweet, simple, guileless, unselfish, retiring, and affectionate; none who knew him as I did could help loving him. No breath of slander ever passed his lips. His mind and thoughts were white and clean as those of a child. He never uttered an unkind word. It is most difficult to convey in words an adequate idea of the simplicity and beauty of Beevor's life [39, p. 1855].

In his talk delivered before the Royal College of Physicians of London in June 1903, Beevor reported a method to access the abdominal wall muscles (Table 11.1):

> I observed some years back a symptom which enables the investigator to tell if there is any weakness of the upper or lower part of the recti. The symptom is the movement of the umbilicus. In health, in the movement of sitting up, the umbilicus does not alter its position, but if from a lesion of the lower part of the spinal cord or its nerves, the part of the recti below the umbilicus be paralyzed, the normal upper part of the recti will draw up the umbilicus, sometimes to the extent of an inch. As the abdominal wall at the level of the umbilicus is supplied by the tenth dorsal root, any marked elevation of the umbilicus in the act of sitting up would show a lesion between the tenth and twelfth dorsal segments of the cord or the roots coming off from them. In the case where I first observed this symptom there was a malignant growth involving the cord at the level of the eleventh and twelfth dorsal roots. In two cases, one a myopathy and the other a case under the care of my colleague, Dr. Ormand, I have seen the umbilicus drawn downwards, due, I have no doubts, to weakness of the part of the recti situated above the umbilicus [44, p. 40].

Thus, Beevor sign refers to the superior movement of the umbilicus when the lower portion of the rectus abdominal muscle is paralyzed.

11.2.9 Ransohoff Sign

Joseph Ransohoff (1853–1921) is the senior of the three generations of Ransohoff physicians. His son was Dr. Joseph Louis Ransohoff (1880–1958), and his grandson was Dr. Joseph Ransohoff (1915–2001) [45]. Joseph Ransohoff (1853–1921) was born in Cincinnati, Ohio, and received his medical degree from the Medical College of Ohio in 1874. He continued his medical studies in Paris, Vienna, Würzburg, Berlin, and London and, on his return, was appointed demonstrator of anatomy in the Medical College of Ohio in 1877 [46–48].

Ransohoff was a professor of anatomy from 1879 to 1891 and anatomy and clinical surgery from 1891 to 1902. When the Medical College of Ohio merged with the University of Cincinnati in 1896 to acquire the new name, the Medical Department of the University of Cincinnati Ransohoff held an appointment of Principles of Surgery from 1902 to 1905, followed by professor of surgery in 1905 [46–49]. He was also on staff as a surgeon at the Cincinnati General Hospital, Good Samaritan, and dean of the Jewish Hospitals in Cincinnati [46, 47].

He was awarded fellow of the Royal College of Surgeons, London, in 1877, a fellow of the American College of Surgeons, and a member of several societies and associations, including the American Medical Association and American Academy of Medicine [47, 49].

As to a glimpse of his character:

> Not only was he a leading physician and surgeon, but he was a public-spired citizen, and he shared a deep and keen interest in his native city, its people, and its institutions. He was exceedingly popular among the members of his profession, and he was especially kind and helpful to the young physicians. He loved his profession and sought no place or preferment outside its limits [49, p. 226].

Ransohoff described a 53-year-old man with a ruptured common bile duct and bile peritonitis (Table 11.1):

> On inspection of the abdomen, attention was called to a marked jaundice of the umbilicus. The navel was of a distinct saffron-yellow color in strong contrast with the rest of the skin over the abdomen. It was the only evidence of jaundice [50, p. 396]. (…) I wish here to call attention to a sign which was referred to in the case of the ruptured duct before the incision was made, and one to which I believe attention has never before been directed. It is the localized jaundice of the umbilicus. Although a single case is not usually sufficient to warrant the assumption that something new has been observed, this feature was so marked that I cannot refrain from believing that further observation will give to this localized jaundice some value as a sign of free bile in the peritoneal cavity. In the case presented, this feature gained in interest as the staining of the subperitoneal fat with bile was observed in the incision through the abdominal wall. The jaundice is probably the result of inhibition. It makes itself manifest first in the integument of the navel, because this part is thinner than the rest of the abdominal wall. It is possible, of course, that by reason of the anatomic relations of the round ligament of the liver to the transverse fissure that is a retrograde flow of bile through the lymphatics toward the navel, just the caput medusa is produced by cirrhosis [50, p. 397].

Thus, Ransohoff sign refers to the saffron-yellow discoloration of the umbilicus in rupture of the common bile duct.

11.2.10   Livierato Sign

Panagino Elenco Livierato (1860–1936) was born in Kefalonia, Greece, and received his medical degree in 1886 [51, 52]. He was appointed ordinary professor of special medical pathology in Genoa, Italy, in 1890 and served at the medical clinic in Palermo, Italy, in 1895 [51, 52].

Livierato observed in a 35-year-old man postprandial chest heaviness and occasional shortness of breath that resolved with activity and was absent with walking up the stair or a hill. An increased pulse rate and right cardiac border extending to the midline of the sternum were found on physical examination. He described a palpatory technique as a means for detecting the early development of right ventricular failure prior to the onset of symptoms. This involved tapping the abdominal wall by placing (Table 11.1):

> [t]he patient in a supine position and delineate the area of absolute obtuseness of the heart. As seen, it has limits: internally, the median line of the sternum; externally, the vertical papilla where the apex beat is perceived; superiorly, the upper border of the fourth left rib on the left margin of the sternum, which curves gradually downwards reaching the region of the cardiac apex; inferiorly, the sixth rib. The pulse has a regular rate and rhythm. Tap repeatedly on the midline of the abdomen, beginning in the epigastrium to the umbilicus along the path of the abdominal aorta. We will determine which cardiac area is modified and can be defined. By delineating the area of the dullness of the heart again, it is seen that its limit has extended considerably to the right. The inner limit reaches the margin to the right of the sternum, while the upper and the exterior are slightly modified. The cardiac dullness extends to the right for about three centimeters. The pulse is increased somewhat in frequency, and the pulmonary component of the second sound is accentuated. I now asked the patient to rise from the bed and walk quickly around the room several times and again delineated the area of cardiac dullness. As is seen, we find this area considerably narrowed. The internal limit reaches the margin to the left of the sternum, the upper area is slightly lowered, almost unchanged, and the left remains the same. The pulse is stronger and more frequent than previously. Moreover, from the subjective point of view, following this movement, the individual, as they see, does not experience any problems with either breathing or palpitations [53, p. 5].

He accounted for the proposed pathogenesis, which he named the abdomino-cardiac reflex:

> In our case, we have seen in a schematic way that the irritation of the abdominal nerves has given rise to the expansion of the right ventricle in an obvious and conspicuous way [53, p. 6]. (…) Usually, a person experiences no subjective feeling because the right ventricle makes up for the increase in energy. However, as soon as the myocardium, due to any cause, is compromised in its potentiality, the impediments that cause reduced pulmonary blood flow explain the dilation of the right ventricle. Thus, we understand why not all individuals were suffering from stomach, liver, or other diseases present with dilation of the heart under the mentioned conditions. The tonicity and energy of the myocardial fiber must decrease for dilatation to occur. In our case, by tapping on the abdomen, we produced excitement due to the sympathetic, which causes a constriction of the pulmonary vessels. We have detected a strengthening of the tones of the lung and the dilation of the dullness of the heart to the right. Our simple observation proves that we did not excite the vagus because the pulse not

only does not slow down but increases in frequency [53, p. 7] (…). The ingested foods produce excitement, starting from the stomach's mucosa, causing the constriction of pulmonary vessels due to the sympathetic. The semiological artifice used by us, which we call the abdominal-cardiac reflex, enables us to explain our patient's bothersome sensation and cure him judiciously. This simple artifice shows that the myocardium of this individual has little energy and tone [53, p. 7].

Thus, Livierato sign refers to the dilation of the right ventricle when tapping the abdominal wall in the midline from the epigastrium to the umbilicus. The phenomenon was believed to be caused by vasoconstriction due to activation of the abdominal sympathetic nerves.

11.2.11 Cruveilhier–Baumgarten Sign

11.2.11.1 Jean Cruveilhier

Jean Cruveilhier (1791–1874) was born near Limoges, France, studied medicine at the University of Paris, and received his medical degree in 1816 based on the thesis *Essai sur l'anatomie pathologique en général* (Essay on Pathological Anatomy in General) [54, 55]. He was appointed professor of anatomy at the medical school of Montpellier, France, in 1825 and later chair of pathological anatomy at the Faculty of Medicine, Paris, from 1835 to 1865 [54–59]. He also served as physician-in-chief and director of the Maternity, Salpêtrière, and Charité Hospitals [54, 57, 58].

Cruveilhier was a member of the French Academy of Medicine of the pathological anatomy section in 1836 and served as president in 1859. He was elected commander of the Legion of Honor in 1863 and an honorary fellow of the Royal Medical-Surgical Society in 1862 [54, 56–58].

His passion in medicine throughout his career was pathological anatomy culminating in his most significant work titled *Anatomie Pathologique du Corps Humain* (first volume published in 1829 and second volume in 1842), which consisted of plates of macroscopic illustration of morbid anatomy [58]. Given his contribution to pathological anatomy, Rudolf Ludwig Carl Virchow (1821–1902) recognized him as "the father and patriarch of pathological anatomy" [59, 60].

As to a description of his character as a eulogy by his friend and pupil M. Bardinet, who was at that time headmaster of the medical school in Limoges:

Cruveilhier was distinguished not only by a superior intellect but also by the noblest qualities of the heart. All men admired his unswerving rectitude, his genuine simplicity, his equanimity of temper, which remained unruffled by the breath of calumny. He was enthusiastically devoted to his patients and science. His industry was unflagging, and he scarcely allowed himself the indispensable repose. (…) Rarely has a man of science been so thoroughly kind and considerate to his patients; rarely have the latter more warmly reciprocated a welcome so sympathizing [57, p. 570].

11.2.11.2   Paul Clemens von Baumgarten

Paul Clemens von Baumgarten (1848–1928) was born in Dresden, Germany, studied medicine at the Universities of Königsberg and Leipzig, and received his medical degree from the latter in 1873 [61, 62]. He served as an assistant anatomist at the Anatomical Institute of the University of Leipzig from 1873 to 1874, an associate professor of pathological anatomy at the University of Königsberg from 1877 to 1881, and a professor from 1881 to 1880 [61, 63]. He was appointed chair of pathological anatomy and general pathology at the University of Tübingen in 1889 [61, 63]. He was a commander second class of the Royal Saxon Order of Albrecht and recipient of the Cross of Honor of the Order of the Württemberg Crown in 1895 [63].

Baumgarten described the case of a 16-year-old man with anemia, splenomegaly ascites, liver cirrhosis, and complete patency of the umbilical vein. He proposed three states of the umbilical vein in liver cirrhosis: i. persistent patency, ii. partial patency, or iii. Complete obliteration (Fig. 11.1):

> If the intra-abdominal part of the umbilical vein remains patent, it abnormally communicates directly at the umbilicus with the epigastric veins. It then extends from the umbilicus, just as in the embryonic state, along the posterior edge of the falciform ligament to the hepatic porta and in a slight curve to the portal venous sinus similar to that occurring in the embryo [64, p. 104]. (…) After this outline of the three modes of vascular connection between the portal vein and the system of deep veins of the anterior abdominal wall, let us look at our case. There can be no doubt that mode 1, a total openness of the intra-abdominal part of the umbilical vein acts [64, p. 105]. (…) The reason for the total openness to be regarded as proven hereafter can be seen in the abnormal direct connection which exists between the umbilical vein and the deep inferior epigastric veins close to the umbilicus. This allows blood to flow through the umbilical vein postpartum along its entire intra–abdominal course, thereby preventing its obliteration along the entire route [64, p. 106].

He compared his case to Cruveilhier's description published in *Anatomie Pathologique du Corps Humain* (Pathological Anatomy of the Human Body) (Table 11.1):

> In Cruveilhier's case, the persistence of the umbilical vein throughout its length from the umbilicus to the portal sinus is, as he rightly says, "a fact beyond dispute"; because the umbilical vein is located on the inferior edge of the falciform ligament, it communicates directly with the umbilicus and vastly expanded epigastric veins (caput medusae). There is no evidence for the obliteration of the umbilical vein trunk. In none of the later observations, apart from ours, has proof of total patency of the umbilical vein been furnished with the same certainty as Cruveilhier. Our case coincides with that of Cruveilhier. Anyone who compares the relevant illustration in Cruveilhier's well-known atlas of pathological anatomy with the illustration of our preparation attached to this treatise will readily admit the essential agreement. Decisive for understanding the large vessel in the inferior edge of the suspensory ligament as an umbilical vein that has remained open is, as already mentioned, the absence of a cord corresponding to the obliterated umbilical vein next to the large open vessel, which has been demonstrated in our case as well as in Cruveilhier's case. The only minor difference is that in Cruveilhier's case, the superficial epigastric veins, not the deep ones, as in ours, flow directly into the umbilical vein. It is fascinating that in Cruveilhier's case, too, atrophy of the liver was associated with the umbilical vein remaining patent, although this was only smooth atrophy, not granular atrophy [64, p. 107].

Thus, Cruveilhier-Baumgarten sign refers to the multiple dilated umbilical and paraumbilical veins on the abdominal wall (caput medusa) in patients with portal hypertension.

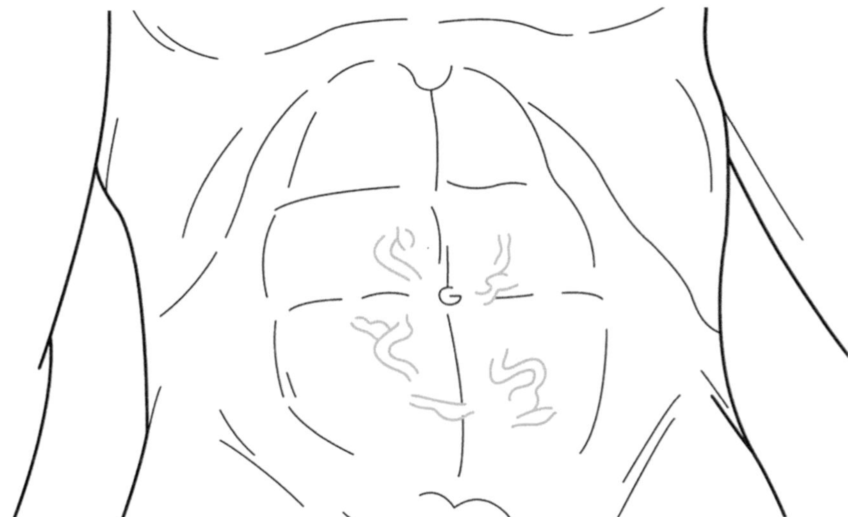

Fig. 11.1 Cruveilhier–Baumgarten sign (by Ryan Yale)

11.2.12 Hofstätter Sign

Robert Wilhelm Ludwig Hofstätter (1883–1970) was born in Vienna, Austria, and received his medical degree from the University of Vienna in 1907. He was the father of Peter Robert Adolf Maria Hofstätter (1913–1994), a social psychologist [65, 66]. He pursued training in gynecology at the second medical university clinic and university women's clinic in Vienna from 1908 to 1910 [65, 66].

Hofstätter was assistant to Heinrich von Peham (1871–1930) at the Vienna General Polyclinic in 1913. He habilitated at the University of Vienna in obstetrics and gynecology in 1919 and was appointed associate professor in 1939 [65]. He was a provisional manager in the Department of Gynecology at the Vienna General Polyclinic, head of the outpatient clinic for gynecological diseases at the Vienna General Hospital from 1936 to 1938, and the women's department of the children's hospital from 1938 to 1940 [65]. He served as a senior physician during World War II and as a German nationalist and Nazi eugenicist [67–69]. After the war, he was in private practice in obstetrics and gynecology and was appointed professor of obstetrics and gynecology at the University of Vienna in 1951. He was a member of the Austrian Cancer Society in 1958 and the German Society of Obstetrics and Gynecology in 1962 [65, 66].

Since eponyms are honorific terms, Hofstätter sign should not be used in medical discourse because of his views and affiliations during National Socialism.

Hofstätter reported the case of a 36-year-old female who developed a "blood discoloration of the skin above the umbilical hernia," later believed to be caused by a ruptured ectopic pregnancy [70, p. 524]. Hofstätter found on the physical examination (Table 11.1):

> The skin above it and a small area around it are suffusion with blood and, in some places, have already turned yellowish. The tumor is moderately firm, has large lobes, and is slightly diffusely sensitive to pressure. There is an empty sound above it; not reducible as a whole and does not change size after coughing or straining [70, p. 524].

Thus, Hofstätter sign refers to a palpable ecchymotic and yellowish discoloration involving the umbilical and periumbilical regions in cases of ectopic pregnancy. Thomas Stephen Cullen (1868–1953) described a similar finding 2 years later (see Cullen sign).

11.2.13   Wynter Sign

Walter Essex Wynter (1860–1945) was born in Brompton, London, England, and received his medical training at the Middlesex and Bartholomew Hospitals, London, qualifying as a member of the Royal College of Surgeons in 1883. He was elected fellow of the Royal College of Surgeons in 1885, medical baccalaureate, London in 1887, and a medical degree in 1888 [71, 72]. Wynter served on staff at Brompton Hospital, the Hospital for Sick Children, and Middlesex Hospital [71]. At the Middlesex Hospital, he was appointed assistant physician in 1891, physician and lecturer in medicine in 1901, and senior physician and consulting physician in 1925 [72]. He was elected fellow of the Royal College of Physicians in 1897. During his retirement in Newbury, he was a consultant at Newbury District Hospital, a town council member, and chairman of the public health committee [71, 72].

As to a description of his character by Taylor:

> Wynter will long be remembered by his contemporaries and pupils for his unvarying kindness and charm; he had a most lovable nature and could not have had an enemy in the world [71, p. 101].

Among his contributions to medicine, he described a sign of acute fibrinous pericarditis secondary to rheumatic heart disease with polyarthritis and, in 1891, a method using a Southey's tube with rubber drainage at the L2 intervertebral space for performing a lumbar puncture. This finding was published five months after Heinrich Irenaeus Quincke (1844–1922) reported a lumbar puncture using a fine needle cannula between the third and fourth lumbar vertebral spaces at the tenth Medical Congress at Wiesbaden in 1891 [73, 74]. According to Wynter, "The first case which the method was tried was February 1889" [74]. This suggests that the attribution to the person who first performed the first lumbar puncture should be attributed to Wynter.

Wynter described a finding he observed in two cases of pericarditis (Table 11.1):

> The sign suggested in this communication is inhibition of the action of the diaphragm, indicated by suppression of normal abdominal respiratory movement, and has probably been hitherto overlooked through examination being unduly restricted to the chest in such cases [75, p. 40]. (…) There is no doubt, however, that when attention is directed to the matter, and a definite note made as to the presence or absence of abdominal movement, this feature will be found fairly constant in acute pericarditis, especially that with fibrinous

exudate. When the front of the body is fully exposed, the stiffness of the abdomen is very striking, suggesting peritonitis, unless as sometimes happens, there is inspiratory recession, which might mislead, unless the want of correspondence with the movement of the upper chest is noted [75, p. 44].

Interestingly, in the discussion regarding this case, Voelcker reported the cases of a child who was initially suspected of having either pericarditis or pneumonia:

> There was absence of abdominal respiratory movement, and there were no definite signs in the chest. Movement though slight in the upper part of the abdomen, was very limited in the lower part of the abdomen, and a diagnosis of appendicitis was afterwards made. At the operation a perforated appendix with general peritonitis was found [75, p. 48].

Thus, Wynter sign refers to the absence of abdominal movement during respiration in patients with pericarditis. Voelcker also noted this sign but in a case of acute appendicitis with peritonitis.

11.2.14 Delbet Sign

Pierre Delbet (1861–1957) was born in La Ferté-Gaucher (Seine-et-Marne), France, and received his medical degree from the University of Paris in 1899 [76]. He was agrégé at the University of Paris in 1892, a surgeon at Hôpitaux de Paris (Hospitals of Paris) in 1893, a professor in 1901, and a full professor of the surgical clinic in the Faculty of Medicine, Paris in 1909 [76–78]. Delbet was chair of the surgical clinic of the Necker Hospital in 1912 and subsequently clinical chair at Cochin Hospital [76, 77].

Among his many accolades, he was an honorary professor of the Faculty of Medicine, Paris, a member of the Academy of Medicine operative medicine section from 1921 to 1957, a founding member along with Drs. Charles Bouchard (1837–1915) and Henri de Rothschild (1872–1947) of the French Association for the Study of Cancer (Currently Société Française du Cancer) in 1906, and commander of the Legion of Honor [76, 77]. He studied and wrote on many diseases and therapeutic areas, including the management of fractures, antisepsis with magnesium chloride solution, mesenteric ischemia, breast cancer, aneurysm, and pleurisy [76].

His character as described by Jean Patel:

> His action, for nearly 30 years, in the clinic and teaching, made people admire his resources as a curious, erudite pathologist, and his talents as an improviser, observer, and teacher [79, p. 139]. (…) One could say that he was as attentive to himself, hungry for study and progress, in love with continuous effort, intoxicated by the greatest thoughts, possessing excellent resources of penetration, analysis, logic, assimilation, memory and reminiscences, very concerned with anticipations, and the most imaginative, the most reformer of his time [79, p. 146].(…) "Finally, he had a fertile imagination, and above all an astonishing memory in which remained engraved, with absolute precision, the memories of his readings, his travels, his clinical observations, his experiences and, at the slightest call, he brought out the facts that came to support his demonstration [79, p. 146].

Delbet in his description of a farmhand kicked in the abdomen by a horse found on physical examination (Table 11.1):

> Palpation everywhere was painless and provoked a weak defense only when one reached an area as wide as the palm located superiorly and the left of the umbilicus. At this location of the trauma, the muscle contraction is caused by the contusion of the wall. (…) [80, p. 370]. The contraction of the muscle and the defense of the wall, as shown by Professor Hartmann, is a reliable sign when present, but its absence does not prove that there has been no damage to the underlying viscera [80, p. 371].

Thus, Delbet sign refers to abdominal wall contraction in abdominal contusion and perforation involving the abdominal viscera.

11.2.15 Ligat Sign

David Ligat (1873–1954) was born near Glasgow, Scotland, and received his Bachelor of Medicine degree from the University of Glasgow in 1894 [81]. He earned his Doctor of Public Health degree in Manchester in 1898 and held a position in the public health service [81]. He then became a surgical clinical assistant at the Evelina Hospital for Sick Children, London [82]. At the Middlesex Hospital, he served as an acting assistant surgeon from 1915 to 1919. He also served as consulting surgeon at St. Leonard's Hospital London. He was appointed to the Buchanan, St. Leonards-on-Sea, and Bexhill Hospitals in 1922. During World War II, he practiced surgery at the Royal Sussex Hospital and suffered injuries that prematurely ended his surgical practice [81, 82].

He obtained a fellowship from the Royal College of Surgeons in 1907 and was a member of the British Medical Association, being selected as chairman of the Hastings Division from 1922 to 1923 and president of the Sussex Branch from 1924 to 1925 [81].

His character, as described by Dr. W.F. Hamilton:

> I had known him for almost 30 years, and had always wondered if enthusiasm were the secret of perpetual youth or if his extreme youthfulness were the source of his abundant enthusiasm. For enthusiasm, courage, honesty, and tenacity of purpose were the keynotes of his character, and kindliness and almost boyish cheerfulness the grace-notes. This enthusiasm was shown in all his activities—his music, his golf, and above all his surgery. But here he never let it interfere with his judgment or allowed it to lead him into an operation which he did not honestly believe was for the good of his patient [83, p. 464].

Ligat described the method for eliciting a viscerosensory reflex (viscera to tissues of body wall comprising muscle, interstitial tissue, and skin):

> I grasp the skin and subcutaneous tissue firmly between finger and thumb and draw them away from deeper layers of the abdominal wall. If a hyperalgesic area be present, the patient winces, and one can tell, by the patient's expression, when such an area is being stimulated [84, p. 107–108]. (…) In this method of examination, the following points should be noted: i) The patient should be made to appreciate a pinch of definitive pressure over a normal point and asked to realize the sensation, the facial expression being watched closely at the

same time, for normal sensation to pinch varies widely in different individuals. ii) An exactly similar pinch is applied at the spot where the maximum response is expected. No downward pressure is made on the abdominal wall, but the skin and subcutaneous tissue are picked up from the abdominal wall and pinched with the same amount of forces that had been applied in the control. iii) The direction and limitation of the extension of hyperalgesia must be carefully noted [84, p. 109].

Ligat noted that the painful regions were not uniformly distributed in a segmental fashion but corresponded to the anatomical subcutaneous innervation of branches of particular nerves. Thus, Ligat sign refers to a functional area of hyperalgesia caused by pressing the skin and subcutaneous tissue between the thumb and finger (Table 11.1).

11.2.16   Handley Sign

William Sampson Handley (1872–1962) was born in Loughborough, England, and qualified with a bachelor of medicine and bachelor of science degrees from Guy Hospital in 1895, earning the London University exhibition and a gold medal [85, 86]. He received his medical degree in 1896, was a house surgeon to William Arbuthnot Lane (1856–1943), and became a fellow of the Royal College of Physicians (FRCP), England, in 1897. He was appointed demonstrator of anatomy for 2 years, followed by serving as a private practitioner in Woolwich, London, England. He received his master's degree in 1899 [85, 86].

Handley was appointed outpatient surgeon at the Samaritan Hospital for Women and Children in 1900. He conducted research at the Middlesex Hospital Cancer Laboratories from 1903 to 1906, where he was instrumental in formulating this theory on the central lymphatic invasion and dissemination of cancer [85]. He was appointed assistant surgeon to the surgical staff at Middlesex Hospital beginning in 1906 under the aegis of Sir John Bland-Sutton (1885–1936) and Eric Lush Pearce Gould (1886–1940); held a consulting practice at Harley Street; and was on the consulting staff at Bolingbroke, Middlesex, and Putney Hospitals [85]. He was a captain in the Royal Academy Medical Corps during World War I from 1914 to 1918, directed the Bournemouth Municipal Cancer Clinic, and was appointed senior consulting surgeon to Middlesex Hospital [85–87].

Handley was the recipient of the Richard Hollins Cancer Research Scholarship at the Middlesex Hospital from 1903 to 1906, the Astley Cooper Prize in 1904, and the Walker Prize from the Royal College of Surgeons in 1911 in recognition of his work advancing the pathology and therapeutics of cancer. He received the Comfort Crookshank Prize for cancer research at the Middlesex Hospital in 1955 [86, 87]. Handley was named an honorary fellow of the American College of Surgeons in 1926, the Medical Society of London in 1944, and the Royal Society of Medicine in 1961 [85]. He was editor of the *Transactions of the British Proctological Society*, associate editor of the *Annals of Surgery*, and vice-president of the Royal College of Surgeons from 1931 to 1933 [85–87].

As to a description of his character as described by Cox:

> Being gentle and earnest in manner, it is not surprising that he should have shared with that grand and kindly physician Dr. Goodall the task of being honorary physician and surgeon to the students. He never ridiculed their fears and phobias, and since his habit was to ponder long before speaking, the student knew that even if his fears be trivial, he would never be considered foolish. Somehow it seems to have been natural that Mr. Handley should have become my lifelong friend and mentor. The dictionary meaning of the word "mentor' is "faithful counsellor," and that is just what Mr. Handley has been to all those who sought his advice and support [88, p. 1082].

Handley described the stage of general peritonitis (Table 11.1):

> If there is a condition in surgery which is stamped with the word hopeless, it is that stage of general peritonitis where, in spite of pelvic drainage, cessation of the passage of flatus and persistent foul vomiting indicate that complete obstruction has supervened. The rigid abdominal muscles have been forced to yield by the pressure of fluid poured out into the paralysed intestine, and the abdomen is uniformly and tightly distended like a drum. The pulse becomes running, the extremities cold, and the patient, measuring his condition by the abnormal clearance of his faculties, only within a few hours of the end realizes with a horrible certainty that he is in the inexorable grasp of death [89, p. 519].

Handley recognized an earlier stage of peritonitis where the inflammation was confined to the pelvis:

> There is a preceding stage in which obstruction is complete, but the pulse is still relatively good, and the vomit has not become offensive. The abdomen is generally distended, but it is absolutely rigid only below the umbilicus. The upper half of both recti is softer than the lower half, and above the umbilicus slight respiratory excursions of the abdomen can still be seen [89, p. 519]. (…) [t]he guts below the horizontal level of the symphysis were paralyzed, while the bowel above, though distended, retained their contractile power. As the pelvis contains both a length of large and a length of small intestines, there are two obstructions to be dealt with, and the name "ileus duplex" was suggested for the condition [89, p. 519].

Handley believed that the operative technique differed depending upon the finding of an ileus duplex or in cases where the peritonitis and intestinal obstruction were confined to the pelvis. In the latter case, he recommended ileo-colostomy to the ascending colon with caecostomy. In cases of general peritonitis, he recommended a jejuno-colostomy to the transverse colon with caecostomy.

Thus, Handley sign refers to the appearance of the abdomen wall in peritonitis confined to the pelvis. Above the umbilicus, the rectus abdominal muscles are soft, move with shallow respiration, and contract.

11.2.17   *Willan Sign*

Robert Joseph Willan (1878–1955) was born in Durham, England, and received his Medical Baccalaureate degree with honors from the University of Durham in 1906 [90]. He was elected fellow in the Royal College of Physicians in 1908 and received his Master of Science degree in 1909 with first-class honors [90]. Willan was appointed house surgeon and surgical registrar at the Royal Victoria Infirmary, senior house surgeon at St. Peter's Hospital London in 1909, an assistant surgeon in 1914, full surgeon in 1922, senior honorary surgeon, and finally, consulting surgeon in 1938 to the Royal Victoria Infirmary, Newcastle-upon-Tyne, in 1914 [90–92]. Other appointments included honorary surgeon at Ingham Infirmary, South Shields, Newcastle-upon-Tyne Dental Hospital, and Whickham and District Cottage Hospital. He served as chair of surgery at Durham University from 1935 to 1942 [92].

Willan was in the Royal Naval Volunteer Reserve (RNVR), rising to the rank of surgeon captain and the King's Honorary Surgeon in 1933. During World War II, he was surgeon Rear-Admiral to the RNVR in 1944 and surgical adviser to the No 1 region of the Ministry of Health [91]. He held the rank of Member of the Victorian Order, Officer of the Most Excellent Order in 1915, Officer of the Most Excellent Order of the British Empire in 1919, and Commander of the Most Excellent Order of the British Empire in 1946 [90]. Willan was an active member of the British Medical Association throughout his career, serving in various positions in this organization's divisions, branches, sections, and committees [90].

As a description of his character by his colleague writes:

> One remembers with affection and gratitude the care and the time he devoted to the guidance and the instruction of surgeon probationers. Professor Willan was a man admired alike for his great personal charm and for his distinguished professional career. He was at all times courteous and modest, yet ready and willing to advice from his superior and expert knowledge. Of upright principles, he was kindness itself, understanding and sympathetic, and would do all in his power—even when physically unfit—to help the sick [93, p. 422].

Willan reported on a finding observed in patients with a perforated duodenal ulcer (Table 11.1):

> The feature about the case most deeply impressed upon my mind was the presence of a transverse ring of constriction across the abdomen at the level of the lower margins of the ribs and extending into the flanks on either side. (…) The constriction is usually present, and does not always disappear with general anesthesia, although it does disappear when the condition has advanced to the stage of general abdominal distention. There is marked hyperesthesia, and the patient is quite unconscious of any feeling of tightness at the site of the constriction. (…) The appearance is as if an invisible rope was constricting the abdomen, dividing it into an upper portion which has a convex aspect centrally, and a normal lower part. Viewed laterally, the region of the "rope" forms the apex of a vertically situated obtuse angle. (…) In passing, it may be mentioned that this line is *below* the level of the transpyloric plane, while it is *above* the level of the umbilicus. The ring of constriction corresponds to that portion of the anterior abdominal wall supplied by the ninth intercostal nerve, and is certainly due to muscular contraction [94, p. 143].

Thus, Willan sign refers to the transverse ring of constriction extending across the abdomen at the level of the lower margins of the ribs bilaterally to the flanks in the case of a perforated duodenal ulcer.

11.2.18 Cullen Sign

Thomas Stephen Cullen (1868–1953) was born in Bridgewater, Ontario, Canada, and received his Bachelor of Medicine degree from Toronto University Medical

School in 1890 [95, 96]. After graduation, he continued his studies under William Henry Welch (1850–1934), followed by an internship with Howard Attwood Kelly (1858–1934) in gynecology. After a brief study at the University of Göttingen, Germany, he returned to Johns Hopkins University and founded the gynecologic pathologic laboratory [95, 96]. He was appointed associate in gynecology in 1897, professor of clinical gynecology in 1919, and professor of gynecology in 1932 [95, 96]. His areas of research focus were endometrial carcinoma and ectopic pregnancy. Cullen was a fellow of the American Gynecological Society and a council member from 1904 to 1914. He served as a consultant and member of the Maryland State Board of Health [97].

Arnaldo de Moraes writes of his fond memory of Cullen:

> This is the life of this famous North American Master that I had the good fortune to meet personally, when I was at Johns Hopkins University, in 1927, thanks to a "fellowship" from the Rockefeller Foundation. I received the most affectionate welcome from him, inviting me to attend the operations of his own private clinic and to participate in the Christmas party at his house that year, where he received me with the hospitality of a true "gentleman" [98, p. 222–223]. In writing these words of nostalgia, I express much of my heart and admiration, grateful for the attention given to that young Brazilian doctor who attended his Service, for whom he was then at the height of fame and prestige, in his country and abroad [98, p. 223].

In the *Transactions of the American Gynecological Society in Philadelphia*, 1918, Cullen described the case of a 38-year-old woman who found on physical examination that (Table 11.1):

> The umbilical region was bluish black, although she gave no account of the abdominal distention. (…) [t]he bluish-black appearance of the umbilicus was due to intraabdominal hemorrhage, and the presence of the nodule to the side of the uterus clinched the diagnosis of extrauterine pregnancy [99, p. 457].

Thus, Cullen sign refers to the bluish-black discoloration of the umbilical area occurring in cases of intra-abdominal hemorrhage (ectopic pregnancy or acute hemorrhagic pancreatitis).

11.2.19   Grey Turner Sign

George Grey Turner (1877–1951) was born in North Shields, England, and received his medical training at Newcastle Medical School of the University of Durham, graduating in 1898 [100]. He completed postgraduate training at King's College Hospital and Vienna. He received his Master of Science with first-class honors in 1901 and was elected fellow of the Royal College of Surgeons in 1903 [101].

He returned to Newcastle-upon-Tyne, where, in addition to being a private practitioner was appointed to the staff of Royal Victoria Infirmary and Newcastle Medical School as a surgeon and lecturer in 1906 [100–102]. During World War I, he served from 1914 to 1918 with the Royal Army Medical Corps. Grey-Turner was a consulting surgeon in Mesopotamia and later a district consulting surgeon and chest disease specialist to the Northern Command in England [101, 102]. He was a professor of surgery at the University of Durham from 1927 to 1934 and accepted an appointment in London as director of surgery at the British Postgraduate Medical School, Hammersmith, and a professorship in London from 1935 to 1946 [101, 102].

He was elected to the council of the Royal College of Surgeons in 1926 and served as an examiner for the Primary Examination of the Royal College of Surgeons' Diploma of FRCS, president of the sections of surgery and proctology, and president-elect of the clinical section [100, 102]. He was president of the Association of Surgeons of Great Britain and Ireland in 1928, president of the Medical Society of London from 1943 to 1944, and president of the 13th Congress of the International Society of Surgery in New Orleans, Louisiana [101].

Among his many accolades, he was awarded the Bigelow Medal for Advancement in Surgery in Boston, Massachusetts, in 1931, an Honorary Doctor of Surgery degree from Durham University, and an L.L.D. degree from the University of Glasgow [101].

A description of his character as articulated by Willan:

> A tenacious memory with an orderly methodical mind were important assets in his makeup. His industry was phenomenal, and he regimented and planned his life—his leisure as well as his work. He was always in pursuit of further knowledge, being willing and anxious to learn from all and sundry, and equally willing to teach. His travels in search of knowledge were worldwide, and he made frequent visits to European and American clinics. A recent air journey included one not free from hazard over the Andes to preside over the International Surgical Congress. He was an outstanding and impressive teacher for students and graduates alike, and was particularly interested in surgical pathology [103, p. 274].

Grey Turner described a cutaneous finding occurring in a 53-year-old male with acute pancreatitis (Table 11.1):

> The tenderness over the gall-bladder region was very marked, and I now noticed two large, discolored areas in the loins. They were about the size of the palm of the hand, slightly raised above the surface, and of a dirty-greenish color. There was little edema, with pitting on pressure, but there was no pain or tenderness [104, p. 394–395].

Interestingly he reported five years earlier the case of a 54-year-old female also with acute pancreatitis and a periumbilical cutaneous finding:

> I was at once struck by the appearance of the abdominal wall surrounding the umbilicus. In this neighborhood there was an area of discoloration about 6 inches in diameter, of a bluish color, very like the early postmortem staining seen on the abdominal wall, or the appearance of the skin in a late case of extravasation of urine. The area was slightly raised, and pitting on pressure [104, p. 394].

Thus, Grey Turner sign refers to the dirty-greenish-colored localized discoloration of the abdominal flank in acute hemorrhagic pancreatitis.

11.2.20 Hellendall Sign

Hugo Hellendall (1872–1954) was born in Münster, North Rhine-Westphalia, Germany, studied medicine in Heidelberg, Munich, and Strasburg, and received his medical degree from the latter in 1896. He founded a private women's clinic in Elisabethstrasse and practiced in Königsallee, Dusseldorf, in 1908 [105]. He was forced to close the practice in 1935 because of harassment by the neighboring steelworks. He re-established a private women's clinic in Dusseldorf until 1938 and emigrated to Switzerland in 1938 and the USA in 1939, where he was involved in cancer research at Columbia University College of Physicians and Surgeons (currently Columbia University Vagelos College of Physicians and Surgeons) [105, 106].

Hellendall described a blushes discoloration of the umbilicus in a case of ectopic pregnancy (Table 11.1):

> I now have an important objective finding in the case of tubal pregnancy—initial bruising in the abdominal wall and free blood intraperitoneally. This finding provides clues to the underlying cause in cases that are difficult to diagnose. As far as I know, this new, not previously described symptom was brought to my attention by the patient herself. The patient told me 1 day before my suspicion of a tubal pregnancy that her navel had changed color and was bluish. I wondered if that finding had any significance. I also noticed that she had a cherry-sized, almost empty umbilical hernia, into which one could insert the index finger, and which was covered by a parchment-thin skin. In fact, something shimmered through this parchment, which immediately reminded me of that peculiar shimmer of color that one so often observes with free bleeding into the abdominal cavity immediately before the opening of the peritoneum. This blue-green shimmer increased while standing, i.e., when the umbilical hernia bulged forward. This finding confirmed my suspicion that it was an ectopic pregnancy. (…) I thought it was important to point out this new symptom of internal bleeding, i.e., also extrauterine pregnancy, since umbilical hernias are not uncommon [107, p. 890–891].

At the time of this publication Hellendall was unaware of Cullen's previous publication. In 1922, he wrote:

> Mr. Thomas S. Cullen in Baltimore recently sent me a reprint of his work entitled with the above heading, which appears in the July 1919 issue of *Contributions to the Medical and Biological Research*. (…) However, my observation does not lose interest, rather it provides further confirmatory evidence regarding the accuracy of this new finding [108, p. 147].

Thus, Hellendall sign refers to the bluish-green discoloration of the umbilicus in cases of ectopic pregnancy.

11.2.21   Schlesinger Sign

Hermann Schlesinger (1866–1934) was born in Pressburg (Bratislava), Slovakia (Austria–Hungary), and received his medical degree from the University of Vienna in 1890 [109, 110]. He was appointed under Theodor Meynert (1833–1892) at the I. Psychiatric and Neurological Clinic of the General Hospital, Vienna, and with Herman Nothnagel (1841–1905) at the I. Vienna Medical University Clinic and General Hospital [109].

He was an assistant physician at the Vienna General Hospital in 1892 and an assistant at the III. Medical Clinic in 1895 [110]. He habilitated in internal medicine in 1895 with the thesis titled *Die Syringomyelie: eine Monagraphie* (Syringomyelia:

A Monograph), followed by appointments as an associate professor at the University of Vienna and assistant physician at III. Medical Clinic of the Vienna General Hospital [109–111]. He was appointed head of the III. Medical Department at the Kaiser-Franz-Josef Hospital in 1901, titular professor in 1902, and extraordinary professor and head of the III. Medical Clinic at the Vienna General Hospital in 1908 [109, 110, 112].

Schlesinger described the finding of the unilateral reflex contraction of the rectus muscle with the displacement of the umbilicus in the case of a peripyloric ulcer. The maneuver is performed as follows (Table 11.1):

> If one asks the patient who is reclining at an angle to strain as if having a bowel movement, one frequently notices a characteristic displacement of the navel. As a rule, the latter rises upwards when the healthy person strains, but if there is a different innervation of the rectus or abdominal wall, the navel also undergoes a lateral displacement at the beginning of the general abdominal wall tension, which resolves after a few seconds. The transitory "lateral umbilical distortion" (as I would like to call this phenomenon) occurs on the diseased side because the more tense abdominal muscles cause this dislocation. The process can be recognized most efficiently when the examiner stands at the foot of the bed. The extent of the dislocation varies significantly in individual cases; sometimes, it is only minimal; in other subjects, the lateral movement is several centimeters (up to 4 cm and more) [113, p. 1].

The finding of unilateral reflex contraction of the rectus muscle with the displacement of the umbilicus occurs on the right side in diseases involving the pylorus, duodenal, or gallbladder and may rarely be found on the left side in gastric ulcers.

11.2.22   Barkman Sign

Limited historical information is available for Ake Barkman. At the time of the publication of his paper titled "Sur les reflexes thoraco-abdominaux normaux et leur localization médullaire" (On Normal Thoraco-abdominal Reflexes and Their Spinal Localization), he served as a physician in the medical department of the Karlstad Hospital under the director Gotthard Söderbergh (1878–1943) [114].

Thoraco-abdominal reflexes refer to superficial cutaneous reflexes originating at the thorax and motor stimulation occurring in the abdominal muscles. Barkman described the method for eliciting the thoraco-abdominal reflexes:

> The patient lies on his back, the muscles relaxed, and the thorax straight. One excites the skin of the thoracic by employing light and rapid brushing, using, for example, a knitting needle which one slides in the intercostal spaces from outside to inside. Start with the first intercostal space and move downward, examining each space separately. The motor effect observed on the abdominal musculature at each excitation is noted [114, p. 367].

Barkman described the three cutaneous tonic reflexes (Table 11.1):

> Excitation of the first three intercostal spaces never caused contraction of the abdominal muscles. The excitation involves the intercostal spaces close to the nipple, generally at the fourth and fifth spaces. In that case, a contraction of the first segment of the rectus muscle and simultaneously a depression, both on the same side, and displacement towards the

excited side of the white line in the portion corresponding to the muscular segment is observed. The depression is formed by the ipsilateral portion adjacent to the midline, with a convex outer edge. The contraction of the muscle segment of the rectus abdominis is recognized both by palpation and sight. We observe, in fact, a very marked finding. The sinking and displacement of the midline attributable to the transversalis muscle. (…) If excitation involves the intercostal space located immediately below, one observes contraction of the first and second segments of the rectus abdominis muscle on the same side and, at the same time, a displacement of the portion of the white line corresponding to these segments with the formation of depression on the excited side (contraction of the transversalis muscle). We will call this reflex the middle thoraco-abdominal reflex. The lower thoraco-abdominal reflex is elicited by stimulating the lower intercostal space. It results in the contraction of the first three segments of the rectus muscle and, by displacement, a depression of the white line corresponding to these three segments [114, p. 367].

Thus, Barkman sign refers to the contraction, depression, and displacement of the first segment of the rectus muscle when the skin just below the nipple is stimulated on that same side.

11.2.23 Jeans Sign

Frank Alexander Galen Jeans (1878–1933) received his medical training at St. John's College in Cambridge, Liverpool University, King's College, and St. Bartholomew's Hospitals. He received his membership in the Royal College of Surgeons (M.R.C.S.) and licentiate of the Royal College of Physicians (L.R.C.P.) in 1904, bachelor of medicine degree in 1906, and fellowship in the Royal College (F.R.C.P.) in 1907 [115].

Jeans was appointed house surgeon to Sir William Mitchell Banks (1842–1904), an assistant surgeon in 1909, and an honorary surgeon in 1924 to the Royal Infirmary, Liverpool. Other appointments included serving as a consulting surgeon to Hoylake and West Cottage Hospitals and the Waterloo and District General Hospitals [115]. He maintained an affiliation with the University of Liverpool and was appointed a lecturer in clinical surgery and vice-president of the Liverpool Medical Institution [115].

During World War I, he was a major in the Liverpool Merchants' Mobile Hospital Surgical Division and a senior surgeon in 1916. He developed a keen interest in the urology specialty serving as a urology consultant at the Liverpool Medical Research Organization [115]. As a description of his character:

> We knew him as a man of great courage, in whom there was nothing mean or paltry, outspoken, fearless, and with a soul full of kindliness. His was a fine, big, generous nature, permeated with that rare quality, the gift of charity. When he spoke it was as a master of happy speech and felicitous phrases, and his friends and students will always remember with pleasure and profit the witty aphorisms with which he enlivened his conversation. But behind the wit and the humour was sound judgement, based on wide knowledge and an uncanny understanding of human nature, and to him to understand was to forgive [116, p. 83].

Jeans described a finding observed in cases of peritonitis (Table 11.1):

In a normal patient the abdomen comes out when the chest comes out (except for the first three or four respiratory movements, which should be ignored because all patients breathe self-consciously when first exposed). If after the first few breaths the abdomen goes in when the chest comes out, then the patient has a diffuse leak, will be found on palpation to have complete rigidity, and on lapratorum to have general peritonitis. (…) Moreover, there is a further refinement. If a transverse crease half an inch above the umbilicus is seen in an abdomen which has the reverse movement described above-or no movement at all, then the patient is likely to have a perforated duodenal or gastric ulcer. If, on the other hand, there is a transverse motionless axis about 2 in. below the umbilicus round which the abdomen "rocks" i.e., the wall goes in below this axis and out above it—then the trouble is probably in the appendix, which is leaking mainly into the pelvis and less so towards the upper abdomen [117, p. 729].

Thus, Jeans sign refers to either the absence of abdominal wall movement or the abdominal wall moving inward during inspiration (reverse respiratory direction) above a transverse crease located half an inch above the umbilicus in cases of perforated duodenal or gastric ulcer.

11.2.24 *Carnett Sign*

John Berton Carnett (1876–1934), father of John Berton Carnett Jr. (1914–1963), was born in Williamsport, Lycoming County, Pennsylvania, USA, and received his medical degree from the University of Pennsylvania Medical School in 1899 [118, 119]. He was appointed surgical assistant to Edward Martin (1859–1938) at the University and Philadelphia General Hospitals and Instructor at the University of Pennsylvania medical school in 1901 [120]. During World War I, he served as chief of the surgical division of the Red Cross Base Hospital No. 20 at the University of Pennsylvania Hospital and as a lieutenant colonel in Château Guyon, France [118, 120]. He received a personal letter of commendation from the American Red Cross and Surgeon General, Washington, D.C., for his exceptionally meritorious and conspicuous services [120].

He was appointed professor of surgery at the Graduate School of Medicine of the University of Pennsylvania, followed by vice-dean of surgery [119]. He became chief surgeon of the Graduate Hospital and the radiologic services at the Philadelphia General Hospital [119]. Carnett served as president of the Board of Trustees of the North American Sanitarium for the Treatment of Surgical Tuberculosis and was a member of the College of Physicians, and the Philadelphia Academy of Surgeons, among others [118].

Carnett described a method for differentiated pain arising from the abdominal wall from an intra-abdominal origin. The maneuver consisted of two stages (A and B) (Table 11.1) (Fig. 11.2):

A. In any patient complaining of abdominal pain and tenderness, the examiner follows the classic advice of gaining the confidence of both the patient and his muscle and then palpates in the usual manner. Irrespective of whether the tenderness is parietal or intra-abdominal the examiner's fingers as a rule, will dip fairly deep into the abdomen before tenderness is elicited. The deep position of the fingers has generally been regarded as proof that the tenderness is intra-abdominal, but in a surprisingly high percentage of cases this assumption will prove to be an error as shown by the next step.
B. The examiner keep his fingers at the most sensitive area he has discovered on deep pressure and requests the patient to make his abdominal muscles rigid by contracting his diaphragm or by raising and holding his head from the pillow; as the patient tenses his muscles, the examiner relaxes his finger pressure so that his fingers rise out of the abdomen; and then with the patient's abdominal muscle tense the examiner reapplies pressure with his finger tips and he also may exert a little twisting motion with them [121, p. 625].

If the origin of the abdominal pain is intra-abdominal, then only the A test will be positive. If the skin and muscles of the abdominal wall are involved, then both A and the B test will be positive. If the parietal peritoneum is involved, the patient will frequently report the pain is less during B than A test. However, if the peritoneal inflammatory process or a local abscess involves the muscles of the anterior abdominal wall both the A and B portions of the tests will be positive. A false negative test may occur in multiparous women who are unable to tense their abdominal muscles.

A positive Carnett sign is when both the A and B test are positive signifying that the pathology involves the cutaneous and subcutaneous tissue and muscles of the abdominal wall. Variation on the how to perform the maneuver has been described by different authors. Suleiman and Johnston (2001) require that the supine patient tense the abdominal wall by lifting the head and shoulders off the examining table [122]. Bailey in contrast stated that the patient is asked to extend both legs and raise the feet from the bed [123].

A positive Carnett sign most commonly occurs in diseases involving the abdominal wall and includes abdominal hernia, entrapment neuropathies (rectus nerve, thoracic lateral cutaneous nerve, ilioinguinal and iliohypogastric nerve), endometriosis, diabetic radiculopathy, and hematoma (abdominal wall and rectus sheath).

Carnett sign has been shown to be useful bedside diagnostic technique for confirming abdominal wall involvement [124, 125]. In a study of 120 patients presenting to the emergency room with abdominal pain, Thomson and Francis (1977) found that of 23 of 24 (96%) with a positive Carnett sign, only one had an abnormal laparotomy [124].

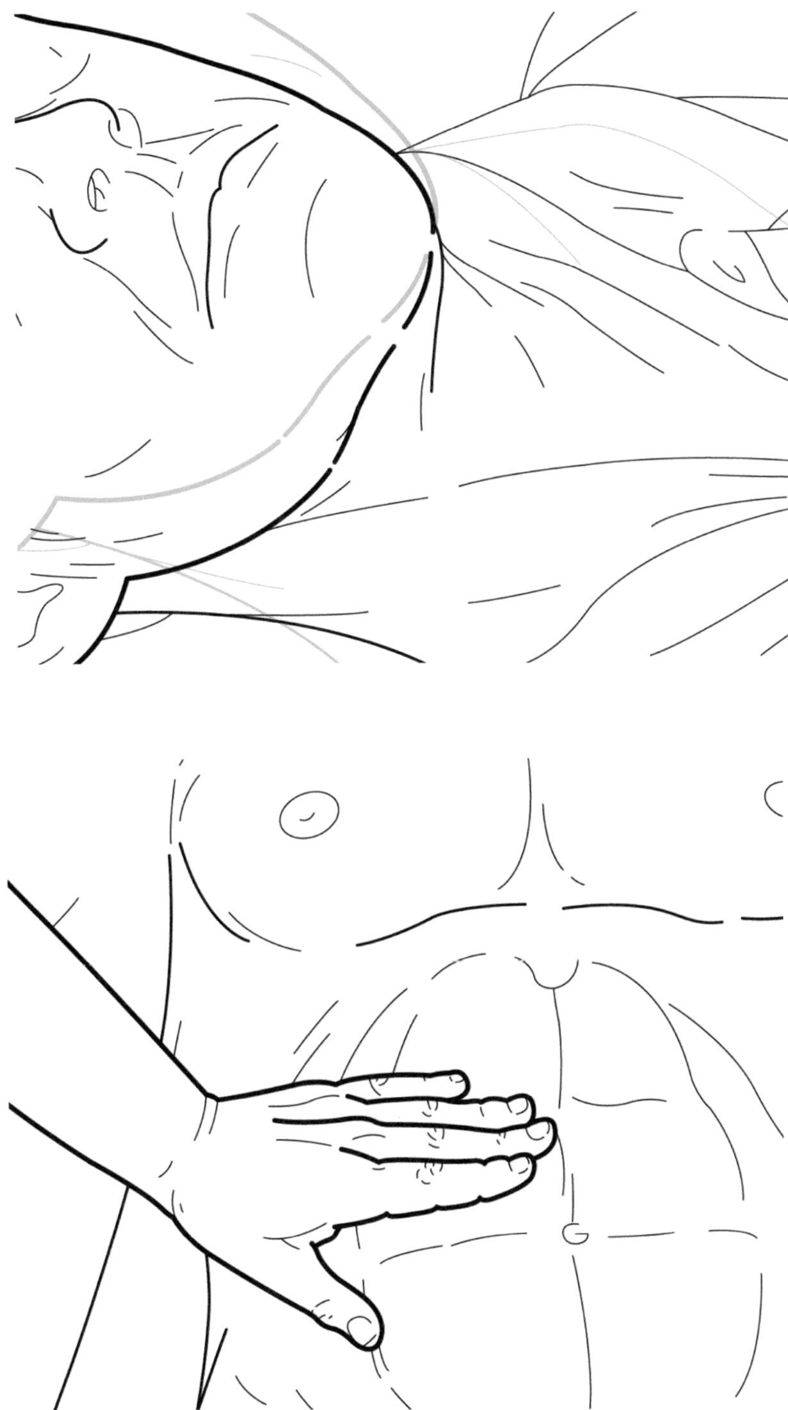

Fig. 11.2   Carnett sign (by Ryan Yale)

11.2.25   *Fothergill Sign*

William Edward Fothergill (1865–1926) was born in Southampton, England, and received his Bachelor of Medicine with distinction (first-class honors and gold medal) from the University of Edinburgh in 1893 [125–129]. He was appointed house physician and clinical assistant to Sir Alexander Russell Simpson (1835–1916), professor of obstetrics in the gynecology wards at the Royal Infirmary, and from 1893 to 1895 in the Royal Maternity Hospital, Edinburgh [126–128]. He received his medical degree in 1897 with a gold medal distinction [127, 130].

In Manchester, he was assistant lecturer to Sir William Japp Sinclair (1846–1912), professor of obstetrics, followed by an appointment as an assistant surgeon at Northern Hospital for Women and Children in 1899 [126]. At the Royal Infirmary, he was instrumental in establishing the first clinical laboratory serving as its director in 1899 [126]. He was appointed as staff to the Southern Hospital in 1904 (Southern Hospital later became incorporated with St. Mary's Hospital). He was named an ordinary fellow of the Edinburgh Obstetrical Society in 1906, an assistant in 1907, and a full surgeon in 1919 at the Manchester Royal Infirmary [128, 131].

At the University of Manchester, he was a lecturer in obstetrics and gynecology in 1901, rose to the ranks of professor of systematic obstetrics and gynecology in 1920, and was later appointed professor of clinical obstetrics and gynecology in 1925 [126]. He also held appointments as a senior surgeon for Women at St. Mary's Hospital and consulting gynecological surgeon at Manchester Royal Infirmary [126].

He wrote the *Manual of Midwifery* (1896), *Lectures to Midwives and Maternity Nurses* (1907), *Golden Rules in Obstetric Practice* (1910), and *Manual of Diseases of Women* (1910), the latter containing a revised classification of diseases afflicting women [127, 132]. He perfected and wrote extensively on the operation for pelvic floor repair originally devised by Archibald Donald (1860–1937), colloquially referred to as the Manchester operation [127].

As described by Fairbairn:

> He was a man we could ill spare, for he had rare force or character and the power of making his influence felt, and it is no exaggeration to say that there is not another of his day and generation who did more to mold gynecological opinion in this country [127, p. 102].

Fothergill described a bedside maneuver for distinguishing a rectus sheath hematoma from an intra-abdominal process (Table 11.1):

> The most interesting thing about these cases is the diagnosis. The patient complains of pain and the medical man finds the swelling. The trouble is that he seldom knows how long the swelling has been present; for patients frequently have masses of various kinds in the pelvis or abdomen whose presence is not suspected until they complain of pain and submit to examination. The main point is the recognition that these swellings are part and parcel of the abdominal wall. This is generally made by noting that they can still be felt when the recti are in action, and that they become fixed as the muscles contract. Another point is that, when a mass in the abdominal wall is not too large, a resonant note may be obtained through it by deep percussion [133, p. 942].

Fothergill sign thus refers to the presence of an abdominal wall mass that is palpable when the abdominal wall is relaxed and tensed, and is fixed in position when the muscle contracts. Additionally, the mass is resonant on percussion. Furthermore, he noted that an intra-abdominal mass adherent to the abdominal wall causes similar findings to those within the abdominal wall.

11.2.26 Co Tui-Meyer Sign

Frank Wang Co Tui (Xu Zhaodui) (1897–1984) was born in Fujian province, China, and received his medical degree from the University of the Philippines [134]. He completed an internship in Chicago from 1923 to 1925 and served as an associate professor of experimental surgery at the surgical laboratories in the Department of Surgery at New York University and Bellevue Hospital Medical College. He earned a professorship at the NY University College of Medicine [134].

He was a member of the American Association of the Advancement of Science American Pharmaceutical Society, chairman of the American Bureau of Medical Aid to China, and a fellow of the NY Academy of Medicine and NY Academy of Science [134].

11.2.26.1 Jacob Meyer

Jacob Meyer (1894–1955) received his medical degree from Rush Medical College in 1916 [135, 136]. He completed his internship at Cook County Hospital from 1916 to 1918 and was appointed instructor in medicine at Loyola University in 1920 [136]. Throughout his career, he maintained several appointments in Chicago, Illinois, including as associate professor of medicine at the University of Illinois College of Medicine, attending physician at Cook County Hospital, associate attending physician at Mt. Sinai Hospital, and senior attending physician at Michael Reese Hospital. He was a member of the internal medicine and pathology and the department of gastrointestinal research and medical chief of the "Stomach Study Group" of the Michael Reese Hospital [136].

Co Tui and Meyer described a finding best observed from either the head or foot of the bed in patients with perforated peptic ulcer disease and acute appendicitis (Table 11.1):

> It is a prolonged displacement of the linea alba and the umbilicus to the affected side with the skin surface disturbance in the form of folds and creases on the side to which the linea alba and the navel are drawn [137, p. 1779]. (…) The umbilicus is located in the median raphe made by the decussation of the fascial fiberes of the rectus sheaths. The sheath in addition to enclosing the rectus muscles, are reinforced by tendinous slips from such powerful muscles as the obliquus externus, the obliquus internus and transverus abdominis. This raphe, the linea alba, is represented on the surface by a pigmented line in the nonhairy abdomen and by the parting of the hairs in the hairy abdomen. (…) A difference in the tension of the two sides of the abdomen would tend to draw the linea alba, and with it the umbilicus, toward the side of greater rigidity. The skin surface changes are due to an effort of the skin to accommodate itself to the contracted underlying surface [137, p. 1779].

Furthermore, they found that the site of greatest rigidity corresponded to the side where the umbilicus was displaced (pointing toward the side of the disease). They believed the sign might be falsely negative in obese patients and those who are either multiparous or have a pendulous abdomen [137].

11.2.27   *Mortola Sign*

We were unable to identify historical information on G.A. Mortola from Buenos Aires, Argentina. Mortola described a method for determining intra-abdominal inflammation.

> The technique is simple but certain details must be studied carefully in order to avoid errors of interpretation. The patient is placed in dorsal decubitus with the abdominal muscle relaxed. The physician takes between the thumbs and index fingers of both hands a large fold of the anterior abdominal wall at the lower right and left quadrants to determine the possible existence of cutaneous hyperesthesia and then exercises traction on the cutaneous folds The same procedure is repeated farther up, and this might be called "aspirating" the anterior wall of the abdomen [138].

If the parietal peritoneum is inflamed, the patient complains of pain when the skin fold is pulled upward. Mortola found this sign useful in acute or subacute forms of appendicitis or tuberculous peritonitis without ascites. This finding represents a somatosensory nerve reflex.

11.2.28   *Raw Sign*

Stanley Collingwood Raw (1910–1994) was born in Spratton, Northamptonshire, England, and received his medical baccalaureate (MB) and bachelor of science (BS) from Durham University, England, in 1934 [139, 140]. He received postgraduate training as a house physician, house surgeon, and resident surgical officer at the Royal Victoria Infirmary, Newcastle-upon-Tyne [139, 140].

He was a member of the Royal Army Medical Corps (RAMC) in 1942 and subsequently a lieutenant colonel in 1945. After World War II, he was appointed consultant at Farnham and Frimley Park Hospitals in 1948 [139, 140].

Raw described a finding for distinguishing diaphragmatic pleurisy from perforated peptic ulcer disease:

> In perforation the onset is nearly always dramatic with little vomiting or change in pulse and temperature. The pain does not vary, and the patient usually lies still. Breathing is short and thoracic in type. In pleurisy, rigidity may sometimes be overcome by holding the breath; in colic, it is commonly removed by breathing; but in perforation it never disappears completely [141, p. 12].

Thus, Raw sign refers to abdominal wall rigidity that does not completely disappear with breath holding in cases of peritonitis.

11.2.29   *Holman Sign*

Emile Frederic Holman (1890–1977) was born in Moberly, Missouri, USA, and received his medical degree from Johns Hopkins School of Medicine in 1918 [142, 143]. He was appointed research fellow at the Hunterian Laboratory for Experimental

Surgery, instructor in surgery at Johns Hopkins University Medical School, and resident surgeon at John Hopkins Hospital. He was a resident surgeon at Peter Bent Brigham Hospital, Boston, from 1922 to 1923 and an assistant professor of surgery at Western Reserve Medical School in 1924 [144].

He served as associate professor of surgery in 1925 and chairman of the Department of Surgery in 1926, a position he held until 1955. He was accepted for Stanford's surgical residency and research during his tenure. He conducted sentinel work in vascular surgery, contributing to understanding an arteriovenous fistula physiology and concepts related to allograft skin grafting rejection [142].

Holman was appointed to the American Board of Thoracic Surgery from 1948 to 1952 [145], elected president of the Society for Vascular Surgery in 1949 and the American Association for Thoracic Surgery from 1953 to 1954, and honorary member of the American Osler Society in 1970 [142, 143, 146, 147]. He was the editor of the *Journal of Thoracic and Cardiovascular Surgery* from 1957 to 1962 [148].

He was awarded the Samuel D. Gross Prize from the Philadelphia Academy of Surgery in 1930 for his work on arteriovenous fistulas and the Rudolph Mattas Medal in vascular surgery, Tulane, in 1954. The Emile F. Holman Chair in Surgery was established in his honor at Stanford University [143].

As a description of his character:

> As a teacher Emile is dynamic, specific and at times a little dramatic if it will emphasize a point. His knowledge of the scientific literature seems to be boundless. He is always available, never too busy to consult and confer with associates or assistants, and he is a slave for work. Meticulous and exacting in his technics, he is never more critical or demanding of others than he is of himself, and he has been a leading example of humanitarianism in his clinical work [149, p. 1089–1090].

Holman emphasized the use of abdominal percussion as a method for diagnosing and determining the location and extent of peritoneal inflammation. He recommends that the patient be asked to cough, followed by gently palpation (Table 11.1):

> The follows light percussion—also begun in presumably unaffected areas—by working downward from epigastrium in lower abdominal discomfort, toward the epigastrium in upper abdominal pain, and from the side of the comfort to the side of pain in unilateral involvement. The area of tenderness is quickly and easily ascertained, its exact extent is determined and, when deemed important, is outlined on the skin by pencil. All degrees of intensity of tenderness are encountered, shading gradually from the mild tenderness at the periphery to the exquisitely painful percussion at the center of the involved areas. The site of greatest tenderness is usually found over the inflammation of longest duration, and this obviously corresponds with the site where the inflammation first began. This may be of real diagnostic importance [150, p. 775].

Thus, Holman sign identifies an area of tenderness by light percussion.

11.2.30   *Fox Sign*

John Adrian Fox (1933–2018) was born in Manchester, UK, and received his medical baccalaureate degree from the University of London in 1957. Fox practiced general surgery at the Royal Free Hospital, London, in 1957. He was a member, followed by a fellow in the Royal College of Physicians in 1962 [151]. He was a consultant surgeon at the Royal Northern Hospital, Clementine Churchill Hospital, and Edgeware General Hospital in Middlesex in 1972 and an honorary consultant surgeon at St. Andrew's Hospital, Doll Hill, London [151, 152].

Fox described in two patients (acute pancreatitis and ruptured abdominal aortic aneurysm) during the latter course of their disease a bluish discoloration located in the upper outer aspect of the thigh(s). He reported on the distinct anatomical, pathological, and physiological mechanisms accounting for this process (Table 11.1):

> Careful examination of the bruised area shows a well-marked upper limit. The straight line runs parellel to and below the inguinal ligament. It corresponds to the attachment of the membranous layer of the superficial fascia (Scarpa's fascia) to the fascial lata of the thigh. (…) It therefore seems likely that the clinical sign seen in the above two case is produced by the tracking of the fluid extraperitoneally along the fascia of the psoas and iliacus beneath the inguinal ligament until it becomes subcutaneous in the upper thigh. Scarpa's fascia prevents the free forward diffusion immediately below the ligament but below its attachment the bruising is more rapidly developed [153, p. 194].

Thus, Fox sign refers to ecchymosis over the inguinal ligament in cases of retroperitoneal hemorrhage.

11.2.31   Tixier Sign

Léon-Eugène-Joseph Tixier (1877–1976) was an extern from 1900 to 1902 and intern from 1902 to 1907 at Hospitals of Paris and received his medical degree from the Faculty of Medicine, Paris, in 1907, followed by an assistant at the pediatric clinic at the Faculty of Medicine from 1907 to 1919 [154, 155].

During World War I, he served as an aide-major in the bacteriology laboratory of the First Army and chief surgeon in the IV. Medical District from 1918 to 1919. He was appointed head of the children's laboratory in the medical clinic of the Faculty of Medicine, Paris, from 1919 to 1920 and a physician at the Charité Hospital in Paris. Tixier was head of the laboratory at the Faculty of Medicine, Paris, in 1939 [155].

We were unable to identify Tixier's original publication on traumatic abdominal shock. As described by Keleman:

> Particularly in shock, when the patient is prostrate at an early stage from rapid exsanguination and his abdominal wall offers poor defense. Tixier sign may point to considerable intra-abdominal hematoma [34, p. 92]. (…) [i]f there is no muscular defense, but a free fluid accumulation in the abdominal cavity, 3–4 impressions, "shakes" performed in quick succession over the left fossa result in palpable and visible undulation in the right fossa (only in cases of greater volume fluid accumulation) [34, p. 59].

Thus, Tixier sign refers to the absence of abdominal guarding in cases of shock in cases of intra-abdominal hemorrhage or hematoma.

Table 11.1 Abdominal wall signs

Name	Year	Description of sign	Significance
Auenbrugger [7]	1761	Epigastric abdominal swelling	Pericardial effusion
Rosenbach [9]	1876	Stroking the abdomen with the fingernail produces a reflex retraction. These indentations are made on one side since the skin stimuli do not cross the midline. The depression occurs most clearly when the nail is quickly run over the abdominal surface, regardless of the direction of the stroke. Contact with cold objects can also often produce the sign. In patients with cerebral hemiplegia, no abdominal reflex occurs on the paralyzed side. In contrast, the same occurs promptly and is unchanged on the other side. If hemiplegia is subacute, the contraction occurs weakly. Even in chronic cases, differences are observed on both sides of the body	Superficial abdominal reflex
Simon [11]	1895	The chest and abdomen in the epigastric region are exposed. Dyssynchronous chest and abdominal wall movements occur during respiration during the first days of meningitis. Additionally, hyperesthesia of the skin causes brief involuntary reflex movements of the chest and stomach	Superficial abdominal reflex
Guinard [15]	1896	1 Prehepatic tympanic sound 2 Contracture of the abdominal muscles prevents deep manual exploration	Intestinal perforation
Demons [21, 22]	1897	Abdominal wall rigidity is sometimes accompanied by either moderate distension, flattening, or concavity of the abdomen	Intestinal perforation
Hartmann [29]	1901	In abdominal contusion, contracture of the abdominal wall is not limited to the contused area in the absence of any other symptoms is a clear indication for an immediate laparotomy	Intestinal perforation
Sergent [33]	1904	A line is traced with the fingernail on the patient's skin. This line grows pale and is outlined, by a whiteness, along the finger's path	Adrenal insufficiency
Beevor [44]	1904	In healthy persons, while sitting up, the position of the umbilicus remains unchanged. If there is a lesion in the lower part of the spinal cord or involves its nerves, the part of the recti below the umbilicus is paralyzed. The normal upper part of the recti draws the umbilicus up, sometimes almost an inch	Superficial abdominal reflex
Ransohoff [50]	1906	The umbilicus is of a distinct saffron-yellow color	Ruptured common bile duct and bile peritonitis

(continued)

Table 11.1 (continued)

Name	Year	Description of sign	Significance
Livierato [53]	1906	The patient is supine on the bed, and the border of the heart is determined through percussion. Internally, it involves the median line of the sternum; externally, the vertical papilla of the apex; superiorly, the upper border of the fourth left rib on the left margin of the sternum curving gradually downwards toward the cardiac apex; and inferiorly at the sixth rib. The pulse has a regular rate and rhythm. Repeatedly tap on the midline of the abdomen, beginning in the epigastrium and extending to the navel. By delineating the area of the dullness of the heart again, it is seen that its limit has extended considerably to the right. The inner limit reaches the margin to the right of the sternum, while the upper and exterior are slightly modified. The cardiac dullness extends to the right for about three centimeters. The pulse is increased, and the pulmonary component of the second sound is accentuated. Ask the patient to rise from the bed, walk quickly around the room several times, and again delineate the area of cardiac dullness. As is seen, we find this area considerably narrowed. The internal limit reaches the margin to the left of the sternum, the upper area is slightly lowered, almost unchanged, and the left remains the same. The pulse is stronger and more frequent than previously. Moreover, from the subjective point of view, following this movement, the patient experiences neither problems with breathing nor palpitation	Right heart failure
Cruveilhier–Baumgarten [64]	1908	The umbilical vein persists and extends from the portal sinus to the umbilicus, with the largest one located in the inferior edge of the falciform ligament. Here it communicates directly to the umbilicus with the vastly expanded superficial or deep epigastric veins (caput medusae)	Caput medusa
Hofstätter [70][a]	1909	The skin above and a small area around the umbilicus contain suffusion with blood and, in some places, turns yellow	Ectopic pregnancy
Wynter [75]	1911	*Exudative pericarditis* The absence of the normal abdominal wall respiratory movement of the chest causes an inspiratory recession between the chest and abdomen *Appendicitis with peritonitis* Absence of abdominal wall respiratory movement and no definite evidence of an inspiratory movement in the chest. However, slight movement in the abdomen's upper part is limited in its lower part	Exudative pericarditis, appendicitis with peritonitis

Delbet [80]	1912	Traumatic muscle contraction caused by abdominal wall contusion is located superiorly and the left of the umbilicus in an area as wide as the palm	Contusion
Ligat [84]	1916	1 The patient is asked to appreciate the sensation elicited by a pinch of absolute pressure over a normal point. The facial expression is watched closely since the sensation of pinching varies widely among individuals 2 A similar pinch is applied at the spot of maximum pain. The skin and subcutaneous tissue are picked up from the abdominal wall and pinched with the same force as the control without applying downward pressure on the abdominal wall 3 The direction and limitation of the extension of hyperalgesia are noted	Viscero-sensory reflex
Handley [89]	1916	The abdominal wall is distended and rigid below the umbilicus. The upper half of both recti is softer than the lower half, and above the umbilicus, slight respiratory excursions of the abdomen are seen. The intestines below the horizontal level of the symphysis are paralyzed, while the bowel above, though distended, retained its contractility. The pelvis contains both a length of large and small intestines. There are two obstructions to be dealt with named "ileus duplex"	Peritonitis
Willan [94]	1918	A transverse ring of constriction travels across the abdominal wall at the level of the lower margins of the ribs, extending into the flanks. There is marked hyperesthesia without a feeling of tightness at the site of the constriction. It appears as if an invisible rope was constricting the abdomen, dividing it into an upper portion with a convex aspect centrally and a normal lower part. Viewed laterally, the region of the "rope" forms the apex of a vertically situated obtuse angle. This line is below the transpyloric plane level and above the umbilicus. The constricting ring corresponds to the portion of the anterior abdominal wall supplied by the ninth intercostal nerve caused by muscular contraction	Perforated duodenal ulcer
Cullen [99]	1918	Bluish-black appearance of the umbilicus	Ectopic pregnancy
Grey-Turner [104]	1919	Large discolored areas in the flanks about the size of the palm, slightly raised above the surface, with a dirty-greenish color, and slight edema, with pitting on pressure but without pain or tenderness	Acute pancreatitis

(continued)

Table 11.1 (continued)

Name	Year	Description of sign	Significance
Hellendall [107]	1921	Bluish discoloration of the umbilicus	Ectopic pregnancy and intra-abdominal hemorrhage
Schlesinger [113]	1921	Asks the patient who is reclining at an angle to strain as if having a bowel movement. The umbilicus is displaced in a superior and lateral direction. This finding resolves after a few seconds. This transitory "lateral umbilical distortion" occurs on the diseased side because the more tense abdominal muscles bring about the dislocation. The process can be recognized most easily when the examiner stands at the foot of the bed. The extent of the dislocation varies significantly in individual cases; sometimes, it is only minimal; in other subjects, the lateral movement is several centimeters ($\geq$ 4 cm). The finding occurs on the right side in cases of disease involving the pylorus, duodenal, or gallbladder and may rarely be found in the left in case of a gastric ulcer	Pyloric, duodenal, or gastric ulcers and gallbladder disease
Barkman [114]	1923	The patient is lying on his back, the muscles are relaxed, and the thorax is straight. One excites the thoracic skin by employing light and rapid frictions, using, for example, a knitting needle which one slides in the intercostal spaces starting laterally and moving medially. Start with the first intercostal space and continue evaluating each intercostal space separately. Observe for contraction and depression of the rectus abdominis muscle on the same side and displacement of the white line (midline)	Thoraco-abdominal reflex
Jeans [117]	1925	1 Normally the abdominal wall protrudes when the chest expands (except for the first three or four respiratory movements, which should be ignored because all patients breathe self-consciously when first exposed). If the abdominal wall contracts when the chest expands after the first few breaths, the patient has a diffuse abdominal perforation, which will be found to be completely rigid on palpation 2 A perforated duodenal or gastric ulcer causes a transverse crease located half an inch above the umbilicus when the abdomen wall expands and the chest retracts or if the abdomen remains motionless. An appendiceal perforation into the pelvis causes a round transverse motionless axis about 2 in. below the umbilicus by which the abdomen "rocks," i.e., the abdominal wall moves in below this axis and out above it	Peritonitis and duodenal ulcer and appendicitis

Carnett [121]	1926	(a) The examiner's fingers are pressed deep into the abdomen before tenderness is elicited (b) The examiner places his fingers at the most sensitive area identified on deep abdominal pressure and requests the patient to make his abdominal muscles rigid by bearing down or by raising and holding his head from the pillow. As the patient tenses his muscles, the examiner relaxes his finger pressure so that his fingers rise out of the abdomen. With the patient's abdominal muscle tense, the examiner reapplies pressure and may exert a slight twisting motion with his fingertips. If the origin of the abdominal pain is intra-abdominal, then only the A test will be positive. If the skin and muscles of the abdominal wall are involved, then both A and B will be positive. If the parietal peritoneum is involved, the patient will frequently report that the pain is less during B than A test. However, if the peritoneal inflammatory process or a local abscess involves the anterior abdominal wall muscles, the A and B portions of the tests will be positive	Abdominal wall versus intra-abdominal origin
Fothergill [133]	1926	An abdominal wall versus an intra-abdominal mass is differentiated by noting that it can still be felt and is fixed when the recti are contracted. When a mass in the abdominal wall is not too large, a resonant note may be heard on deep percussion	Abdominal wall mass
Co-Tui and Meyer [137]	1928	Displacement of the linea alba and the umbilicus to the affected side. Skin folds and creases occur on the side where the linea alba and the navel are drawn	Superficial abdominal reflex
Mortola [138]	1937	The patient is placed in a dorsal decubitus position with the abdominal muscle relaxed. The physician using the thumbs and index fingers of both hands takes a large fold of the anterior abdominal wall at the lower right and left quadrants and then exercises traction on the cutaneous folds to determine the possible existence of cutaneous hyperesthesia. The same procedure is repeated upward	Viscero-sensory reflex
Raw [141]	1944	In intestinal perforation, abdominal wall rigidity persists even with breath holding	Peritonitis

(continued)

Table 11.1 (continued)

Name	Year	Description of sign	Significance
Holman [150]	1951	Cough following light percussion should begin at presumably unaffected areas. Move downward from the epigastrium in lower abdominal discomfort, upward toward the epigastrium in upper abdominal pain, and from the side of the comfort to the side of pain in unilateral involvement. The area of tenderness is quickly and easily ascertained, its exact extent determined, and outlined on the skin by pencil. All degrees of intensity of tenderness are encountered, from mild tenderness at the periphery to the exquisitely painful percussion at the center of the involved areas. The greatest tenderness is usually found over the site of inflammation of the most prolonged duration, which corresponds to the area of initial inflammation	Viscerosensory reflex
Fox [153]	1966	A bluish discoloration is located in the upper outer aspect of the thigh(s)	Ruptured abdominal aortic aneurysm and acute pancreatitis
Tixier [34]	[n.a.]	There is no abdominal wall guarding when the patient is in shock during the early stage of rapid exsanguination	Intrabdominal hemorrhage

[a] *Denotes an individual who supported anti-Semitism, racial acts, or committed crimes against humanity*

11.3 Conclusion

There is an overlap of the signs affecting the abdominal wall. Delbet, Guinard, Demons, and Hartmann described abdominal rigidity or involuntary guarding secondary to intestinal perforation from intra-abdominal trauma. Other signs secondarily involving the abdominal wall were reported by several authors as a means to better define the underlying organ responsible for intestinal perforation. Hofstätter, Cullen, and Hellendall described bruising of the umbilicus occurring in extrauterine pregnancy. Except for Carnett sign, these signs have not been well studied, and their significance in clinical medicine remains unknown. We believe they are important to learn as their presence provides clues to the potential cause of the underlying disease.

References

1. Dock G. Leopold Auenbrugger and the history of percussion: an address given at the opening exercises of the department of Medicine. Ann Arbor: University of Michigan; 1898.
2. Walsh JJ. Auenbrugger, the inventor of percussion. In: Makers of modern medicine. New York: Fordham University Press; 1907. p. 55–85.
3. Willius FA, Keys TE. Joseph Leopold Auenbrugger. In: Classics of cardiology, vol. 1. New York: Dover Publications; 1941. p. 191–2.
4. Smith JJ. The Inventum Novum of Joseph Leopold Auenbrugger. Bull N York Acad M. 1962;38:691–701.
5. Bedford DE. Auenbrugger's contribution to cardiology: history of percussion of the heart. Br Heart J. 1971;33:817–21.
6. Clar F. Leopold Auenbrugger, der Erfinder der Percussion des Brustkorbes, geb. zu Graz 1722, gest. zu Wien 1809, und sein Inventum novum. Graz: Leuschner & Lubensky; 1867.
7. Auenbrugger L. Text and documents on percussion of the chest being a translation of Auenbrugger's original treatis entitled "Inventum novum ex percussion thoracis humani, ut singo abstrsos interni perectoris morbos detegendi" [Vienna 1761]. Forbes J, trans. London: The Johns Hopkins Press; 1824. p. 373–403.
8. Guttmann W. Zum Andenken an Ottomar Rosenbach. Leipzig: Verlag von J.A. Barth; 1908.
9. Rosenbach O. Ein Beitrag zur Symptomatologie cerebraler Hemiplegieen. Arch Psychiat Nerven. 1876;6:845–51.
10. Merklen P. Discours prononcé au nom de la Société par M. Merklen aux obsèques de M. Jules Simon. Bull Soc Méd Hôp Paris. 1899;16:769–70.
11. Simon J. Sur un signe constant de la méningite au début. Gaz Hôp Paris. 1895;26:250–1.
12. Simon J. Record of medical progress: a constant early symptom in meningitis. North Am J Homoeop. 1895;43:769.
13. Guinard B. L'assassinat du docteur Aimé Guinard, chirurgien des Hôpitaux de Paris (1856–1911). http://www.bernard-guinard.com/arcticles%20divers/docteur%20Guinard/docteur_Guinard.html. Accessed 20 Oct 2022.
14. Mouchet A. Nécrologie: Le docteur Aimé Guinard (1856–1911). Paris méd. 1911;2:99–101.
15. Guinard A. De la laparotomie dans les contusions de l'abdomen. Rev Chir. 1896;16:873–4.
16. [No author]. Death of professor Demons. JAMA. 1920;75:118.
17. Laveran A, Janes J. Demons, Jean octave Albert. Comité des travaux historiques et scientifiques. https://cths.fr/an/savant.php?id=3385. Accessed 27 Oct 2022.
18. [No author]. Nécrologie: Albert Demons (1842–1920). Paris Méd. 1920;38:410.

19. Demons A. Mémoires. Acad méd. 1895;37:17.
20. A. Demons (Bordeaux). Archives franco-bulges de chirurgie, 1904. https://www.google.com/books/edition/Archives_franco_belges_de_chirurgie/Sgo0AQAAMAAJ?hl=en&gbpv=1&dq=Demons+and+Bordeaux&pg=PP9&printsec=frontcover. Accessed 30 Oct 2022.
21. Demons A. Des contusions de l'abdomen. Rev chir. 1897;17:974–9.
22. Binnie JF. The discussion of contusions of the abdomen at the recent French Congress of Surgery. Ann Surg. 1898;27:384–94.
23. Hartmann, Henri (1860–1952). Royal College of Surgeons of England. Plarr's lives of the fellows. https://livesonline.rcseng.ac.uk/client/en_GB/lives/search/detailnonmodal/ent:$002f$002fSD_ASSET$002f0$002fSD_ASSET:377221/one?qu=%22rcs%3A+E005038%22&rt=false%7C%7C%7CIDENTIFIER%7C%7C%7CResource+Identifier. Accessed 22 Oct 2022.
24. [No author]. Henri Hartmann. Br Med J 1952;1:167.
25. Karamanou M, Abid L, Zografos G, Androutsos G. Henri Hartmann (1860–1952): grand maître de la chirurgie colorectale du 20e siècle. Presse Méd. 2017;46:620–4.
26. Moulonguet P. Henri Hartmann (1860–1952). J Chir (Paris). 1952;68:169–76.
27. Hartmann, Henri Albert Charles Antoine. Comité des travaux historiques et scientifiques. https://cths.fr/an/savant.php?id=112478#. Accessed 22 Oct 2022.
28. Cope VZ. Henri Hartmann MD, FRCS. Br Med J. 1952;1:167.
29. Hartmann H. Rapport par M. Hartmann. Bull Soc Méd Chir. 1901;27:234–6.
30. Balthazard V, Ribadeau-Dumas L, Floderer A, Wauthier A. Sergent, Émile Eugène Joseph. Comité des travaux historiques et scientifiques. https://cths.fr/an/savant.php?id=4744. Accessed 4 Nov 2022.
31. Émile Sergent (1867–1943). Bibliothèque nationale de France. https://data.bnf.fr/fr/12374807/emile_sergent/. Accessed 4 Nov 2022
32. Ribadeau-Dumas L. Docteur Emile Sergent (1867–1943). Bulletin de l'Académie nationale de médecine 1943. Paris, séance du 29 juin 1943. Société d'Histoire du Vesinet. http://www.histoire-vesinet.org/docteursergent.htm. Accessed 4 Nov 2022.
33. Sergent E. Le diagnostic du syndrome d'insuffisance surrénale pure et la ligne blanche surré. Bull Mém Soc Méd Hôp Paris. 1904;3:380–4.
34. Keleman E. Physical diagnosis of acute abdominal diseases and injuries. Budapest: Akadémiai Kiadó; 1964.
35. Birrer RB, Birrer CD. Medical diagnostic signs: a reference collection of eponymic bedside signs. Springfield: Charles C. Thomas; 1982.
36. No author]. Obituary: Charles Edward Beevor, MD, FRCO Lond. Br Med J. 1908;2:1785–6.
37. [No author]. Charles Edward Beevor, MD. Boston M & S J. 1908;159:916.
38. Brown GH. Charles Edward Beevor. Royal College of Physicians. https://history.rcplondon.ac.uk/inspiring-physicians/charles-edward-beevor. Accessed 5 Nov 2022.
39. [No author]. Obituary: Charles Edward Beevor MD Lond, MRCS Eng; FRCP Lond. Lancet. 1908;4:1854–5.
40. Beevor CE. Diseases of the nervous system: a handbook for students and practitioners. London: H.K. Lewis; 1898.
41. Guthrie LG. Beevor, Charles Edward. Dictionary of National Biography. 1912. https://en.wikisource.org/wiki/Dictionary_of_National_Biography,_1912_supplement/Beevor,_Charles_Edward. Accessed 22 Oct 2022.
42. [No author]. The Lettsomian lectures on the diagnosis and localization of cerebral tumours. Lancet. 1907;169:491–7.
43. Beevor CE. On the distribution of the different arteries supplying the human brain. Philos Trans R Soc Lond. 1909;200:1–55.
44. Beevor CE. The Croonian lectures on muscular movements and their representation in the central nervous system: delivered before the Royal College of Physicians of London, June, 1903. London: Adlard; 1904.
45. [No author]. Dr. Louis Ransohoff dies; noted Cincinnati surgeon. The Cincinnati Enquirer. 1958:28.

46. [No author]. Obituary: Doctor Joseph Ransohoff. Radium. 1921;17–18:16.
47. Ransohoff, Joseph (1853–1921). Plarr's lives of the fellows. Royal College of Surgeons of England. https://livesonline.rcseng.ac.uk/client/en_GB/lives/search/detailnonmodal/ent:$002f$002fSD_ASSET$002f0$002fSD_ASSET:375211/one?qu=%22rcs%3A+E003028%22&rt=false%7C%7C%7CIDENTIFIER%7C%7C%7CResource+Identifier. Accessed 22 Oct 2022.
48. [No author]. Report of Committee on necrology: Dr. Joseph Ransohoff. Trans Meet Am Surg Assoc. 1922;39:xliii–iv.
49. Cutter WR. Dr. Joseph Ransohoff. American biography: a new cyclopedia, vol. 27. New York: American Historical Society; 1926. p. 225–226.
50. Ransohoff J. Gangrene of the gallbladder: rupture of the common bile duct, with a new sign. JAMA. 1906;45:395–7.
51. [No author]. Obituary: Dr. Panagino Livierato. Br Med J. 1936;12:1278.
52. [No author]. Necrologio: Panagino Livierato L'università italiana rivista dell'istruzione superiore. 1936;2:148.
53. De Rossi L. Riflesso addomino-cardiaco: lezione del Prof. Livierato. Napoli: G. Civelli; 1906.
54. McGuire ER. Transactions of the historical section of the Buffalo Medical Journal Club. Med Libr Hist J. 1905;3:155–6.
55. [No author]. Obituary Dr. Jean Cruveilhier. Int Rec Med Gen Pract Clin. 1874;19:559–60.
56. [No author]. Jean Cruveilhier. Proc R Soc Med. 1875;7:317–9.
57. [No author]. Jean Cruveilhier. Lancet. 1874;1:570.
58. Collective. Cruveilhier, Jean. In: The American Annual Cyclopedia and Register of Important Events of the Year 1874, vol. 14. New York: D. Appleton; 1875. p. 254.
59. Després A. Nécrologie: Cruveilhier. Rev Sci Par. 1874;2:908.
60. [No author]. Professor Jean Cruveilhier. J Nerv Ment Dis. 1874;1:227.
61. Paul Clemens von Baumgarten. Gastroenterología. http://articulos.sld.cu/gastroenterologia/archives/6876. Accessed 17 Oct 2022.
62. Baumgarten, Paul Clemens von. Deutsche Biographie. https://www.deutsche–biographie.de/pnd116091444.html. Accessed 17 Oct 2022.
63. Fischer M. Actors and agents. In: Bibliographic encyclopedia of pharmacologists between Germany and Russia in the 19th century. Aachen: Shaker Verlag; 2014. p. 11–4.
64. Baumgarten PC. Über vollständiges Offenbleiben der Vena umbilicalis; zugleich ein Beitrag zur Frage des Morbus Bantil. In: Arbeiten auf dem Gebiete der pathologischen Anatomie und Bacteriologie aus dem Pathologisch-Anatomischen Institut zu Tübingen, Bd. 6. Leipzig: Verlag von S. Hirzel; 1908. p. 93–110.
65. Hofstätter VR. Robert (Wilhelm). In: Deutsche biographische Enzyklopädie, Hitz – Kozub, Bd. 5. München: K.G. Saur Verlag; 2011. p. 81.
66. Taylor SS. Hofstätter, Robert. In: Who's who in Austria 1959/1960. Vienna: Intercontinental Book & Publishing; 1961. p. 230.
67. Turda M. The history of East-Central European eugenics, 1900–1945: sources and commentaries. London: Bloomsbury Publishing; 2015.
68. Moscucci O. Gender and cancer in England, 1860–1948. London: Palgrave Macmillan; 2017.
69. Samaan AE. From a race of masters to a master race: 1948 to 1848. [New York]: Library without Walls; 2020.
70. Hofstätter R. Ueber einen Fall von durch Tubargravidität komplizierter akkreter Nabelhernie. Wien klin Wochenschr. 1909;22:524–5.
71. [No author]. Walter Essex Wynter MD, FRCP. Br Med J. 1945;1:100–1.
72. Brown GH. Walter Essex Wynter. Royal College of Physicians. https://history.rcplondon.ac.uk/inspiring-physicians/walter-essex-wynter. Accessed 22 Oct 2022.
73. Quincke HI. Ueber hydrocephalus. In: Leyden E, Pfeiffer E, editors. Verhandlungen des Congresses für innere Medicin, Bd. 10. Wiesbaden: Verlag von J.F. Bergmann; 1891. p. 321–39.
74. Wynter WE. Four cases of tubercular meningitis in which paracentesis of the theca vertebralis was performed for the relief of fluid pressure. Lancet. 1891;1:981–2.

75. Wynter E. Absence of abdominal respiratory movement as an indication of pericarditis. Proc R Soc Med. 1911;4:40–50.
76. François M, Dosso D, Lévy-Solal E. Pierre Delbet (1861–1957). Bibliothèque nationale de France. https://data.bnf.fr/de/14629849/pierre_delbet/. Accessed 22 Oct 2022.
77. Prat D. Profesor Pierre Delbet. Bol Soc Cir Uruguay. 1957;28:123–131.
78. Delbet Pierre Louis Ernest. Comité des travaux historiques et scientifiques. https://cths.fr/an/savant.php?id=112306. Accessed 4 Nov 2022.
79. Patel J. Pierre Delbet (1861–1957). Mém Acad Chir. 1962;88:133–52.
80. Delbet P. Contusion abdominale sans plaie extérieure. Paris Chir. 1912;4:370–1.
81. [No author]. Obituary: David Ligat, MB, FRCS, DPH. Br Med J. 1954;1:339.
82. Ligat, David (1873–1954). Plarr's lives of the fellows. Royal College of Surgeons of England. https://livesonline.rcseng.ac.uk/client/en_GB/lives/search/detailnonmodal/ent:$002f$002fSD_ASSET$002f0$002fSD_ASSET:377448/one?qu=%22rcs%3A+E005265%22&rt=false%7C%7C%7CIDENTIFIER%7C%7C%7CResource+Identifier. Accessed 4 Nov 2022.
83. Hamilton WF. Obituary [David Ligat]. Br Med J. 1954;1:464.
84. Ligat D. Hyperalgesia in abdominal disease: preliminary notes on the diagnostic value of maximal points of hyperalgesia of the skin and subcutaneous tissue of the abdominal wall in affections of the abdominal viscera. Practitioner. 1916;97:106–36.
85. [No author]. Obituary: W. Sampson Handley MD, MS, FRCS. Br Med J. 1962;1:948.
86. [No author]. In memoriam: William Sampson Handley. Ann R Coll Surg Engl. 1962;30:344–6.
87. Handley, William Sampson (1872–1962). Royal College of Surgeons of England. Plarr's lives of the fellows. https://livesonline.rcseng.ac.uk/client/en_GB/lives/search/detailnon-modal/ent:$002f$002fSD_ASSET$002f0$002fSD_ASSET:377198/one?qu=%22rcs%3A+E005015%22&rt=false%7C%7C%7CIDENTIFIER%7C%7C%7CResource+Identifier. Accessed 15 Oct 2022.
88. [No author]. W. Sampson Handley, MD, MS, FRCS Hon FACS. Br Med J. 1962;1:1082–3.
89. Handley WS. A method of treating general peritonitis with obstruction: its application in military surgery. Br Med J. 1916;1:519–22.
90. [No author]. Obituary: R. J Willan. Br Med J. 1955;1:231–2.
91. [No author]. Royal Victoria infirmary, Newcastle-upon-Tyne. Lancet. 1915;1:43.
92. [No author]. University of Durham College of Medicine. Chem Drug. 1909;75:23.
93. [No author]. Obituary: R.J. Willan, CBE, MVO; MS, FRCS. Br Med J. 1955;1:422.
94. Willan RJ. Note upon a helpful diagnostic sign in ruptured digestive ulcers. Br Med J. 1918;1:142–3.
95. Thomas S. Cullen collection. Chesney archives. Johns Hopkins Medicine Nursing Public Health. https://medicalarchives.jhmi.edu/collection/thomas-s-cullen-collection/. Accessed 22 Oct 2022.
96. Thomas Stephen Cullen. The Alan Mason Chesney Medical Archives of The Johns Hopkins Medical Institutions. https://portraitcollection.jhmi.edu/portraits/cullen-thomas-stephen. Accessed 22 Oct 2022.
97. One hundred and thirty-eighth annual report of the Department of Health, 1952. City of Baltimore. https://health.baltimorecity.gov/sites/default/files/City%20of%20Baltimore%20138th%20Annual%20Report%20of%20The%20Department%20of%20Health.pdf. Accessed 22 Oct 2022.
98. De Moraes A. Prof. Dr. Thomas Stephen Cullen; 1869–1953. An Bras Ginecol. 1953;36:222–223.
99. Cullen S. A new sign in ruptured extrauterine pregnancy. Am J Obstet. 1918;78:457.
100. George G. Turner, surgeon. The University of Leeds. https://explore.library.leeds.ac.uk/special-collectionsexplore/participant/5157%20%20%20%20Accessed%2022%20Aug%202022. Accessed 22 Oct 2022.
101. Turner, Professor George Grey. Welcome collection. https://wellcomecollection.org/works/j8u8vyzc. Accessed 22 Oct 2022.

102. George Grey Turner (1877–1951). Plarr's lives of the fellows. Royal College of Surgeons of England. https://livesonline.rcseng.ac.uk/client/en_GB/lives/search/detailnonmodal/ent:$002f$002fSD_ASSET$002f0$002fSD_ASSET:376907/one?qu=%22rcs%3A+E004724%22&rt=false%7C%7C%7CIDENTIFIER%7C%7C%7CResource+Identifier. Accessed 22 Oct 2022.

103. Willan RJ. George Grey Turner. Ann R Coll Surg Engl. 1951;9:274–6.

104. Turner GG. Local discoloration of the abdominal wall as a sign of acute pancreatitis. Br J Surg. 1919;7:394–5.

105. Düwell K. Hugo Hellendall. In: Vertreibung jüdischer Künstler und Wissenschaftler aus Düsseldorf, 1933–1945. Düsseldorf: Droste; 1998. p. 188–9.

106. [No author]. Personalien und Notizen. Gynaek Rundscha. 1908;2:284.

107. Hellendall H. Ein neues Symptom der Extrauterinschwangerschaft. Zentralblatt Gyn. 1921;45:890–1.

108. Hellendall H. Blutige Verfärbung des Nabels als diagnostisches Zeichen von Extrauteringravidität. Zentralblatt Gyn. 1922;46:147.

109. Hermann Schlesinger (1866–1934). Deutsch Gesellschaft für Gastroenterologie, Verdauungs– und Stoffwechselkrankheiten. https://www.dgvs–gegendas-vergessen.de/en/biografie/hermann-schlesinger/. Accessed 3 Nov 2022.

110. Collective. Schlesinger Hermann. Österreichisches Biographisches Lexikon, Bd. 10. Wien: Verlag der Österreichischer Akademie der Wissenschaften; 1991. p. 191.

111. Schlesinger H. Die Syringomyelie: eine Monographie. Leipzig: Franz Deuticke Verlag; 1895.

112. Rosenbach H. Obituary [Hermann Schlesinger]. Br Med J. 1934;2:496.

113. Schlesinger H. Die "Nabelverziehung" bei Ulcus ventriculi und anderen Abdominalaffektionen. Wien klin Wochenschr. 1921;34:1.

114. Barkman A. Sur les réflexes thoraco-abdominaux normaux et leur localisation médullaire. Acta Med Scand. 1923;58:364–371.

115. [No author]. Obituary: Frank Jeans, FRCS. Br Med J. 1933;2:37.

116. [No author]. The late Mr. Frank Jeans. Br Med J. 1933;1:83.

117. Jeans F. Treatment of acute peritonitis. Lancet. 1925;2:729–30.

118. [No author]. Dr. John B. Carnett, surgeon, dies at 57. Philadelphia: The Philadelphia Inquirer; 1934. p. 2.

119. [No author]. Memoir of Dr John Berton Carnett. Trans Coll Phys Phila. 1934;1–2:xx–ii.

120. Collective. Philadelphia in the World War, 1914–1919. New York: Wynkoop Hallenbeck Crawford Company; 1922.

121. Carnett JB. Intercostal neuralgia as a cause of abdominal pain and tenderness. Surg Gyn Obst. 1926;42:625–32.

122. Suleiman S, Johnston DE. The abdominal wall: an overlooked source of pain. Am Fam Phys. 2001;64:431–8.

123. Bailey H. Non-acute abdominal conditions: general principles in the consideration of the abdomen. In: Physical signs in clinical surgery. 11th ed. Baltimore: Williams & Wilkins; 1949. p. 204.

124. Thomson H, Francis DMA. Abdominal-wall tenderness: a useful sign in the acute abdomen. Lancet. 1977;2:1053–4.

125. Thomson WHF, Dawes RFH, Carter SST. Abdominal wall tenderness: a useful sign in chronic abdominal pain. Br J Surg. 1991;78:223–5.

126. [No author]. William Edward Fothergill, MA, MD. Br Med J. 1926;2:913–4.

127. Fairbairn JS. Obituary: William Edward Fothergill. Br J Obs Gyn. 1927;34:102–6.

128. Elwood WJ, Tuxford AF. Archibald Donald, 1860–1937 MA, MD, FRCP. Hon FRCOG, hon LLD, and William Edward Fothergill, 1865–1926 MA, BSc, MD. In: Some Manchester doctors: a biographical collection to Mark the 150th anniversary of the Manchester medical society 1834-1984. Manchester: Manchester University Press; 1984. p. 116–25.

129. [No author]. Medical news: William Edward Fothergill, MA, BSc. Lancet. 1897;3:427.

130. [No author]. William Edward Fothergill. Lancet. 1897;3:426–7.

131. [No author]. The Transaction of the Edinburgh Obstetrical Society, vol. 31. Edinburgh: Oliver and Boyd, Publisher to the Society; 1906.
132. [No author]. Book reviews: manual of diseases of women by W.E. Fothergill, MA, BSc, MD. Med Rec. 1911;79:1070.
133. Fothergill WE. Haematoma in the abdominal wall simulating pelvic new growth. Br Med J. 1926;1:941–2.
134. Gully P. Sisters of heaven: China's barnstorming aviatrixes—modernity, feminism, and popular imagination in Asia and the west. San Francisco: Long River Press; 2008.
135. Kagan SR. Dr. Jacob Meyer. In: Jewish Contributions to Medicine in America (1656–1934). Boston: Boston Medical Publishing; 1934. p. 124.
136. No author]. Jacob Meyer—Department of Medicine Catalogue. Bulletin of Loyola University. Chicago: Loyola University; 1917. p. 81.
137. Co Tui F, Meyer J. Umbilical displacement and deviation of linea alba in acute abdominal conditions. JAMA. 1928;90:1779.
138. Mortola GA. Abdominal examination: a new method of abdominal exploration. In: International surveys of recent advances in medicine, vol. 1. Washington, D.C.: Washington Institute of Medicine; 1937.
139. Raw, Stanley Collingwood, 1910–1994. Royal College of Surgeons of England. Plarr's Lives of the Fellows Published. https://livesonline.rcseng.ac.uk/client/en_GB/lives/search/detail-nonmodal/ent:$002f$002fSD_ASSET$002f0$002fSD_ASSET:380466/one. Accessed 10 Oct 2022.
140. Raw AJ. Stanley Collingwood Raw, MS, FRCS. Br Med J. 1994;308:1565.
141. Raw SC. Perforation of gastric and duodenal ulcers a series of 312 cases. Lancet. 1944;243:12–4.
142. About Emile Frederic Holman, MD. Stanford Medicine, Surgery. https://surgery.stanford.edu/holman.html. Accessed 27 July 2022.
143. Mark JBD. Historical perspective of the American Association for Thoracic Surgery: Emile Frederic Holman, MD (1890–1977). J Thorac Cardiovasc Surg. 2005;130:206–7.
144. Emile Frederic Holman: on oral history. National Library of Medicine. General History of Medicine. https://oculus.nlm.nih.gov/cgi/t/text/text-idx?c=oralhist;cc=oralhist;rgn=main;view=text;idno=2935115r. Accessed 27 Oct 2022.
145. Emile Holman, 1948–1952. American Board of Thoracic Surgery. https://www.abts.org/ABTS/Public/About/Emeritus_Directors.aspx. Accessed 27 Oct 2022.
146. History of AOS. American Osler Society. http://www.americanosler.org/about/history-of-the-aos.php. Accessed 27 Oct 2022.
147. SVS Past Presidents. Society for Vascular Surgery. https://vascular.org/about/history/svs-past-presidents. Accessed 27 Oct 2022.
148. [No author]. Emile Holman. J Thorac Cardiovasc Surg. 2005;129:28.
149. Chandler LR. Emile Frederic Holman. Am J Surg. 1955;89:1089–90.
150. Holman E. The art of abdominal percussion in the presence of inflammation. Surg Gyn Obst. 1951;9:775–7.
151. Fox, Mr. John Adrian. Medical Directory, vol. 154, part 1. 1998. https://www.google.com/books/edition/The_Medical_Directory/k_8fAQAAMAAJ?hl=en&gbpv=0. Accessed 20 Oct 2022.
152. Maringot R. John Adrian Fox, MB, BS, FRCS (Eng). Abdominal operations. 1974;1:viii.
153. Fox JA. A diagnostic sign of extraperitoneal haemorrhage. Br J Surg. 1966;53:193–5.
154. [No author]. Tixier L-E. Progrès Méd. 1902;15–16:296.
155. [No author]. Tixier (Léon-Eugène-Joseph). J off répub fr. [n.a.]; 1909. p. 8348.

Chapter 12
Hernia Signs

12.1 Introduction

A hernia is the Latin term for a rupture or protrusion. The suffix "cele" remained in use in the 1800s in connotation to a hernia [1]. The word "bubonocele" is an archaic term coined by the Roman medical writer Aulus Cornelius Celsus (c. 25 BC–c. 50 AD) in reference to an inguinal hernia, and "enterocele" is an old term coined by the Greeks of antiquity and used today when referring to a hernia containing the intestines [1]. Celsus apologetically used the term hernia to describe a protrusion of an internal organ in the first century AD [2]. In a translation of his work in *De Medicina* (On Medicine) on inguinal hernia:

> Now under this several diseases occur; sometimes arising from a rupture of the tunica, which I have stated to take their origin from the groins; and sometimes happening while these remain entire. Indeed, sometimes inflammation takes place from disease, and then a rupture from a weight of the parts; or that tunic *peritoneum*, which is designed to separate the intestines from the lower parts, the *genitals,* is ruptured at ounce by some violence: then either the omentum alone, or that and the intestine together, protrude into that part by their own weight, and by this a passage formed, they press down gradually from the groin into the inferior parts, and by degrees separate the nervous-*membranous*-coats, which naturally yield to this dilation. The Greeks term a descent of the intestines *enterocele*, the omentum *epiplocele*: with us the term *hernia* is in becoming, but common to them both [2, p. 269].

In addition to an inguinal hernia, Celsus described eight others, both umbilical and intestinal, and omental in the abdomen. Covered are signs of a hernia: enterocele, obturator, vitelline, and inguinal hernia. Their methods of diagnosis are named eponymously in honor of the person and their discovery.

© The Author(s), under exclusive license to Springer Nature
Switzerland AG 2023
S. H. Yale et al., *Gastrointestinal Eponymic Signs*,
https://doi.org/10.1007/978-3-031-33673-7_12

12.2 Eponymous Signs

12.2.1 Laugier Sign

Stanislas Laugier (1799–1872) was born in Paris, France, and received his medical degree in 1828 [3]. He was an intern under the auspices of Baron Guillaume Dupuytren (1777–1835) at the Hôtel-Dieu and appointed associate professor of the Faculty of Medicine, Paris, in 1830, a surgeon at the central surgical office in 1831, Necker Hospital in 1832, and Beaujon Hospital in 1835 [3, 4]. He was selected as professor and chair of the surgical clinic at La Pitié Hospital in 1848 and the Hôtel-Dieu in 1854 [3, 4]. Laugier was elected member of the French National Academy of Medicine in 1844, president in 1848, and to the Academy of Sciences in 1868 [3]. His name is eponymously associated with a hernia, fractures, and sign [5, 6].

As to a description of his character:

> He was full of good sense and a gifted speaker who sought neither success from either the Academy or his patients. He wrote with elegance; as shown in his *Tribute to Jean-Louis Petit,* in the articles in the 30 volumes of *Dictionary of Medical Sciences,* and in the *New Dictionary of Practical Medicine and Surgery* [4, p. 545].

Laugier described a method for distinguishing a small and large bowel hernia and differentiated it from a hernia involving the epiploic appendages (Table 12.1):

> The extent, form, and cause of meteorism of the abdomen occurring during a strangulated hernia vary depending upon whether the hernia is epiploic or intestinal, as the latter contains fat and small or large intestines. Its extent also varies depending upon whether the incarcerated portion of the small intestine lies close to the stomach. In an epiploic hernia, before the development of peritonitis, the abdomen is soft even in the vicinity of the hernia without meteorism. The meteorism is present within the first hours of the strangulated intestinal hernia. When the hernia contains the large intestine, the proximal portion of the intestine of the meteorism causes the abdomen to assume a cylindrical shape. If the small intestine or omentum is within the hernial sac, the flanks and epigastric regions are supple and depressed. The bloated abdomen occupies the hypogastric and umbilical regions. It is spherical, or nearly so in shape, like an encysted tumor or pregnancy at six or seven months. (…) When the strangulation of the small intestines occurs near the stomach, abdominal distention is less pronounced for the same duration of the disease because the upper end is shorter [7, p. 370–371].

Thus, Laugier sign refers to the appearance of the abdomen in small and large intestinal hernias. The hernia is cylindrical when the large bowel is involved, while the flanks and epigastric regions are depressed in small intestinal or omental hernias.

12.2.2 Howship–Romberg Sign

12.2.2.1 John Howship

John Howship (1781–1841) was born in London, England, and attended medical school in 1799. He was appointed assistant surgeon at St. George's Infirmary,

London, in 1805, and served as an assistant surgeon in 1834 and chief surgeon in 1836 to the Charing Cross Hospital [8]. He was a member of the Royal College of Surgeons from 1828 to 1841 and delivered the Hunterian Oration at the Royal College of Surgeons in 1833. Howship was a member of the Royal Medico-Chirurgical Society of London; Medico-Chirurgical Society and Royal Medical Society of Edinburgh, England; Copenhagen Royal Academy of Medicine; Society for Natural and Medical Sciences, Dresden; German Academy of Natural Sciences, Bonn; and corresponding member of the Paris Emulation Medical Society [9].

His contributions spanned the fields of gastroenterology, genitourinary, and disorder of bone. Another eponym attributed to his namesake is the Howship lacunae, the histological findings of the groove or pit containing osteoclast cells indicative of bone resorption [10].

In his book *Practical Remarks on the Discrimination and Appearance of Surgical Disease*, Howship described the symptoms in a case titled "Strangulated thyroidal hernia, diagnostic symptom, appearances on dissection," involving an aged female under the care of Mr. Weatherfield:

> In November she was seized with violent spasmodic pain in the left side of the abdomen, running down the left leg, with sickness, vomiting, and, as she said diarrhea [11, p. 323]. March 23, 1839—Mr. W[eatherfield] found her again suffering under extreme pain and tenderness in the abdomen, especially in the left side, with constant vomiting, preceded by diarrhea, and attended with the same pain as before, down the left leg. The symptoms, those of strangulated hernia, Mr. W. made a careful inquiry and examination but could nowhere ascertain outward tumor [11, p. 324].

On postmortem examination, he found:

> On opening the abdomen, a portion of small intestine was seen stretched towards the left obturator foramen, where a knuckle was firmly impacted, forming a small hernia, no larger than a nutmeg, protruding through the opening. The intestine, high inflamed, was almost gangrenous. The parts were carefully removed and admirably dissected; demonstrating the hernia to the best advantage [11, p. 324].

Thus, Howship described the symptoms in patients with an obturator hernia (Table 12.1).

12.2.2.2 Moritz Romberg

Moritz Heinrich Romberg (1795–1873) was born in Meiningen, Saxony, Germany, in 1795 and received his medical degree from the University of Berlin in 1817 [12]. He was appointed a medical officer for the poor in 1820 and was associate professor in 1830. He served as director of the Cholera Hospitals in Berlin in 1830, 1836, and 1838. Romberg was appointed extraordinary professor of medicine and director of the university polyclinic in 1838 and an ordinary professor at the University of Berlin in 1845 [13, 14].

Ramberg's most widely recognized work, published from 1840 to 1846 and translated into English in 1853, was a treatise on the nervous system of man where he described another better-known neurological sign involving the dorsal column of the spinal cord in patients with tabes dorsalis. He authored other works on cholera and respiratory paralysis [15]. He described the significance of his findings of an obturator hernia in 1847 (Table 12.1):

> What gives this case a special interest is not that it is rare, but elucidating the diagnosis by its neurologic phenomenon. Pressure and distortion of the obturator nerve may be found in every obturator hernia and if the content of the hernia is bowel, symptoms of nerve entrapment is associated with the intestinal entrapment. Both the sensory fibers of the obturator nerve, which spread as cutaneous nerves on the inner side of the thigh as well as the motorfibers, destined for the gracilis and adductors of the thigh, confirm this disorder by the presence of severe pain located in the inner thigh, paresthesia, and the inability to adduct the thigh. In some older observations, we find mention of this pain accompanying an existing ileus, without any value placed in diagnosis [16, p. 624].

He explained the diagnostic criteria for an obturator hernia:

> For the obturator hernia is a diagnostic criterion as it is associated with pain, disturbed movement of the thigh, and altered intestinal movement. Most important, because this condition is chronic it rarely forms a tumor visible from the outside, and is subjected to temporary, repeated incarceration. Circumstances occurring in the female sexes, where this hernia is more likely to occur, may lead one to misinterpret that this pain represent a nervous, hysterical affection. Knowing that the pain on the thigh is a neuralgic assist in confirming the diagnosis [16, p. 625].

Hence, Howship was the first to describe the clinical syndrome, while Romberg reported on the diagnostic criteria and explained the pathophysiology of an incarcerated obturator hernia (Table 12.1). The Howship–Romberg sign was identified in 11 of 30 (37%) of patients with obturator hernia [17]. In another small study, the Howship–Romberg sign was present in only 3 of 13 (23%) patients [18]. It has been shown to be present in 15–50% of cases of obturator hernia [19].

The obturator hernia may follow the route of the branch of the anterior or posterior obturator nerve or between the internal and external obturator membranes. The different route that the obturator hernia takes as it enters the obturator canal explains the lower detection rate of this sign in some patients. The sign was shown to occur more commonly in patients when the hernia follows the anterior branch of the obturator nerve, which innervates the muscles of the pectineus, adductor brevis and longus, and gracilis [20].

In a study of 43 patients, comparing those with obturator hernia before and after the advent of computed tomography (CT) of the pelvis showed a better preoperative diagnostic accuracy and a lower rate of intestinal resection and surgical mortality with preoperative CT scan [21]. In another small study, no difference was found in the time to operation, length of stay, need for bowel resection, and mortality rate, regardless of whether a patient received a preoperative CT scan [17].

The Howship–Romberg sign refers to pain at the medial side of the thigh in an obturator hernia.

12.2.3 Ladd Sign

William Eduard Ladd (1880–1967) was born in Milton, Norfolk County, Massachusetts, USA, and received his medical degree from Harvard Medical School in 1906 [22–26]. He completed a surgical internship at Boston City Hospital from 1906 to 1908. He was appointed assistant visiting surgeon to the Infants and Children's Hospital from 1909 to 1913, assistant visiting surgeon to the Boston City Hospital from 1910 to 1913, and visiting surgeon to Milton Hospital beginning in 1910 [23]. He was an assistant in surgery beginning in 1912, an instructor in 1917 at the Harvard Graduate School of Medicine, and a surgeon-in-chief at Boston Children's Hospital in 1927 [23]. He served as a clinical professor of surgery at Harvard Medical School in 1931 [22, 25]. The William E. Ladd Professor of Child Surgery was named in his honor at Harvard Medical School from 1941 to 1947 [22, 25, 26]. He cofounded the American Board of Surgery, the Surgical Section of the American Board of Surgery, and the American Board of Plastic Surgery [22, 25]. He is credited for writing with his colleague Robert Edward Gross (1905–1988) the book *Abdominal Surgery of Infancy and Childhood* in 1941 [26, 27].

As to a description of his character by Donald Watson:

> At the patient's bedside, in the operating room, and the informal surroundings of the surgeon's dressing room or private office, there have been few teachers as effective as this kindly, impressive, stimulating man. A whole generation of surgeons and untold numbers of children will forever be in his debt [22, p. 296].

His name is eponymously recognized in association with congenital fibrous bands that cause the cecum to attach to the posterior abdominal wall leading to duodenal obstruction (Ladd bands) and the surgical procedure used to resolve the intestinal malrotation (Ladd procedure).

Ladd described a method for examining an inguinal hernia in infants (Table 12.1):

> When an infant is presented with this complaint, a method of examination different from that employed in the older child or adult is used. The practice used in the adult of inverting the scrotum, palpating the external ring and the impulse on coughing is almost valueless. Instead of this, the cord is palpated as it emerges from the external ring and, if hernia be present, it will be found to be thicker than that of the other side. If the hernia extends only part way down the canal, the finger is placed flat over the inguinal canal and the cord rolled back and forth underneath it. If hernia be present, this give a sensation to the finger of thickening of the cord, which is quite unmistakable to the trained finger [28, p. 235].

Ladd sign is the palpatory method of examining an infant for an inguinal hernia.

12.2.4 Hannington-Kiff Sign

There is limited historical information on John. Garfield Hannington-Kiff. He was appointed consultant anesthetist and director of the Pain Relief Centre at the Frimley

Park Hospital in Surrey, England, in the 1980s [29]. Hannington-Kiff was the recipient of the Jacksonian Prize from the Royal College of Surgeons of England in 1981 for his dissertation titled "The relief of dystrophic inflammatory and spastic conditions of limbs by the local deposition of high doses of drugs administered during regional circulatory occlusion with a tourniquet" [30]. He was the first anesthetist to receive this award. The commendation is given to fellows and members who "aspire to high place in surgery, dentistry, and anesthetics" [30].

His areas of medical practice and research interest were pain management and anesthesia. He developed a stellate ganglion block technique and a regional intravenous sympathetic block using guanethidine [31, 32].

Hannington-Kiff described the percussion method, the thigh adductor stretch reflex, for diagnosing a strangulated obturator hernia (Table 12.1) (Fig. 12.1):

> A firm blow from a patellar hammer over the thumb or index finger laid at right angles across the adductor muscle about 5 cm above the medial epicondyle of the femur. In this way any contraction of the adductor muscle can be felt as well as seen, and the patient will be saved some discomfort from the blow of the hammer [29, p. 180].

Thus, Hannington-Kiff described the percussion method for detecting the adductor stretch reflex used for the diagnosis of an obturator hernia. A positive sign is due to the pressure exerted on the irritated obturator nerve by the obturator hernia.

Table 12.1 Hernia signs

Name	Year	Description of sign	Significance
Laugier [7]	1840	When the hernia contains the proximal portion of the large intestine, the meteorism gives the abdomen an almost cylindrical shape. If the small intestine or omentum is within the hernial sac, the flanks and epigastric region are supple and depressed. At the same time, the bloated abdomen occupies the hypogastric and umbilical regions and is spherical	Small and large bowel hernia (enterocele)
Howship–Romberg [11, 16]	1840 1847	Severe pain located in the inner thigh, paresthesia, and the inability to adduct the thigh. An ileus may also be present	Obturator hernia
Ladd [28]	1941	The cord is palpated as it emerges from the external ring. If a hernia is present, it is thicker compared to the other side. If the hernia extends only part way down the canal, the finger is placed flat across the inguinal canal, and the cord is rolled back and forth. If a hernia is present, a thick cord is palpated	Inguinal hernia (infants)
Hannington-Kiff [29]	1980	A firm blow is delivered from a patellar hammer over the thumb or index finger placed at a right angle to the adductor muscle about 5 cm above the medial epicondyle of the femur. Contraction of the adductor muscle is observed or palpated	Strangulated obturator hernia

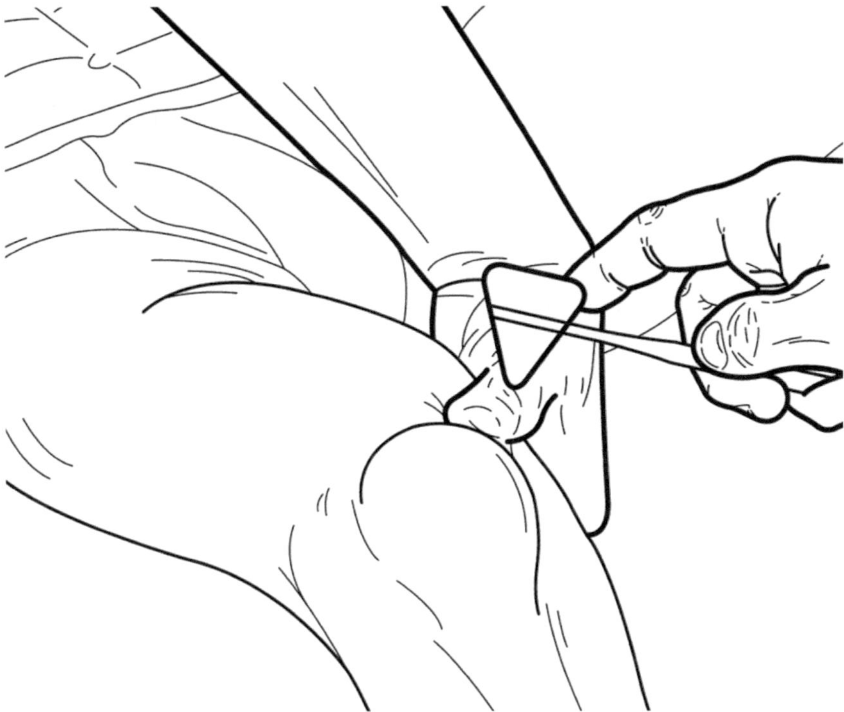

Fig. 12.1 Hannington-Kief sign (by Ryan Yale)

12.3 **Conclusion**

There are four eponymic named hernia signs, one of which (Ladd) is found in infants. These signs employ the physical examination skills of observation, palpation, and percussion as the method for eliciting these diagnostic findings. Howship–Romberg and Hannington-Kiff signs are used to assist in the diagnosis of obturator hernia. The Hannington-Kiff sign, unlike the Howship–Romberg, represents an objective means for diagnosing a strangulated obturator hernia. The Howship–Romberg sign is the best well-studied of these signs, found in only 15–50% of cases. The lack of description of what constitutes a positive test limits the ability to interpret findings from these studies. Despite these limitations, we contend that the signs should be taught as they provide a more in-depth understanding of the pathophysiologic process and anatomical variations, which may account for the inability to elicit a positive sign.

References

1. Skinner HA. The origin of medical terms. Baltimore: Williams & Wilkins; 1949.
2. Celsus AC. On medicine in eight books, vol. 1. (trans: L. Targa). Lee A, editor. London: E. Cox; 1831.

3. Broca P. Laugier, Stanislas. Comité des travaux historiques et scientifiques. 2020. https://cths.fr/an/savant.php?id=124583#. Accessed 15 Nov 2022.

4. [No author]. Nécrologie scientifique: Stanislas Laugier. L'Année scientifique et industrielle. 1873;16:544–5.

5. Marcucci L. Handbook of medical eponyms. Philadelphia: Lippincott Williams & Wilkins; 2002.

6. Birrer RB, Birrer CD. Medical diagnostic signs: a reference collection of eponymic bedside signs. Springfield: Charles C. Thomas; 1982.

7. Laugier S. Sur un signe nouveau dans l'histoire des hernies étranglées. C R Acad Sci. 1840;10:370–1.

8. Royal College of Surgeons of England. Howship, John (1781–1841). https://aim25.com/cats/9/10031.htm. Accessed 25 Nov 2022.

9. Howship J. Practical observation in surgery and morbid anatomy. London: Longman, Hurst, Rees, Orme and Brown; 1816.

10. Bir SC, Kalakoti P, Notarianni C, Nanda A. John Howship (1781–1841) and growing skull fracture: historical perspective. J Neurosurg Pediatr. 2015;16:472–6.

11. Howship J. Practical remarks on the discrimination and appearance of surgical disease. London: John Churchill; 1840.

12. Firkin BG, Whitworth JA. Dictionary of medical eponyms. Boca Raton: Parthenon Publishing; 2002.

13. [No author]. Obituary record: Romberg M. Med News. 1873;31–32:135.

14. [No author]. Obituary: Moritz Heinrich Romberg. Med Times Gaz. 1873;2:81.

15. [No author]. News and miscellany: death of Romberg. Med Surg Rep. 1873;29:88.

16. Romberg MH. Die Operation des eingeklemmten Bruches des eirunden Loches: Operatio herniae foraminis ovalis incarceratae. In: Dieffenbach JF, editor. Die operative Chirurgie, Bd. 2. Leipzig: F.A. Brockhaus; 1847. p. 619–25.

17. Nasir BS, Zendejas B, Ali SM, Groenewald CB, Heller SF, Farley DR. Obturator hernia: the mayo clinic experience. Hernia. 2012;16:315–9.

18. Yip AWC, AhChong AK, Lam KH. Obturator hernia: a continuing diagnostic challenge. Surgery. 1993;113:266–9.

19. Mantoo SK, Mak K, Tan TJ. Obturator hernia: diagnosis and treatment in the modern era. Singap Med J. 2009;50:866–70.

20. Karasaki T, Nakagawa T, Tanaka N. Obturator hernia: the relationship between anatomical classification and the Howship–Romberg sign. Hernia. 2014;18:413–6.

21. Kammori M, Mafune KI, Hirashima T, Kawahara M, et al. Forty-three cases of obturator hernia. Am J Surg. 2004;187:549–52.

22. Watson D. Dr. William E. Ladd. J Pediatr Surg. 1967;2:295–6.

23. [No author]. William Edward Ladd. In: Harvard college, class of 1902—Secretary's fifth report. Cambridge: Harvard University Press; 1917. p. 184–5.

24. Lim PW, Martin ND, Hicks BA, Yeo CJ, Cowan SW. William Edwards Ladd, MD (1880–1967): the description of his bands. Am Surg. 2013;79:11–3.

25. Bill H, William E, Ladd MD. Great pioneer of north American pediatric society. Progr Pediatr Surg. 1986;20:52–9.

26. Wiedermann HRK. William E. Ladd (1880–1967). Eur J Pediatr. 1990;149:669.

27. Ladd WE, Gross RE. Abdominal surgery of infancy and childhood. Philadelphia: W.B. Saunders; 1941.

28. Ladd WE. Hernia in infancy and childhood. Nebraska Med J. 1941;26:235–9.

29. Hannington-Kiff JG. Absent thigh adductor reflex in obturator hernia. Lancet. 1980;315:180.

30. [No author]. News and notices: award of the Jacksonian prize of the Royal College of Surgeons of England. Anaesthesia. 1981;36:731–6.

31. Hannington-Kiff JG. Intravenous regional sympathetic block with guanethidine. Lancet. 1974;303:1019–20.

32. Hannington-Kiff JG. Relief of causalgia in limbs by regional intravenous guanethidine. Br Med J. 1979;2:367–8.

Epilogue

The current book follows in the steps of the authors' first book, *Cardiovascular Eponymic Signs* (2021), which received international acclaim among clinicians, researchers, medical students, and medical historians for its unique approach uncovering otherwise dormant first-hand accounts that should continue to serve a role in modern medical practice.

Index

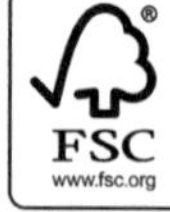